Ophthalmology at a Glance

Ophthalmology at a Glance

Edited by **Ray George**

hayle
medical

New York

Published by Hayle Medical,
30 West, 37th Street, Suite 612,
New York, NY 10018, USA
www.haylemedical.com

Ophthalmology at a Glance
Edited by Ray George

International Standard Book Number: 978-1-63241-393-2 (Hardback)

The publisher's policy is to use permanent paper from mills that operate a sustainable forestry policy. Furthermore, the publisher ensures that the text paper and cover boards used have met acceptable environmental accreditation standards.

Trademark Notice: Registered trademark of products or corporate names are used only for explanation and identification without intent to infringe.

Printed in the United States of America.

Contents

Preface

This book has been a concerted effort by a group of academicians, researchers and scientists, who have contributed their research works for the realization of the book. This book has materialized in the wake of emerging advancements and innovations in this field. Therefore, the need of the hour was to compile all the required researches and disseminate the knowledge to a broad spectrum of people comprising of students, researchers and specialists of the field.

Ophthalmology is the branch of medical science that studies the structure of the eye and deals with the diagnosis and treatment of diseases and disorders related to it. This field has advanced over the years to include different categories of surgeries for diseases such as cataract, glaucoma, refractive surgery, vitreo-retinal surgery, etc. This book unravels the recent studies in the area of ophthalmology. As this field is emerging at a rapid pace, the contents of this book will help the readers understand the modern concepts and applications of the subject. It will help the readers in keeping pace with the rapid changes in this discipline. Those in search of information to further their knowledge in the field of opthalmology will be greatly assisted by this book.

At the end of the preface, I would like to thank the authors for their brilliant chapters and the publisher for guiding us all-through the making of the book till its final stage. Also, I would like to thank my family for providing the support and encouragement throughout my academic career and research projects.

Editor

A Comparative Study of Retinal Function in Rabbits after Panretinal Selective Retina Therapy versus Conventional Panretinal Photocoagulation

Young Gun Park,[1] Seungbum Kang,[1] Ralf Brinkmann,[2] and Young-Jung Roh[1]

[1]*Department of Ophthalmology, Yeouido St. Mary's Hospital, College of Medicine, The Catholic University of Korea, No. 10, 63-ro Yeongdeungpo-gu, Seoul 07345, Republic of Korea*
[2]*Medical Laser Center Lübeck GmbH, Lübeck, Germany*

Correspondence should be addressed to Young-Jung Roh; youngjungroh@hanmail.net

Academic Editor: Theodore Leng

Purpose. This study evaluates functional changes in electroretinographic findings after selective retina therapy (SRT) compared to panretinal photocoagulation (PRP) in rabbits. *Methods.* The right eyes of 12 Chinchilla rabbits received 200 laser treatment spots. The right eyes of six rabbits received SRT (SRT group), whereas the other six animals were treated using PRP on the right eye (PRP group). The eyes were investigated using full-field ERG 1 hour and 3 weeks after treatment. Histologic exam to assess the tissue response of lasers was performed on 3 weeks. *Results.* No significant changes in the mean ROD or CR b-wave amplitudes of the SRT lesions were evident, compared to baseline, 1 h after laser treatment ($p = 0.372$ and 0.278, resp.). In addition, the OPs and 30 Hz flickers of the SRT lesions were not significantly altered ($p = 0.17$ and 0.243, resp.). At 3 weeks, similar results were found. Comparing the two groups, the ROD b-wave amplitude was reduced in the PRP and SRT groups to $60.04 \pm 4.2\%$ and $92.32 \pm 6.43\%$ of baseline ($p < 0.001$). Histologically, there was no visible photoreceptor alterations on week 3. *Conclusions.* SRT in rabbit eyes induced less functional loss than PRP in both rod-mediated retinal function and cone-mediated retinal function. In addition, SRT irradiated eyes had no functional loss compared to its control.

1. Introduction

Retinal photocoagulation is a major therapeutic method for various retinal and choroidal diseases. After irradiation, the laser energy is converted into heat in the retina, which leads to thermal damage of the RPE and photoreceptors. In addition, secondary damage in the neuroretina and choroid can occur [1]. The complications of laser photocoagulation such as visual field defects, loss of color vision, and lower night vision after panretinal treatment can be related to photoreceptor destruction [2–4]. Previous studies showed that laser photocoagulation induced destruction of the outer retina histologically and a decreased retinal function on electroretinogram [5, 6].

Selective retina therapy (SRT) was introduced as a new laser treatment for retinal diseases using the concept, which

is associated with RPE degradation. The purpose of the irradiation is to selectively damage the RPE without affecting the surrounding tissue such as the neural retina, photoreceptors, and choroid. The treatment goal is to stimulate RPE cell migration and proliferation into the irradiated areas and to improve the metabolism at the diseased lesions [7]. SRT has already been performed in patients with various retinal diseases, such as drusen, due to age-related macular degeneration, diabetic macular edema, and central serous chorioretinopathy [8–10]. With the laser parameters (pulse duration: 1.7 μs; repetition rate: 100 Hz; maximum number of pulses in a burst: 30; maximum adjustable pulse energy: 400 μJ) used, no bleeding or scotoma was observed, as confirmed by microperimetry, thus demonstrating no adverse effects to the choroid or photoreceptors, respectively [7, 11]. Considering the photoreceptor-sparing effect of SRT, it could be another treatment option for aforementioned retinal diseases.

SRT spots are invisible on ophthalmoscopy. However, these spots can be visualized by fluorescein angiography. So, dosimetry like reflectometry can be useful to prevent thermal damage to adjacent cells and to monitor the irradiated laser energy. This technique will allow an adequate treatment of retinal diseases for each individual with different pigmented fundus.

An optoacoustic (OA) device has been used as a dosimetry tool in previous SRT studies. The OA device is an instrument that detects pressure waves according to the collapse of microbubbles induced in the melanosome of RPE cells by laser irradiation. This device generally consists of an ultrasonic transducer embedded in an ophthalmologic contact lens. In contrast, reflectometry is a real-time controlled method for determining changes in the reflectance properties without embedding transducers. We previously reported the safety of SRT by using feedback controlled reflectometry in animal study, demonstrating that SRT of the rabbit eye induced selective RPE damage, as confirmed by both optical coherence tomography (OCT) and histological evaluation [12]. However, no detailed analysis of retinal function after SRT using real-time automated reflectometry in an experimental setting has been performed. In the present study, we investigated whether SRT preserved general retinal function compared to conventional panretinal photocoagulation (PRP). We used standardized protocols for full-field electroretinography (ERG) and histologic evaluation.

2. Materials and Methods

2.1. Animals. Twelve Chinchilla Bastard rabbits were used in this study, because pigmentations in RPEs in the retina are considerably similar to those in the human eye. We designed to use animals (4–6 months old, 2.0–2.5 kg) to have the similar levels of retinal maturation. The animals were used in accordance with the Association for Research in Vision and Ophthalmology (ARVO) statement for the use of animals in ophthalmic and vision research. The experiment was approved by the Institutional Animal Care and Use Committee of the Catholic University of Korea (Permit Number: YEO20131704FA). The animals were randomly assigned to two groups (both $n = 6$) and were treated using either an SRT laser (SRT group) or a PRP laser (PRP group). Only the right eyes were treated and the left eyes served as controls.

2.2. Laser Treatment. In the SRT group, the animals were treated using an SRT Laser (Q-switched Nd:YLF Laser: wavelength: 527 nm; pulse duration: 1.7 μs; repetition rate: 100 Hz; maximum number of pulses in a burst: 30; maximum adjustable pulse energy: 40 μJ; number of spots: 200; laser spot diameter: 200 μm). In contrast, eyes of the PRP group received conventional PRP by using Zeiss (VISULAS 532s, Carl Zeiss, Dublin, CA, USA; pulse duration: 200 ms; laser power: 100 mW; number of spots: 200; laser spot diameter: 200 μm), inducing ophthalmoscopically visible lesions. All laser photocoagulation using contact lens (TransEquator;

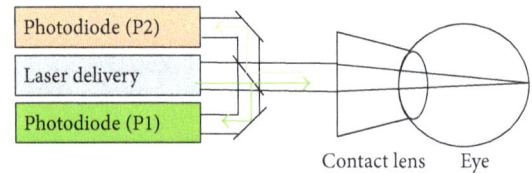

FIGURE 1: Schematic sketch of the reflectometry. The system contained two photodiodes; one of them (P1) detects the laser pulses applied to the fundus, and the other (P2) detects reflected and backscattered light from the retina. As a result, reflectometry can stop laser irradiation appropriately for selective RPE damage.

Volk Optical Inc., USA) was done below the optic nerve head along a horizontal marker to the medullary rays after the animals were sufficiently anesthetized by 0.2 mg/kg of Zoletil (250 mg of tiletamine and 250 mg of zolazepam; Virbac, Carros, France) administered intramuscularly.

2.3. Reflectometry. We used the same reflectometry system as previously described [12]. Briefly, reflectometry contained two photodiodes: one of them (P1) detects the laser pulses applied to the fundus and the other (P2) detects reflected and backscattered light from the retina. SRT emits 30 micropulses increasing stepwise by 3% of the dynamic range. However, reflectometry can stop laser irradiation when it detects microbubble formation in RPE. Given that microbubbles are the origin of instantaneous selective RPE damage, the backscattered light in the signal of P2 can be used as useful indicator (Figure 1). SRT provides that the pulse energy is increased stepwise from subthreshold intensity to a point of the selective RPE cell damage. For this purpose, the reflectometry system can adequately stop the laser emission as soon as microbubbles occur.

2.4. Electrophysiological Tests. The pupils of both eyes in each animal were dilated with topical 0.5% tropicamide and 0.5% phenylephrine hydrochloride (Mydrin-P ophthalmic solution; Santen Pharmaceutical Co., Ltd., Osaka, Japan). The animals were sufficiently anesthetized as aforementioned by 0.2 mg/kg of Zoletil (250 mg of tiletamine and 250 mg of zolazepam; Virbac, Carros, France) administered intramuscularly. The rabbits were dark-adapted for more than 1 hour, and a Burian-Allen bipolar contact lens electrode (Hansen Laboratories, Iowa City, Iowa, USA) was placed on the cornea. A needle ground electrode was inserted subcutaneously behind the ear.

Full-field electroretinograms were recorded and analyzed using the UTAS-E3000 system (LKC Technologies, Inc., Gaithersburg, MD), based on the protocols recommended by International Society for Clinical Electrophysiology of Vision. According to the protocols that have been described in detail previously [13], the dark-adapted rod responses were recorded with single flashes (20 μs) on dim blue light background. On the other hand, combined rod and cone responses were measured using white light (0.8 cd s/m^2). A 30 Hz flickering white light averaged from 20 sweeps was adequate to acquire light-adapted cone responses.

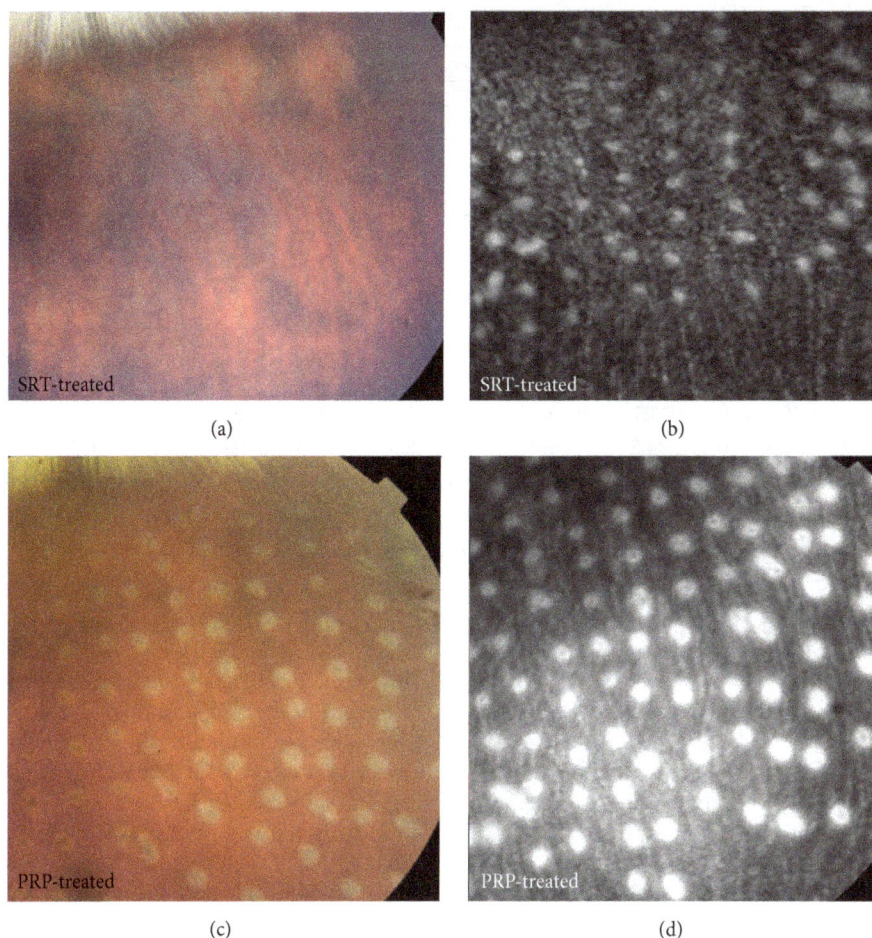

FIGURE 2: (a) A fundus image obtained 1 h after selective retina therapy (SRT) revealed no visible SRT spots. (b) Fluorescein angiography (FA) performed 1 hr after the irradiation showed hyperfluorescence on SRT spots. (c) A fundus photograph taken 1 hr after conventional PRP showed whitish spots. (d) FA performed 1 hr after PRP showed larger hyperfluorescence than that of SRT, although the same spot size (200 μm) was applied.

The amplitude of the b-wave measured from the trough of the a-wave to the following peak of the b-wave. And the implicit time measured from flash onset to the peak of the b-wave. Data are expressed as means ± standard deviation. Paired t-tests were performed to compare responses, and p values less than 0.05 indicated statistical significance.

2.5. Histologic Evaluation. On week 3, the animals were anesthetized as aforementioned and sacrificed by an overdose with KCL in the unconscious state to evaluate permanent changes of irradiated lesions rather than temporary changes. For immersion fixation in 4% glutaraldehyde, following removal of the anterior parts of the eyes, the rest of the eye was prepared within 15 minutes immediately. The tissue was trimmed to block size after fixation for 12–24 hours in 4°C cold room. After dehydration in ethanol, the tissue was embedded. Sections with five micron thick were stained with hematoxylin and eosin. Histopathology was performed based on landmarks such as the optic nerve head and medullary rays to include the SRT lesions.

3. Results

3.1. Fundus Examination and Angiography. In the SRT group, a total of 200 SRT laser spots were created in each rabbit (range, 10–40 μJ), and most of the test lesions were invisible. The representative fundus photographs obtained 1 hour after irradiation using SRT are shown in Figure 2(a). Table 1 showed the energy levels of all lesions produced by SRT using reflectometric dosimetry. 1197 of total 1200 laser spots were evaluable.

Because these SRT lesions were invisible on ophthalmoscopy, SRT lesion can be detected by hyperfluorescence on fluorescein angiography (Figure 2(b)). In contrast, whitening lesions were immediately observed in the PRP group (range 100 mW) and were detected by fluorescein angiography. Although the same size of laser diameter (200 μm) was used in both SRT and PRP groups, the lesion size of PRP is larger than that of SRT on FA (Figures 2(c) and 2(d)).

3.2. Electrophysiological Tests. The ERG recording results demonstrated general functional changes in the laser-induced retinal lesions after SRT and PRP. In the control

TABLE 1: The results of automatic turn-off in the selective retina therapy groups.

Energy of SRT[a] (0–40 μJ)	Number of SRT[a] lesions	Fundoscopically visible lesions (%)	FA[b]-positive lesions	Automatic turn-off
0–19	515	2 (0.39%)	515	510
20–39	674	5 (0.74%)	674	669
40	8	0	8	8
Total	1197	7 (0.58%)	1197	1190

[a]SRT, selective retina therapy; [b]FA, fluorescein angiography.

TABLE 2: Full-field electroretinography (ERG).

Parameter	Control	PRP groups ($n = 6$)				SRT groups ($n = 6$)			
		1 h	p value	3 weeks	p value	1 h	p value	3 weeks	p value
Blue light (rod)	106.3 ± 49.7	63.8 ± 33.5	$<0.0001^*$	77.3 ± 22.8	$<0.0001^*$	98.2 ± 32.3	0.372	101.2 ± 31.9	0.142
White light (CR)	157.6 ± 34.8	109.5 ± 34.5	$<0.0001^*$	111.3 ± 28.5	$<0.0001^*$	138.7 ± 29.4	0.278	151.4 ± 23.0	0.187
Oscillatory potential	84.4 ± 23.4	48.6 ± 28.4	0.023^*	43.5 ± 21.5	0.031^*	81.5 ± 31.4	0.170	89.5 ± 42.5	0.435
30 Hz flicker (cone)	49.4 ± 17.8	26.8 ± 18.5	$<0.0001^*$	24.4 ± 18.5	0.012^*	47.6 ± 15.2	0.243	46.3 ± 21.5	0.272

*Averaged values ± two standard deviations of the b-wave amplitudes (μV). The two-tailed paired t-test was used to calculate p value, and $^*p < 0.05$ was considered to mean the significance.

groups, the mean ROD b-wave and combined response (CR) b-wave amplitudes were $106.3 \pm 49.7\,\mu V$ and $157.6 \pm 34.8\,\mu V$, respectively. The mean oscillatory potential (OP) and 30 Hz flicker amplitude were $84.4 \pm 23.4\,\mu V$ and $49.4 \pm 17.8\,\mu V$, respectively. At 1 hour and 3 weeks after SRT, the mean ROD b-wave amplitude of the SRT lesions was $98.2 \pm 32.3\,\mu V$ and $101.2 \pm 31.9\,\mu V$, respectively, and the mean CR b-wave amplitude was $138.7 \pm 29.4\,\mu V$ and $151.4 \pm 23.0\,\mu V$, respectively. The mean (OP) and 30 Hz flicker amplitude was $81.5 \pm 31.4\,\mu V$ and $89.5 \pm 42.5\,\mu V$, respectively, at 1 h, and $47.6 \pm 15.2\,\mu V$ and $46.3 \pm 21.5\,\mu V$, respectively, after 3 weeks (Table 2).

No significant changes in the mean ROD and CR b-wave amplitudes of the SRT lesions were evident 1 hour after laser treatment compared to baseline ($p = 0.372$ and 0.278, resp.). In addition, the OPs and 30 Hz flickers of the SRT lesions were not significantly altered 1 hour after SRT compared to baseline ($p = 0.17$ and 0.243, resp.). At 3 weeks, similar results were found for the ROD and CR b-wave amplitudes, OPs, and 30 Hz flickers ($p = 0.142$, 0.187, 0.435, and 0.272, resp.).

In contrast, at 1 hour and 3 weeks after conventional PRP, the mean ROD b-wave amplitude was $63.8 \pm 33.5\,\mu V$ and $77.3 \pm 22.8\,\mu V$, respectively, and the CR b-wave amplitude was $109.5 \pm 34.5\,\mu V$ and $111.3 \pm 28.5\,\mu V$, respectively. The mean OP and 30 Hz flicker amplitude at 1 hour were $48.6 \pm 28.4\,\mu V$ and $43.5 \pm 21.5\,\mu V$, respectively, and on week 3 they were $26.8 \pm 18.5\,\mu V$ and $14.4 \pm 18.5\,\mu V$, respectively. The ROD and CR b-wave amplitudes, OP, and 30 Hz flickers all significantly decreased 1 hour after conventional laser treatment compared to baseline ($p < 0.0001$, $p < 0.0001$, $p = 0.023$, and $p < 0.0001$, resp.). Similar results were also found on week 3 ($p < 0.0001$, $p < 0.0001$, $p = 0.031$, and $p = 0.012$, resp.). In the PRP group, apparent reductions in amplitudes were demonstrated 1 hour after SRT compared to baseline. These showed moderate recovery at 3 weeks but did not attain baseline values and remained significantly different.

Comparing the two groups, the ROD b-wave amplitudes in the PRP and SRT groups 1 h after irradiation were reduced to $60.0 \pm 4.2\%$ and $92.3 \pm 6.4\%$ of the baseline, respectively. This reduction was significantly greater in the PRP group compared to the SRT group ($p < 0.001$). The dark-adapted CR b-wave amplitude also showed similar results, which were a reduction in the PRP and SRT groups at 1 h (compared to baseline values) of $69.5 \pm 5.4\%$ and $88.0 \pm 7.6\%$, respectively. The PRP group significantly decreased more than the SRT group ($p < 0.05$). OPs, cone single flash, and 30 Hz flicker responses were also significantly decreased in the PRP group, whereas the SRT group showed no statistically significant decrease. No statistically significant change in the ERG implicit time was observed after treatment in both groups.

At 3 weeks after treatment, similar results were observed. All parameters improved slightly compared to the values measured at the previous time point (1 h after irradiation), but the PRP group amplitudes were significantly reduced in comparison with those of the control group. Otherwise, no significant difference was noted between the SRT group and controls (Figures 3 and 4).

3.3. Histologic Evaluation. In addition to the irradiation-outcome evaluation using ERG, a histologic examination was performed in order to access the extent of the laser lesions. At 3 weeks after irradiation, full-thickness retinal structures and arrangement were lost in the PRP group. In contrast, condensed focally proliferated RPE with preserved photoreceptors in the SRT lesions was observed. And the surrounding tissues such as Bruch's membrane and choriocapillaris were not affected by the SRT (Figure 5).

4. Discussion

Although conventional PRP is an effective treatment to reduce the risk of severe visual loss in Diabetic Retinopathy Study (DRS), it may cause visual acuity and peripheral visual field constriction due to neuroretinal damages [14, 15]. Moreover, conventional laser treatment develops irreversible damage on retinal tissue because the laser energy which is

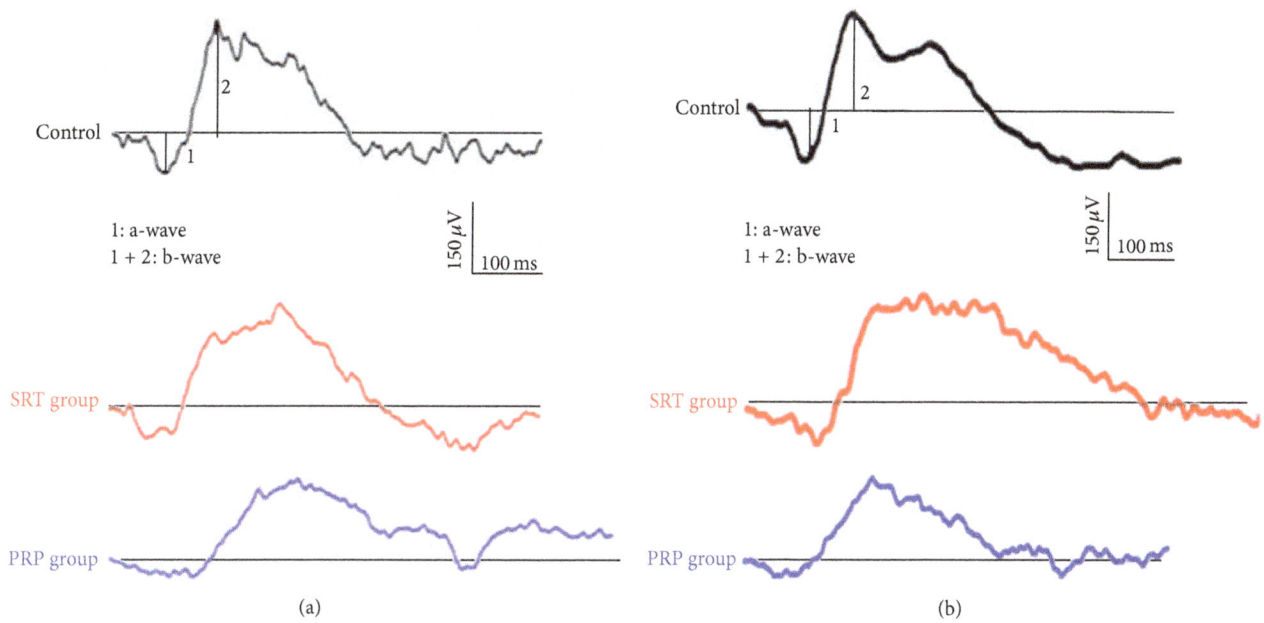

FIGURE 3: Dark-adapted ERG in the control group (top). ERG responses in the SRT groups were not significantly different from those of the control groups at either 1 h or 3 weeks after irradiation. (a, b, middle) However, the amplitudes of the conventional PRP group were significantly lower at these two time points (a, b, bottom).

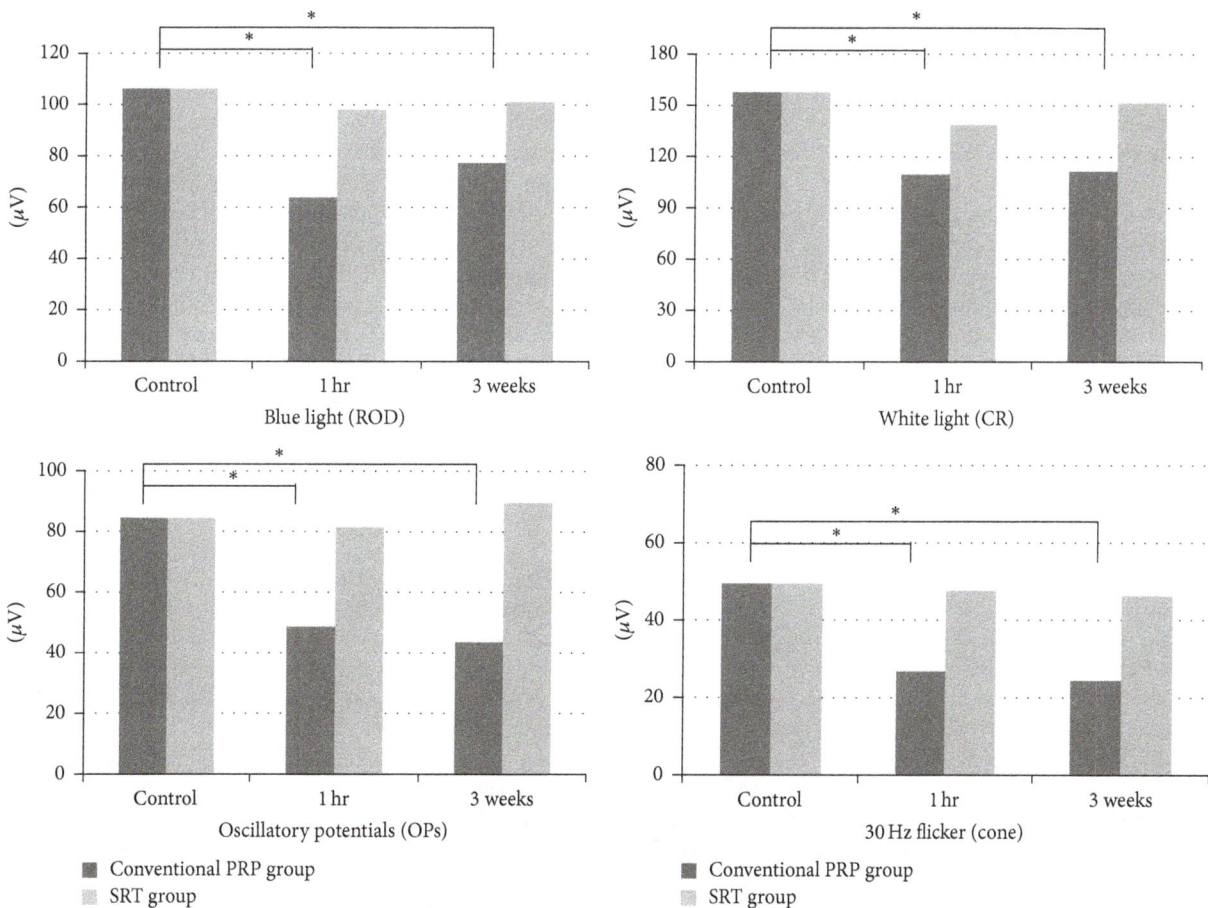

FIGURE 4: None of the b-wave amplitudes of the rods, CR, the amplitudes of the oscillatory potentials, or the 30-Hz flicker of the SRT group was significantly decreased. However, those of the conventional PRP group were significantly less than the control group.

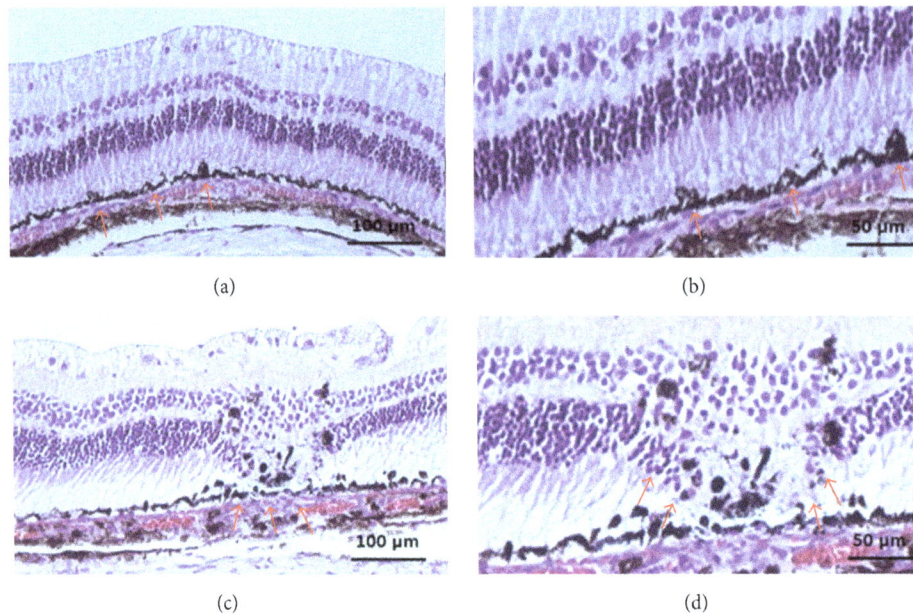

FIGURE 5: (a, b) The photoreceptor inner segments were preserved, and the distal ends of the photoreceptor outer segments were slightly relaxed. The RPE layer proliferated focally along the SRT lesion, and Bruch's membrane was intact. Histology of conventional laser lesions after 3 weeks. (c, d) The full-thickness structure of the retina involving the photoreceptors was disrupted and disorganized (magnification 200x; a, c) (magnification 400x; b, d) (red arrow, irradiated lesion).

absorbed primarily by melanin in RPE conducts heat not only to RPE cells but also to the adjacent neurosensory retina.

SRT is a new laser technology that selectively damages the RPE while sparing neurosensory retinal tissue [16]. SRT was proved to reduce the risk of laser-induced scotoma induced by excessive thermal damage and has already been performed in patients with a range of retinal diseases [17–20]. In previous studies, preservation of the retinal anatomy was confirmed from histological findings and OCT images [12, 21]. However, the preservation of retinal function after SRT has not yet been evaluated, with the exception of one previous study that used microperimetry [11].

ERG is a useful examination method for study retinal function. The ERG b-wave is obtained primarily from the maximal combined response and reflects photoreceptor function. Physiologically, the b-wave results from the current flow along Muller cells in response to an increased extracellular potassium ion concentration. ERG is highly dependent on bipolar cells within the inner nuclear layer and hence on the retinal circulation. In the current study, we described retinal function using ERG and investigated whether SRT is associated with less retinal functional loss than PRP treatment.

In our study, the ERG of the SRT groups was not significantly changed at either 1 h or 3 weeks and generally recovered to baseline over 3 weeks. The subtle reduction in mean amplitudes measured 1 hr after SRT was not statistically significant. It was correlated well with the histopathological results showing no manifestation of retinal damage. This suggests that temporary RPE anatomical changes at the sites of SRT lesions become gradually resolved based on the histologic finding at 3 weeks. Histologically, we noted

a focally proliferated RPE with relatively intact photoreceptors in the regions of irradiation at 3 weeks after irradiation. These findings support that SRT feedback controlled by reflectometry could induce RPE proliferation at irradiated lesions without photoreceptor damage as we published before [12]. In sections, Bruch's membrane and choriocapillaris were well preserved. The outer segments of the photoreceptors that were in contact with the RPE remained unaffected and it meant intact photoreceptor structure. In contrast, all of those of conventional PRP were significantly decreased at both time points, and these results also corresponded with the histologic findings. In conventional PRP lesions, full-thickness retinal layers were destroyed and disoriented. In addition, the decreased amplitude of OP and 30 Hz flickers at week 3 compared to 1 hour might reflect that both inner and outer retinal damages were intensified with permanent scarring process.

Anatomical changes in retinal tissue after SRT have been investigated in several previous studies [7, 12, 22, 23]. Selective RPE damage has been confirmed by histological findings and OCT images. To the best of our knowledge, this is the first electrophysiological study to compare SRT with conventional PRP using full-field ERG. The results of this study suggest that SRT using micropulsed duration and repeated pulses accompanied by real-time automated feedback dosimetry is fundamentally safe.

Roider et al. [24] found that multiple short laser pulses could selectively coagulate the RPE but with sparing of the adjacent neural retina and choroid. During the healing period, the epithelium reformed from a single sheet of hypertrophic retinal pigment epithelial cells that exhibited clear signs of viability, in that the cells phagocytized outer segments. The local edema of the photoreceptor layer and subretinal space evident at early stages disappeared when the blood-retinal barrier was reestablished and no subsequent damage to the photoreceptors was evident. In addition, many previous studies using SRT also reported temporary relaxation of the photoreceptor outer segment with subsequent restoration of the normal structure [12, 25, 26]. In the present study, preservation of the photoreceptor layer was noted in histological findings, which is in accordance with previous results. Therefore our work demonstrates that SRT did not significantly affect retinal tissue anatomy and function but rather induced reversible and temporary changes. These results suggest that SRT is a safe method for treating central macular disease, because the risk of laser-induced scotoma caused by irreversible thermal damage can be avoided and because any change to retinal function after SRT was reversible according to ERG.

Our study had several limitations. Full-field ERG cannot explore the functionality of each SRT spot but rather overall retinal functioning. Although multifocal ERG might be a better option for evaluation of individual SRT spots, the full-field ERG can be more suitable to examine an overall retinal function. Because of invisibility of SRT spot and the short distances between the spots, the spatial resolution would be far more below to see the specific laser-induced scotoma. Second, as the rabbit does not have a macula, our results are relevant to the effect of SRT on functioning of the overall retina, not the macula. Third, due to the tendency of laser effects which remain for a long period, a future study should be conducted to investigate the long-term effects of SRT.

In conclusion, SRT of microsecond duration featuring repeated pulses controlled by real-time automated reflectometry could preserve retinal function after laser irradiation compared to conventional PRP treatment, as verified by the ERG results. ERG can be an effective tool to evaluate the retinal function impairment and to comprehend the new treatment methods for the safety of SRT. In addition, retinal structures studied were not significantly damaged at 3 weeks after SRT. Furthermore, the changes in anatomy and function of retinal tissue after SRT were interrelated. The use of reflectometry as a dosimetry tool could avoid irreversible thermal damage during SRT by ensuring the appropriate energy delivery. Further studies are required to improve the safety of SRT by evaluating the functionalities of SRT lesions and to verify the efficacy of SRT applied to treat patients with various macular diseases.

Conflict of Interests

The authors declare that there is no conflict of interests regarding the publication of this paper.

Acknowledgment

This study was supported by the South Korean government-affiliated ministry of Trade, Industry and Energy (M000004912-00192937).

References

[1] J. Marshall, "Structural aspects of laser-induced damage and their functional implications," *Health Physics*, vol. 56, no. 5, pp. 617–624, 1989.

[2] V. C. Greenstein, H. Chen, D. C. Hood, K. Holopigian, W. Seiple, and R. E. Carr, "Retinal function in diabetic macular edema after focal laser photocoagulation," *Investigative Ophthalmology and Visual Science*, vol. 41, no. 11, pp. 3655–3664, 2000.

[3] M. Henricsson and A. Heijl, "The effect of panretinal laser photocoagulation on visual acuity, visual fields and on subjective visual impairment in preproliferative and early proliferative diabetic retinopathy," *Acta Ophthalmologica*, vol. 72, no. 5, pp. 570–575, 1994.

[4] P. K. Khosla, V. Rao, H. K. Tewari, and A. Kumar, "Contrast sensitivity in diabetic retinopathy after panretinal photocoagulation," *Ophthalmic Surgery*, vol. 25, no. 8, pp. 516–520, 1994.

[5] H.-C. Chuang, S. Kawano, M. Arai et al., "The influence of argon laser panretinal photocoagulation on the rabbit ERG c-wave," *Acta Ophthalmologica*, vol. 70, no. 3, pp. 303–307, 1992.

[6] R. Schechner, M. Gdal-on, D. Cohen, E. Meyer, S. Zonis, and I. Perlman, "Recovery of the electroretinogram in rabbits after argon laser photocoagulation," *Investigative Ophthalmology & Visual Science*, vol. 28, no. 9, pp. 1605–1613, 1987.

[7] B. Brinkmann, T. D. Maines, M. J. Naughton, J. M. Stebbins, and A. Weimerskirch, "Bridging the gap. Catholic health care organizations need concrete ways to connect social principles to practice," *Health Progress*, vol. 87, no. 6, pp. 43–50, 2006.

[8] J. Roider, R. Brinkmann, C. Wirbelauer, R. Birngruber, and H. Laqua, "Variability of RPE reaction in two cases after selective RPE laser effects in prophylactic treatment of drusen," *Graefe's Archive for Clinical and Experimental Ophthalmology*, vol. 237, no. 1, pp. 45–50, 1999.

[9] J. Roider, S. H. M. Liew, C. Klatt et al., "Selective retina therapy (SRT) for clinically significant diabetic macular edema," *Graefe's Archive for Clinical and Experimental Ophthalmology*, vol. 248, no. 9, pp. 1263–1272, 2010.

[10] C. Klatt, M. Saeger, T. Oppermann et al., "Selective retina therapy for acute central serous chorioretinopathy," *British Journal of Ophthalmology*, vol. 95, no. 1, pp. 83–88, 2011.

[11] J. Roider, R. Brinkmann, C. Wirbelauer, H. Laqua, and R. Birngruber, "Retinal sparing by selective retinal pigment epithelial photocoagulation," *Archives of Ophthalmology*, vol. 117, no. 8, pp. 1028–1034, 1999.

[12] Y.-G. Park, E. Seifert, Y. J. Roh, D. Theisen-Kunde, S. Kang, and R. Brinkmann, "Tissue response of selective retina therapy by means of a feedback-controlled energy ramping mode," *Clinical and Experimental Ophthalmology*, vol. 42, no. 9, pp. 846–855, 2014.

[13] K. G. Wallentén, M. Malmsjö, S. Andréasson, A. Wackenfors, K. Johansson, and F. Ghosh, "Retinal function and PKC alpha expression after focal laser photocoagulation," *Graefe's Archive for Clinical and Experimental Ophthalmology*, vol. 245, no. 12, pp. 1815–1824, 2007.

[14] Early Treatment Diabetic Retinopathy Study Research Group, "Early photocoagulation for diabetic retinopathy. ETDRS report number 9," *Ophthalmology*, vol. 98, no. 5, supplement, pp. 766–785, 1991.

[15] The Diabetic Retinopathy Study Research Group, "Photocoagulation treatment of proliferative diabetic retinopathy: the second report of diabetic retinopathy study findings," *Ophthalmology*, vol. 85, no. 1, pp. 82–106, 1978.

[16] R. Brinkmann, G. Schüle, J. Neumann et al., "Selective retina therapy: methods, technique, and online dosimetry," *Ophthalmologe*, vol. 103, no. 10, pp. 839–849, 2006.

[17] C. Framme, G. Schuele, K. Kobuch, B. Flucke, R. Birngruber, and R. Brinkmann, "Investigation of selective retina treatment (SRT) by means of 8 ns laser pulses in a rabbit model," *Lasers in Surgery and Medicine*, vol. 40, no. 1, pp. 20–27, 2008.

[18] H. Elsner, C. Klatt, S. H. M. Liew et al., "Selective retina therapy in patients with diabetic maculopathy," *Ophthalmologe*, vol. 103, no. 10, pp. 856–860, 2006.

[19] H. Elsner, E. Pörksen, C. Klatt et al., "Selective retina therapy in patients with central serous chorioretinopathy," *Graefe's Archive for Clinical and Experimental Ophthalmology*, vol. 244, no. 12, pp. 1638–1645, 2006.

[20] S. Koinzer, H. Elsner, C. Klatt et al., "Selective retina therapy (SRT) of chronic subfoveal fluid after surgery of rhegmatogenous retinal detachment: three case reports," *Graefe's Archive for Clinical and Experimental Ophthalmology*, vol. 246, no. 10, pp. 1373–1378, 2008.

[21] R. Brinkmann, G. Hüttmann, J. Rögener, J. Roider, R. Birngruber, and C. P. Lin, "Origin of retinal pigment epithelium cell damage by pulsed laser irradiance in the nanosecond to microsecond time regimen," *Lasers in Surgery and Medicine*, vol. 27, no. 5, pp. 451–464, 2000.

[22] C. Framme, A. Walter, P. Prahs et al., "Structural changes of the retina after conventional laser photocoagulation and selective retina treatment (SRT) in spectral domain OCT," *Current Eye Research*, vol. 34, no. 7, pp. 568–579, 2009.

[23] H. D. Kim, J. W. Han, Y.-H. Ohn, R. Brinkmann, and T. K. Park, "Functional evaluation using multifocal electroretinogram after selective retina therapy with a microsecond-pulsed laser," *Investigative Ophthalmology and Visual Science*, vol. 56, no. 1, pp. 122–131, 2015.

[24] J. Roider, N. A. Michaud, T. J. Flotte, and R. Birngruber, "Response of the retinal pigment epithelium to selective photocoagulation," *Archives of Ophthalmology*, vol. 110, no. 12, pp. 1786–1792, 1992.

[25] C. Framme, C. Alt, S. Schnell, M. Sherwood, R. Brinkmann, and C. P. Lin, "Selective targeting of the retinal pigment epithelium in rabbit eyes with a scanning laser beam," *Investigative Ophthalmology & Visual Science*, vol. 48, no. 4, pp. 1782–1792, 2007.

[26] C. Alt, C. Framme, S. Schnell, H. Lee, R. Brinkmann, and C. P. Lin, "Selective targeting of the retinal pigment epithelium using an acousto-optic laser scanner," *Journal of Biomedical Optics*, vol. 10, no. 6, Article ID 064014, 2005.

Wavefront-Guided Photorefractive Keratectomy with the Use of a New Hartmann-Shack Aberrometer in Patients with Myopia and Compound Myopic Astigmatism

Steven C. Schallhorn,[1] **Jan A. Venter,**[2] **Stephen J. Hannan,**[2] **and Keith A. Hettinger**[3]

[1]*University of California, San Francisco, 11730 Caminito Prenticia, San Diego, CA 92131, USA*
[2]*Optical Express, 5 Deerdykes Road, Cumbernauld G68 9HF, UK*
[3]*Optical Express, 9820 Willow Creek Road, Suite 260, San Diego, CA 92131, USA*

Correspondence should be addressed to Steven C. Schallhorn; scschallhorn@yahoo.com

Academic Editor: David P. Piñero

Purpose. To assess refractive and visual outcomes and patient satisfaction of wavefront-guided photorefractive keratectomy (PRK) in eyes with myopia and compound myopic astigmatism, with the ablation profile derived from a new Hartmann-Shack aberrometer. *Methods.* In this retrospective study, 662 eyes that underwent wavefront-guided PRK with a treatment profile derived from a new generation Hartmann-Shack aberrometer (iDesign aberrometer, Abbott Medical Optics, Inc., Santa Ana, CA) were analyzed. The preoperative manifest sphere ranged from −0.25 to −10.75 D, and preoperative manifest cylinder was between 0.00 and −5.25 D. Refractive and visual outcomes, vector analysis of the change in refractive cylinder, and patient satisfaction were evaluated. *Results.* At 3 months, 91.1% of eyes had manifest spherical equivalent within 0.50 D. The percentage of eyes achieving uncorrected distance visual acuity 20/20 or better was 89.4% monocularly and 96.5% binocularly. The mean correction ratio of refractive cylinder was 1.02 ± 0.43, and the mean error of angle was 0.00 ± 14.86° at 3 months postoperatively. Self-reported scores for optical side effects, such as starburst, glare, halo, ghosting, and double vision, were low. *Conclusion.* The use of a new Hartmann-Shack aberrometer for wavefront-guided photorefractive keratectomy resulted in high predictability, efficacy, and patient satisfaction.

1. Introduction

Although laser in situ keratomileusis (LASIK) outperforms photorefractive keratectomy in early postoperative stages [1], there are patients where the choice of surface ablation over the flap creation is well justified [2, 3]. These include eyes with thinner corneas, superficial scars, and epithelial basement membrane dystrophy and eyes where ocular pathology might create concerns for increased intraocular pressure during femtosecond flap creation or simply patients who wish to preserve corneal integrity due to the increased risk of trauma in their profession.

Since the advent of PRK over two decades ago, several improvements were introduced to maximize the postoperative visual quality, one of them being the use of wavefront-guided ablation profiles. When it comes to the higher order aberrations treatment, some studies even suggest that PRK might offer an advantage over LASIK [4–6]. Corneal flap creation induces its own aberrations that are unaccounted for in preoperative planning, although this risk has significantly decreased with the introduction of femtosecond lasers [7]. Wavefront-guided ablation profiles as such undergo continuous improvements, with more sophisticated wavefront mapping devices being introduced. In this study, we evaluate the results of a large consecutive cohort of patients with myopia/myopic astigmatism undergoing the wavefront-guided surface ablation with the ablation profile derived from the new Hartmann-Shack aberrometer (iDesign Advanced Wavescan Studio, Abbott Medical Optics, Inc., Santa Ana, CA). Accuracy of refractive and astigmatic correction, visual acuities, and patient satisfaction, including self-reported night vision disturbances, are evaluated up to 3 months postoperatively.

2. Patients and Methods

This retrospective, noncomparative study was deemed exempt from full review by the Committee on Human Research at the University of California, San Francisco, because it used only retrospective, deidentified patient data. Informed consent to undergo PRK procedure was obtained from all patients.

The deidentified patients records were extracted from an electronic database with the following criteria: cases that underwent primary photorefractive keratectomy targeted for emmetropia and were available for 1 week, 1 month, and 3 months following operative examination; preoperative myopic refraction with less than 12.00 D of spherical myopia, less than 6.00 D of refractive astigmatism, and no more than 12.00 D of manifest spherical equivalent; surgeries performed with the Visx Star S4 IR excimer laser (Abbott Medical Optics, Santa Ana, CA) using a wavefront-guided ablation profile derived from a new diagnostic device (iDesign System); visual acuity correctable to 20/32 or better in both eyes and age of 18 years or older. Data extraction techniques have been previously described [8].

Exclusion criteria for treatment were active ophthalmic disease, abnormal corneal shape, concurrent medications or medical conditions that could impair healing, and the final calculated stromal bed thickness less than $350\,\mu m$. Soft contact lens wearers were asked to discontinue use at least 7 days prior to the procedure. Hard contact lens users (PMMA or rigid gas permeable lenses) removed their lenses at least 3 weeks prior to baseline measurements and had two central keratometry readings and two manifest refraction values taken at least 1 week apart that did not differ by more than 0.50 D in either meridian.

Preoperative examination included manifest and cycloplegic refraction, monocular and binocular uncorrected distance visual acuity (UDVA), corrected distance visual acuity (CDVA) using a calibrated projected eye chart, low-light pupil diameter, slit-lamp biomicroscopy, dilated fundus examination, applanation tonometry, corneal topography, ultrasound pachymetry, and wavefront aberration measurement.

Postoperative examinations were conducted at 1 day, 4 days, 1 week, 1 month, and 3 months. On the first and fourth postoperative day, a detailed slit-lamp examination of the cornea was performed and unaided visual acuity checked. On the fourth day, the bandage contact lens was removed, if the process of reepithelization was completed. At the subsequent postoperative visits, the same preoperative examination protocol (excluding cycloplegic refraction, pupil diameter, topography, aberrometry, and pachymetry) was used. As part of current practice, all patients were asked to complete a questionnaire et each postoperative visit. The questionnaire from the last available visit was used for analysis. It was self-administered by the patient using a password protected and secure computer terminal in an isolated area of the clinic. The questionnaire responses were stored in the secured Optical Express central database, which is compliant with ISO 27001 for information security management systems. The questionnaire was derived from the Joint LASIK Study Task

Force [9] (Table 1). All response fields utilized a Likert scale to obtain the patient's preferences or degree of agreement. Night vision phenomena such as starburst, glare, halo, ghosting, and double vision and difficulty with dry eyes were rated on the scale from 1 (no difficulty) to 7 (severe difficulty).

2.1. Surgical Technique. All PRK procedures were performed by experienced surgeons certified to use the equipment. The eye was first anaesthetized with topical proxymetacaine hydrochloride 0.5%, and a 9 mm well was placed on the cornea and filled with 20% ethanol. Following a 30–40 seconds' application, the alcohol was carefully drained with a surgical spear and the epithelium removed with a blunt spatula. Wavefront-guided excimer laser ablation was performed using the Visx Star S4 IR laser system (Abbott Medical Optics) with iris registration. The ablation algorithm was derived from the iDesign aberrometer. For all treatments, the optical zone diameter was 6.0 mm with a transition zone of 8.0 mm. In patients with astigmatism, 6.0 mm was the size of the minor axis of the elliptical ablation. A nomogram was used to adjust the sphere according to the magnitude of the aberrometer-derived cylinder to avoid overcorrection of sphere when treating high cylinder (Table 2).

For stromal ablations greater than $70\,\mu m$, a circular sponge soaked in mitomycin C 0.02% was applied for 20 seconds. The ocular surface was then thoroughly rinsed with 15 mL of balanced salt solution. A bandage contact lens (PureVision, Bausch & Lomb) was placed on the eye and left in place until the cornea reepithelialized.

Postoperative medications consisted of topical levofloxacin 0.5%, 4 times a day for one week, and 4 weeks of tapering dose of topical fluorometholone ophthalmic solution 0.1% in the following sequence: 4 times a day for 1 week, 3 times a day for 1 week, 2 times a day for one week, and once a day for one week.

2.2. Wavefront Sensor. The iDesign System is a new generation high definition Hartmann-Shack aberrometer that has greater dynamic range (−16.0 to +12.0 D with up to +8.0 D of cylinder and up to $8\,\mu m$ of HOA RMS) and higher resolution than previous generation Hartmann-Shack devices. Refraction measured by this wavefront sensor was found to have high repeatability [10]. The data reconstruction is done by Fourier algorithms, using up to 1,257 data points over a 7 mm pupil diameter. The device performs five ocular measurements within a single capture sequence: topography, autorefractometry, pupillometry, and keratometry.

2.3. Statistical Analysis. Snellen visual acuity was converted into logMAR for statistical analysis, and all continuous variables were described with mean, standard deviation, and range. Paired Student's t-test was used for comparisons between consecutive visits. Correlation coefficients were calculated to assess the correlation between different variables. To evaluate the change in refractive cylinder, vector analysis was performed, using a previously described technique [11]. All data were analysed using Microsoft Office Excel 2007 program (Microsoft Corp.) and STATISTICA (StatSoft Inc.)

TABLE 1: Patient satisfaction questionnaire (follow-up: 3.1 ± 0.9 months, $n = 296$ patients).

Questions	Responses
Thinking about your vision during the last week, how satisfied are you with your vision? (without the use of glasses or contact lenses)	
Very satisfied	58.1%
Satisfied	36.7%
Neither	2.9%
Dissatisfied	1.8%
Very dissatisfied	0.5%
Because of your eyesight, how much difficulty do you have driving at night?	
No difficulty at all	61.0%
A little difficulty	23.6%
Moderate difficulty	5.9%
A lot of difficulty	0.4%
I am unable to drive at night because of my vision	0.4%
I do not drive at night for other reasons	8.8%
Would you recommend vision correction surgery to your friends and relatives?	
Yes	95.5%
No	4.5%
Visual phenomena	Mean ± SD (median)
Night vision phenomena scores measured on scale from 1 (no difficulty) to 7 (severe difficulty)	
Starburst	1.55 ± 0.99 (1)
Glare	1.57 ± 0.95 (1)
Halo	1.50 ± 0.92 (1)
Ghosting/double vision	1.38 ± 0.89 (1)
Dry eye symptoms rated on scan from 1 (no difficulty) to 7 (severe difficulty)	
Dry eye score (mean ± SD (median))	2.17 ± 1.31 (2)

TABLE 2: Nomogram for physician adjustment based on preoperative cylinder values obtained with the aberrometer. D: diopters.

Preoperative cylinder on aberrometry (D) (range)	Physician adjustment for sphere (D)
0 to 0.25	−0.25
0.26 to 0.75	−0.13
0.76 to 1.00	0.00
1.01 to 2.00	0.20
2.01 to 3.00	0.40
3.01 to 4.00	0.60
4.01 to 5.00	0.80
5.01 to 6.00	1.00
6.01 to 7.00	1.20
7.01 to 8.00	1.40

on a personal computer. A level of significance of $P = .05$ was used.

3. Results

This study comprised 662 consecutive eyes of 352 patients that underwent primary myopic wavefront-guided photorefractive keratectomy between December 2013 and June 2014. Demographics of the study group, as well as the main preoperative and 3 months' postoperative outcomes, are summarized in Table 3.

3.1. *Refractive and Visual Outcomes.* Figure 1 displays the predictability of the manifest spherical equivalent (MSE) at 3 months postoperatively. There was a strong and statistically significant correlation between the attempted and achieved MSE ($r = 0.99$, $P < .01$). The percentages of eyes with the 3 months' postoperative MSE within ±0.50 D and within ±1.00 D were 91.1% (603 eyes) and 97.6% (646 eyes), respectively. There was a statistically significant reduction in sphere, cylinder, and MSE postoperatively (Table 3). Table 4 shows the stability of manifest refraction between consecutive visits. There was no statistically significant change in manifest sphere between 1-week and 1-month and between 1-month and 3-month examinations. Manifest cylinder reduced significantly between 1-month and 3-month visits (change by 0.19 D, $P < .01$), which resulted in a slight increase of MSE

TABLE 3: Demographics and preoperative and 3 months' postoperative outcomes ($n = 662$ eyes).

	Preoperative	3 months' postoperative	P value
Age (years)			
Mean ± SD	32.3 ± 9.4	—	—
Range	(18 to 62)		
Gender			
Male/female	54%/46%	—	—
Eye			
Right/left	51%/49%	—	—
Sphere [D]			
Mean ± SD	−3.26 ± 2.18	+0.14 ± 0.38	<.01
Range	(−10.75 to −0.25)	(−1.75 to +2.25)	
Cylinder [D]			
Mean ± SD	−0.86 ± 0.83	−0.22 ± 0.28	<.01
Range	(−5.25 to 0.00)	(−2.00 to 0.00)	
MSE [D]			
Mean ± SD	−3.69 ± 2.20	+0.03 ± 0.38	<.01
Range	(−11.00 to −0.50)	(−2.50 to +2.00)	
UDVA [logMAR]			
Mean ± SD	0.90 ± 0.40	−0.05 ± 0.11	<.01
Range	(0.10 to 1.60)	(−0.20 to 0.60)	
CDVA [logMAR]			
Mean ± SD	−0.07 ± 0.05	−0.08 ± 0.06	<.01
Range	(−0.20 to 0.22)	(−0.20 to 0.40)	

TABLE 4: Stability of refraction ($n = 662$).

	1 week to 1 month	1 month to 3 months
Change in sphere by ≤0.5	82.9% (549 eyes)	92.1% (610 eyes)
Change in sphere by ≤1.0 D	95.0% (629 eyes)	98.9% (655 eyes)
Mean change in sphere ± SD	−0.01 ± 0.53	−0.02 ± 0.35
(P value)	(P = .50)	(P = .16)
95% CI	−0.05 to 0.03	−0.05 to 0.01
Change in Cyl by ≤0.5 D	74.9% (496 eyes)	87.0% (576 eyes)
Change in Cyl by ≤1.0 D	93.5% (619 eyes)	98.8% (654 eyes)
Mean change in Cyl ± SD	−0.02 ± 0.66*	+0.19 ± 0.38*
(P value)	(P = .48)	(P < .01)
95% CI	−0.07 to 0.03	0.16 to 0.22
Change in MSE by ≤0.5 D	82.8% (548 eyes)	89.3% (591 eyes)
Change in MSE by ≤1.0 D	96.7% (640 eyes)	99.1% (656 eyes)
Mean change in MSE ± SD	−0.02 ± 0.48	+0.07 ± 0.34
(P value)	(P = .35)	(P < .01)
95% CI	−0.06 to 0.02	0.04 to 0.10

MSE: manifest spherical equivalent; D: diopter; SD: standard deviation; CI: confidence interval; Cyl: cylinder.
* Cylinder recorded in "minus" form. Positive change means reduction in manifest cylinder.

between 1-month and 3-month visits (change by +0.07 D, $P <$ .01). Figure 2 shows the change in MSE, UDVA, and CDVA over 3-month postoperative period.

Figure 3 displays the 3 months' postoperative monocular and binocular cumulative UDVA. The percentage of eyes with monocular UDVA 20/20 or better was 89.4% (592 eyes). In patients that had both eyes treated, the percentage of patients achieving binocular UDVA 20/20 or better was 96.5% (299 patients). Figure 4 depicts safety, the change between preoperative and postoperative CDVA. At 3 months postoperatively, 1.1% (7 eyes) lost 2 or more lines of CDVA, whereas 27.5% (182 eyes) gained 1 or more lines. The loss of

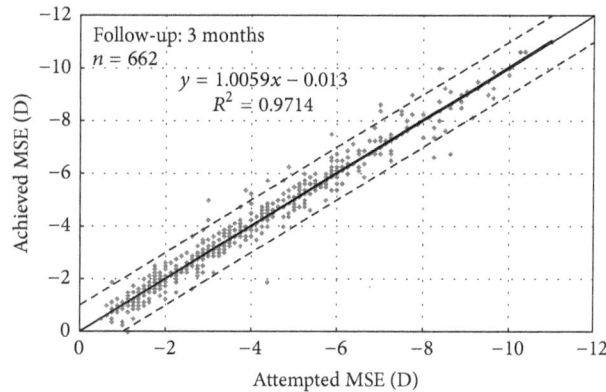

FIGURE 1: Predictability of manifest spherical equivalent (MSE). The area between two dotted lines is the postoperative MSE within ±1.00 D. The solid black line represents linear regression.

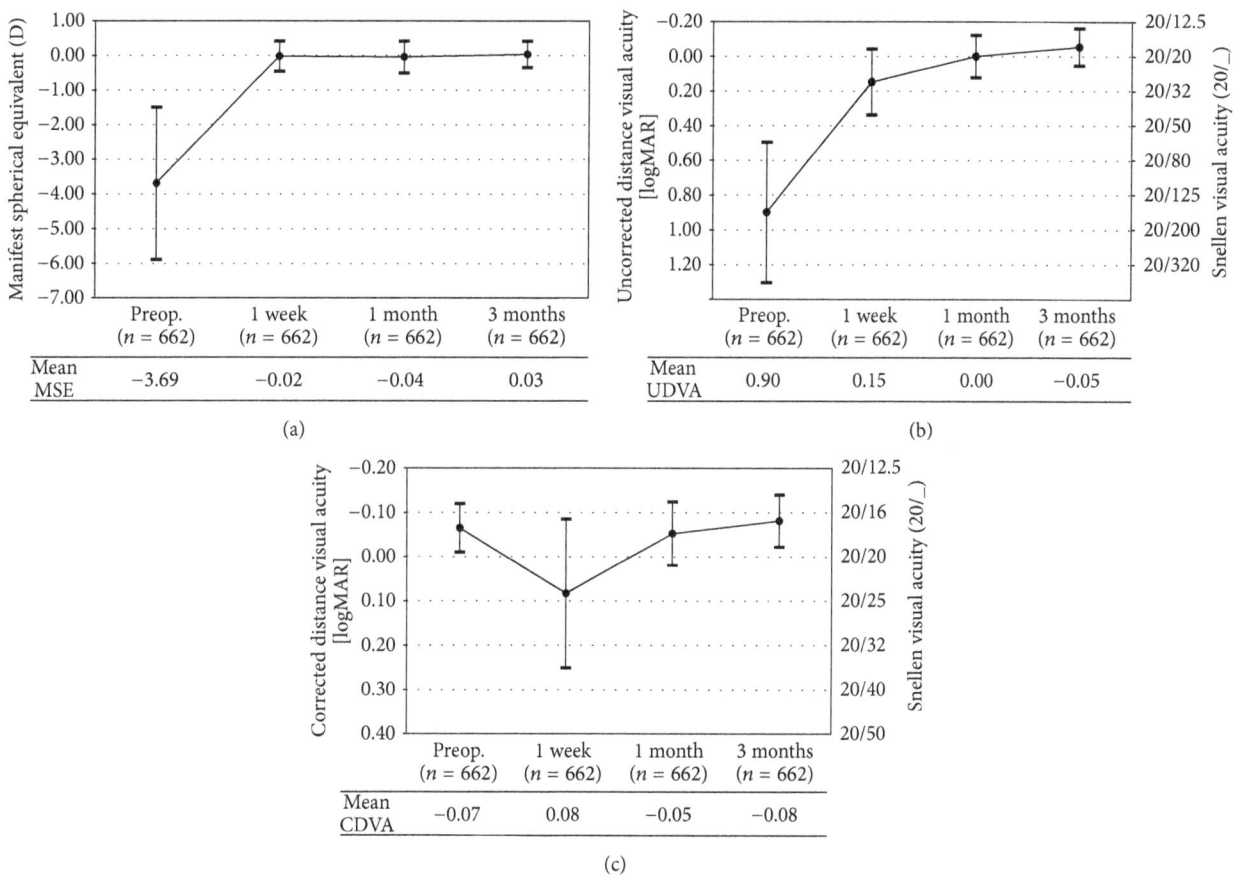

| Mean MSE | −3.69 | −0.02 | −0.04 | 0.03 |

(a)

| Mean UDVA | 0.90 | 0.15 | 0.00 | −0.05 |

(b)

| Mean CDVA | −0.07 | 0.08 | −0.05 | −0.08 |

(c)

FIGURE 2: Change in refraction and visual acuities over time: (a) change in manifest spherical equivalent (MSE), (b) change in uncorrected distance visual acuity (UDVA), and (c) change in corrected distance visual acuity (CDVA). Error bars represent ± one standard deviation.

2 lines of CDVA was due to ocular surface issues, such as reduced tear break-up time and the presence of superficial punctate keratitis (4 eyes) and unresolved haze (3 eyes).

3.2. Vector Analyses of Refractive Astigmatism. Table 5 summarizes the mean values for vector analysis of the change in refractive astigmatism. At 3 months, 93.6% of eyes had a mean error of magnitude (difference between SIRC and IRC)

within 0.50 D. The mean correction ratio (|SIRC|/|IRC|) was 1.02 ± 0.43, and the mean error of angle was 0.00 ± 14.86°. Figure 5 plots the surgically induced refractive correction (SIRC) against intended refractive correction (IRC). Strong and statistically significant correlation was found between IRC and SIRC (r = 0.95, P < .01, Figure 5). The linear regression of IRC versus SIRC had a slope of 0.88 and intercept of 0.07 (Figure 5).

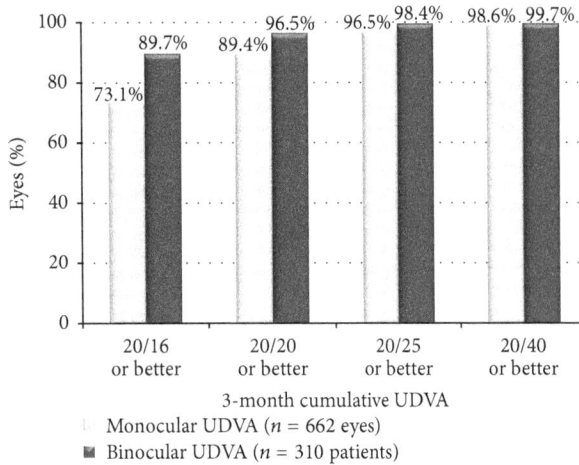

FIGURE 3: Cumulative monocular and binocular uncorrected distance visual acuity (UDVA) at 3 months postoperatively.

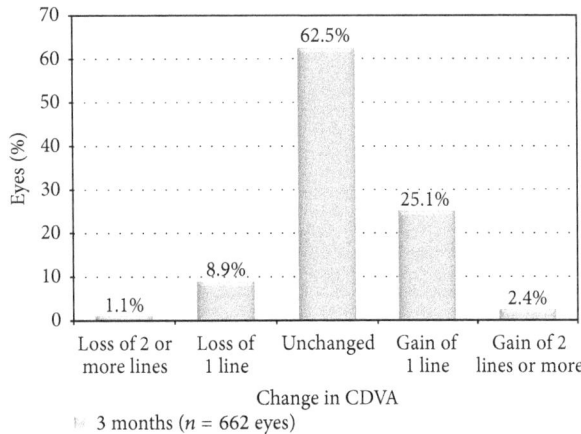

FIGURE 4: Safety comparison of preoperative and postoperative corrected distance visual acuity (CDVA) at 3 months postoperatively.

3.3. Patient Reported Outcomes.

Out of 352 patients, 296 (84.1%) completed the postoperative patient satisfaction questionnaire with the mean follow-up of 3.1 ± 0.9 months. The percentage of patients willing to recommend the procedure to their friends and relatives was 95.5%. All scores for night vision disturbances had a median of 1 (no difficulty). A small percentage of patients (0.4%) claimed to have a lot of difficulty with night driving, and 0.4% felt unable to drive at night because of their vision. The percentage of patients being "dissatisfied" or "very dissatisfied" with their uncorrected vision was 2.3%. There was a statistically significant correlation between the magnitude of postoperative MSE, postoperative UDVA, and patients' satisfaction with visual outcomes (MSE versus satisfaction: $r = 0.10$, $P = .01$; UDVA versus satisfaction: $r = 0.20$, $P < .01$). Postoperative UDVA was also correlated to the scores for night vision disturbances and night driving (starburst: $r = 0.08$, $P = .03$; glare: $r = 0.14$, $P < .01$; halo: $r = 0.12$, $P < .01$; ghosting/double vision: $r = 0.13$, $P < .01$; night driving: $r = 0.08$, $P = .03$).

TABLE 5: Vector analysis of refractive astigmatism (follow-up: 3 months, $n = 662$).

Vector parameter	Mean ± SD (range)
Intended refractive correction [D]	0.86 ± 0.83 (0 to 5.25)
Surgically induced refractive correction [D]	0.92 ± 0.76 (0 to 5.71)
Error vector [D]	0.23 ± 0.29 (0 to 2.00)
Correction ratio	1.02 ± 0.43 (0 to 4.12)
Error of magnitude [D]	0.04 ± 0.27 (−1.25 to 1.25)
Error of angle [°]	0.00 ± 14.86 (−85.15 to 84.03)
Absolute error of angle [°]	4.97 ± 14.00 (0 to 84.03)
Axis shift [°]	0.13 ± 28.52 (−89.00 to 89.00)

SD: standard deviation; D: diopters.

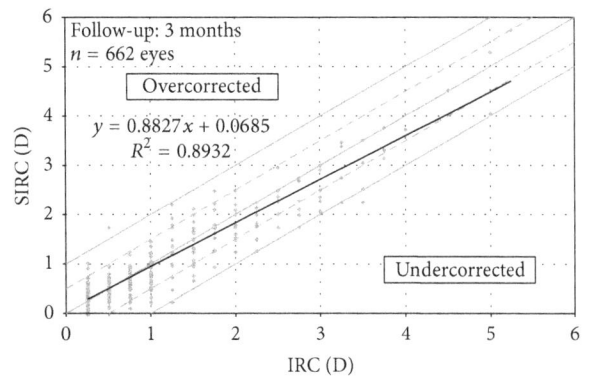

FIGURE 5: Intended refractive correction (IRC) versus surgically induced refractive correction (SIRC) at 3 months postoperatively. Solid black line is the linear regression.

4. Discussion

Outcomes of wavefront-guided keratorefractive procedures, developed to target eye's preexisting lower and higher order aberrations, can be influenced by several factors. These include quality, resolution, and repeatability of the preoperative diagnostic equipment [12, 13], as well as the technology engaged in precise alignment of ablation profile on patient's cornea during the excimer laser procedure [14]. The new iDesign System has the highest resolution of any Hartmann-Shack aberrometer available in clinical practice. The device can capture up to 1257 data points, depending on pupil size, allowing more precise determination of true ocular wavefront and better accuracy of aberrometer-derived refraction, including magnitude and axis of astigmatism. Another feature of this new device is an enhanced iris registration system, which may improve rotational and directional alignment

TABLE 6: Summary of published results of wavefront-guided photorefractive keratectomy.

Author (year)	Number of eyes	Follow-up (months)	Laser	Preoperative MSE [D] Mean ± SD (range)	Preoperative Magnitude of cylinder [D] Mean ± SD (range)	Postoperative MSE [D] Mean ± SD (range)	Postoperative Magnitude of cylinder [D] Mean ± SD (range)	Postoperative MSE within ±0.50 D	Postoperative MSE within ±1.00 D	Postop. UDVA 20/20 or better	Loss of 2 or more lines of CDVA
Vinciguerra et al. (2007) [15]	68	3	NIDEK EC-5000 CX II	−5.73 ± 2.03 (−2.50 to −11.25)	0.66 ± 0.59 (0 to 2.50)	−0.02 ± 0.78 (—)	—	92%	98%	100%	0%
Durrie et al. (2008) [16]	50	6	Alcon LADARVision 4000	−3.99 (—)	0.63 (0 to 2.75)	+0.08 (—)	0.26 (—)	—	—	94%	—
Karimian et al. (2010) [17]	28	8.1 ± 3.3	Technolas 217z	−4.92 ± 1.60 (−1.13 to −7.87)	0.93 ± 1.10 (—)	+0.19 ± 0.60 (−0.63 to +1.38)	0.57 ± 0.40 (0 to 1.50)	60.7%	100%	67.9%	—
Moshirfar et al. (2010) [5]	101	6	Visx Star S4 IR	−4.31 ± 2.01 (−1.53 to −8.07)	0.96 ± 0.78 (0 to 3.00)	+0.08 ± 0.35 (−0.75 to 1.50)	0.36 ± 0.37 (0 to 1.25)	77%	—	75%	2%
Manche and Haw (2011) [18]	34	12	Visx Star S4 IR	−4.39 ± 2.02 (−0.75 to −8.00)	0.85 ± 0.62 (0.0 to 2.50)	−0.17 ± 0.41 (—)	0.25 ± 0.25 (—)	91%	97%	97%	0%
Joosse et al. (2011) [19]	60	12	Technolas 217z	−6.05 ± 0.77 (−4.25 to −7.63)	0.88 ± 0.56 (0 to 2.25)	−0.02 ± 0.47 (−1.50 to 0.88)	0.32 ± 0.32 (0 to 1.25)	80%	96.7%	80%	6.7%
van Philips (2011) [20]	27	10	Technolas 217z100	−5.72 ± 0.88 (−4.25 to −7.50)	0.84 ± 0.59 *(0 to 2.25)	−0.03 ± 0.42 (−0.75 to +1.00)	0.32 ± 0.33 (0 to 1.25)	82%	100%	78%	0%
Bababeygy and Manche (2011) [21]	146	12	Visx Star S4 IR	−5.70 ± 2.54 (−0.13 to −10.30)	0.96 ± 0.81 (0 to 3.25)	−0.26 ± 0.31 (—)	0.30 ± 0.35 (0 to 1.50)	81.5%	96.6%	—	0%
Moshirfar et al. (2011) [22]	23	3	Visx Star S4 IR	−3.34 ± 1.75 (+1.0 to −8.50)	0.47 ± 0.35 (0 to 2.75)	+0.14 ± 0.31 (−0.38 to +0.88)	0.27 ± 0.25 (0 to 0.75)	96%	100%	91%	0%
Mifflin et al. (2012) [23]	40	12	Visx Star S4 IR	−3.22 ± 1.86 (+0.38 to −7.13)	0.72 ± 0.64 (0 to 2.50)	−0.08 ± 0.35 (−0.63 to +0.75)	0.31 ± 0.40 (0 to 1.25)	88.6%	94.3%	88.6%	0%
Ryan and O'Keefe (2012) [6]	38	12	Technolas 217z100	−3.99 ± 1.26 (−2.04 to −6.52)	1.01 ± 1.23 (−0.25 to 5.80)	−0.26 ± 0.31 (—)	0.47 ± 0.51 (—)	89.2%	97.3%	87%	0%
Current study	662	3	Visx Star S4 IR	−3.69 ± 2.20 (−0.50 to −11.00)	0.86 ± 0.83 (0 to 5.25)	+0.03 ± 0.38 (−2.50 to +2.00)	0.22 ± 0.28 (0 to 2.00)	91.1%	97.6%	89.4%	1.1%

*Cylinder change in the table: positive change in cylinder means reduction of cylinder.

of the ablation profile. Correct alignment of ablation on patient's cornea is critical when the treatment of higher order aberrations is attempted. Wavefront-guided ablations tend to be more sensitive to any misalignment (whether caused by an initial placement error or by intraoperative eye movement) than standard spherocylindrical corrections [24, 25]. In this study, we analyzed the outcomes of wavefront-guided photorefractive keratotomy in a large cohort of consecutive patients with a new generation Hartmann-Shack aberrometer used in preoperative planning. To our knowledge, this is the first study evaluating the use of this new device in treatment planning of surface ablations.

In this study, we observed the mean MSE of +0.03 ± 0.38 D at 3 months postoperatively, which is an excellent result considering the wide range of preoperative spherical equivalents (−0.50 to −11.00 D). The percentage of eyes with postoperative MSE within 0.50 D and 1.00 D was 91.1% and 97.6%, respectively. At 3 months, 89.4% of eyes had monocular UDVA of 20/20 or better, and the percentage of patients achieving binocular UDVA 20/20 or better was 96.5%. The change in manifest sphere was relatively stable between 1-week and 1-month and between 1-month and 3-month visits. However, manifest cylinder improved significantly between the 1-month and 3-month postoperative examinations (Table 4). Table 6 presents a summary of the literature [5, 6, 15–23] with refractive and visual outcomes of wavefront-guided PRK using different laser platforms and aberrometers. Most of the studies were performed with a small number of subjects, which makes the comparison difficult. Despite this, our results are comparable or superior to the studies in this review.

When it comes to the astigmatic correction, we achieved a mean correction ratio (ratio of the magnitude of SIRC to IRC) of 1.02 ± 0.43 at 3 months, which is comparable to the previous report on the use of the same aberrometer (iDesign System) in eyes undergoing wavefront-guided LASIK (1.02 ± 0.30, n = 243) [23]. The mean error of magnitude was +0.04 ± 0.27 D (arithmetic difference of the magnitudes between SIRC and IRC), and the mean error of angle was 0.00 ± 14.86° (angular difference between attempted treatment and achieved treatment). Hardly did any studies of wavefront-guided surface ablation report detailed vector analysis of astigmatic correction; however, Table 6 shows the magnitude of residual cylinder in each study found in the literature [5, 6, 15–23]. We achieved the lowest magnitude of postoperative cylinder (0.22 D) and one of the lowest standard deviations (0.28) despite having the largest cohort of patients and the widest range cylindrical correction (0 to 5.25 D). In addition, the scattergram of IRC versus SIRC shows undercorrection for higher values of preoperative cylinder (linear regression slope of 0.88, Figure 5), which could potentially be further improved with nomogram refinement.

One of the main reasons for considering the use of WFG ablation is its ability to minimize the induction of higher order aberrations (HOAs). The induction of HOA typically observed when using standard spherocylindrical corrections can result in unwanted optical side effects, as well as reduced patient satisfaction. The postoperative satisfaction with visual outcomes in our study was correlated to the amount of residual refractive error. We measured scores for night vision disturbances on the scale from 1 (no difficulty) to 7 (severe difficulty) and achieved mean scores of 1.55 ± 0.99 for starburst, 1.57 ± 0.95 for glare, 1.50 ± 0.92 for halos, and 1.38 ± 0.89 for ghosting and double vision at the 3.1 ± 0.9 months' follow-up visits. A prospective study by He and Manche [26] reports postoperative scores for night vision phenomena for WFG PRK, using a scale from 0 (no symptoms) to 10 (disabling symptoms) as follows: between 1 and 1.5 for night time glare and halos and close to 0.5 at 12 months postoperatively for diplopia/ghosting. Another study [18] found similar scores (1 to 1.5 for glare and halos at 12 months) measured on the same scale from 0 to 10, with the highest peak of symptoms at 1 month postoperatively (both night time glare and halos close to 2.5).

We found favorable outcomes with wavefront-guided PRK with ablation profiles derived from the new generation Hartmann-Shack aberrometer. Although LASIK is the preferred surgical choice in our practice, there are still a reasonable number of patients where surface ablation is selected, following surgeon/patient discussion. Many studies confirmed that the two techniques have similar efficacy, predictability, and safety, with the important exception of the slower visual recovery for PRK [1]. Some studies even found that PRK might induce fewer higher order aberrations compared to LASIK. Review of the literature regarding the impact of flap creation on postoperative higher order aberrations is mixed. For example, the study of Barreto Jr. et al. [27] found no difference in postoperative HOA between WFG LASIK and PRK, as far as the microkeratome flap creation is concerned, whereas other studies [4, 6] found fewer HOAs being induced with the surface ablation technique. Femtosecond flap is known to have minimal impact on HOA [7]. However, a study by Moshirfar et al. [5] found statistically significantly higher induction of HOAs with femtosecond LASIK (increase factor 1.74) than with PRK (increase factor 1.22), with wavefront-guided ablation used in both cases.

Our study has several limitations. Firstly, it is retrospective, and no comparison of preoperative and postoperative higher order aberrations was conducted. Secondly, refractive outcomes are evaluated over a 3-month period; long-term data might be necessary to confirm refractive stability. Despite the limitations, results of a large consecutive cohort of patients are presented in this study. The use of a new generation Hartmann-Shack aberrometer resulted in high predictability, efficacy, and safety, in a wide range of refractive errors undergoing a surface ablation treatment. Preoperative to postoperative changes in higher order aberrations should be further investigated.

Conflict of Interests

Steven C. Schallhorn, M.D., is a consultant for Abbott Medical Optics and Zeiss and global medical director for Optical Express. None of the other authors have a financial or proprietary interest in the products and materials presented in this paper.

References

[1] A. J. Shortt, B. D. S. Allan, and J. R. Evans, "Laser-assisted in-situ keratomileusis (LASIK) versus photorefractive keratectomy (PRK) for myopia," *Cochrane Database of Systematic Reviews*, vol. 1, Article ID CD005135, 2013.

[2] R. Ambrósio Jr. and S. E. Wilson, "LASIK vs LASEk vs PRK: advantages and indications," *Seminars in Ophthalmology*, vol. 18, no. 1, pp. 2–10, 2003.

[3] K. Kamiya, K. Shimizu, and F. Ohmoto, "Comparison of the changes in corneal biomechanical properties after photorefractive keratectomy and laser in situ keratomileusis," *Cornea*, vol. 28, no. 7, pp. 765–769, 2009.

[4] A. D. Wallau and M. Campos, "One-year outcomes of a bilateral randomised prospective clinical trial comparing PRK with mitomycin C and LASIK," *British Journal of Ophthalmology*, vol. 93, no. 12, pp. 1634–1638, 2009.

[5] M. Moshirfar, J. A. Schliesser, J. C. Chang et al., "Visual outcomes after wavefront-guided photorefractive keratectomy and wavefront-guided laser in situ keratomileusis: prospective comparison," *Journal of Cataract & Refractive Surgery*, vol. 36, no. 8, pp. 1336–1343, 2010.

[6] A. Ryan and M. O'Keefe, "Wavefront-guided and aspheric ablation for myopia—one-year results of the zyoptix personalized treatment advanced algorithm," *American Journal of Ophthalmology*, vol. 153, no. 6, pp. 1169–1177, 2012.

[7] C. T. Hood, R. R. Krueger, and S. E. Wilson, "The association between femtosecond laser flap parameters and ocular aberrations after uncomplicated custom myopic LASIK," *Graefe's Archive for Clinical and Experimental Ophthalmology*, vol. 251, no. 9, pp. 2155–2162, 2013.

[8] K. A. Hettinger, "The role of biostatistics in the quality improvement of refractive surgery," *Journal of Refractive Surgery*, vol. 25, no. 7, supplement, pp. S651–S654, 2009.

[9] K. D. Solomon, L. E. F. de Castro, H. P. Sandoval et al., "LASIK world literature review: quality of life and patient satisfaction," *Ophthalmology*, vol. 116, no. 4, pp. 691–701, 2009.

[10] C. E. Charles, T. D. Raymond, C. D. Baer, and D. R. Neal, "Comparison of repeatability of manifest refraction and instrument-based refraction," in *Proceedings of the ARVO Annual Meeting*, Orlando, Fla, USA, May 2012.

[11] M. B. Eydelman, B. Drum, J. Holladay et al., "Standardized analyses of correction of astigmatism by laser systems that reshape the cornea," *Journal of Refractive Surgery*, vol. 22, no. 1, pp. 81–95, 2006.

[12] M. Lombardo and G. Lombardo, "New methods and techniques for sensing the wave aberrations of human eyes," *Clinical and Experimental Optometry*, vol. 92, no. 3, pp. 176–186, 2009.

[13] G. R. Mello, K. M. Rocha, M. R. Santhiago, D. Smadja, and R. R. Krueger, "Applications of wavefront technology," *Journal of Cataract and Refractive Surgery*, vol. 38, no. 9, pp. 1671–1683, 2012.

[14] M. Khalifa, M. El-Kateb, and M. S. Shaheen, "Iris registration in wavefront-guided LASIK to correct mixed astigmatism," *Journal of Cataract and Refractive Surgery*, vol. 35, no. 3, pp. 433–437, 2009.

[15] P. Vinciguerra, E. Albè, F. I. Camesasca, S. Trazza, and D. Epstein, "Wavefront- versus topography-guided customized ablations with the NIDEK EC-5000 CX II in surface ablation treatment: refractive and aberrometric outcomes," *Journal of Refractive Surgery*, vol. 23, supplement 9, pp. S1029–S1036, 2007.

[16] D. S. Durrie, S. G. Slade, and J. Marshall, "Wavefront-guided excimer laser ablation using photorefractive keratectomy and sub-Bowman's keratomileusis: a contralateral eye study," *Journal of Refractive Surgery*, vol. 24, no. 1, pp. S77–S84, 2008.

[17] F. Karimian, S. Feizi, and M. R. Jafarinasab, "Conventional versus custom ablation in photorefractive keratectomy: randomized clinical trial," *Journal of Cataract and Refractive Surgery*, vol. 36, no. 4, pp. 637–643, 2010.

[18] E. E. Manche and W. W. Haw, "Wavefront-guided laser *in situ* keratomileusis (LASIK) versus wavefront-guided photorefractive keratectomy (PRK): a prospective randomized eye-to-eye comparison," *Transactions of the American Ophthalmological Society*, vol. 109, pp. 201–220, 2011.

[19] M. V. Joosse, C. Snoek, and H. M. van Minderhout, "Comparison of wavefront-guided photorefractive keratectomy and foldable iris-fixated phakic intraocular lens implantation for low to moderate myopia," *Journal of Cataract and Refractive Surgery*, vol. 37, no. 2, pp. 370–377, 2011.

[20] L. A. M. van Philips, "Higher-order aberrations after iris-fixated foldable phakic intraocular lens implantation and wavefront-guided photorefractive keratectomy for the correction of myopia," *Journal of Cataract and Refractive Surgery*, vol. 37, no. 2, pp. 284–294, 2011.

[21] S. R. Bababeygy and E. E. Manche, "Wavefront-guided photorefractive keratectomy with the VISX platform for myopia," *Journal of Refractive Surgery*, vol. 27, no. 3, pp. 173–180, 2011.

[22] M. Moshirfar, D. S. Churgin, B. S. Betts et al., "Prospective, randomized, fellow eye comparison of WaveLight Allegretto Wave Eye-Q versus VISX CustomVueTM STAR S4 IRTM in photorefractive keratectomy: analysis of visual outcomes and higher-order aberrations," *Clinical Ophthalmology*, vol. 5, no. 1, pp. 1185–1193, 2011.

[23] M. D. Mifflin, B. B. Hatch, S. Sikder, J. Bell, C. J. Kurz, and M. Moshirfar, "Custom vs conventional PRK: a prospective, randomized, contralateral eye comparison of postoperative visual function," *Journal of Refractive Surgery*, vol. 28, no. 2, pp. 127–132, 2012.

[24] M. Bueeler, M. Mrochen, and T. Seiler, "Maximum permissible lateral decentration in aberration-sensing and wavefront-guided corneal ablation," *Journal of Cataract and Refractive Surgery*, vol. 29, no. 2, pp. 257–263, 2003.

[25] L. Wang and D. D. Koch, "Residual higher-order aberrations caused by clinically measured cyclotorsional misalignment or decentration during wavefront-guided excimer laser corneal ablation," *Journal of Cataract and Refractive Surgery*, vol. 34, no. 12, pp. 2057–2062, 2008.

[26] L. He and E. E. Manche, "Prospective randomized contralateral eye evaluation of subjective quality of vision after wavefront-guided or wavefront-optimized photorefractive keratectomy," *Journal of Refractive Surgery*, vol. 30, no. 1, pp. 6–12, 2014.

[27] J. Barreto Jr., M. T. S. Barboni, C. Feitosa-Santana et al., "Intraocular straylight and contrast sensitivity after contralateral wavefront-guided LASIK and wavefront-guided PRK for myopia," *Journal of Refractive Surgery*, vol. 26, no. 8, pp. 588–593, 2010.

3

Choroidal Thickness in Eyes with Unilateral Ocular Ischemic Syndrome

Dong Yoon Kim,[1] **Soo Geun Joe,**[2] **Joo Yong Lee,**[3] **June-Gone Kim,**[3] **and Sung Jae Yang**[2]

[1]*Department of Ophthalmology, College of Medicine, Chungbuk National University, Cheongju, Republic of Korea*
[2]*Department of Ophthalmology, Gangneung Asan Hospital, College of Medicine, University of Ulsan,*
Gangneung 210-711, Republic of Korea
[3]*Department of Ophthalmology, Asan Medical Center, College of Medicine, University of Ulsan, Seoul, Republic of Korea*

Correspondence should be addressed to Sung Jae Yang; d001065@naver.com

Academic Editor: Ireneusz Grulkowski

Aim. To analyze the subfoveal choroid thickness and choroidal volume in unilateral ocular ischemic syndrome (OIS). *Methods.* A retrospective review was conducted for all patients with unilateral OIS from October 2010 through June 2014. The subfoveal choroidal thickness (SFChT) and choroidal volume of both eyes were compared. *Results.* 19 unilateral OIS patients were included in this study. The mean SFChT of OIS eyes was significantly lower than that of fellow eyes (OIS eyes: 208.89 ± 82.62 μm and fellow eyes: 265.31 ± 82.77 μm, $P < 0.001$). The choroidal volume of OIS eyes was significantly smaller than that of fellow eyes (OIS eyes: 0.16 ± 0.05 mm^3 and fellow eyes: 0.21 ± 0.05 mm^3, $P < 0.001$). *Conclusion.* The choroidal thickness and volume of OIS eyes were smaller than those of unaffected fellow eyes. Decreased choroidal circulation caused by carotid artery stenosis might affect the discordance of choroidal thickness and choroidal volume.

1. Introduction

Ocular ischemic syndrome (OIS) is a potentially vision-threatening disorder caused by ocular hypoperfusion resulting from stenosis or occlusion of the common or internal carotid arteries [1]. OIS manifests as visual loss, orbital pain, and changes of the visual field. Chronic progressive ocular ischemia may lead to permanent blindness secondary to neovascular glaucoma and optic atrophy [2, 3].

Stenosis or occlusion of the common or internal carotid arteries affects not only retinal blood flow but also choroidal blood flow. Because the choroid is a vascular tissue layer encasing a cavernous space, certain characteristics of the choroid, particularly its thickness, have been challenging to study histologically. Recent studies reported that the subfoveal choroidal thickness can be measured noninvasively by enhanced depth imaging OCT (EDI-OCT) [4, 5]. The choroid plays an important role in the physiology of healthy eyes and in the pathogenesis of a variety of ocular diseases. Because the choroidal thickness changes with specific pathologies, measurements of choroidal thickness are

becoming more common, and it is an accepted procedure in the clinic and in research [6–9].

A previous study reported 3 cases of OIS patients who showed lower choroidal thickness in affected eye [10]. We postulated that ocular hypoperfusion may affect choroidal thickness and tried to demonstrate a difference in choroidal thickness in ocular ischemic syndrome with a large number of patients. To our knowledge, subfoveal choroidal thickness has not been fully investigated in a large number of patients. Here, we compared the subfoveal choroid thickness and choroidal volume between eyes with OIS and healthy contralateral eyes in 19 patients.

2. Patients and Methods

2.1. Study Design and Participants. A retrospective review was conducted of all patients who were diagnosed with OIS at Asan Medical Center in Seoul, Korea, and Gangneung Asan Hospital in Gangneung, Korea, from October 2010 through June 2014. We diagnosed OIS in eyes with at least four of

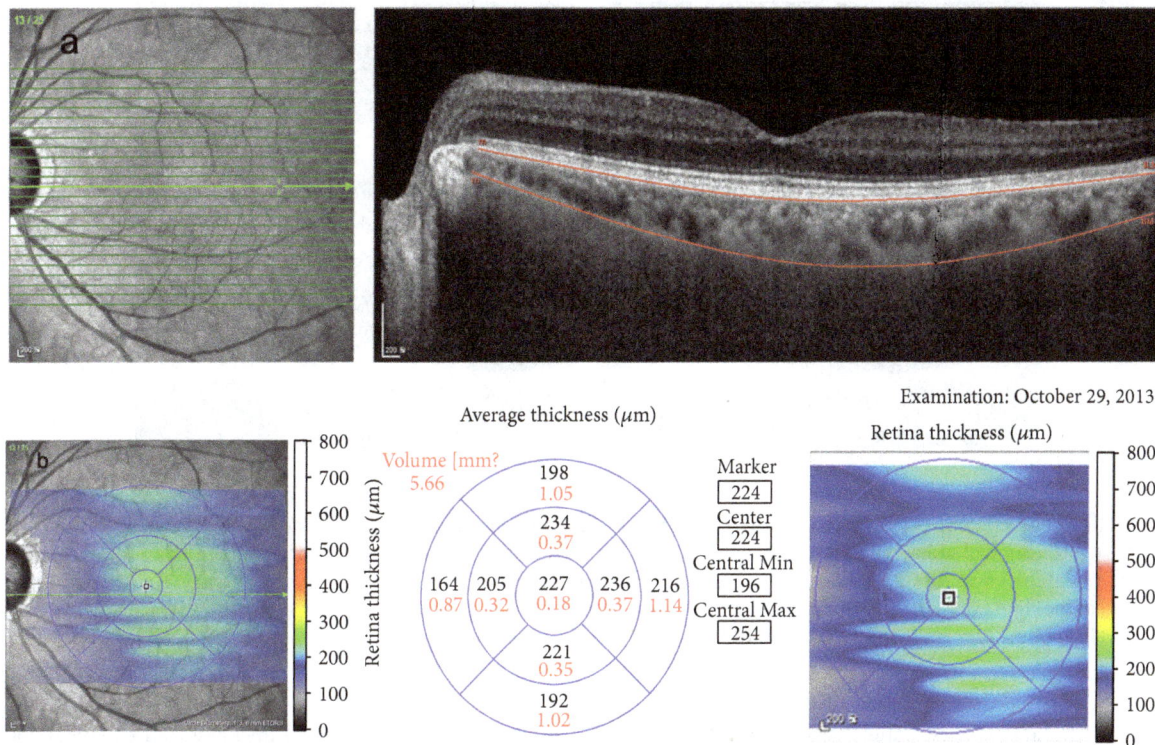

FIGURE 1: Choroidal volume measurement. For choroidal volume measurement, we manually moved the automatically segmented internal limiting membrane line to the retinal pigment epithelium and the automatically segmented retinal pigment epithelium lint to the chorioscleral junction. Once we changed the automatically segmented line, the choroidal volume was automatically calculated and displayed within the ETDRS grid.

the following symptoms and signs: (1) visual loss, abrupt or gradual; (2) ocular pain; (3) iris rubeosis; (4) narrow retinal arteries; (5) dilated, nontortuous retinal veins; (6) midperipheral retinal hemorrhages; and (7) neovascularization of the optic disc in the posterior segment, in addition to two or more of the following fluorescein angiographic signs: (1) patchy, delayed choroidal filling; (2) increased retinal arteriovenous transit time; and (3) late retinal artery staining and definite stenosis of carotid artery in carotid doppler examination [11, 12]. Exclusion criteria included bilateral OIS eyes, presence of refractive error > ±4.0 diopters, choroidal neovascularization or other macular diseases that might affect vision, active intraocular inflammation and/or infection, or a history of any type of intraocular surgery (except cataract surgery), and diabetic retinopathy. We also excluded patients who underwent carotid endarterectomy before SD-OCT examination. The study was approved by the Institutional Review Board of Asan Medical Center and Gangneung Asan Hospital and this study followed the tenets of the Declaration of Helsinki.

2.2. Ophthalmic Examinations. All patients received a complete bilateral ophthalmic examination, including best corrected visual acuity (BCVA), by using the Snellen eye chart. All BCVA results were converted to the LogMAR scale. All patients also underwent refractive error assessment, biomicroscopic examination, fundus examination, fundus photography, FA (fluorescein angiography), and SD-OCT. A Heidelberg Spectralis device (Heidelberg Engineering,

Heidelberg, Germany) was used to obtain SD-OCT images of the macula by applying a custom 25° × 25° volume acquisition protocol to obtain a set of high-speed scans from each eye. Using this protocol, 25 cross-sectional B-scan images were obtained, each of which was composed of 512 A-scans. Choroidal images were also obtained using the EDI technique.

SFChT was manually measured by two retina specialists (Dong Yoon Kim and Sung Jae Yang) using calipers and Heidelberg Eye Explorer software. For choroidal volume measurement, we manually moved the automatically segmented internal limiting membrane line to the retinal pigment epithelium and the automatically segmented retinal pigment epithelium line to the chorioscleral junction. Once we changed the automatically segmented line, the choroidal volume was automatically calculated and displayed within the ETDRS grid. We obtained five choroidal volume data points within 3000 μm in the EDTRS grid (foveal center, superior, nasal, inferior, temporal) (Figure 1). Choroidal volume measurement was also conducted by two retina specialists (Dong Yoon Kim and Sung Jae Yang). From these data, we analyzed differences in SFChT and choroidal volume between the OIS eye and fellow eye.

2.3. Statistical Analysis. The independent t-test was used to compare OCT parameters between OIS eyes and fellow eyes. To assess the interrater reproducibility of the SFChT and choroidal volume measurements, a Bland-Altman plot was

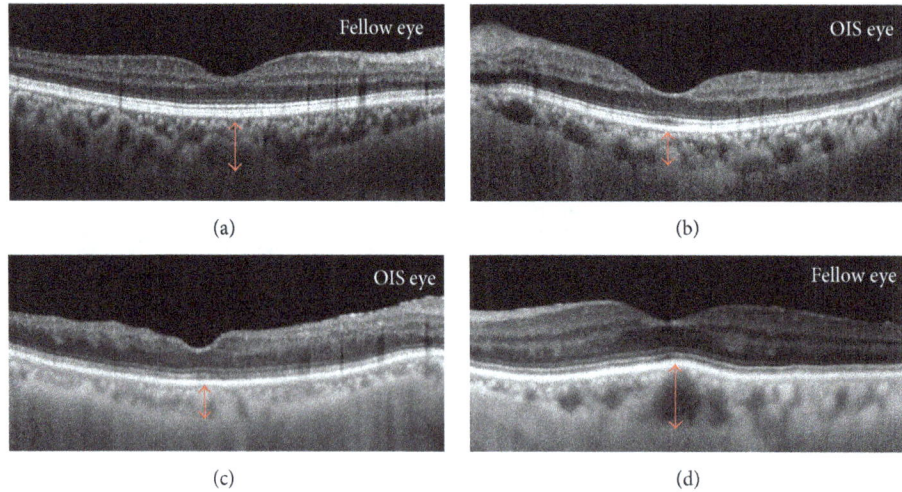

(a)

(b)

(c)

(d)

Figure 2: Optical coherent tomography (OCT) findings, choroidal volume, and fundus image of ocular ischemic syndrome (OIS) and fellow eyes. A 59-year-old man had unilateral OIS in the left eye (a, b). The visual acuity of his right and left eye was 1.0 and 0.4, respectively. The subfoveal choroidal thickness (SFChT) of the OIS eye (b) and fellow eye (a) was 204 μm and 302 μm, respectively. An 82-year-old man had unilateral OIS in the right eye (c, d). The visual acuity of his right and left eye was counting finger and 0.4, respectively. The subfoveal choroidal thickness (SFChT) of the OIS eye (c) and fellow eye (d) was 155 μm and 279 μm, respectively.

Table 1: Clinical characteristics of unilateral ocular ischemic syndrome.

Characteristic	OIS eyes	Fellow eyes	P value
Number of eyes	19		
Age (year)	68.79 ± 8.08		
Sex (male/female)	15/4		
Right/left	13/6		
Carotid stenosis (%)	79.8 (%)	47.3 (%)	<0.001[a]
Refractive error (SE)	0.46 ± 1.26	0.57 ± 1.20	0.689[a]
Baseline BCVA (LogMAR)	0.97 ± 0.75	0.16 ± 0.17	<0.001[a]
IOP (mm Hg)	19.47 ± 9.32	15.21 ± 3.24	0.082[a]

OIS: ocular ischemic syndrome; BCVA: best corrected visual acuity; SE: spherical equivalent; IOP: intraocular pressure.
[a]Independent t-test.

Table 2: Subfoveal choroidal thickness and choroidal volume in unilateral ocular ischemic syndrome.

	OIS eyes	Fellow eyes	P value[a]
Baseline SFChT (μm)	208.89 ± 82.62	265.31 ± 82.77	<0.001
Choroidal volume			
Foveal center (mm^3)	0.16 ± 0.05	0.21 ± 0.05	<0.001
Superior (mm^3)	0.33 ± 0.10	0.40 ± 0.10	0.002
Nasal (mm^3)	0.30 ± 0.11	0.37 ± 0.10	0.001
Inferior (mm^3)	0.32 ± 0.11	0.39 ± 0.10	0.001
Temporal (mm^3)	0.32 ± 0.09	0.41 ± 0.08	<0.001

OIS: ocular ischemic syndrome; SFChT: subfoveal choroidal thickness.
[a]Independent t-test.

generated for each subject. SPSS version 21.0 (SPSS Inc., Chicago, IL) was used to perform all analyses, and $P < 0.05$ was considered statistically significant.

3. Results

19 patients were diagnosed with unilateral OIS at the Asan Medical Center and Gangneung Asan Hospital from October 2010 through June 2014.

Table 1 shows the clinical characteristics of unilateral ocular ischemic syndrome. The mean age of all included eyes was 68.79 ± 8.08 years. Among 19 patients, 15 and 4 patients were male and female, respectively. Among 19 OIS eyes, 13 and 6 eyes developed OIS in the right and left eye, respectively. The proportion of carotid stenosis of the OIS eye and fellow eye was 79.8% and 47.3%, respectively. The baseline LogMAR BCVA was significantly worse in OIS eyes than in the fellow eyes (OIS eye: 0.97 ± 0.75 and fellow eye: 0.16 ± 0.17,

$P < 0.001$). The mean SFChT of OIS eyes was significantly lower than that of fellow eyes (OIS eyes: 208.89 ± 82.62 μm and fellow eyes: 265.31 ± 82.77 μm, $P < 0.001$). At foveal center, the choroidal volume of OIS eyes was significantly smaller than those of fellow eyes (Table 2, OIS eyes: 0.16 ± 0.05 mm^3 and fellow eyes: 0.21 ± 0.05 mm^3, $P < 0.001$), and the choroidal volume was also significantly smaller in OIS eyes than in the fellow eyes in the superior, nasal, inferior, and temporal quadrants within a 1000 μm ETDRS grid.

Two representative patients are described as follows. A 59-year-old man had unilateral OIS in the left eye. The visual acuity of his right and left eye was 1.0 and 0.4, respectively. On slit lamp examination, rubeosis at the iris and angle was found. SFChT and choroidal volume were larger in OIS eyes than in fellow eyes (Figures 2(a) and 2(b)). The patient underwent carotid endarterectomy because of severe carotid arterial stenosis. At 2 days after carotid endarterectomy, the intraocular pressure in the left eye was increased to the 30 mmHg. Because of the uncontrolled intraocular pressure,

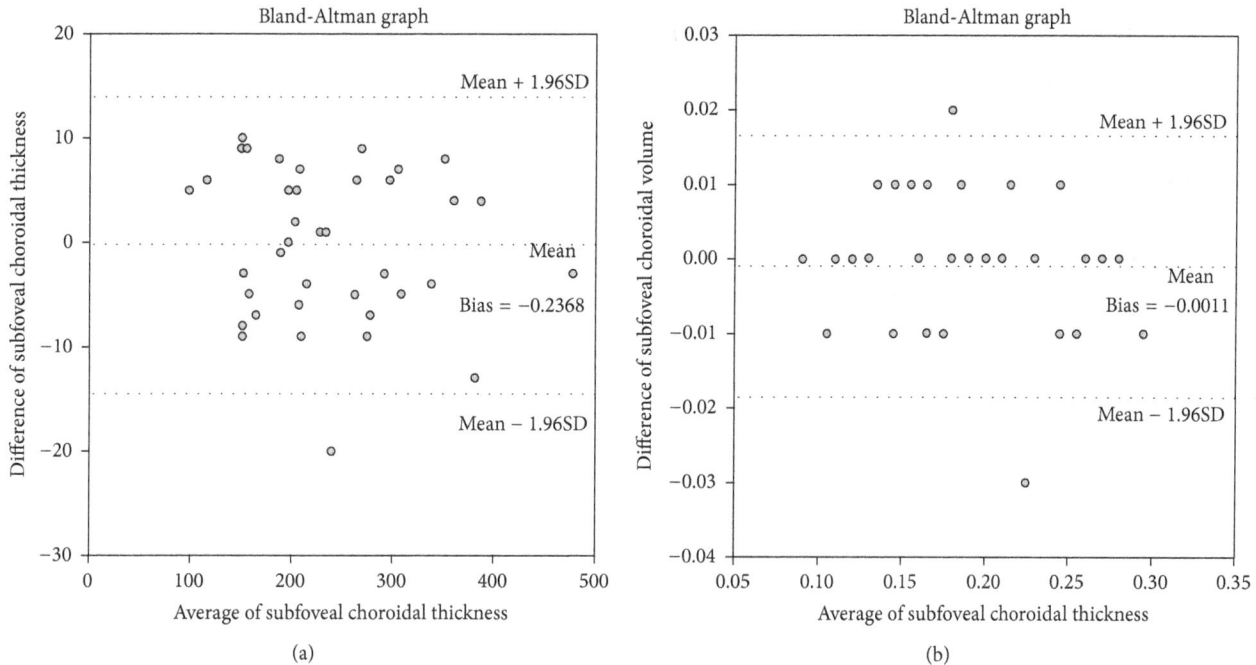

Figure 3: Bland-Altman plot of subfoveal choroidal thickness (SFChT) and choroidal volume. (a) Bland-Altman plot of SFChT measurements taken by two independent retina specialists. No substantial bias was found between the two sets of measurements. The 95% limit of agreement for the SFChT ranged from −14.40 to 13.93. (b) Bland-Altman plot of choroidal volume measurements showing no substantial bias between the two sets of measurements. The 95% limit of agreement for the choroidal volume measurement ranged from −0.186 to 0.165.

a drainage implant was inserted to control intraocular pressure. An 82-year-old man had unilateral OIS in the right eye. The visual acuity of his right and left eye was counting finger and 0.4, respectively. The SFChT and choroidal volume were larger in the fellow eye than in the fellow eye (Figures 2(c) and 2(d)).

To evaluate interobserver reliability of SFChT and choroidal volume measure, Bland-Altman plots were generated and good agreement between the two sets of SFChT and choroidal volume measurements was observed (Figure 3).

4. Discussion

In this study, we compared the subfoveal choroid thickness and choroidal volume between eyes with OIS and healthy fellow eyes in 19 patients. Kang et al. reported that, compared with fellow eyes, the choroidal thickness of OIS eyes was significantly decreased [10]. In this study, we have demonstrated that unilateral OIS eyes have a thinner subfoveal choroid and lower choroidal volume than fellow eyes, indicating impaired choroidal circulation in patients with OIS.

Posterior segment changes, such as narrowed retinal arteries, dilated retinal veins, midperipheral retinal hemorrhages, microaneurysms, retinal neovascularization, and vitreous hemorrhage, are characteristic in OIS. These findings are associated with retinal ischemia and it is unclear how choroidal ischemia would affect the retinal ischemia and vice versa. It is also not certain whether the choroidal thickness change occurs earlier than retinal changes with the development of OIS. It is also not possible to know when the retina and choroid change occurs and whether choroidal thinning

occurred before retinal changes or whether retinal changes occurred before choroidal thinning with the progression of OIS.

The BCVA was also significantly different between OIS eyes and fellow eyes. The baseline LogMAR BCVA was significantly worse in OIS eyes than in fellow eyes (OIS eye: 0.97 ± 0.75 and fellow eye: 0.16 ± 0.17, $P < 0.001$).

To our knowledge, subfoveal choroidal thickness and choroidal volume have not been fully investigated in a large number of patients. The strength of our current study is that it is the first to analyze choroidal volume and thickness difference in unilateral OIS eyes in a larger number of patients. However, our present study has limitations that are inherent to its retrospective design. The sample size of this study was also relatively small, which may have limited the statistical strength of the analysis. Therefore, future studies that examine a larger number of patients are needed to confirm the difference in choroidal thickness in unilateral OIS eyes, and it will be also necessary to observe how retina and choroid change with the progression of OIS by serial evaluation.

In conclusion, the choroidal thickness and volume of OIS eyes were smaller than those of unaffected fellow eyes. Decreased choroidal circulation caused by carotid artery stenosis may affect the discordance of choroidal thickness and choroidal volume.

Conflict of Interests

The authors have no financial or conflict of interests to disclose.

Acknowledgment

This study was funded by Gangneung Asan Hospital (Biomedical Research Center Promotion Fund).

References

[1] V. Biousse, "Carotid disease and the eye," *Current Opinion in Ophthalmology*, vol. 8, no. 6, pp. 16–26, 1997.

[2] J. B. Mizener, P. Podhajsky, and S. S. Hayreh, "Ocular ischemic syndrome," *Ophthalmology*, vol. 104, no. 5, pp. 859–864, 1997.

[3] L. H. Y. Young and R. E. Appen, "Ischemic oculopathy. A manifestation of carotid artery disease," *Archives of Neurology*, vol. 38, no. 6, pp. 358–361, 1981.

[4] R. F. Spaide, H. Koizumi, and M. C. Pozonni, "Enhanced depth imaging spectral-domain optical coherence tomography," *The American Journal of Ophthalmology*, vol. 146, no. 4, pp. 496–500, 2008.

[5] R. Margolis and R. F. Spaide, "A pilot study of enhanced depth imaging optical coherence tomography of the choroid in normal eyes," *American Journal of Ophthalmology*, vol. 147, no. 5, pp. 811–815, 2009.

[6] I. Maruko, T. Iida, Y. Sugano, A. Ojima, and T. Sekiryu, "Subfoveal choroidal thickness in fellow eyes of patients with central serous chorioretinopathy," *Retina*, vol. 31, no. 8, pp. 1603–1608, 2011.

[7] M. Nakayama, H. Keino, A. A. Okada et al., "Enhanced depth imaging optical coherence tomography of the choroid in Vogt-Koyanagi-Harada disease," *Retina*, vol. 32, no. 10, pp. 2061–2069, 2012.

[8] T. Fujiwara, Y. Imamura, R. Margolis, J. S. Slakter, and R. F. Spaide, "Enhanced depth imaging optical coherence tomography of the choroid in highly myopic eyes," *American Journal of Ophthalmology*, vol. 148, no. 3, pp. 445–450, 2009.

[9] V. Manjunath, J. Goren, J. G. Fujimoto, and J. S. Duker, "Analysis of choroidal thickness in age-related macular degeneration using spectral-domain optical coherence tomography," *American Journal of Ophthalmology*, vol. 152, no. 4, pp. 663–668, 2011.

[10] H. M. Kang, C. S. Lee, and S. C. Lee, "Thinner subfoveal choroidal thickness in eyes with ocular ischemic syndrome than in unaffected contralateral eyes," *Graefe's Archive for Clinical and Experimental Ophthalmology*, vol. 252, no. 5, pp. 851–852, 2014.

[11] G. C. Brown and L. E. Magargal, "The ocular ischemic syndrome. Clinical, fluorescein angiographic and carotid angiographic features," *International Ophthalmology*, vol. 11, no. 4, pp. 239–251, 1988.

[12] P. K. Kofoed, I. C. Munch, B. Sander et al., "Prolonged multifocal electroretinographic implicit times in the ocular ischemic syndrome," *Investigative Ophthalmology and Visual Science*, vol. 51, no. 4, pp. 1806–1810, 2010.

4

Correlation of Vitreous Vascular Endothelial Growth Factor and Uric Acid Concentration Using Optical Coherence Tomography in Diabetic Macular Edema

Libuse Krizova,[1,2] **Marta Kalousova,**[1] **Ales Antonin Kubena,**[1] **Oldrich Chrapek,**[3] **Barbora Chrapkova,**[3] **Martin Sin,**[3] **and Tomas Zima**[1]

[1]*Institute of Medical Biochemistry and Laboratory Diagnostics, First Faculty of Medicine, Charles University in Prague and General University Hospital, U Nemocnice 2, 128 08 Prague 2, Czech Republic*
[2]*Augenzentrum Augsburg, Prinzregentenstraße 25, 86150 Augsburg, Germany*
[3]*Department of Ophthalmology, Faculty of Medicine and Dentistry, Palacky University Olomouc, I. P. Pavlova 6, 775 20 Olomouc, Czech Republic*

Correspondence should be addressed to Oldrich Chrapek; olchrapek@gmail.com

Academic Editor: Vicente Zanon-Moreno

Purpose. We investigated two factors linked to diabetic macular edema (DME), vitreous and serum levels of vascular endothelial growth factor (VEGF) and uric acid (UA) in patients with DME, and compared the results with changes in optical coherence tomography (OCT) and visual acuity (VA). *Methods.* A prospective study of 29 eyes, 16 cystoid DME and nonproliferative diabetic retinopathy (DR) and 13 nondiabetic controls. Biochemical analysis of vitreous and serum samples was performed and OCT scans were graded according to central retinal thickness (CRT), cube volume (CV), cube average thickness (CAT), and serous retinal detachment (SRD). *Results.* In DME group, intravitreal concentrations of VEGF ($p < 0.001$), UA ($p = 0.038$), and total protein ($p < 0.001$) were significantly higher than in control group. In DME subjects, intravitreal UA correlated significantly with intravitreal VEGF ($\varrho = 0.559$, $p = 0.03$) but not with total vitreous protein and serum UA. Increased intravitreal VEGF in DME group correlated with increase in CV ($\varrho = 0.515/p = 0.041$). None of the OCT parameters correlated with the VA. *Conclusions.* The results suggest that the CV might be assessor of anti-VEGF therapy efficacy. Second, apart from VEGF, the role of UA in the pathogenesis and progression of DR should be considered.

1. Introduction

Diabetic macular edema (DME) is a common complication of diabetic retinopathy (DR) and a leading cause of visual loss in this population [1, 2]. Major components of DME are retinal microvascular dysfunction and blood-retinal barrier (BRB) breakdown with consequent increase in vascular permeability that allows plasma compounds to leak into the retina [3–5]. There is evidence that upregulation of angiogenic and inflammatory factors, including vascular endothelial growth factor (VEGF), and downregulation of antiangiogenic factors as well as redox shift contribute to the breakdown of the BRB in DR [5–10]. Oxidative stress and inflammation also play an important role in the pathogenesis of DR and DME [5].

VEGF causes conformational changes in the tight junctions of the retinal vascular endothelial cells and plays a major role in the increased vascular permeability and BRB breakdown in diabetic eyes [5, 7, 11, 12]. Vitreous VEGF levels correlate significantly with the severity of DR [13], but DME can occur in nonproliferative DR (NPDR) as well as proliferative DR (PDR). Interventional studies on ranibizumab, a monoclonal antibody against VEGF, have shown that intraocular injections of ranibizumab significantly reduce foveal thickness and improve visual acuity in patients with DME [14, 15]. This demonstrates that VEGF is an important therapeutic target in DME. However, the conclusions of the studies were not based on the comparison of the real intravitreal concentration of VEGF with the foveal

---

TABLE 1: Clinical and laboratory characteristic of diabetic subjects and nondiabetic controls.

Parameter	DME ($n = 16$)	Control ($n = 13$)	p
Number of patients (men/women)	4/12	1/12	ns
Age (years)	71 (61–77)	71 (66–74)	ns
LogMAR BCVA	1.0 (0.6–1.0)	0.5 (0.5–0.6)	**
Chronic kidney disease	1 (6.2%)	0 (0.0%)	ns
Dyslipidemia	8 (50.0%)	4 (30.8%)	ns
Hypertension	14 (87.5%)	10 (76.9%)	ns
HbA$_{1c}$ (mmol/mol)	51.5 (43.0–63.3)	NA	NA
Serum albumin (g/L)	42.7 (41.1–44.6)	44.4 (39.6–45.2)	ns
CRP (mg/L)	1.6 (1.0–3.7)	2.0 (0.8–3.6)	ns

Data are expressed as median ± interquartile range or total number and %. ns: not significant; $^{*}p < 0.05$, $^{**}p < 0.01$, and $^{***}p < 0.001$ DME versus control patients; BCVA: best corrected visual acuity; CRP: C-reactive protein; HbA$_{1c}$: glycated haemoglobin; logMAR: logarithm of the minimal angle of resolution; and NA: not assessed; chronic kidney disease was defined as either structural kidney damage or glomerular filtration rate $< 1.0 \, \mathrm{mL \cdot s^{-1} \cdot 1.73 \, m^{-2}}$ for ≥ 3 months.

thickness in OCT; they only asses the retinal thickness before and after therapy.

In our earlier study, we found that also the intravitreal uric acid (UA) concentrations correlated significantly with degree of DR [16]. We suspect that UA may play a role in the pathogenesis of DR and DME: studies of UA strongly suggest that its redox potential affects endothelial function [17] and might contribute to the BRB breakdown. The correlation of intravitreal UA with VEGF in NPDR and DME has not been studied yet.

Optical coherence tomography (OCT) has enabled clinicians to noninvasively evaluate the effect of DR on retinal thickness in a standard clinical setting [18, 19]. However, there are very limited data on how OCT parameters in DME correlate with vitreous levels of VEGF and other biochemical parameters.

The aim of our study was to analyse the vitreous and serum of diabetic patients with DME and severe NPDR and compare them to nondiabetic controls. The analysis focused on VEGF and UA as two possible pathogenetic factors in the development of DME. We compared blood and vitreous levels of VEGF, UA, and protein between the two study groups and describe their correlation with the changes seen in OCT.

2. Materials and Methods

2.1. Subjects.
This consecutive, prospective study involved 29 patients divided into two groups. First group involved 16 subjects with type 2 diabetes mellitus (DM) with NPDR and cystoid DME. In this group, the mean duration of DM was 18.6 ± 8.3 years and 15 patients (93.75%) were treated with

insulin and 1 patient (6.25%) was treated with peroral antidiabetics. A group of 13 nondiabetic subjects with idiopathic epiretinal membrane and diffuse retinal thickening served as control. Characteristics of all subjects are listed in Table 1.

The diagnosis of DM was based on the WHO criteria [20]. DM duration was defined as the duration from the first diagnosis of DM to the time of vitreous sampling. All patients underwent a standard ophthalmologic examination including measurement of best corrected visual acuity, slit-lamp biomicroscopy, indirect ophthalmoscopy, and OCT. The retinopathy was graded according to the Early Treatment Diabetic Retinopathy Study Research Group and patients enrolled in the study had moderate to severe nonproliferative DR (NPDR) [21]. The center involving DME was defined clinically and confirmed by retinal thickening in cross-sectional spectral domain (SD) OCT scans. The indications for vitrectomy in this study were macular edema and preoperative best corrected visual acuity (BCVA) more than 0.3 logMAR (logarithm of the minimum angle of resolution) and in the diabetic group no or poor response to previous therapy with photocoagulation or intravitreal injection. Exclusion criteria were as follows: (a) history of intraocular haemorrhage, (b) prior vitreoretinal surgery, (c) other ocular surgeries or laser coagulation less than 6 months prior to the operation, (d) history of ocular inflammation, (e) proliferative DR or other retinal conditions causing neovascularisation, (f) ophthalmic disorders associated with macular edema, and (g) treatment with intravitreal anti-VEGF or steroid injections (e.g., triamcinolone, dexamethasone, bevacizumab, ranibizumab, and aflibercept) less than 6 months prior to the operation.

At the time of the study, all patients were in a stable clinical condition without clinical or laboratory signs of acute inflammation. The research was approved by the Local Institutional Ethics Committee, Faculty of Medicine and Dentistry, Palacky University Olomouc, Czech Republic. Data and sample collection was independent of all treatment decisions. It did not affect a patient's access to treatment and fully complied with all ethical and legal requirements for noninterventional data collection in the Czech Republic. All patients gave written informed consent to the treatment, as well as data collection. The reported investigations were in accordance with the principles of the current version of the Declaration of Helsinki.

2.2. Methods.
OCT examinations were performed one day before vitrectomy with spectral domain OCT (Cirrus HD-OCT, Carl Zeiss Meditec AG, Jena, Germany) using macular cube acquisition according to the manufacturer's protocol. The macular cube 512 × 128 scan consists of 128 raster scans with 512 A-scans, within a 6 × 6 mm macular area. The mean central retinal thickness (CRT, i.e., central subfield thickness) from the internal limiting membrane to the retinal pigment epithelium at the fovea was defined as the mean retinal thickness in a 1 mm diameter circular zone concentred on the fovea. Also cube volume (CV) and cube average thickness (CAT) of the scanned area were calculated by Cirrus HD-OCT software and checked for accuracy. The CV is calculated from the 1 mm diameter zone and CAT from the central 6 mm diameter zone concentred on the fovea.

Based on previous studies that evaluated morphological changes in DME [22, 23], the central scan through the fovea was assessed for the presence of intraretinal cysts and serous retinal detachment (SRD) by an independent examiner.

Vitrectomy was performed to improve visual acuity and to decrease retinal thickness in the macula. Each patient underwent standard three-port therapeutic pars plana vitrectomy using current surgical techniques (the Alcon CONSTELLATION Vision System). Before opening the infusion port at the start of the vitrectomy, undiluted vitreous samples were obtained and collected in sterile tubes (cca. 0.3 mL). Overnight fasting blood samples were drawn from the antecubital vein at the time of vitrectomy and used for biochemical assay. Samples of vitreous and serum were rapidly frozen after collection at $-80°C$.

Routine biochemical parameters of serum were determined by standard clinical-chemistry methods. The concentration of UA was estimated using enzymatic methods (uricase-peroxidase) with photometric detection (Modular, Roche, Germany). The low detection limit of the method was $30\,\mu mol/L$. HbA_{1c} was measured by high performance liquid chromatography and calibration was traced to the reference method of the International Federation of Clinical Chemistry (Variant II, Bio-Rad; http://www.bio-rad.com/). The concentration of VEGF was quantified by enzyme linked immunosorbent assay (ELISA) using a commercial human VEGF Kit (R and D Systems, Minneapolis, MN, USA) according to the manufacturer's protocol. The limits of Quantification for VEGF were min = 31.2 pg/mL and max = 1000 pg/mL, respectively.

2.3. Statistical Analysis. All statistical analyses were performed using the SPSS version 16 (SPSS Inc., Chicago, IL, USA). We calculated the median with 1st and 3rd quartile (IQR, interquartile range). In 16 subjects, the intravitreal VEGF and in 3 subjects the intravitreal UA concentration were under the detection limit; these subjects were included in the statistical analysis to avoid selection bias. Hence, we used the nonparametric analysis for ordinal variables, and the concentrations under the detection limit were assigned "minor than other." The comparison between DME group and control group was done by Mann-Whitney U test and Fisher's exact test. To examine correlations, Spearman rank correlation coefficients were calculated. Two-tailed p values of less than 0.05 were considered significant.

3. Results and Discussion

3.1. Results

3.1.1. Biochemical Analysis of Serum and Vitreous. Biochemical analysis of the vitreous showed significant differences between DM and control group in the concentration of VEGF, UA, and total protein but not albumin as shown in Table 2 and Figures 1–3. In all nondiabetic control subjects, the concentration of VEGF in vitreous was under the detection limit of 31.2 pg/mL.

In the diabetic group, UA concentration in vitreous correlated significantly with vitreous VEGF concentration

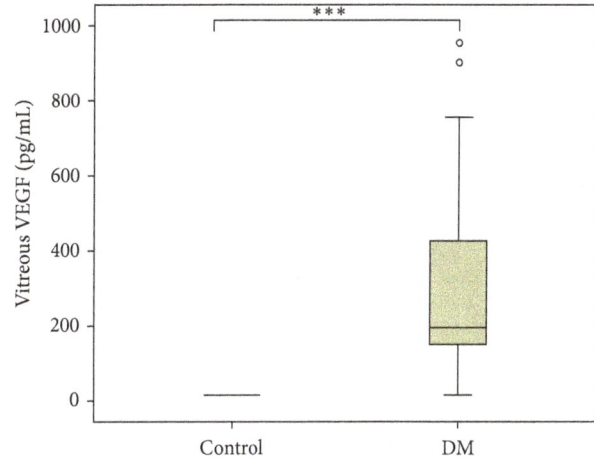

FIGURE 1: Vitreous concentrations of VEGF in diabetic versus control group. DM group n = 16, control group n = 13, and $^{***}p < 0.001$ DM versus control patients.

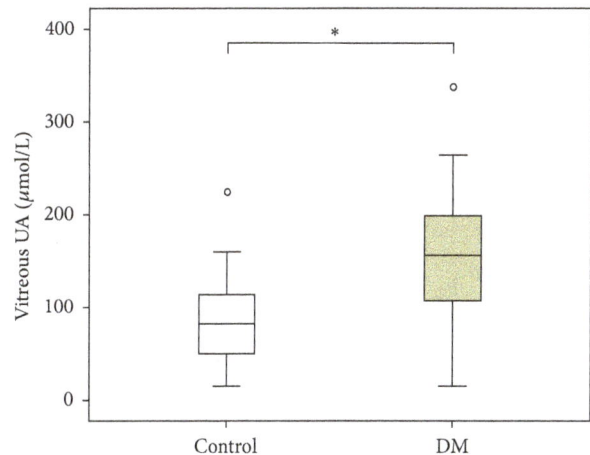

FIGURE 2: Vitreous concentrations of uric acid in diabetic versus control group. DM group n = 16, control group n = 13, and $^{*}p = 0.038$ DM versus control patients.

TABLE 2: Laboratory analysis of vitreous of diabetic subjects and nondiabetic controls.

Parameter	DME ($n = 16$)	Control ($n = 13$)	p
VEGF (pg/mL)	192.7 (140.9–523.5)	<LOD	* * *
UA ($\mu mol/L$)	156.0 (86.0–209.0)	70.0 (48.5–138.0)	*
Albumin (mg/L)	1050 (618–1780)	550 (295–1495)	ns
Total protein (g/L)	6.3 (4.9–9.1)	3.6 (3.1–4.2)	* * *

Data are expressed as median with interquartile range.
ns: not significant, $^{*}p < 0.05$, $^{**}p < 0.01$, and $^{***}p < 0.001$ DME versus control patients.
LOD: limit of detection (31.2 pg/mL).

($\varrho = 0.559$, $p = 0.03$). However, in DME vitreous VEGF and UA did not correlate with the total vitreous protein. Further, in the control group, no significant correlation between the biochemical analytes in vitreous was found. Figure 4 shows

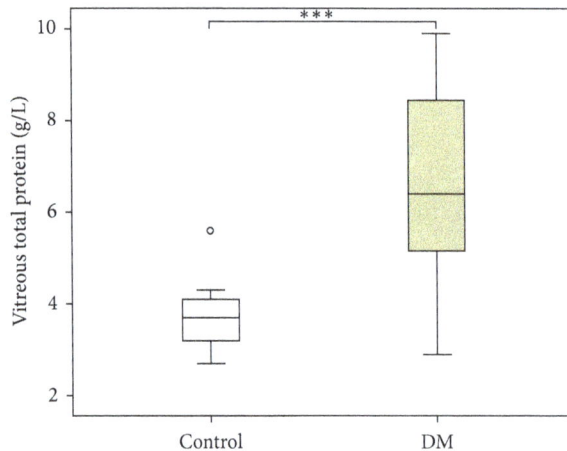

FIGURE 3: Vitreous concentrations of total protein in diabetic versus control group. DM group $n = 16$, control group $n = 13$, and $^{***}p < 0.001$ DM versus control patients.

TABLE 3: OCT parameters of diabetic subjects and nondiabetic controls.

Parameter	DME ($n = 16$)	Control ($n = 13$)	p
CRT (μm)	479.0 (421.5–661.3)	498.0 (374.5–540.5)	ns
CAT (μmL)	392.0 (329.8–414.3)	332.0 (316.0–346.5)	ns
CV (mm^3)	14.2 (11.9–15.0)	12.0 (11.4–12.5)	ns
SRD	6 (37.5%)	0 (0%)	*

Data are expressed as median with interquartile range or total number and %.
ns: not significant, $^{*}p < 0.05$, $^{**}p < 0.01$, and $^{***}p < 0.001$ DME versus control patients.
CAT: cube average thickness, CRT: central retinal thickness, CV: cube volume, and SRD: serous retinal detachment.

There was a significant correlation between UA concentrations in serum and vitreous ($\varrho = 0.652$, $p = 0.016$) in the control group but not in DME. Further, no significant correlation between concentrations of VEGF in serum and vitreous was found in both groups.

3.1.2. OCT Parameters. The median CRT, CAT, and CV did not differ significantly between both groups and are listed in Table 3. Significant difference was found in presence of SRD between the groups as shown in Table 3.

In the diabetic group, there was a significant correlation between CRT and CAT ($\varrho = 0.589$, $p = 0.016$). The CRT of DM subjects also correlated significantly with the CV ($\varrho = 0.581$, $p = 0.018$). However, the strongest correlation in the DM group was between CAT and CV ($\varrho = 0.999$, $p < 0.001$). The SRD was found in the OCT scans of 6 diabetic eyes, but its presence did not correlate with any of the other OCT parameters.

Further, among all OCT parameters, only CV correlated significantly with the concentration of vitreous VEGF in the DM group ($\varrho = 0.515$, $p = 0.041$). The CRT, CAT, CV, and SRD show in DM and control subjects no significant correlation to vitreous concentrations of UA, albumin, or total protein.

The correlation of logMAR BCVA with changes in OCT parameters and vitreous content was also evaluated and we found it to be nonsignificant in both groups. There was also no correlation between OCT parameters and serous concentrations of UA or VEGF.

3.2. Discussion. The results demonstrate that biochemical analysis of the vitreous showed significant higher concentrations of VEGF, UA, and total protein in DM and control group. Moreover, in patients with DME intravitreal levels of UA correlate significantly with intravitreal levels of VEGF. Furthermore, we found that the CV measured with Cirrus HD-OCT correlate significantly with the concentration of VEGF in the vitreous of patients with NPDR and DME.

In our earlier study, we showed that the levels of intravitreal UA correlated significantly with the degree of DR [16] and recently also serum UA concentration has been found to be associated with increase in severity of DR [24]. Finding significant higher UA concentration in vitreous of DM compared to controls and a correlation between UA and VEGF in the vitreous of NPDR patients supports our

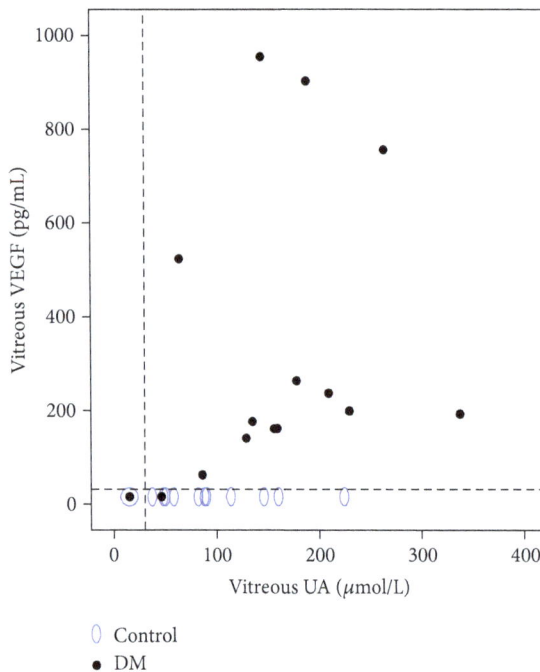

FIGURE 4: Relationship between vitreous VEGF and vitreous UA concentrations in diabetic versus control group. Dashed lines represent limits of detection (VEGF = 31.2 pg/mL, UA = 30 μmol/L).

the relationship between vitreous VEGF and vitreous UA of DME and control group.

Median of serum concentration of UA in diabetic patients was significantly elevated compared with the control group (337.0 μmol/L, IQR: 324.0–407.0 μmol/L in DM group versus 259.5 μmol/L, IQR: 220.0–334.8 μmol/L in control group; $p = 0.025$). Also median concentration of VEGF in serum of diabetic patients (414.3 pg/mL, IQR: 293.1–512.0 pg/mL) was higher than in controls (332.7 pg/mL, IQR: 149.4–551.8 pg/mL), but the difference was not significant.

assumption that UA too may be one contributing causal factor in the pathogenesis of DR.

UA is a degradation product of metabolism and under normal conditions UA acts as an antioxidant. In diabetics, hyperglycaemia induces redox stress, which leads to consumption of the naturally occurring local antioxidants protecting capillary endothelium [17]. This results in urate redox shuttle, meaning that UA paradoxically becomes prooxidant and contributes to endothelial dysfunction through oxidative-redox stress [17]. Johnson et al. showed that local ischemia results, via enzymatic activation, in increased UA production as well as oxidant formation [25]. Decreased total antioxidant status was shown to contribute to the progression of PDR via induction of VEGF [26].

On the other side, high UA concentration in the vitreous of diabetic patients may also be a compensatory protective factor. Under experimental conditions, the VEGF-induced production of reactive oxygen species was attenuated by urate; however, it did not modify the VEGF-induced changes in permeability of monolayers [27]. This could explain the correlation of UA and VEGF in the vitreous of diabetic group found in the present study.

It has to be elucidated whether UA is originating from leakage of retinal vessels, which is increased in DR, or from local production. Although total vitreous protein was significantly higher in the diabetic group compared to controls, its level did not correlate with both UA and VEGF. Furthermore, in the diabetic subjects we found no correlation between serum and vitreous level of UA. These findings support the local production of UA in DR. However, to be able to distinguish the origin of increased UA in the vitreous, further analyses, for example, with tagged UA, should be done.

Since there was a correlation between vitreous UA and VEGF but no correlation between vitreous UA and OCT parameters, we conclude that UA has a probable relation with diabetic microangiopathy and accordingly DR but not directly with the development of DME.

Recent studies have shown that VEGF causes conformational changes in the tight junctions of retinal vascular endothelial cells and plays a major role in the elevated vascular permeability in diabetic eyes with DME. It is well known that the vitreous VEGF levels correlate significantly with the severity of DR [11–13, 28]. Few authors have also found a significant correlation between retinal thickness at the fovea measured on OCT and VEGF concentrations in the vitreous [29, 30] and aqueous [31]. The association of vitreous VEGF levels and DME morphology was studied by Sonoda et al. [32] and these authors showed no significant differences in VEGF concentrations in cystoid versus diffuse aspect of DME.

In the present study, there was no significant correlation between vitreous VEGF levels and CRT of diabetic patients. However, the results show that in DME increase in CV correlated with increased concentration of VEGF in the vitreous. Nevertheless, one caveat is that previous studies defined central retinal thickness differently. The retinal thickness at the central fovea in Funatsu et al. [29] was calculated as average foveal thickness from 4 manual measurements per patient. Shimada et al. [30] used the average thickness of the central

area with 1000 μm in diameter calculated by Humphrey OCT. Javanmard et al. [31] defined the central macular thickness as the average thickness of the central 500 μm in diameter.

The mean CRT in DME is widely accepted as the new surrogate marker for evaluating treatment efficacy [33]. This is also because the changes in the fovea are deciding for the visual acuity. In our study, the CRT, CAT, and CV in both DM and control group did not correlate with the logMAR BCVA. There are also studies evaluating the effect of the anti-VEGF therapy using both the mean foveal thickness and CV [34]. On the other hand, since DME usually affects the macular area and not only the foveal region, assessment of VEGF concentration in clinical practice using the CV is comprehensible.

Like us, Sonoda et al. showed that there was no significant correlation between intravitreal VEGF levels and the amount of subretinal fluid in DME [35]. Other studies have reported that eyes with serous retinal detachment often have a poor prognosis after treatment [22, 36].

The strength of the study described here is that it determined the relationship between the levels of intravitreal biochemical parameters and retinal morphology at the same time. The limitation was the small sample size (29 eyes). This was caused by decreasing use of vitrectomy for DME and this curtailed collection of vitreous samples. Although our vitrectomy for DME might be considered overtreatment, it was a comparatively effective method as it stabilized the intraocular condition of DME and the efficacy was maintained for a long period [37]. In interpreting or generalizing our results, it should be remembered that the findings demonstrate association of VEGF levels in the vitreous with the cube volume, but they do not prove cause and effect. Further, the study was focused on VEGF and UA; however, the pathogenesis of the DME is complex and still not fully understood.

4. Conclusions

Vitreous concentrations of uric acid and VEGF were significantly higher in DM subjects than in controls. Moreover, vitreous UA concentration correlated significantly with the vitreous VEGF concentrations in patients with NPDR and cystoid DME. Increased VEGF concentrations are known to be involved in the pathogenesis of DME. Our results suggest that, apart from VEGF, the role of UA in the pathogenesis and progression of DR should also be considered.

Comparing OCT parameters to the vitreous levels of UA and VEGF, we found that increased concentration of intravitreal VEGF in patients with NPDR and cystoid DME correlated with increase of cube volume calculated by Cirrus HD-OCT. Since DME usually affects the macular area and not only the foveal region, the assessment of the VEGF concentration in clinical practice using the cube volume is comprehensible. This OCT parameter could be used to assess the efficacy of anti-VEGF therapy.

Disclosure

No financial relationship with the organisation that sponsored the research exists.

Conflict of Interests

The authors declare that there is no conflict of interests regarding the publication of this paper.

Acknowledgments

This study was supported by research Projects DRO VFN64165, Prvouk P25/LF1/2, and SVV 260032-2015. The authors thank the laboratory staff for technical assistance.

References

[1] S. Sivaprasad, B. Gupta, R. Crosby-Nwaobi, and J. Evans, "Prevalence of diabetic retinopathy in various ethnic groups: a worldwide perspective," *Survey of Ophthalmology*, vol. 57, no. 4, pp. 347–370, 2012.

[2] S. E. Moss, R. Klein, and B. E. K. Klein, "The 14-year incidence of visual loss in a diabetic population," *Ophthalmology*, vol. 105, no. 6, pp. 998–1003, 1998.

[3] M. J. Sheetz and G. L. King, "Molecular understanding of hyperglycemia's adverse effects for diabetic complications," *The Journal of the American Medical Association*, vol. 288, no. 20, pp. 2579–2588, 2002.

[4] T. W. Gardner, D. A. Antonetti, A. J. Barber, K. F. LaNoue, and S. W. Levison, "Diabetic retinopathy: more than meets the eye," *Survey of Ophthalmology*, vol. 47, supplement 2, pp. S253–S262, 2002.

[5] E. S. Shin, C. M. Sorenson, and N. Sheibani, "Diabetes and retinal vascular dysfunction," *Journal of Ophthalmic and Vision Research*, vol. 9, no. 3, pp. 362–373, 2014.

[6] A. M. Joussen, V. Poulaki, M. L. Le et al., "A central role for inflammation in the pathogenesis of diabetic retinopathy," *The FASEB Journal*, vol. 18, no. 12, pp. 1450–1452, 2004.

[7] R. A. Kowluru and P.-S. Chan, "Oxidative stress and diabetic retinopathy," *Experimental Diabetes Research*, vol. 2007, Article ID 43603, 12 pages, 2007.

[8] R. Simó, E. Carrasco, M. García-Ramírez, and C. Hernández, "Angiogenic and antiangiogenic factors in proliferative diabetic retinopathy," *Current Diabetes Reviews*, vol. 2, no. 1, pp. 71–98, 2006.

[9] A. Praidou, S. Androudi, P. Brazitikos, G. Karakiulakis, E. Papakonstantinou, and S. Dimitrakos, "Angiogenic growth factors and their inhibitors in diabetic retinopathy," *Current Diabetes Reviews*, vol. 6, no. 5, pp. 304–312, 2010.

[10] J. M. Tarr, K. Kaul, M. Chopra, E. M. Kohner, and R. Chibber, "Pathophysiology of diabetic retinopathy," *ISRN Ophthalmology*, vol. 2013, Article ID 343560, 13 pages, 2013.

[11] T. Quam, Q. Xu, A. M. Joussen et al., "VEGF-initiated blood-retinal barrier breakdown in early diabetes," *Investigative Ophthalmology & Visual Science*, vol. 42, no. 10, pp. 2480–2513, 2001.

[12] J. S. Penn, A. Madan, R. B. Caldwell, M. Bartoli, R. W. Caldwell, and M. E. Hartnett, "Vascular endothelial growth factor in eye disease," *Progress in Retinal and Eye Research*, vol. 27, no. 4, pp. 331–371, 2008.

[13] R. B. Caldwell, M. Bartoli, M. A. Behzadian et al., "Vascular endothelial growth factor and diabetic retinopathy: pathophysiological mechanisms and treatment perspectives," *Diabetes/Metabolism Research and Reviews*, vol. 19, no. 6, pp. 442–455, 2003.

[14] P. Massin, F. Bandello, J. G. Garweg et al., "Safety and efficacy of ranibizumab in diabetic macular edema (RESOLVE study): a 12-month, randomized, controlled, double-masked, multicenter phase II study," *Diabetes Care*, vol. 33, no. 11, pp. 2399–2405, 2010.

[15] P. Mitchell, F. Bandello, U. Schmidt-Erfurth et al., "The RESTORE Study: ranibizumab monotherapy or combined with laser versus laser monotherapy for diabetic macular edema," *Ophthalmology*, vol. 118, no. 4, pp. 615–625, 2011.

[16] L. Krizova, M. Kalousova, A. Kubena et al., "Increased uric acid and glucose concentrations in vitreous and serum of patients with diabetic macular oedema," *Ophthalmic Research*, vol. 46, no. 2, pp. 73–79, 2011.

[17] M. R. Hayden and S. C. Tyagi, "Uric acid: a new look at an old risk marker for cardiovascular disease, metabolic syndrome, and type 2 diabetes mellitus: the urate redox shuttle," *Nutrition and Metabolism*, vol. 1, no. 1, article 10, 2004.

[18] P. Massin, A. Girach, A. Erginay, and A. Gaudric, "Optical coherence tomography: a key to the future management of patients with diabetic macular edema," *Acta Ophthalmologica Scandinavica*, vol. 84, no. 4, pp. 466–474, 2006.

[19] B. Mushtaq, N. J. Crosby, A. T. Dimopoulos et al., "Effect of initial retinal thickness on outcome of intravitreal bevacizumab therapy for diabetic macular edema," *Clinical Ophthalmology*, vol. 8, pp. 807–812, 2014.

[20] World Health Organization, *Definition, Diagnosis and Classification of Diabetes Mellitus and Its Complications: Report of a WHO Consultation. Part 1: Diagnosis and Classification of Diabetes Mellitus*, World Health Organization, Geneva, Switzerland, 1999.

[21] C. P. Wilkinson, F. L. Ferris III, R. E. Klein et al., "Proposed international clinical diabetic retinopathy and diabetic macular edema disease severity scales," *Ophthalmology*, vol. 110, no. 9, pp. 1677–1682, 2003.

[22] G. G. Deák, M. Bolz, M. Ritter, S. Prager, T. Benesch, and U. Schmidt-Erfurth, "A systematic correlation between morphology and functional alterations in diabetic macular edema," *Investigative Ophthalmology and Visual Science*, vol. 51, no. 12, pp. 6710–6714, 2010.

[23] L. Reznicek, S. Cserhati, F. Seidensticker et al., "Functional and morphological changes in diabetic macular edema over the course of anti-vascular endothelial growth factor treatment," *Acta Ophthalmologica*, vol. 91, no. 7, pp. e529–e536, 2013.

[24] J.-J. Lee, I.-H. Yang, H.-K. Kuo et al., "Serum uric acid concentration is associated with worsening in severity of diabetic retinopathy among type 2 diabetic patients in Taiwan—a 3-year prospective study," *Diabetes Research and Clinical Practice*, vol. 106, no. 2, pp. 366–372, 2014.

[25] R. J. Johnson, D.-H. Kang, S. Kivlighn et al., "Is there a pathogenic role for uric acid in hypertension and cardiovascular and renal disease?" *Hypertension*, vol. 41, no. 6, pp. 1183–1190, 2003.

[26] M. Yokoi, S.-I. Yamagishi, M. Takeuchi et al., "Elevations of AGE and vascular endothelial growth factor with decreased total antioxidant status in the vitreous fluid of diabetic patients with retinopathy," *British Journal of Ophthalmology*, vol. 89, no. 6, pp. 673–675, 2005.

[27] T. Marumo, T. Noll, V. B. Schini-Kerth et al., "Significance of nitric oxide and peroxynitrite in permeability changes of the retinal microvascular endothelial cell monolayer induced by vascular endothelial growth factor," *Journal of Vascular Research*, vol. 36, no. 6, pp. 510–515, 1999.

[28] X. Zhang, H. Zeng, S. Bao, N. Wang, and M. C. Gillies, "Diabetic macular edema: new concepts in patho-physiology and treatment," *Cell & Bioscience*, vol. 4, article 27, 2014.

[29] H. Funatsu, H. Yamashita, S. Nakamura et al., "Vitreous levels of pigment epithelium-derived factor and vascular endothelial growth factor are related to diabetic macular edema," *Ophthalmology*, vol. 113, no. 2, pp. 294–301, 2006.

[30] H. Shimada, E. Akaza, M. Yuzawa, and M. Kawashima, "Concentration gradient of vascular endothelial growth factor in the vitreous of eyes with diabetic macular edema," *Investigative Ophthalmology and Visual Science*, vol. 50, no. 6, pp. 2953–2955, 2009.

[31] S. H. Javanmard, Z. Hasanpour, Z. Abbaspoor, G. A. Naderian, and M. Jahanmard, "Aqueous concentrations of VEGF and soluble VEGF receptor-1 in diabetic retinopathy patients," *Journal of Research in Medical Sciences*, vol. 17, no. 12, pp. 1124–1127, 2012.

[32] S. Sonoda, T. Sakamoto, T. Yamashita, M. Shirasawa, H. Otsuka, and Y. Sonoda, "Retinal morphologic changes and concentrations of cytokines in eyes with diabetic macular EDEMA," *Retina*, vol. 34, no. 4, pp. 741–748, 2014.

[33] Diabetic Retinopathy Clinical Research Network, "Relationship between optical coherence tomography-measured central thickness and visual acuity in diabetic macular edema," *Ophthalmology*, vol. 114, no. 3, pp. 525–536, 2007.

[34] Q. D. Nguyen, S. Tatlipinar, S. M. Shah et al., "Vascular endothelial growth factor is a critical stimulus for diabetic macular edema," *American Journal of Ophthalmology*, vol. 142, no. 6, pp. 961–969, 2006.

[35] S. Sonoda, T. Sakamoto, M. Shirasawa, T. Yamashita, H. Otsuka, and H. Terasaki, "Correlation between reflectivity of subretinal fluid in OCT images and concentration of intravitreal VEGF in eyes with diabetic macular edema," *Investigative Ophthalmology & Visual Science*, vol. 54, no. 8, pp. 5367–5374, 2013.

[36] M. Ota, K. Nishijima, A. Sakamoto et al., "Optical coherence tomographic evaluation of foveal hard exudates in patients with diabetic maculopathy accompanying macular detachment," *Ophthalmology*, vol. 117, no. 10, pp. 1996–2002, 2010.

[37] K. Kumagai, M. Furukawa, N. Ogino, E. Larson, M. Iwaki, and N. Tachi, "Long-term follow-up of vitrectomy for diffuse nontractional diabetic macular edema," *Retina*, vol. 29, no. 4, pp. 464–472, 2009.

5

Evaluation of Central Corneal Thickness Using Corneal Dynamic Scheimpflug Analyzer Corvis ST and Comparison with Pentacam Rotating Scheimpflug System and Ultrasound Pachymetry in Normal Eyes

Ayong Yu,[1,2] **Weiqi Zhao,**[1,2] **Giacomo Savini,**[3] **Zixu Huang,**[1] **Fangjun Bao,**[1,2] **Weicong Lu,**[1,2] **Qinmei Wang,**[1,2] **and Jinhai Huang**[1,2]

[1]*School of Ophthalmology and Optometry, Wenzhou Medical University, 270 West Xueyuan Road, Wenzhou, Zhejiang 325027, China*
[2]*Key Laboratory of Vision Science, Ministry of Health of the People's Republic of China, Wenzhou, Zhejiang, China*
[3]*G. B. Bietti Foundation IRCCS, Rome, Italy*

Correspondence should be addressed to Qinmei Wang; wqm6@mail.eye.ac.cn and Jinhai Huang; vip999vip@163.com

Academic Editor: David P. Piñero

Purpose. To assess the repeatability and reproducibility of central corneal thickness (CCT) measurements by corneal dynamic Scheimpflug analyzer Corvis ST in normal eyes and compare the agreement with Pentacam rotating Scheimpflug System and ultrasound pachymetry. *Methods.* 84 right eyes underwent Corvis ST measurements performed by two operators. The test-retest repeatability (TRT), within-subject coefficient of variation (CoV), and intraclass correlation coefficient (ICC) were used to evaluate the intraoperator repeatability and interoperator reproducibility. CCT measurements also were obtained from Pentacam and ultrasound pachymetry by the first operator. The agreement between the three devices was evaluated with 95% limits of agreement (LoA) and Bland-Altman plots. *Results.* Corvis ST showed high repeatability as indicated by TRT $\leq 13.0\,\mu$m, CoV $< 0.9\%$, and ICC > 0.97. The interoperator reproducibility was also excellent. The CoV was $<0.9\%$, and ICC was >0.97. Corvis ST showed significantly lower values than Pentacam and ultrasound pachymetry ($P < 0.001$). The 95% LoA between Corvis ST and Pentacam or ultrasound pachymetry were -15.8 to $9.5\,\mu$m and -27.9 to $12.3\,\mu$m, respectively. *Conclusions.* Corvis ST showed excellent repeatability and interoperator reproducibility of CCT measurements in normal eyes. Corvis ST is interchangeable with Pentacam but not with ultrasound pachymetry.

1. Introduction

Accurate assessment of the central corneal thickness (CCT) has become extremely important in ophthalmologic examinations. Preoperatively, it helps the ophthalmologist to safely plan corneal refractive procedures and screen for refractive surgery candidates, in order to reduce the risk of postoperative complications [1]. Besides, CCT measurements play a crucial role in the diagnosis and management of glaucoma because the value of intraocular pressure should be adjusted in accordance with CCT [2]. CCT measurements also play an important role in the diagnosis of corneal diseases, such as Fuchs' corneal dystrophy and keratoconus [3, 4].

For many years, ultrasound pachymetry has been the most frequently used method to measure CCT because it is relatively inexpensive and easy to use and has high intraoperator repeatability [2, 5]. Nevertheless, ultrasound pachymetry has certain disadvantages, such as corneal-probe contact, the need for topical anesthesia, and the risk for transmission of infections and corneal epithelial lesions [6]. Besides, the reliability of ultrasound pachymetry results depends on the operator's skill when placing the probe perpendicularly to the cornea. Over the last decade, many noncontact devices have been developed. Among these, Scheimpflug technology plays a major role, including Pentacam (Oculus, Wetzlar, Germany), Sirius (Costruzione Strumenti Oftalmici,

Florence, Italy), Galilei (Ziemer, Port, Switzerland), and TMS-5 (Tomey, Nagoya, Japan). Previous studies have shown that common used device Pentacam has high intraoperator repeatability and interoperator reproducibility for CCT measurements [7–9].

The corneal dynamic Scheimpflug analyzer Corvis ST (Oculus Optikgeräte, Inc., Wetzlar, Germany) is relatively new, noncontact corneal biomechanics equipment, which is composed of an air puff indentation system and ultra-high-speed Scheimpflug technology. The ultra-high-speed Scheimpflug camera has a blue light LED and acquires the deformation process at 4330 frames/s with an 8 mm horizontal coverage. Because of the air impulse, the cornea experiences three stages: first applanation, highest concavity, and second applanation. Furthermore, CCT is obtained by the corneal initial state of the central horizontal cross-section diagram through the Scheimpflug technology. Few studies [10–12] have evaluated the intraoperator repeatability of CCT measurements obtained by this device in normal population. Ali et al. [10] evaluated the intersession reproducibility of the CCT at different times of the day with this device. Chen et al. [13] assessed the intraoperator repeatability and interobserver reproducibility in virgin and post-PRK eyes but only applied single value to evaluate interobserver reproducibility. However, to our knowledge, the interoperator reproducibility of Corvis ST for CCT measurements using both single and average measurement value methods in normal eyes has not yet been evaluated.

The purpose of the present study was to prospectively assess the intraoperator repeatability and interoperator reproducibility of CCT measurements using both single and average methods acquired from the Corvis ST in normal eyes and compare the agreement with Pentacam and ultrasound pachymetry.

2. Subjects and Methods

This prospective study was conducted on normal subjects recruited from the staff and students of the Eye Hospital of Wenzhou Medical University. The research protocol conformed to the tenets of the Declaration of Helsinki and was approved by the Office of Research Ethics, Eye Hospital of Wenzhou Medical University. Informed consent was acquired from all subjects after explaining the purpose of the study.

The exclusion criteria were active ocular pathology, any history of ocular surgery or trauma, recent contact lens wear (soft contact lens within two weeks and rigid contact lens within four weeks), systemic diseases with eye symptoms, and intraocular pressure >21 mmHg.

All subjects underwent a comprehensive ophthalmic examination, including uncorrected distance visual acuity, best-corrected visual acuity, slit-lamp microscopy, noncontact tonometer, and fundus examinations. Subsequently, we applied Pentacam, Corvis ST, and ultrasound pachymetry to measure CCT. To avoid any effect of the ultrasound probe and topical anesthetic on the cornea, the two noncontact pieces of equipment were used first. The sequence of

measurements with Pentacam and Corvis ST was randomly chosen. Measurements were acquired from the right eyes of subjects to avoid structural similarities between fellow eyes [14]. In order to minimize the diurnal variation on CCT readings, all measurements were performed from 10:00 to 17:00. The subjects were required to completely blink twice before measurements, in order to form an optically smooth tear film on the cornea.

Corvis ST examination applies four red alignment marks to position the center of the cornea on the computer screen. Once positioned successfully, a puff of air with a pressure of 25 kPa is emitted automatically from the instrument aimed at the cornea at a distance of 11 mm. During the examination, the Scheimpflug camera records corneal deformation process and CCT. The process was repeated until three acceptable readings were obtained. The three CCT measurements obtained by each examiner were used to evaluate the intraoperator repeatability. The mean value of three successive measurements and the first measurement by each examiner were used to analyze the interoperator reproducibility.

The Pentacam was used as previously described [8, 9]. Briefly, the subject was instructed to sit, open both eyes, and fixate on a target within the device. The real-time image of the subject's eye on the computer screen was adjusted according to the pupil edge, center, and the corneal apex by moving the joystick. To avoid operator-dependent variables, the automatic release mode was applied. The Pentacam would automatically measure when correct alignment with the corneal apex and focus was achieved. Only when the "examination quality specification" reading showed OK, it was recorded; otherwise it was excluded and remeasured until three valid readings were obtained.

After the CCT measurements were obtained by Pentacam and Corvis ST, an A-scan ultrasound pachymetry (SP-3000, Tomey Inc., Nagoya, Japan) was used. Before the measurements, the instrument was calibrated by an experienced technician. First, the cornea was anesthetized with topical 0.5% proparacaine hydrochloride (Alcaine; Alcon Laboratories, TX, USA). Then, the subject in the supine position was asked to fixate on a target on the ceiling. The examiner placed the pachymeter probe on the central cornea as perpendicularly as possible. Then, five consecutive measurements were obtained, of which the highest and lowest were excluded, and the remaining three were recorded.

Statistical Analysis. Statistical analysis was performed using SPSS software for Windows version 21 (IBM Corporation, USA) and Microsoft Office Excel (Microsoft Corp., WA, USA). $P < 0.05$ was considered to be statistically significant. The distributions were checked by Kolmogorov-Smirnov test, which showed that the data were normally distributed ($P > 0.05$). Results were presented as means ± standard deviations.

To assess the intraoperator repeatability of Corvis ST, within-subject standard deviation (S_w), test-retest repeatability (TRT), within-subject coefficient of variation (CoV), and intraclass correlation coefficient (ICC) were calculated for the three successive measurements obtained by the two operators. The TRT is 2.77 times S_w, which represents an interval within which 95% of the differences between

TABLE 1: Intraobserver repeatability of the corneal dynamic Scheimpflug analyzer Corvis ST in measuring central corneal thickness ($N = 84$).

Operator	Mean (μm) $\pm$ SD	S_w (μm)	TRT (μm)	CoV (%)	ICC (95% CI)
1st	535.9 $\pm$ 27.0	4.8	13.0	0.87	0.971 (0.958 to 0.980)
2nd	537.4 $\pm$ 27.6	4.7	13.0	0.87	0.972 (0.960 to 0.981)

SD = standard deviation, S_w = within-subject standard deviation, TRT = test-retest repeatability ($2.77S_w$), CoV = within-subject coefficient of variation, and ICC = intraclass correlation coefficient.

TABLE 2: Interobserver reproducibility of central corneal thickness readings using average (from average of 3 consecutive readings from each observer) and single (from the first reading from each observer) measurement by the corneal dynamic Scheimpflug analyzer Corvis ST.

Parameter	Mean (μm) $\pm$ SD	S_w (μm)	TRT (μm)	CoV (%)	ICC (95% CI)
Average	536.6 $\pm$ 27.2	3.5	9.7	0.65	0.984 (0.973 to 0.990)
Single	536.4 $\pm$ 27.5	4.5	12.6	0.85	0.973 (0.958 to 0.982)

SD = standard deviation, S_w = within-subject standard deviation, TRT = test-retest repeatability ($2.77S_w$), CoV = within-subject coefficient of variation, and ICC = intraclass correlation coefficient.

TABLE 3: Comparison of the central corneal thickness readings obtained using the corneal dynamic Scheimpflug analyzer Corvis ST, Pentacam rotating Scheimpflug system, and ultrasound pachymetry.

Device pairings	Mean difference (μm) $\pm$ SD	95% LoA (μm)	P value
Corvis-Pentacam	-3.2 ± 6.5	-15.8 to 9.5	<0.001
Corvis-USP	-7.8 ± 10.3	-27.9 to 12.3	<0.001

USP = ultrasound pachymetry, SD = standard deviation.

measurements are expected to lie [15]. The CoV is defined as the ratio of S_w to the overall mean. A lower CoV is closely related to higher repeatability. The ICC represents the consistency of measurement. The closer the ICC is to 1, the better the consistency of measurement is. To evaluate the interoperator reproducibility of Corvis ST, the average method (the difference between the mean of the three successive measurements obtained by the two operators) and the single method (the first measurement of each operator) were used. Then, the interoperator S_w, TRT, CoV, and ICC were also calculated.

For multiple comparisons between CCT measurements obtained by Corvis ST and Pentacam or ultrasound pachymetry, the repeated-measures analysis of variance (ANOVA) with Bonferroni post hoc comparison test was used. Furthermore, the 95% limits of agreement (LoA) were calculated and Bland-Altman plots were produced to evaluate the agreement on the CCT measurements between Corvis ST versus Pentacam and Corvis ST versus ultrasound pachymetry [16]. The 95% LoA are defined as mean $\pm$ 1.96 SD, which represent an interval within which 95% of the differences between readings are expected to lie [8].

3. Results

This study enrolled 84 right eyes of 84 subjects (38 males and 46 females). The mean age of the subjects was 27.30 $\pm$ 6.06 years (range 18 to 49 years). The mean spherical equivalent refraction was -4.12 ± 2.66 D (range -10.50 to $+0.50$ D).

3.1. Intraoperator Repeatability. The CCT measurements obtained using Corvis ST showed excellent intraoperator repeatability for both operators (Table 1). The TRT values were $\leq$13 μm, the CoV values were <0.9%, and the ICC values were >0.97.

3.2. Interoperator Reproducibility. The mean $\pm$ SD of CCT, S_w, TRT, CoV, and ICC of Corvis ST are shown in Table 2, which demonstrate high interoperator reproducibility. In the average method, the TRT was 9.7 μm, the CoV was 0.65%, and the ICC was 0.98. In the single method, the TRT was 12.6 μm, the CoV was 0.85%, and the ICC was 0.97. Obviously, the error of the average method was smaller than the single method.

3.3. Agreement between Corvis ST, Pentacam, and Ultrasound Pachymetry. The mean CCT readings using Corvis ST, Pentacam, and ultrasound pachymetry were 535.9 $\pm$ 27.0 μm, 539.0 $\pm$ 25.70 μm, and 543.7 $\pm$ 27.52 μm, respectively. The CCT readings measured by Corvis ST were significantly thinner than Pentacam ($P < 0.001$). Bland-Altman analysis confirmed these results (Table 3 and Figure 1). The mean difference was -3.2μm (95% LoA, -15.8 to 9.5 μm).

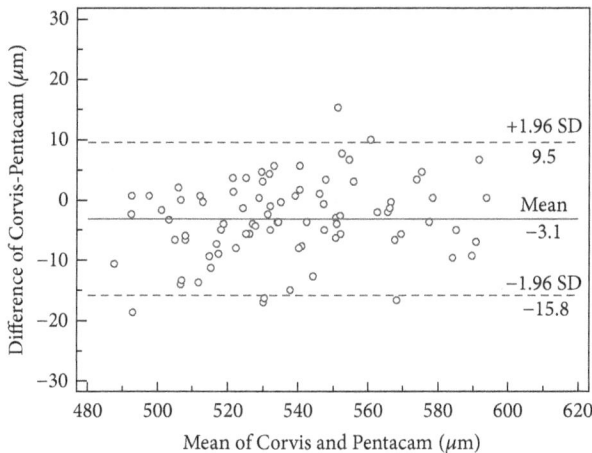

FIGURE 1: Bland-Altman plot demonstrating central corneal thickness measurements obtained using corneal dynamic Scheimpflug analyzer Corvis ST and Pentacam rotating Scheimpflug system against the mean values for both devices. The 95% limits of agreement are represented as the upper and lower lines.

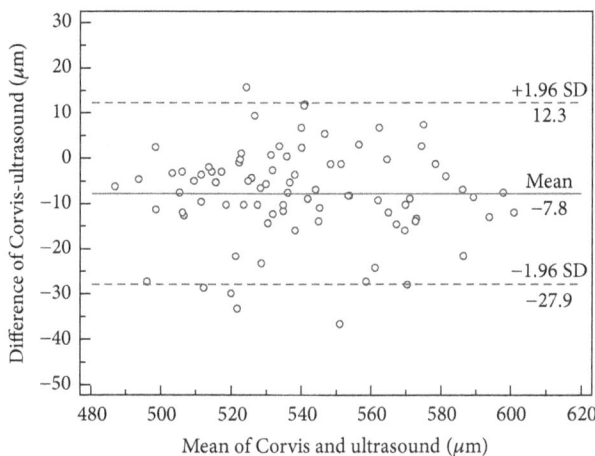

FIGURE 2: Bland-Altman plot demonstrating central corneal thickness measurements obtained using corneal dynamic Scheimpflug analyzer Corvis ST and ultrasound pachymetry against the mean values for both devices. The 95% limits of agreement are represented as the upper and lower lines.

CCT measurements between Corvis ST and ultrasound pachymetry were significantly different ($P < 0.001$). The mean difference was $-7.8\,\mu$m (95% LoA, -27.9 to $12.3\,\mu$m) (Table 3 and Figure 2).

4. Discussion

The present study was prospectively designed to assess (1) the intraoperator repeatability and (2) the interoperator reproducibility by applying the single and average methods on CCT measurements obtained from Corvis ST in normal eyes and (3) to evaluate the agreement between Corvis ST, Pentacam, and ultrasound pachymetry. The TRT was $\leq 13.0\,\mu$m, the CoV was $<0.90\%$, and the ICC was >0.97,

which represented high intraoperator repeatability in CCT readings using Corvis ST in normal eyes. Ali et al. [10] obtained similar results in normal eyes, with TRT, CoV, and ICC of $27\,\mu$m, 1.83%, and 0.95, respectively. Hon and Lam [11] reported TRT, CoV, and ICC of $15.34\,\mu$m, 1.01%, and 0.96, respectively, in normal subjects. Nemeth et al. [12] obtained similar ICC of 0.97 and CoV of 0.8% for CCT in normal eyes. Salvetat et al. [17] reported ICC of 0.99 in normal subjects and primary open-angle glaucoma patients. Chen et al. [13] obtained similar results in virgin eyes, with TRT, CoV, and ICC of $12.56\,\mu$m, 0.69%, and 0.99, respectively. However, they reported worse results in post-PRK eyes, with TRT and CoV of $22.61\,\mu$m and 2.29%, respectively.

Previous studies had assessed the intraoperator repeatability of CCT values using other Scheimpflug systems and specular microscopes, such as Pentacam, Sirius, Galilei, Orbscan II (Bausch & Lomb, Rochester, NY, USA), and SP-02 (Costruzione Strumenti Oftalmici, Italy). Huang et al. [7] evaluated the intraoperator repeatability of Sirius and Pentacam, a rotating Scheimpflug camera combined with a Placido disk corneal topographer and a rotating Scheimpflug camera, respectively, in normal subjects. They indicated that the TRT values were $8.79\,\mu$m and $9.65\,\mu$m, the CoV values were 0.59% and 0.65%, and the ICC values were 0.98 and 0.98, respectively. These results were slightly better than our results with Corvis ST. Al-Mohtaseb et al. [18] assessed the intraoperator repeatability of the Galilei, a dual rotating Scheimpflug camera combined with a Placido disk, in normal eyes. The CoV was 0.36% and the ICC was 0.99, which were also slightly better than our results with Corvis ST. Maldonado et al. [19] studied the intraoperator repeatability of the Orbscan II, a scanning-slit combined with Placido disc topography, with TRT and CoV of $20.2\,\mu$m and 1.5%, respectively, which were worse than our results. Bao et al. [20] assessed the intraoperator repeatability of SP-02, a noncontact specular microscope, in normal eyes with TRT, CoV, and ICC of $18.67\,\mu$m, 1.23%, and 0.97, respectively, which were worse than our results with Corvis ST. These indirect comparisons indicate that the above-mentioned devices have high intraoperator repeatability, with Galilei being the best. The Galilei has two opposite Scheimpflug cameras and can calculate the average value of the CCT obtained by the two cameras. This reduces the artifact error caused by ocular movements and increases repeatability [21]. Therefore, future studies should compare Corvis ST, Galilei, and Sirius.

In the present study, we analyzed the interoperator reproducibility of CCT measurements acquired with Corvis ST by applying the single and average methods. The TRT and CoV of the mean values were smaller than the single values. Chen and Lam [22, 23] demonstrated that the width of 95% LoA was reduced by using an averaged result rather than the first result of each visit. Ali et al. [10] assessed the reproducibility of the CCT with the device in normal eyes, which was intersession reproducibility at different times of the day. In their study, TRT, CoV, and ICC were $11.0\,\mu$m, 7.41%, and 0.995, respectively, while they were $9.70\,\mu$m, 0.65%, and 0.984 in the current study, respectively. Our results were obviously better than their results because our results were accomplished within 30 minutes, which eliminated the effects of different

TABLE 4: Summary of previous studies for the agreement of CCT measurements obtained by other Scheimpflug systems, Orbscan II and specular microscopes in comparison to Pentacam or ultrasound pachymetry.

Author (year)	Patients/eyes	Device pairings	Mean difference (μm) $\pm$ SD	P value	95% LoA (μm)
Lanza et al. [27] (2015)	102/102	Pentacam-Orbscan II	13.66 $\pm$ 16.53	<0.0001	−18.74 to 46.06
		Sirius-Orbscan II	15.18 $\pm$ 17.16	<0.0001	−18.45 to 48.81
		Sirius-Pentacam	1.52 $\pm$ 6.21	0.015	−10.65 to 13.69
Khaja et al. [28] (2015)	32/32	USP-Orbscan II	2.8 $\pm$ 0.28	NA	−30.15 to 24.40
		USP-specular microscopy	8.69 $\pm$ 1.24	NA	−8.82 to 27.4
Smedowski et al. [29] (2014)	76/152	Corvis ST-Pentacam	NA	>0.05	NA
		Corvis ST-USP	NA	>0.05	NA
Huang et al. [30] (2014)	66/66	Pentacam-Sirius	−3.3 $\pm$ 5.2	<0.001	−13.6 to 6.9
		Pentacam-Galilei	−9.3 $\pm$ 3.7	<0.001	−16.6 to −2.0
		Sirius-Galilei	−6.0 $\pm$ 4.0	<0.001	−13.8 to 1.9
Anayol et al. [31] (2014)	32/32	Galilei-Pentacam	13.93 $\pm$ 0.88	<0.001	11.74 to 16.12
		Galilei-Sirius	14.66 $\pm$ 0.69	<0.001	12.96 to 16.37
		Pentacam-Sirius	0.73 $\pm$ 0.93	1.0	−1.50 to 3.02
Maresca et al. [32] (2014)	35/35	Sirius-USP	−13.9 $\pm$ 14.4	<0.001	−42.2 to 14.4
Feizi et al. [33] (2014)	88/88	USP-Orbscan	−14.5 $\pm$ 22.9	<0.001	−59.4 to 30.4
		USP-Galilei	−16.0 $\pm$ 19.6	<0.001	−54.5 to 22.5
		Orbscan-Galilei	−1.5 $\pm$ 17.0	0.99	−34.8 to 31.9
De La Parra-Colín et al. [34] (2014)	16/16	Sirius-Pentacam	−10.1 $\pm$ 9.0	NA	−27.7 to 7.5
Jorgel et al. [35] (2013)	50/50	Sirius-USP	4.68 $\pm$ 10.47	0.003	−15.84 to 25.20
Bayhan et al. [36] (2014)	50/50	USP-Sirius	17.58 $\pm$ 8.13	<0.001	15.27 to 19.89
Huang et al. [37] (2013)	43/43	Sirius-USP	6.88 $\pm$ 6.77	0.000	−6.39 to 20.14
Nassiri et al. [38] (2014)	32/61	Pentacam-USP	−1 $\pm$ 9	0.32	−20 to 17
		Orbscan II-USP	6 $\pm$ 14	<0.001	−21 to 33
Al Farhan et al. [39] (2013)	30/30	USP-specular microscopy	−2.40 $\pm$ 9.10	0.16	−38.70 to 39.90
Tai et al. [40] (2013)	92/184	Pentacam-USP	10.08 $\pm$ 10.96	0.012	−11.40 to 31.56
		Specular microscopy-USP	−20.49 $\pm$ 8.91	<0.001	−37.95 to −3.04
		Specular microscopy-Pentacam	−30.57 $\pm$ 10.26	<0.001	−59.69 to −10.45
Chen et al. [41] (2012)	35/35	Pentacam-USP	5.27 $\pm$ 9.55	0.007	−24.0 to −13.4
Aramberri et al. [42] (2012)	35/35	Pentacam-Galilei	−2.76 $\pm$ 4.52	<0.01	−6.1 to 11.6
González-Pérez et al. [43] (2011)	22/22	USP-Pentacam	3 $\pm$ 10	0.233	−16.2 to 21.2
		USP-Orbscan II	32 $\pm$ 15	<0.001	3.1 to 60.8
		USP-specular microscopy	26 $\pm$ 37	0.004	−46.2 to 97.8
		Pentacam-Orbscan II	29 $\pm$ 11	<0.001	7.2 to 51.6
		Pentacam-specular microscopy	23 $\pm$ 32	0.003	−40.2 to 86.2
		Orbscan II-specular microscopy	−6 $\pm$ 35	0.399	−74.8 to 62.0
		USP-Orbscan II	−15 $\pm$ 17	0.001	−47.9 to 18.7
		Pentacam-Orbscan II	−17 $\pm$ 14	<0.001	−43.9 to 9.8

times on the CCT. Chen et al. [13] measured the interoperator reproducibility of the CCT by the single method in virgin and post-PRK eyes, and the TRT, CoV, and ICC were 13.24 μm, 0.72%, and 0.98 in virgin eyes and 9.89 μm, 0.58%, and 1.00 in post-PRK eyes, respectively, which were similar to our results using the single method. Salvetat et al. [17] only applied ICC to assess the interoperator reproducibility, which was 0.99 in normal subjects and primary open-angle glaucoma

patients. We believe that ours is the first study to evaluate the interoperator reproducibility of Corvis ST using the average and single methods with TRT, CoV, and ICC.

In addition, we compared the CCT readings between Corvis ST, Pentacam, and ultrasound pachymetry in normal eyes. Corvis ST had a slightly lower CCT measurement as compared to Pentacam with a mean of 3.2 μm. Meanwhile, Corvis ST significantly underestimated CCT as compared to ultrasound pachymetry with an average of 7.8 μm. The 95% LoA between Corvis ST and Pentacam were narrow and comparable, with the CCT diurnal pachymetric variation range of -11 to $11\,\mu$m [24]. Therefore, Corvis ST and Pentacam could be interchangeably used in normal eyes in most clinical applications. However, Corvis ST cannot be interchangeably used with ultrasound pachymetry in normal eyes because of broad 95% LoA between the two devices. Our results were similar to or better than those previously reported when investigating agreement of CCT measurements obtained from other Scheimpflug systems, Orbscan II, and specular microscopes with respect to Pentacam or ultrasound pachymetry (Table 4). Several reasons may explain the difference in CCT readings between Corvis ST and ultrasound pachymetry. Firstly, topical 0.5% proparacaine hydrochloride may cause corneal thickness to increase by 8.6 μm in 80 seconds [25]. Secondly, the accuracy of ultrasound pachymetry depends on the operator's proficiency and whether the corneal probe is perpendicularly placed on the center of the cornea. Thirdly, if the posterior surface reflection point is closer to the anterior chamber, the CCT measurement is thicker than the actual value [26].

The present study had some limitations. First, we only assessed the intraoperator repeatability and interoperator reproducibility in normal subjects and did not include keratoconus, glaucoma, or postrefractive surgery patients. Further research is needed to assess the intraoperator repeatability and interoperator reproducibility in the above-mentioned patients. Second, our study is restricted by the different algorithms each device uses for obtaining the CCT. The CCT obtained by Corvis ST and Pentacam are derived from the corneal apex. However, ultrasound pachymetry is performed over the pupil center, and its position depends on the operator's experience.

In conclusion, Corvis ST showed high intraoperator repeatability and interoperator reproducibility of CCT measurements in normal eyes. Corvis ST and Pentacam showed excellent agreement, which suggests that the two devices may be interchangeably used for CCT measurements in the clinical setting. However, the CCT readings between Corvis ST and ultrasound pachymetry are not directly interchangeable owing to the relatively wide 95% LoA.

Conflict of Interests

The authors have no proprietary or commercial interest in any materials discussed in this paper.

Authors' Contribution

Ayong Yu and Weiqi Zhao have contributed equally as first authors.

Acknowledgments

This work is supported in part by the National Natural Science Foundation of China (81300807); Foundation of Wenzhou City Science & Technology Bureau (J20140014 and Y20140619); Health Bureau of Zhejiang Province (2016RCB013); Zhejiang Provincial & Ministry of Health Research Fund for Medical Sciences (WKJ-ZJ-1530); National Science and Technology Major Project (2014ZX09303301). The contribution of G. B. Bietti Foundation IRCCS was supported by the Italian Ministry of Health and Fondazione Roma.

References

[1] Z. Wang, J. Chen, and B. Yang, "Posterior corneal surface topographic changes after laser in situ keratomileusis are related to residual corneal bed thickness," *Ophthalmology*, vol. 106, no. 2, pp. 406–410, 1999.

[2] M. J. Doughty and M. L. Zaman, "Human corneal thickness and its impact on intraocular pressure measures: a review and meta-analysis approach," *Survey of Ophthalmology*, vol. 44, no. 5, pp. 367–408, 2000.

[3] G. U. Auffarth, L. Wang, and H. E. Völcker, "Keratoconus evaluation using the Orbscan Topography System," *Journal of Cataract and Refractive Surgery*, vol. 26, no. 2, pp. 222–228, 2000.

[4] Ö. Ö. Uçakhan, M. Özkan, and A. Kanpolat, "Corneal thickness measurements in normal and keratoconic eyes: pentacam comprehensive eye scanner versus noncontact specular microscopy and ultrasound pachymetry," *Journal of Cataract and Refractive Surgery*, vol. 32, no. 6, pp. 970–977, 2006.

[5] H. A. Swarbrick, G. Wong, and D. J. O'Leary, "Corneal response to orthokeratology," *Optometry and Vision Science*, vol. 75, no. 11, pp. 791–799, 1998.

[6] Y. Barkana, Y. Gerber, U. Elbaz et al., "Central corneal thickness measurement with the Pentacam Scheimpflug system, optical low-coherence reflectometry pachymeter, and ultrasound pachymetry," *Journal of Cataract and Refractive Surgery*, vol. 31, no. 9, pp. 1729–1735, 2005.

[7] J. Huang, X. Ding, G. Savini et al., "A comparison between scheimpflug imaging and optical coherence tomography in measuring corneal thickness," *Ophthalmology*, vol. 120, no. 10, pp. 1951–1958, 2013.

[8] J. Huang, K. Pesudovs, A. Yu et al., "A comprehensive comparison of central corneal thickness measurement," *Optometry and Vision Science*, vol. 88, no. 8, pp. 940–949, 2011.

[9] R. Khoramnia, T. M. Rabsilber, and G. U. Auffarth, "Central and peripheral pachymetry measurements according to age using the Pentacam rotating Scheimpflug camera," *Journal of Cataract and Refractive Surgery*, vol. 33, no. 5, pp. 830–836, 2007.

[10] N. Q. Ali, D. V. Patel, and C. N. J. McGhee, "Biomechanical responses of healthy and keratoconic corneas measured using a noncontact scheimpflug-based tonometer," *Investigative Ophthalmology and Visual Science*, vol. 55, no. 6, pp. 3651–3659, 2014.

[11] Y. Hon and A. K. C. Lam, "Corneal deformation measurement using Scheimpflug noncontact tonometry," *Optometry and Vision Science*, vol. 90, no. 1, pp. e1–e8, 2013.

[12] G. Nemeth, Z. Hassan, A. Csutak, E. Szalai, A. Berta, and L. Modis Jr., "Repeatability of ocular biomechanical data measurements with a scheimpflug-based noncontact device on normal corneas," *Journal of Refractive Surgery*, vol. 29, no. 8, pp. 558–563, 2013.

[13] X. Chen, A. Stojanovic, Y. Hua et al., "Reliability of corneal dynamic scheimpflug analyser measurements in virgin and post-PRK eyes," *PLoS ONE*, vol. 9, no. 10, Article ID e109577, 2014.

[14] J. Katz, S. Zeger, and K.-Y. Liang, "Appropriate statistical methods to account for similarities in binary outcomes between fellow eyes," *Investigative Ophthalmology and Visual Science*, vol. 35, no. 5, pp. 2461–2465, 1994.

[15] J. M. Bland and D. G. Altman, "Measurement error," *British Medical Journal*, vol. 313, no. 7059, article 744, 1996.

[16] J. M. Bland and D. G. Altman, "Statistical methods for assessing agreement between two methods of clinical measurement," *The Lancet*, vol. 1, no. 8476, pp. 307–310, 1986.

[17] M. L. Salvetat, M. Zeppieri, C. Tosoni, M. Felletti, L. Grasso, and P. Brusini, "Corneal deformation parameters provided by the Corvis-ST Pachy-Tonometer in healthy subjects and glaucoma patients," *Journal of Glaucoma*, vol. 24, no. 8, pp. 568–574, 2015.

[18] Z. N. Al-Mohtaseb, L. Wang, and M. P. Weikert, "Repeatability and comparability of corneal thickness measurements obtained from Dual Scheimpflug Analyzer and from ultrasonic pachymetry," *Graefe's Archive for Clinical and Experimental Ophthalmology*, vol. 251, no. 7, pp. 1855–1860, 2013.

[19] M. J. Maldonado, A. López-Miguel, J. C. Nieto, J. Cano-Parra, B. Calvo, and J. L. Alió, "Reliability of noncontact pachymetry after laser in situ keratomileusis," *Investigative Ophthalmology and Visual Science*, vol. 50, no. 9, pp. 4135–4141, 2009.

[20] F. Bao, Q. Wang, S. Cheng et al., "Comparison and evaluation of central corneal thickness using 2 new noncontact specular microscopes and conventional pachymetry devices," *Cornea*, vol. 33, no. 6, pp. 576–581, 2014.

[21] N. Menassa, C. Kaufmann, M. Goggin, O. M. Job, L. M. Bachmann, and M. A. Thiel, "Comparison and reproducibility of corneal thickness and curvature readings obtained by the Galilei and the Orbscan II analysis systems," *Journal of Cataract and Refractive Surgery*, vol. 34, no. 10, pp. 1742–1747, 2008.

[22] D. Chen and A. K. C. Lam, "Intrasession and intersession repeatability of the Pentacam system on posterior corneal assessment in the normal human eye," *Journal of Cataract and Refractive Surgery*, vol. 33, no. 3, pp. 448–454, 2007.

[23] D. Chen and A. K. C. Lam, "Reliability and repeatability of the Pentacam on corneal curvatures," *Clinical and Experimental Optometry*, vol. 92, no. 2, pp. 110–118, 2009.

[24] M. R. Lattimore Jr., S. Kaupp, S. Schallhorn, and Rt. Lewis, "Orbscan pachymetry: implications of a repeated measures and diurnal variation analysis," *Ophthalmology*, vol. 106, no. 5, pp. 977–981, 1999.

[25] S. M. Nam, H. K. Lee, E. K. Kim, and K. Y. Seo, "Comparison of corneal thickness after the instillation of topical anesthetics: proparacaine versus oxybuprocaine," *Cornea*, vol. 25, no. 1, pp. 51–54, 2006.

[26] S. Amano, N. Honda, Y. Amano et al., "Comparison of central corneal thickness measurements by rotating scheimpflug camera, ultrasonic pachymetry, and scanning-slit corneal topography," *Ophthalmology*, vol. 113, no. 6, pp. 937–941, 2006.

[27] M. Lanza, E. Paolillo, U. A. Gironi Carnevale et al., "Central corneal thickness evaluation in healthy eyes with three different optical devices," *Contact Lens and Anterior Eye*, vol. 38, no. 6, pp. 409–413, 2015.

[28] W. A. Khaja, S. Grover, A. T. Kelmenson, L. R. Ferguson, K. Sambhav, and K. V. Chalam, "Comparison of central corneal thickness: ultrasound pachymetry versus slit-lamp optical coherence tomography, specular microscopy, and Orbscan," *Clinical Ophthalmology*, vol. 9, pp. 1065–1070, 2015.

[29] A. Smedowski, B. Weglarz, D. Tarnawska, K. Kaarniranta, and E. Wylegala, "Comparison of three intraocular pressure measurement methods including biomechanical properties of the cornea," *Investigative Ophthalmology and Visual Science*, vol. 55, no. 2, pp. 666–673, 2014.

[30] J. Huang, X. Ding, G. Savini et al., "Central and midperipheral corneal thickness measured with Scheimpflug imaging and optical coherence tomography," *PLoS ONE*, vol. 9, no. 5, Article ID e98316, 2014.

[31] M. A. Anayol, E. Güler, R. Yağci et al., "Comparison of central corneal thickness, thinnest corneal thickness, anterior chamber depth, and simulated keratometry using galilei, Pentacam, and Sirius devices," *Cornea*, vol. 33, no. 6, pp. 582–586, 2014.

[32] N. Maresca, F. Zeri, P. Palumbo, and A. Calossi, "Agreement and reliability in measuring central corneal thickness with a rotating Scheimpflug-Placido system and ultrasound pachymetry," *Contact Lens and Anterior Eye*, vol. 37, no. 6, pp. 442–446, 2014.

[33] S. Feizi, M. R. Jafarinasab, F. Karimian, H. Hasanpour, and A. Masudi, "Central and peripheral corneal thickness measurement in normal and keratoconic eyes using three corneal pachymeters," *Journal of Ophthalmic & Vision Research*, vol. 9, pp. 296–304, 2014.

[34] P. De La Parra-Colín, M. Garza-León, and T. Barrientos-Gutierrez, "Repeatability and comparability of anterior segment biometry obtained by the Sirius and the Pentacam analyzers," *International Ophthalmology*, vol. 34, no. 1, pp. 27–33, 2014.

[35] J. Jorgel, J. Rosado, J. Diaz-Rey, and J. Gonzalez-Meijome, "Central corneal thickness and anterior chamber depth measurement by Sirius Scheimpflug tomography and ultrasound," *Clinical Ophthalmology*, vol. 7, pp. 417–422, 2013.

[36] H. A. Bayhan, S. A. Bayhan, and I. Can, "Comparison of central corneal thickness measurements with three new optical devices and a standard ultrasonic pachymeter," *International Journal of Ophthalmology*, vol. 7, no. 2, pp. 302–308, 2014.

[37] J. Huang, G. Savini, L. Hu et al., "Precision of a new Scheimpflug and Placido-disk analyzer in measuring corneal thickness and agreement with ultrasound pachymetry," *Journal of Cataract and Refractive Surgery*, vol. 39, no. 2, pp. 219–224, 2013.

[38] N. Nassiri, K. Sheibani, S. Safi et al., "Central corneal thickness in highly myopic eyes: Inter-device agreement of ultrasonic pachymetry, Pentacam and Orbscan II before and after photorefractive keratectomy," *Journal of Ophthalmic & Vision Research*, vol. 9, no. 1, pp. 14–21, 2014.

[39] H. M. Al Farhan, W. M. Al Otaibi, H. M. Al Razqan, and A. A. Al Harqan, "Assessment of central corneal thickness and corneal endothelial morphology using ultrasound pachymetry, non-contact specular microscopy, and Confoscan 4 confocal microscopy," *BMC Ophthalmology*, vol. 13, no. 1, article 73, 2013.

[40] L.-Y. Tai, K.-W. Khaw, C.-M. Ng, and V. Subrayan, "Central corneal thickness measurements with different imaging devices and ultrasound pachymetry," *Cornea*, vol. 32, no. 6, pp. 766–771, 2013.

[41] S. Chen, J. Huang, D. Wen, W. Chen, D. Huang, and Q. Wang, "Measurement of central corneal thickness by high-resolution Scheimpflug imaging, Fourier-domain optical coherence tomography and ultrasound pachymetry," *Acta Ophthalmologica*, vol. 90, no. 5, pp. 449–455, 2012.

[42] J. Aramberri, L. Araiz, A. Garcia et al., "Dual versus single Scheimpflug camera for anterior segment analysis: Precision

and agreement," *Journal of Cataract and Refractive Surgery*, vol. 38, no. 11, pp. 1934–1949, 2012.

[43] J. González-Pérez, J. M. González-Méijome, M. T. Rodríguez Ares, and M. Á. Parafita, "Central corneal thickness measured with three optical devices and ultrasound pachometry," *Eye & Contact Lens*, vol. 37, no. 2, pp. 66–70, 2011.

6

The Arclight Ophthalmoscope: A Reliable Low-Cost Alternative to the Standard Direct Ophthalmoscope

James Lowe,[1] Charles R. Cleland,[2] Evarista Mgaya,[2] Godfrey Furahini,[2] Clare E. Gilbert,[3] Matthew J. Burton,[3] and Heiko Philippin[2,3]

[1]Eastbourne District General Hospital, Kings Drive, Eastbourne BN21 2UD, UK
[2]Kilimanjaro Christian Medical Centre Eye Department, P.O. Box 3010, Moshi, Tanzania
[3]International Centre for Eye Health, London School of Hygiene & Tropical Medicine, Keppel Street, London WC1E 7HT, UK

Correspondence should be addressed to Charles R. Cleland; crcleland87@gmail.com

Academic Editor: Van C. Lansingh

Background. The Arclight ophthalmoscope is a low-cost alternative to standard direct ophthalmoscopes. This study compared the Arclight ophthalmoscope with the Heine K180 direct ophthalmoscope to evaluate its reliability in assessing the vertical cup disc ratio (VCDR) and its ease of use (EOU). *Methods.* Eight medical students used both the Arclight and the Heine ophthalmoscopes to examine the optic disc in 9 subjects. An EOU score was provided after every examination (a higher score indicating that the ophthalmoscope is easier to use). A consultant ophthalmologist provided the reference standard VCDR. *Results.* 288 examinations were performed. The number of examinations that yielded an estimation of the VCDR was significantly higher for the Arclight ophthalmoscope (125/144, 85%) compared to the Heine ophthalmoscope (88/144, 61%) ($p < 0.001$). The mean difference from the reference standard VCDR was similar for both instruments, with a mean of −0.078 (95% CI: −0.10 to −0.056) for the Arclight and −0.072 (95% CI: −0.097 to −0.046) for Heine ($p = 0.69$). The overall EOU score was significantly higher for the Arclight ophthalmoscope ($p < 0.001$). *Conclusion.* The Arclight ophthalmoscope performs as well as, and is easier to use than, a standard direct ophthalmoscope, suggesting it is a reliable, low-cost alternative.

1. Introduction

Vision 2020 is the global initiative, launched in 1999 by the World Health Organization (WHO) and the International Agency for the Prevention of Blindness (IAPB), with the aim of eliminating avoidable blindness. In the African region, WHO estimates that 26 million people are visually impaired and 6 million people are blind [1]. Significant progress has already been made in treating or preventing anterior segment eye diseases such as cataract and trachoma and an increasing proportion of the remaining burden of avoidable blindness in sub-Saharan Africa (SSA) is attributable to diseases of the back of the eye, particularly glaucoma and diabetic retinopathy [2].

The International Diabetes Federation predicts that the number of adults with diabetes in Africa will double from 12 million in 2010 to 24 million in 2030 [3]. Diabetic retinopathy is the commonest microvascular complication of diabetes [4]

and, globally, is the leading cause of blindness in adults of working age [5]. The number of people in SSA with glaucoma was estimated to be 6.5 million in 2010 and is anticipated to increase to 8.4 million by 2020 [6]. Although no cure exists for glaucoma or diabetic retinopathy, early detection and timely management can help slow progression and improve prognosis [7, 8].

In many SSA countries the *per capita* number of ophthalmologists and the prevalence of blindness are inversely correlated; the former concentrated in major urban areas and the latter in poorer rural regions [9]. In addition to this, the overall numbers of eye health personnel are below that which is needed. The regional ratio of ophthalmologists in SSA is 2.3 per million population [10]. For example, in Malawi there are seven consultant ophthalmologists serving a population of 15.2 million [11]. Therefore, general healthcare workers, opticians, and allied eye care professionals often review patients with eye diseases. These groups need access to equipment and adequate training to allow them to examine and detect pathology in the posterior segment of the eye. However, standard direct ophthalmoscopes are expensive, ranging from USD $200 to 600 per instrument.

The Arclight ophthalmoscope (http://www.arclightscope .com; Figure 1) provides a low-cost alternative to standard direct ophthalmoscopes. It is marketed at USD $7.50 when sold in bulk. It has a small direct ophthalmoscope at one end with an illuminating magnifying loupe (allowing examination of the anterior segment) and a detachable otoscope at the other end. It weighs 18 grams, uses three LED light sources, and has an inbuilt rechargeable battery powered by either an integrated solar panel (useful for mobile clinics in sub-Saharan Africa) or a USB port. The device has an adjustable lens slider with three different lenses, allowing for a rough correction of the patient's or examiner's refractive error. The device also incorporates a small colour vision test, a near visual acuity chart, a ruler, and a pupil size gauge.

The aim of this study was to assess if the Arclight ophthalmoscope performs as well as a conventional direct ophthalmoscope in the hands of final-year medical students (representative of nonspecialist users) in terms of estimating the vertical cup : disc ratio (VCDR) and its ease of use (EOU), in order to evaluate Arclight as an alternative to the standard direct ophthalmoscope. The VCDR was chosen as it is a clinically important measure in the assessment of glaucoma. The disc is a central and easily identifiable structure with sufficient variation in cup : disc ratios to provide numerical data for formal analysis [12, 13].

2. Materials and Methods

The study was approved by the Research Ethics Review Committee at Kilimanjaro Christian Medical University College (KCMUC), Moshi, Tanzania. It was conducted in the Department of Ophthalmology at Kilimanjaro Christian Medical Centre (KCMC). Written informed consent was provided by all participants.

In this study we compared the Arclight ophthalmoscope to the Heine K180 in terms of four measures: (1) accuracy of VCDR assessment, (2) ease of use (EOU) for the examiner using a score of 1–8 (Table 1), (3) the level of glare experienced by the subject using a score of 1–4 (Table 1), and (4) the perceived duration of the assessment using a score of 1–4 (Table 1) and scored by the subject as well. For measures (2) to (4) higher scores indicated better results.

Eight final-year medical students performed the examinations. To ensure a similar level of experience in ophthalmology, students who had taken more than one undergraduate course in ophthalmology were excluded. Students with a refractive error exceeding the corrective lenses of Arclight (−6 to +4) were also excluded. An introductory "refresher" session on direct ophthalmoscopy with particular reference to examination of the optic disc and assessment of the VCDR was provided. Following this, the examiners had a short practice session to familiarize themselves with both devices.

Nine healthy volunteers (18 eyes) acted as subjects and each was examined by the eight medical students. All subjects had one eye dilated at random using tropicamide 1% eye

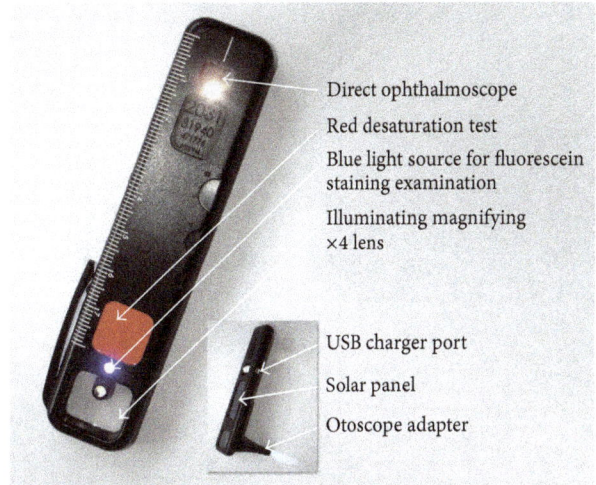

FIGURE 1: The Arclight direct ophthalmoscope with selected features highlighted.

TABLE 1: Examination scales: (a) ease of use (examiner), (b) comfort scale (subject) and (c) length of examination (subject).

	(1) Could not use at all
	(2) Could not see the red reflex to even begin with
	(3) Could identify red reflex
	(4) Could see vessels but not disc
(a) Ease of use	(5) Could identify disc but not vertical CD-ratio (VCDR)
	(6) Could determine VCDR with a high level of difficulty
	(7) Could determine VCDR with a medium level of difficulty
	(8) Could determine VCDR with a low level of difficulty
(b) Comfort scale	(1) Uncomfortable glare
	(2) Significant glare
	(3) Some glare
	(4) No glare
(c) Length of examination	(1) Uncomfortably long
	(2) Long examination time
	(3) Average examination time
	(4) Short examination time

drops. Therefore, half of the examinations were performed on a dilated pupil. Each examiner assessed both eyes of each volunteer subject with both devices. They were randomly assigned to start with an Arclight or Heine ophthalmoscope. Examinations were conducted in two circuits. In the first circuit the examiners examined both eyes of each subject using either the Arclight or the Heine ophthalmoscope. In the second circuit the examiners changed ophthalmoscopes and reexamined both eyes of each subject. Within each circuit, all the right eyes were examined first, followed by all the left eyes. This was done as we recognized that there could be a tendency, because of the normal symmetry between eyes, not

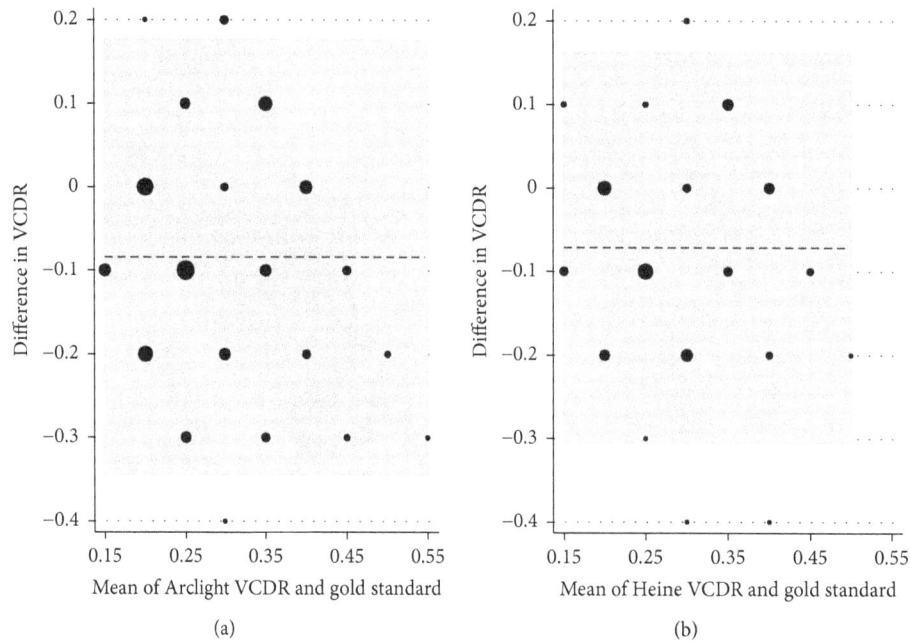

FIGURE 2: Bland-Altman plots showing the difference between the examiner's estimate of vertical cup : disc ratio (VCDR) and the reference standard, split by instrument. Plot (a) represents the Arclight direct ophthalmoscope and plot (b) represents the Heine K180 direct ophthalmoscope. Where there is exact agreement between the examiner and the reference standard the difference in VCDR is noted as 0. Any deviation from 0 represents underestimation (if negative) or overestimation (if positive) of the VCDR compared with the reference standard. The horizontal dotted line represents the mean of all observations (i.e., their mean deviation from the reference standard), and the grey area represents the proportion of all observations lying within 95% of the normal distribution for each of the two ophthalmoscopes. The size of each black dot is proportional to the number of observations it represents.

to grade the eyes in an independent manner [14]. A consultant ophthalmologist (HP), with a specialty interest in glaucoma, examined each subject with the Heine direct ophthalmoscope to provide the "reference standard" for VCDR measurement.

Data were recorded at the end of each examination by both the examiner and the subject. The examiner recorded the VCDR (range: 0.0 to 1.0) and an ease of use score (Table 1). The subject recorded the level of glare experienced and an impression of the length of the examination (Table 1).

Statistical analysis was performed using Student's t-test to compare differences between examiners' VCDR measurements and the reference standard. A Bland-Altman plot was calculated for both devices to provide a visual guide to the differences between examiners' VCDR scores and the "reference standard." STATA version 13 was used to compute statistics and graphs. A chi-squared test was used to compare the proportion of examinations that yielded an estimation of the VCDR with the Arclight versus the Heine ophthalmoscope. Ease of use, "glare," and "length of examination" were analyzed using chi-squared and Wilcoxon rank-sum tests.

3. Results and Discussion

3.1. Results

3.1.1. VCDR Estimation. Each examiner performed 36 examinations (18 with the Arclight ophthalmoscope and 18 with

the Heine ophthalmoscope, 9 dilated and 9 undilated eyes each), resulting in a total of 288 examinations. In total, 213 (74%) examinations resulted in an estimate of the VCDR. Significantly more of the Arclight examinations (125/144 [85%]) compared to the Heine ophthalmoscopes examinations (88/144 [61%]) produced a VCDR measure (χ^2, $p <$ 0.001). For both devices significantly more VCDR estimates were possible through examination of dilated pupils: 71/125 (57%) for the Arclight (χ^2, $p < 0.001$) and 58/88 (66%) for the Heine (χ^2, $p < 0.001$).

There was a very small difference between the reference standard VCDR measure and the Arclight measurements: mean difference −0.078 (95% CI: −0.10 to −0.056). There was a similar, very small difference for the comparison between the reference standard and Heine ophthalmoscope measurements: mean difference −0.072 (95% CI: −0.097 to −0.046). There was no difference in this mean performance between the two measures (p = 0.69). Bland-Altman plots were constructed for the difference in VCDR estimates between examiners and the reference standard (Figure 2).

Separate subanalyses of dilated and undilated pupils had similar results. For dilated pupils, the mean difference between the reference standard VCDR and the Arclight measurement was −0.087 (95% CI: −0.057 to −0.12) compared to −0.084 (95% CI: −0.053 to −0.12) for the Heine ophthalmoscope, with no difference between ophthalmoscopes (p = 0.9). For undilated pupils, the mean difference between the Arclight measurement and the reference standard was

−0.067 (95% CI: −0.033 to −0.10) compared to −0.047 (95% CI: −0.004 to −0.089) for the Heine ophthalmoscope, with no difference between ophthalmoscopes ($p = 0.47$).

The total number of examinations that yielded a ≥0.2 difference in the VCDR from the reference standard was 37/125 (29.6%) and 25/88 (28.4%) for the Arclight and Heine ophthalmoscopes, respectively (χ^2, $p = 0.85$). A random effects model was performed which showed no significant between-cluster variation between the two eyes.

3.1.2. Ease of Use.
An ease of use score was obtained for all 288 examinations. The overall median score was significantly higher (Wilcoxon rank-sum, $p < 0.001$) for the Arclight (median 7, IQR 6 to 8) than the Heine (median 6, IQR 5 to 7), Figure 3. Both devices had higher EOU scores for dilated pupils: Arclight median score 7 (IQR 7-8) for dilated eyes versus 7 (IQR 5.75-7) for undilated pupils (Wilcoxon rank-sum, $p < 0.001$) and Heine median score 7 (IQR 6-7) versus 5 (IQR 5-6) (Wilcoxon rank-sum, $p < 0.001$) for dilated and undilated eyes, respectively. There were no significant differences in EOU scores between the first and second circuits.

3.1.3. Examination Comfort.
Subject-rated "glare" and perceived "length of examination" data were obtained for 285/288 examinations. Responses were missing for three examinations. Participants reported significantly more "glare" from the Heine ophthalmoscope ($p = 0.046$): Arclight median score 3 (IQR 3-3), Heine median score 3 (IQR 2-3) (Figure 4). Similarly, participants reported significantly longer examinations for the Heine ophthalmoscope ($p < 0.001$): Arclight median score 3 (IQR 3-4), Heine median score 3 (IQR 2-3) (Figure 5). There were no significant differences in subject-rated "glare" between dilated and undilated pupils. However, subjects reported a significantly shorter "length of examination" when dilated pupils versus undilated pupils were examined ($p < 0.001$). This difference was also apparent when each device was compared separately.

3.2. Discussion.
The Arclight ophthalmoscope aims to provide a reliable, low-cost alternative to the standard direct ophthalmoscope. We found no evidence of a difference between the Arclight ophthalmoscope and the Heine K180 direct ophthalmoscope in terms of accuracy of the VCDR measurement, performed by final-year medical students. However, the students found the Arclight significantly easier to use. We also found no clinically significant differences between the devices, with a similar proportion of examinations yielding a ≥0.2 difference in the VCDR compared to the reference standard for both the Arclight and Heine ophthalmoscopes.

Importantly, 85% of Arclight examinations yielded a VCDR estimation, compared to 61% with the Heine ophthalmoscope. This provides an additional indication that the Arclight ophthalmoscope is easier to use with added clinical benefits. From a patient perspective, the LED bulb in the Arclight ophthalmoscope resulted in a subjectively more

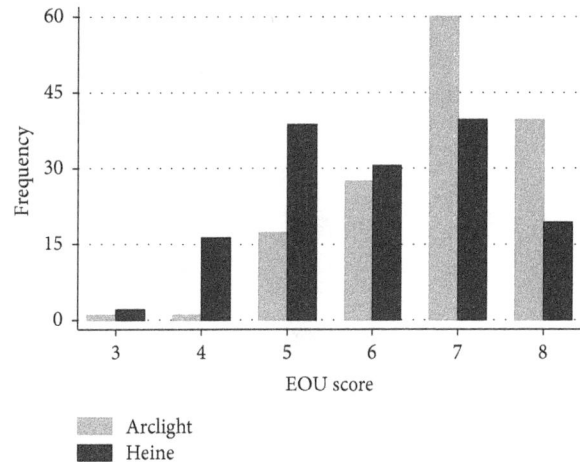

FIGURE 3: A histogram of the frequency of ease of use score for the Arclight and Heine direct ophthalmoscopes. 3: could identify red reflex. 4: could see vessels but not disc. 5: could identify disc but not vertical CD-ratio (VCDR). 6: could determine VCDR with a high level of difficulty. 7: could determine VCDR with a medium level of difficulty. 8: could determine VCDR with a low level of difficulty.

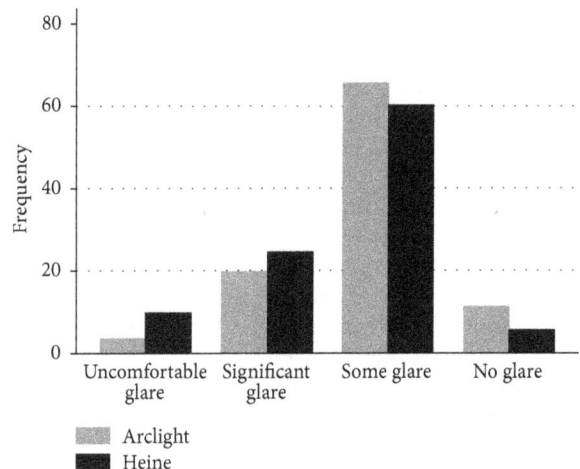

FIGURE 4: A histogram of the frequency of brightness reported by those examined for the Arclight and Heine direct ophthalmoscopes.

comfortable examination, with significantly lower scores for both "glare" and "length of examination."

The cost of an Arclight ophthalmoscope is considerably lower than Heine K180 direct ophthalmoscope or comparable instruments. For the current price of Heine direct ophthalmoscope (USD $365), one can buy 48 Arclight ophthalmoscopes at their marketed bulk order price (USD $7.5).

Arclight is the first direct ophthalmoscope to be specifically designed for low-income settings. However, it also has a potential application to training and education globally by providing a more affordable direct ophthalmoscope for students. In contrast to other low-cost direct ophthalmoscopes [13, 15], the Arclight has an adjustable lens power with three settings (+4, −3, and −6 dioptres). This simple adjustment will compensate for most patient and examiner refractive error. It also has an additional function as an

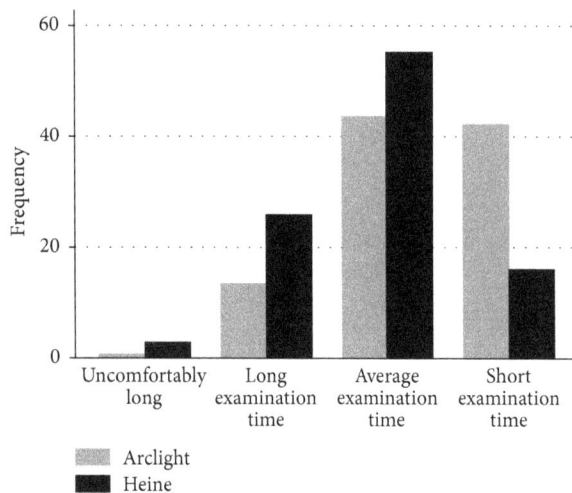

FIGURE 5: A histogram showing the subjective length of examination reported by those examined for the Arclight and Heine direct ophthalmoscopes.

otoscope in combination with the provided attachable device (Figure 1).

The human resources situation in SSA means that large numbers of patients are seen in rural areas or in mobile clinics by allied eye health professionals who often have limited access to equipment and training, making examination of the posterior segment of the eye impossible [10]. Due to its low cost, Arclight has the potential to be much more widely available, hence improving training opportunities and allowing examination of the optic disc more routinely. This will aid the early detection of glaucomatous disc changes. The earlier the glaucoma is detected and managed the better the prognosis with a reduced likelihood of progression to blindness is. The solar powered battery of the Arclight ophthalmoscope offers a further advantage for remote, rural clinics enabling the Arclight ophthalmoscope to be easily recharged in rural areas without access to power and also avoiding the expense of replacing batteries.

Although this study did not assess the accuracy of the Arclight ophthalmoscope in detecting abnormalities in the retina, it is possible that it could be used to detect diabetic retinopathy. The effective management of diabetic retinopathy in SSA will need a coordinated effort and faces multiple challenges. Burgess et al. highlighted a number of these including lack of training for opticians and other eye care workers in fundoscopy as well as poor equipment [11]. Arclight has the potential to help with both these challenges through greater access to direct ophthalmoscopes; however, this will need to be formally evaluated.

One of the limitations of our study was that all the eyes examined were healthy. It is therefore not possible to comment on how Arclight will perform in the presence of pathology. In everyday clinical practice it is clear that pathology such as cataract will be common, especially in low-income settings, and will generally make the examination of the posterior segment more difficult.

In conclusion, the Arclight ophthalmoscope provides a low-cost alternative to the standard direct ophthalmoscope.

It is easier to use and more comfortable for the subject. It appears to provide comparable results when examining the VCDR. It has the potential to significantly improve access to equipment in low-income settings around the world. This could improve fundoscopy amongst eye care workers and enable routine examination of the posterior segment of the eye, which is an area that is becoming increasingly important in SSA. Further studies assessing the reliability of the Arclight ophthalmoscope in diabetic retinopathy detection and in the presence of other pathology would be useful.

Conflict of Interests

The authors declare that there is no conflict of interests regarding the publication of this paper.

Acknowledgments

The authors would like to thank the students and volunteers who took part in the study and also the staff of Kilimanjaro Christian Medical Centre Eye Department who helped with the arrangements for the study. Matthew J. Burton is supported by Wellcome Trust (Grant no. 098481/Z/12/Z). Heiko Philippin is supported by CBM and Seeing is Believing.

References

[1] D. Pascolini and S. P. Mariotti, "Global estimates of visual impairment: 2010," British Journal of Ophthalmology, vol. 96, no. 5, pp. 614–618, 2012.

[2] A. Bastawrous, P. I. Burgess, A. M. Mahdi, F. Kyari, M. J. Burton, and H. Kuper, "Posterior segment eye disease in sub-Saharan Africa: review of recent population-based studies," Tropical Medicine & International Health, vol. 19, no. 5, pp. 600–609, 2014.

[3] J. E. Shaw, R. A. Sicree, and P. Z. Zimmet, "Global estimates of the prevalence of diabetes for 2010 and 2030," Diabetes Research and Clinical Practice, vol. 87, no. 1, pp. 4–14, 2010.

[4] S. Sivaprasad, B. Gupta, M. C. Gulliford et al., "Ethnic variations in the prevalence of diabetic retinopathy in people with diabetes attending screening in the United Kingdom (DRIVE UK)," PLoS ONE, vol. 7, no. 3, Article ID e32182, 2012.

[5] B. E. K. Klein, "Overview of epidemiologic studies of diabetic retinopathy," Ophthalmic Epidemiology, vol. 14, no. 4, pp. 179–183, 2007.

[6] H. Quigley and A. T. Broman, "The number of people with glaucoma worldwide in 2010 and 2020," British Journal of Ophthalmology, vol. 90, no. 3, pp. 262–267, 2006.

[7] A. Heijl, M. C. Leske, B. Bengtsson, L. Hyman, B. Bengtsson, and M. Hussein, "Reduction of intraocular pressure and glaucoma progression: results from the Early Manifest Glaucoma Trial," Archives of Ophthalmology, vol. 120, no. 10, pp. 1268–1279, 2002.

[8] The Diabetes Control and Complications Trial Research Group, "The effect of intensive treatment of diabetes on the development and progression of long-term complications in insulin-dependent diabetes mellitus," The New England Journal of Medicine, vol. 329, no. 14, pp. 977–986, 1993.

[9] A. Bastawrous and B. D. Hennig, "The global inverse care law: a distorted map of blindness," *British Journal of Ophthalmology*, vol. 96, no. 10, pp. 1357–1358, 2012.

[10] J. J. Palmer, F. Chinanayi, A. Gilbert et al., "Mapping human resources for eye health in 21 countries of sub-Saharan Africa: current progress towards VISION 2020," *Human Resources for Health*, vol. 12, no. 1, article 44, 2014.

[11] P. I. Burgess, G. Msukwa, and N. A. V. Beare, "Diabetic retinopathy in sub-Saharan Africa: meeting the challenges of an emerging epidemic," *BMC Medicine*, vol. 11, no. 1, article 157, 2013.

[12] N. Mandal, P. Harborne, S. Bradley et al., "Comparison of two ophthalmoscopes for direct ophthalmoscopy," *Clinical and Experimental Ophthalmology*, vol. 39, no. 1, pp. 30–36, 2011.

[13] J. E. McComiskie, R. M. Greer, and G. A. Gole, "Panoptic versus conventional ophthalmoscope," *Clinical & Experimental Ophthalmology*, vol. 32, no. 3, pp. 238–242, 2004.

[14] H. Li, P. R. Healey, Y. M. Tariq, E. Teber, and P. Mitchell, "Symmetry of optic nerve head parameters measured by the heidelberg retina tomograph 3 in healthy eyes: the blue mountains eye study," *American Journal of Ophthalmology*, vol. 155, no. 3, pp. 518.e1–523.e1, 2013.

[15] R. H. Armour, "Manufacture and use of home made ophthalmoscopes: a 150th anniversary tribute to Helmholtz," *British Medical Journal*, vol. 321, no. 7276, pp. 1557–1559, 2000.

7

Evaluation of Agreement between HRT III and iVue OCT in Glaucoma and Ocular Hypertension Patients

A. Perdicchi,[1] M. Iester,[2] D. Iacovello,[1] A. Cutini,[1] M. Balestrieri,[1] M. G. Mutolo,[1] A. Ferreras,[3] M. T. Contestabile,[1] and S. M. Recupero[1]

[1]*Department of Ophthalmology II, Faculty of Medicine and Psychology, "Sapienza" University of Rome, Sant'Andrea Hospital, 00100 Rome, Italy*

[2]*Anatomical-Clinical Laboratory for the Diagnosis and Treatment of Glaucoma and Neuroophthalmology, Eye Clinic, DINOGMI, University of Genoa, Viale Benedetto XV 5, 16132 Genoa, Italy*

[3]*Department of Ophthalmology, Miguel Servet University Hospital, Aragon Health Research Institute, 50009 Zaragoza, Spain*

Correspondence should be addressed to M. Balestrieri; marco.balestrieri@me.com

Academic Editor: Bartosz Sikorski

Purpose. To determine the agreement between Moorfields Regression Analysis (MRA), Glaucoma Probability Score (GPS) of Heidelberg retinal tomograph (HRT III), and peripapillary nerve fibers thickness by iVue Optical Coherence Tomography (OCT). *Methods.* 72 eyes with ocular hypertension or primary open angle glaucoma (POAG) were included in the study: 54 eyes had normal visual fields (VF) and 18 had VF damage. All subjects performed achromatic 30° VF by Octopus Program G1X dynamic strategy and were imaged with HRT III and iVue OCT. Sectorial and global MRA, GPS, and OCT parameters were used for the analysis. Kappa statistic was used to assess the agreement between methods. *Results.* A significant agreement between iVue OCT and GPS for the inferotemporal quadrant (κ: 0.555) was found in patients with abnormal VF. A good overall agreement between GPS and MRA was found in all the eyes tested (κ: 0.511). A good agreement between iVue OCT and MRA was shown in the superonasal (κ: 0.656) and nasal (κ: 0.627) quadrants followed by the superotemporal (κ: 0.602) and inferotemporal (κ: 0.586) sectors in all the studied eyes. *Conclusion.* The highest percentages of agreement were found per quadrant of the MRA and the iVue OCT confirming that in glaucoma damage starts from the temporal hemiretina.

1. Introduction

Glaucoma is an optic neuropathy characterized by progressive damage of the retinal nerve fiber layer (RNFL) and the nerve head (ONH). It often precedes perimetric damage and in its most advanced stages leads to atrophy of the ONH [1–5]. Various diagnostic instruments have been used for evaluating RNFL thickness (RNFLt) and the morphometry of the ONH. Optic Coherence Tomography (OCT) and the Heidelberg Retina Tomograph (HRT; Heidelberg Engineering GMBH, Heidelberg, Germany) are the most used systems.

OCT is a high resolution imaging technique that permits direct measurement of retinal thickness [2] and monitoring treatment in retinal pathology. Numerous studies have shown a good correlation between RNFLt measured with this technique and that calculated on histological preparations [3].

The HRT is a confocal laser system that acquires three-dimensional topographic images of the ONH and the peripapillary area [4, 5]. Moorfields Regression Analysis (MRA) and Glaucoma Probability Score (GPS) are able to distinguish normal from glaucomatous eyes with a good diagnostic precision [6].

Numerous studies have been carried out for calculating the degree of correlation between RNFLt obtained with the first generation "Time Domain" OCT and ONH parameters calculated by HRT [7–11]. In recent years OCT has greatly developed with the introduction of the "spectral domain" technique for acquiring images. The spectral domain OCT system has a greater resolution power, allowing a more accurate analysis of anatomical structures which do not always agree with the information obtained with the time domain OCT [12–14]. One of the latest spectral domain OCT tools is the iVue OCT which has shown its value in the study of numerous retinal pathologies and in glaucoma.

The aim of this study was to assess agreement among HRT MRA and HRT GPS and RNFLt measurement with the iVue OCT in ocular hypertension (OH) and primary open angle glaucoma (POAG) patients.

2. Material and Methods

This was a prospectively cross-sectional study. The research followed the tenets of the Declaration of Helsinki and informed consent was obtained from all the patients included.

Patients were recruited from the clinics of one glaucoma specialist (AP), and they were not excluded on the basis of sex, age, or race. Seventy-two eyes of 40 patients were included in this study [15]. All the eyes were classified as OH or POAG. OH patients had a normal VF, ophthalmoscopically normal ONH, and an intraocular pressure (IOP) greater than 21 mmHg without therapy measured by i-Care tonometry [16], while POAG patients had abnormal VF with corresponding ONH damage by ophthalmoscopy and an IOP greater than 21 mmHg without therapy.

All patients had carried out a two-phase white on white dynamic strategy perimetry Octopus 1-2-3 Program G1X [17]. Mean Defect (MD) and Loss Variance (LV) values were taken to distinguish the visual fields between normal and pathological. After any phase all patients had performed IOP measurement to evaluate any IOP changes [18]. Visual fields with MD values between +2 dB and −2 dB and LV between 0 and 6 dB^2 were considered normal and those with MD < −2 dB and LV > 6 dB^2 were considered pathological. None of the patients had a MD > −10 dB and a LV > 10 dB^2. The entire group was then divided into two subgroups based on the VF classification: normal VF subgroup and abnormal VF subgroup.

Each included eye underwent ONH analysis by HRT III and the RNFLt assessment by iVue OCT. The imaging examinations were performed on the same day, while the perimetric test was performed within 7 days.

2.1. iVue OCT.
The ONH protocol of iVue OCT consists of 12 radial scans of 3.4 mm in length (452 A scans each) and 6 concentric ring scans ranging from 2.5 to 4.0 mm in diameter (587 to 775 A scans each), all centred on the optic disc. All the images were reprocessed with three-dimensional/video baseline. ONH parameters measured by the software included optic disc area, optic cup area, neuroretinal rim area, nerve head volume, cup volume, rim volume, cup-disc area ratio, horizontal cup-disc ratio, and vertical cup-disc ratio. The ONH protocol also generates a polar RNFL thickness map, measured along a circle 3.45 mm in diameter centred on the optic disc. It gives the average RNFLt in the temporal, superior, nasal, and inferior quadrants as well as the overall average along the entire measurement circle [19].

The software automatically calculates the disc margins, along the six radial scans, and uses an algorithm to automatically differentiate the microstructures of the retina that form part of the same RNFL [20, 21]. This automated computer algorithm separates the anterior and posterior margins of

the identifying reflection group of the RNFL [22], making it possible to quantify thickness. These measurements can be compared with a database included in the iVue OCT.

2.1.1. HRT.
HRT is able to scan the retinal and optic nerve area surface at multiple consecutive parallel focal planes. These parameters have been shown to have a good sensitivity and specificity to detect glaucomatous ONH changes [23, 24].

However, there are 2 weak points in the HRT methodology: the reference plane and the contour line [25, 26] that are related to the capacity of the operator to detect the right size of the peripapillary area to be analyzed. The results obtained can be processed by several methods of analysis. One of the most used and significant is the MRA which has an extensive and specific database for various ethnic groups. It is formed of 948 eyes of which 733 belonged to Caucasians and 215 to blacks. In order to increase the diagnostic capacity of HRT, in 2000 Swindale et al. [27] published a new method to analyze ONHs without using a contour line by evaluating the shape of the ganglion cells when they cross the scleral canal. A good sensitivity and specificity was obtained and recently this new method called Glaucoma Probability Score (GPS) was applied to the HRT III [14].

For every single imaging test the values of the different quadrants were assessed; in particular the *inferotemporal* (IT), *inferonasal* (IN), *superotemporal* (ST), *superonasal* (SN), *nasal* (N), and *temporal* (T) ONH and RNFLt were considered. Furthermore, for MRA and GPS, a global (GLOBAL) index was calculated.

2.2. Statistical Analysis.
In our study the percentages of concordance (n-n; b-b; a-a), relative concordance (n-b; b-a), and discordance (a-n) obtained with the different methods were calculated in relation to the VF damage classification (normal or abnormal VF). For the three devices six different sectors were considered, while for HRT MRA and GPS global indices were also considered.

Kappa statistic (κ) was used to study the agreement among the 3 different methods (MRA and GPS for HRT and OHN protocol for iVue) and between the methods. κ measures the change-corrected agreement on a scale of −1.0 to 1.0, with 1.0 indicating perfect agreement. We used the indications suggested by Landis and Koch: κ's of 0.0 or less were considered to indicate poor; 0.0 to 0.2, slight; 0.21 to 0.4, fair; 0.41 to 0.6, moderate; 0.61 to 0.8, substantial; and 0.81 to 1, almost perfect agreement. In κ analysis only the agreement between normality and abnormality for the different methods was considered.

3. Results

On the basis of the results of VF examination, 72 eyes were recruited in the study and in particular 54 eyes had normal achromatic perimetry (MD between +2 and −2 dB and LV between 0 and 6 dB^2) and 18 had visual field damage. Refractive error was −2.3 ± 3.2 diopters. Besides in the subgroup with normal VF the mean MD was 0.08 ± 0.98 dB

TABLE 1: (%) Normal VF.

	IT	IN	ST	SN	N	T	Global
GPS versus iVue							
Concordance	39	35.3	39	37.1	29	28.5	
Relative concordance	29.5	31.4	40.7	33.2	33.5	29	
Discordance	31.5	33.3	20.3	29.7	37.5	42.5	
MRA versus GPS							
Concordance	50	55	42.5	46	39.5	29.5	44.5
Relative concordance	37	26	39	39	40.5	46	39
Discordance	13	19	18.5	15	20	24.5	16.5
iVue versus MRA							
Concordance	61	50	64.5	63	55.5	74	
Relative concordance	26	31.5	26	24	24.5	24	
Discordance	13	18.5	9.5	13	20	2	

TABLE 2: (%) Glaucoma VF damage.

	IT	IN	ST	SN	N	T	Global
GPS versus iVue							
Concordance	55.3	33.4	50	27.8	27.5	16.7	
Relative concordance	33.5	50	39	50	39	39	
Discordance	11.2	16.6	11	22.2	33.5	44.3	
MRA versus GPS							
Concordance	55.3	55.4	66.2	55.3	44.5	39	66.5
Relative concordance	39.5	33.3	22.5	33.7	33.2	39	27.6
Discordance	5.2	11.3	11.3	11	22.3	22	5.9
iVue versus MRA							
Concordance	72.1	39	50	50.2	50	50	
Relative concordance	16.2	39	39	27.5	27.5	24	
Discordance	11.7	22	11	22.3	22.5	26	

and LV was 2.2 ± 0.93, while in the subgroup with abnormal VF the mean MD was −5.85 ± 5.82 dB and LV was 5.87 ± 2.39.

In the normal VF group the global index of HRT III classified 63% subjects as normal by using MRA and 28.5% by GPS, and borderline results were 24% and 28.5%, respectively, and abnormal results 11% and 41%, respectively, while in the glaucoma VF damage group, percentages were, respectively, 16.6% and 33.3% for normal, 27.7% and 33.3% for borderline, and 55.5% and 33.3% for abnormal.

Tables 1 and 2 show the percentage of concordance, relative concordance, and discordance for each single sector and globally (only HRT) among MRA, GPS, and iVue in patients with normal VF (Table 1) and abnormal VF (Table 2).

When iVue OCT and GPS data were compared, the κ statistic indicated in the eyes with abnormal VF a good agreement especially of the inferotemporal quadrant (κ: 0.555), while a low agreement was indicated for all the other sectors considered both in patients with normal and in patients with altered VF (Table 3).

TABLE 3: Inferotemporal (IT), inferonasal (IN), superotemporal (ST), superonasal (SN), nasal (N), and temporal (T) quadrants.

iVue versus GPS	Kappa test (SE) All patients	Kappa test (SE) Normal VF	Kappa test (SE) Abnormal VF
IT	0.225 (0.136)	0.059 (0.171)	0.555 (0.286)
IN	0.105 (0.134)	0.044 (0.150)	0.333 (0.304)
ST	0.404 (0.136)	0.225 (0.186)	0.173 (0.632)
SN	0.202 (0.133)	0.182 (0.152)	0.250 (0.279)
N	0.060 (0.125)	0.134 (0.152)	0.153 (0.232)
T	−0.015 (0.124)	−0.059 (0.161)	0.043 (0.176)

When GPS and MRA data were compared, the κ statistic showed a good agreement in the global analysis (κ: 0.511). The agreement was more significant in the inferotemporal (κ: 0.618), inferonasal (κ: 0.527), and superonasal (κ: 0.519) quadrants. This result was confirmed also in the normal VF

TABLE 4: Inferotemporal (IT), inferonasal (IN), superotemporal (ST), superonasal (SN), nasal (N), and temporal (T) quadrants.

GPS versus MRA	κ-test (SE) All patients	κ-test (SE) Normal VF	κ-test (SE) Abnormal VF
IT	0.618 (0.121)	0.516 (0.160)	0.792 (0.197)
IN	0.527 (0.123)	0.503 (0.142)	0.526 (0.295)
ST	0.448 (0.134)	0.314 (0.178)	0.560 (0.281)
SN	0.519 (0.131)	0.508 (0.161)	0.476 (0.257)
N	0.333 (0.139)	0.299 (0.169)	0.400 (0.244)
T	0.143 (0.154)	0.211 (0.203)	0.310 (0.267)
Global	0.511 (0.133)	0.391 (0.168)	0.782 (0.206)

TABLE 5: Inferotemporal (IT), inferonasal (IN), superotemporal (ST), superonasal (SN), nasal (N), and temporal (T) quadrants.

iVue versus MRA	Kappa test (SE) All patients	Kappa test (SE) Normal VF	Kappa test (SE) Abnormal VF
IT	0.585 (0.117)	0.465 (0.181)	0.545 (0.234)
IN	0.265 (0.165)	0.152 (0.270)	0.400 (0.244)
ST	0.602 (0.139)	0.370 (0.262)	0.607 (0.251)
SN	0.656 (0.132)	0.845 (0.106)	0.225 (0.316)
N	0.627 (0.142)	0.843 (0.107)	−0.200 (0.489)
T	−0.050 (0.405)	−0.023 (0.706)	−0.130 (0.470)

subgroup (inferotemporal κ: 0.516, inferonasal κ: 0.503, and superonasal κ: 0.508). A slightly different distribution was noted in patients with an abnormal VF where the global agreement between GPS and MRA was high (κ: 0.782) with greater significance that decreased from the inferotemporal (κ: 0.792), superotemporal (κ: 0.560), and inferonasal (κ: 0.526) to the superonasal (κ: 0.476) quadrant (Table 4).

When iVue and MRA data were compared, there was a good agreement in the superonasal (κ: 0.656) and nasal (κ: 0.627) quadrants followed by the superotemporal (κ: 0.602) and inferotemporal (κ: 0.585) sectors. When the normal VF subgroup was considered, it was found that the superonasal quadrant had the highest agreement (κ: 0.845) followed by the nasal quadrant (κ: 0.843), while when the abnormal VF subgroup was considered, a moderate significance was shown in the inferotemporal (κ: 0.545) and superotemporal (κ: 0.607) quadrants (Table 5).

4. Discussion

Glaucoma is an optic neuropathy characterized by specific and progressive ONH and RNFL damage. Consequently the ability to identify these alterations at the earliest possible stage is fundamental to start the treatment and to decrease the loss of ganglion cells which could carry to the atrophy of the ONH with functional loss and serious visual disability [1–4].

It is well known how time domain OCT appears to be highly sensitive and specific in identifying anatomic damage in the presence of manifest VF damage [8–11, 28] and these

results were subsequently confirmed by studies done with spectral domain OCT [29–31].

The aim of our study was to determine if the parameters provided by a new instrument, a spectral domain OCT (iVue OCT), were in agreement, and to what extent, with those provided by the HRT III, more specifically with the GPS and with the MRA, in eyes with OH and/or glaucoma, both in the presence and in the absence of perimetric damage.

The comparison between iVue and GPS, two automatic methods of classification of the anatomical ONH and peripapillary RNFL damage, did not show a satisfactory agreement except for the inferotemporal (κ: 0.555) quadrant and only in eyes with an abnormal VF.

The comparison between GPS and MRA showed a good agreement in all the eyes examined, both those with normal VF and those with altered VF (κ: 0.511). In the abnormal VF subgroup this result increased (κ: 0.782) and the inferotemporal sector had the highest agreement (κ: 0.792). Similarly in the normal VF subgroup, the agreement between GPS and MRA was not significant when considered globally (κ: 0.391) but became significant when the inferotemporal (κ: 0.516) quadrant was considered. In the abnormal VF subgroup, better agreement was found between GPS and MRA outlining that GPS had similar sensitivity and specificity to MRA. This result is different from those of other studies in which MRA and linear regression analysis had higher ROC curves than GPS. In this study we did not evaluate the diagnostic capacity but only if the classification was similar and for this reason we probably obtained better results because no healthy normal subjects were included where usually GPS has a low specificity.

When the agreement between iVue OCT and MRA was considered, it was significant in eyes both with normal and with abnormal VF especially in the superonasal (κ: 0.656), nasal (κ: 0.627), and inferotemporal (κ: 0.585) quadrants. This tendency was confirmed in an analysis of eyes with both a normal and with an abnormal VF, even if in the latter the agreement was less significant.

Finally the agreement was good in the superonasal and nasal quadrant probably because these areas are the last to be involved in glaucoma, while the inferotemporal is the first to change.

In conclusion, the automatic methods of ONH analysis by GPS and peripapillary RNFL with the ONH protocol of the iVue OCT offer interesting application ideas but appear to have little agreement with one another. This weakness mainly regards eyes with a normal VF, where evidence of early anatomical damage is certainly of greatest interest. Moreover, our results suggest that the measurement of the RNFL using the HRT III and the iVue OCT is not interchangeable with the automatic methods (GPS), outlining that the computerized devices are able to analyze different anatomical structures. It has not yet been determined how useful and reliable these new objective techniques are for measuring anatomical damage when it comes to evaluating the progression of glaucoma over time. This is still the main goal to pursue in order to preserve good sight and consequently an acceptable quality of life for glaucoma patients.

Disclosure

Part of this study was presented at 2012 ARVO Annual Meeting, Fort Lauderdale, Florida, USA, May 6–10, 2012.

Conflict of Interests

The authors declare that there is no conflict of interests regarding the publication of this paper.

References

[1] A. Tuulonen, J. Lehtola, P. J. Airaksinen, and D. R. Anderson, "Nerve fiber layer defects with normal visual fields. Do normal optic disc and normal visual field indicate absence of glaucomatous abnormality?" *Ophthalmology*, vol. 100, no. 5, pp. 587–597, 1993.

[2] M. T. Contestabile, S. M. Recupero, D. Palladino et al., "A new method of biofeedback in the management of low vision," *Eye*, vol. 16, no. 4, pp. 472–480, 2002.

[3] Y. Huang, A. V. Cideciyan, G. I. Papastergiou et al., "Relation of optical coherence tomography to microanatomy in normal and rd chickens," *Investigative Ophthalmology and Visual Science*, vol. 39, no. 12, pp. 2405–2416, 1998.

[4] K. Rohrschneider, R. O. W. Burk, F. E. Kruse, and H. E. Volcker, "Reproducibility of the optic nerve head topography with a new laser tomographic scanning device," *Ophthalmology*, vol. 101, no. 6, pp. 1044–1049, 1994.

[5] P. Janknecht and J. Funk, "Optic nerve head analyser and Heidelberg retina tomograph: accuracy and reproducibility of topographic measurements in a model eye and in volunteers," *British Journal of Ophthalmology*, vol. 78, no. 10, pp. 760–768, 1994.

[6] M. Iester, A. Perdicchi, E. Capris, A. Siniscalco, G. Calabria, and S. M. Recupero, "Comparison between discriminant analysis models and 'glaucoma probability score' for the detection of glaucomatous optic nerve head changes," *Journal of Glaucoma*, vol. 17, no. 7, pp. 535–540, 2008.

[7] J. Moreno-Montañés, A. Antón, N. García, N. Olmo, A. Morilla, and M. Fallon, "Comparison of retinal nerve fiber layer thickness values using stratus optical coherence tomography and Heidelberg retina tomograph-III," *Journal of Glaucoma*, vol. 18, no. 7, pp. 528–534, 2009.

[8] O. J. Knight, R. T. Chang, W. J. Feuer, and D. L. Budenz, "Comparison of retinal nerve fiber layer measurements using time domain and spectral domain optical coherent tomography," *Ophthalmology*, vol. 116, no. 7, pp. 1271–1277, 2009.

[9] E. Z. Blumenthal, J. M. Williams, R. N. Weinreb, C. A. Girkin, C. C. Berry, and L. M. Zangwill, "Reproducibility of nerve fiber layer thickness measurements by use of optical coherence tomography," *Ophthalmology*, vol. 107, no. 12, pp. 2278–2282, 2000.

[10] J. S. Schuman, "Spectral domain optical coherence tomography for glaucoma (an AOS thesis)," *Transactions of the American Ophthalmological Society*, vol. 106, pp. 426–458, 2008.

[11] H. A. Quigley, E. M. Addicks, and W. R. Green, "Optic nerve damage in human glaucoma. III. Quantitative correlation of nerve fiber loss and visual field defect in glaucoma, ischemic neuropathy, papilledema, and toxic neuropathy," *Archives of Ophthalmology*, vol. 100, no. 1, pp. 135–146, 1982.

[12] C. Cukras, Y. D. Wang, C. B. Meyerle, F. Forooghian, E. Y. Chew, and W. T. Wong, "Optical coherence tomography-based decision making in exudative age-related macular degeneration: comparison of time- vs spectral-domain devices," *Eye*, vol. 24, no. 5, pp. 775–783, 2010.

[13] G. Savini, P. Barboni, M. Carbonelli, A. Sbreglia, G. Deluigi, and V. Parisi, "Comparison of optic nerve head parameter measurements obtained by time-domain and spectral-domain optical coherence tomography," *Journal of Glaucoma*, vol. 22, no. 5, pp. 384–389, 2013.

[14] S. Hong, G. J. Seong, S. S. Kim, S. Y. Kang, and C. Y. Kim, "Comparison of peripapillary retinal nerve fiber layer thickness measured by spectral vs. time domain optical coherence tomography," *Current Eye Research*, vol. 36, no. 2, pp. 125–134, 2011.

[15] G. Scuderi, M. Pompili, M. Innamorati et al., "Affective temperaments are associated with higher hopelessness and perceived disability in patients with open-angle glaucoma," *International Journal of Clinical Practice*, vol. 65, no. 9, pp. 976–984, 2011.

[16] G. L. Scuderi, N. C. Cascone, F. Regine, A. Perdicchi, A. Cerulli, and S. M. Recupero, "Validity and limits of the rebound tonometer (ICare): clinical study," *European Journal of Ophthalmology*, vol. 21, no. 3, pp. 251–257, 2011.

[17] G. L. Scuderi, M. Cesareo, A. Perdicchi, and S. M. Recupero, "Standard automated perimetry and algorithms for monitoring glaucoma progression," *Progress in Brain Research*, vol. 173, pp. 77–99, 2008.

[18] S. M. Recupero, M. T. Contestabile, L. Taverniti, G. M. Villani, and V. Recupero, "Open-angle glaucoma: variations in the intraocular pressure after visual field examination," *Journal of Glaucoma*, vol. 12, no. 2, pp. 114–118, 2003.

[19] Optovue Inc, *User's Manual Vers 1.9*, Optovue Inc, Fremont, Calif, USA, 2011.

[20] M. R. Hee, J. A. Izatt, E. A. Swanson et al., "Optical coherence tomography of the human retina," *Archives of Ophthalmology*, vol. 113, no. 3, pp. 325–332, 1995.

[21] D. S. Chauhan and J. Marshall, "The interpretation of optical coherence tomography images of the retina," *Investigative Ophthalmology and Visual Science*, vol. 40, no. 10, pp. 2332–2342, 1999.

[22] D. L. Budenz, M.-J. Fredette, W. J. Feuer, and D. R. Anderson, "Reproducibility of peripapillary retinal nerve fiber thickness measurements with stratus OCT in glaucomatous eyes," *Ophthalmology*, vol. 115, no. 4, pp. 661–666.e4, 2008.

[23] H. Uchida, L. Brigatti, and J. Caprioli, "Detection of structural damage from glaucoma with confocal laser image analysis," *Investigative Ophthalmology & Visual Science*, vol. 37, no. 12, pp. 2393–2401, 1996.

[24] M. Iester, F. S. Mikelberg, N. V. Swindale, and S. M. Drance, "ROC analysis of Heidelberg Retina Tomograph optic disc shape measures in glaucoma," *Canadian Journal of Ophthalmology*, vol. 32, no. 6, pp. 382–388, 1997.

[25] M. Iester, F. S. Mikelberg, P. Courtright et al., "Interobserver variability of optic disk variables measured by confocal scanning laser tomography," *American Journal of Ophthalmology*, vol. 132, no. 1, pp. 57–62, 2001.

[26] M. Iester, V. Mariotti, F. Lanza, and G. Calabria, "The effect of contour line position on optic nerve head analysis by Heidelberg Retina Tomograph," *European Journal of Ophthalmology*, vol. 19, no. 6, pp. 942–948, 2009.

[27] N. V. Swindale, G. Stjepanovic, A. Chin, and F. S. Mikelberg, "Automated analysis of normal and glaucomatous optic nerve

head topography images," *Investigative Ophthalmology and Visual Science*, vol. 41, no. 7, pp. 1730–1742, 2000.

[28] D. L. Budenz, R. T. Chang, X. Huang, R. W. Knighton, and J. M. Tielsch, "Reproducibility of retinal nerve fiber thickness measurements using the stratus OCT in normal and glaucomatous eyes," *Investigative Ophthalmology and Visual Science*, vol. 46, no. 7, pp. 2440–2443, 2005.

[29] C. K.-S. Leung, C. Ye, R. N. Weinreb et al., "Retinal nerve fiber layer imaging with spectral-domain optical coherence tomography: a study on diagnostic agreement with Heidelberg Retinal Tomograph," *Ophthalmology*, vol. 117, no. 2, pp. 267–274, 2010.

[30] A. W. Hewitt, A. J. Chappell, T. Straga, J. Landers, R. A. Mills, and J. E. Craig, "Sensitivity of confocal laser tomography versus optical coherence tomography in detecting advanced glaucoma," *Clinical and Experimental Ophthalmology*, vol. 37, no. 9, pp. 836–841, 2009.

[31] M. T. Leite, H. L. Rao, L. M. Zangwill, R. N. Weinreb, and F. A. Medeiros, "Comparison of the diagnostic accuracies of the spectralis, cirrus, and RTVue optical coherence tomography devices in glaucoma," *Ophthalmology*, vol. 118, no. 7, pp. 1334–1339, 2011.

8

Excimer versus Femtosecond Laser Assisted Penetrating Keratoplasty in Keratoconus and Fuchs Dystrophy: Intraoperative Pitfalls

Moatasem El-Husseiny,[1] Berthold Seitz,[1] Achim Langenbucher,[2] Elena Akhmedova,[1] Nora Szentmary,[1] Tobias Hager,[1] Themistoklis Tsintarakis,[1] and Edgar Janunts[2]

[1]*Department of Ophthalmology, Saarland University Medical Center UKS, Homburg/Saar, Germany*
[2]*Experimental Ophthalmology, University of Saarland, Homburg/Saar, Germany*

Correspondence should be addressed to Berthold Seitz; berthold.seitz@uks.eu

Academic Editor: José L. Güell

Purpose. To assess the intraoperative results comparing two non-mechanical laser assisted penetrating keratoplasty approaches in keratoconus and Fuchs dystrophy. *Patients and Methods.* 68 patients (age 18 to 87 years) with keratoconus or Fuchs dystrophy were randomly distributed to 4 groups. 35 eyes with keratoconus and 33 eyes with Fuchs dystrophy were treated with either excimer laser ([Exc] groups I and II) or femtosecond laser-assisted ([FLAK] groups III and IV) penetrating keratoplasty. Main intraoperative outcome measures included intraoperative decentration, need for additional interrupted sutures, alignment of orientation markers, and intraocular positive pressure (vis a tergo). *Results.* Intraoperative recipient decentration occurred in 4 eyes of groups III/IV but in none of groups I/II. Additional interrupted sutures were not necessary in groups I/II but in 5 eyes of groups III/IV. Orientation markers were all aligned in groups I/II but were partly misaligned in 8 eyes of groups III/IV. Intraocular positive pressure grade was recognized in 12 eyes of groups I/II and in 19 eyes of groups III/IV. In particular, in group III, severe vis a tergo occurred in 8 eyes. *Conclusions.* Intraoperative decentration, misalignment of the donor in the recipient bed, and need for additional interrupted sutures as well as high percentage of severe intraocular positive pressure were predominantly present in the femtosecond laser in keratoconus eyes.

1. Introduction

Keratoconus (KC) and Fuchs' dystrophy (Fuchs) are the leading indications for penetrating keratoplasty (PKP) [1]. The cornea surgeon's main attention in corneal transplantation has shifted from preserving a "clear graft" to achieving a good refractive outcome.

The nonmechanical excimer laser trephination (Exc) has been first introduced in 1989 at the University Eye Hospital of Erlangen (Germany) [1–3]. It has been frequently reported that this technique yielded a better refractive outcome in comparison to manual trephination, particularly lower postoperative keratometric astigmatism, higher regularity of topography, and improved visual acuity [4, 5]. It ensures an outstanding perpendicular incision profile. Such cut edges in combination with "orientation teeth" (Figure 1) potentially reduce "vertical tilt" and "horizontal torsion" of the graft in the recipient bed, thus improving the visual performance after transplantation [5].

However, despite the promising results, the Exc PKP did not get widely spread, because corneal surgeons did not have an excimer laser in their operating theater. Instead, newer technologies were introduced, particularly femtosecond laser-assisted keratoplasty (FLAK), which got spread more widely since 2006 [6–8]. Historically, the femtosecond laser has been mainly used in refractive surgery, for example, for flap preparation in LASIK, intracorneal ring segment implantation in keratoconus patients, or antistigmatic incisions following PKP [9–11].

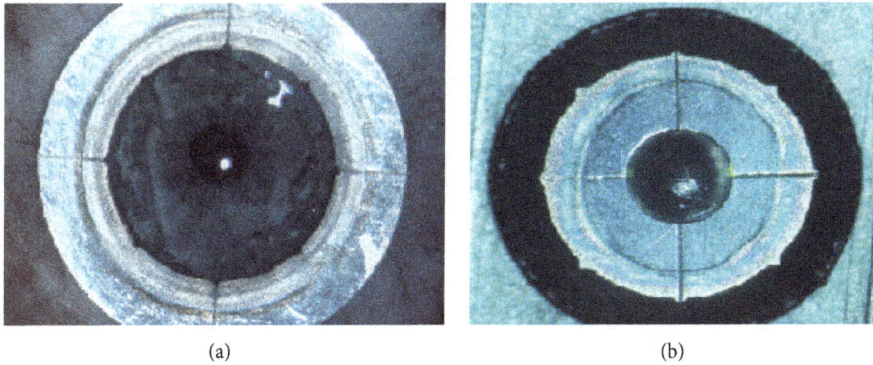

(a)   (b)

FIGURE 1: Left: 8 "orientation notches" at the recipient mask lying on a patient's cornea. Right: 8 "orientation teeth" at the donor mask lying on a corneoscleral button in an artificial anterior chamber.

This new technique allowed creating reproducible, customized trephination patterns. The most common trephination profiles are the "mushroom" and the "top hat" profile [12] as well as the more complex "zig-zag" profile [13]. These shaped wound configurations offer the advantages of better donor-recipient fit and increased donor-host junction surface area contact, both resulting in faster wound healing and earlier suture removal, thus potentially promoting rapid visual recovery [14]. In addition, in vivo confocal microscopy (IVCM) after FLAK showed earlier regrowth of corneal nerves in both the peripheral and central stroma compared to conventional PKP [15].

To the best of our knowledge, this is the first study to compare two nonmechanical (excimer and femtosecond laser) laser-assisted PKP in keratoconus and Fuchs dystrophy. The purpose of this work is to demonstrate the intraoperative results regarding the centration of the graft, necessity of completion of graft and donor incisions with scissors, anterior stepping, gaping, necessity of additional interrupted sutures, positive pressure during the surgery (vis a tergo), and the proper alignment of the orientation markers in host and graft.

2. Patients and Methods

In this prospective randomized clinical single-center study, 68 patients (age 18 to 87 years) with keratoconus or Fuchs dystrophy (phakic or pseudophakic eyes that underwent a primary central PKP) were randomly distributed to 4 groups: 35 eyes with keratoconus and 33 eyes with Fuchs dystrophy were treated either with excimer laser ([Exc] groups I and II) and with femtosecond laser-assisted ([FLAK] groups III and IV) penetrating keratoplasty. Exclusion criteria were repeated PKP and simultaneous cataract surgery because during the triple procedure, the iris-lens diaphragm is not stable and, therefore, might influence the main outcome measures of this study. All patients agreed to the informed consent. The study was approved from the Ethics Committee of the Saarland University, Germany.

All surgical procedures were carried out by one surgeon (BS) and under general anesthesia. In the study, a 193 nm excimer laser (MEL 70, Carl Zeiss Meditec, Jena, Germany) with a 35 Hz repetition rate and spot size of 1.2 mm, in

combination with conventional donor/recipient masks, and the 60 KHz IntraLase FS Laser [AMO (Abbott Medical Optics), Abbott Park, IL, USA] have been used.

2.1. Indications. Exc and FLAK were performed in patients with keratoconus and with Fuchs' endothelial dystrophy (if they presented advanced stages of the disease including scarring, thus they were not suitable for lamellar techniques such as DSAEK or DMEK).

2.2. Main Outcome Measures. Main intraoperative outcome measures included ultrasound pachymetry AL-3000 (Tomey, Nagoya, Japan) at the center and in 4 midperipheral points at $0°$, $90°$, $180°$, and $270°$ of the donor, complications of laser trephination, trephination time, anterior gaping, graft override, need for additional interrupted sutures to achieve proper donor-host alignment, and alignment of orientation markers and positive vitreous pressure (vis a tergo) depicted in three grades (0 = no intraoperative pressure, 1 = iris prolapse till the level of the corneal incision, and 2 = iris prolapse beyond the level of corneal incision). Graft decentration was measured at the end of the operation by measuring the distance between limbus and graft with calipers at the 12- and 6-o'clock position. Decentration was considered if the difference between the two distances was more than 0.5 mm. A measurement prior to incision was not possible because of the suction ring for the femtolaser which prevents view on the limbus area.

2.3. Excimer Laser Trephination. Trephination was performed using the 193 nm excimer laser along metal masks with eight orientation teeth/notches. Mean patient age in keratoconus was 37.4 ± 14.2 and in Fuchs 69.8 ± 8.9 years. For donor trephination from the epithelial side using the 193 nm excimer laser MEL 70, a circular metal aperture mask (diameter: 8.1 mm; central opening: 3.0 mm for centration; thickness: 0.5 mm; weight: 0.173 g; eight orientation teeth: 0.15×0.3 mm, Figure 1) was positioned on a corneoscleral button (16 mm diameter) fixed in an artificial anterior chamber under microscopic control (Figure 2). After perforation, the remaining stromal lamellae and Descemet's membrane were cut with curved corneal microscissors. The donor oversize was 0.1 mm in all cases.

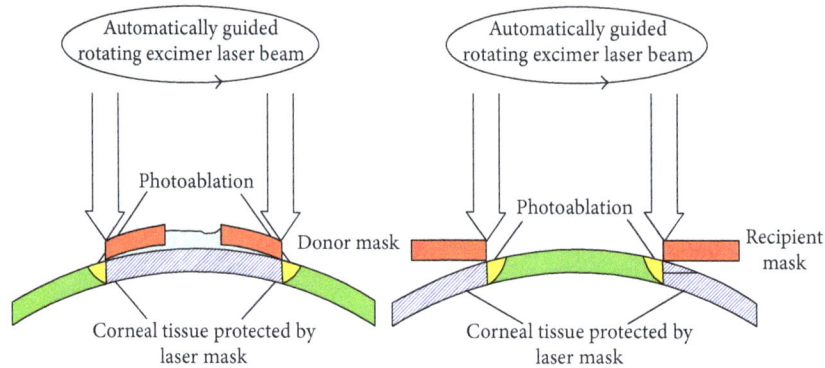

FIGURE 2: Donor and recipient trephination through rotating excimer laser beam.

For recipient trephination, a corresponding circular metal mask was used (diameter: 12.5 mm; central opening: 8.0 mm; thickness: 0.5 mm; weight: 0.29 g; eight orientation notches: 0.15×0.3 mm, Figures 1 and 2). The mask holds without additional stabilization because of the horizontal orientation of the patient's head. The laser beam is guided automatically along the edge of the mask without ablating the central cornea. After focal corneal perforation, the remaining deep stromal lamellae and Descemet's membrane were cut with curved corneal microscissors.

2.4. Femtosecond Laser Trephination and Profiles. Mean patient age in keratoconus group was 40.2 ± 14.0 years and in the Fuchs group it was 69.2 ± 12.0 years. In all cases, we used energy of $0.1 \mu J$ less than the maximum energy in the posterior side cut, $0.5 \mu J$ less than the maximum energy in the anterior side cut, and $0.4 \mu J$ less than the maximum energy in the ring lamellar cut (2.3 to $2.9 \mu J$). The 8 alignment incisions in both the donor and recipient were created as follows: energy of $1.5 \mu J$, length of $1000 \mu m$, width of $50 \mu m$, spot separation of $6 \mu m$, line separation of $6 \mu m$, and layer separation of $5 \mu m$. The radial offsets were +2 in all recipients (meaning that all the alignment incisions were outside the trephination) and −2 in all donors (meaning that all the alignment incisions were inside the trephination).

On the anterior side cuts, the spot separation and the layer separation were $3 \mu m$; in the ring lamellar cut (spiral pattern), the tangential spot separation was $5 \mu m$ and the radial spot separation was $4 \mu m$; on the posterior side cut, the spot separation was $3 \mu m$ and the layer separation was $2 \mu m$. The depth of the lamellar cut of the donor and recipient was 2/3 of the mean corneal thickness of the graft and recipient's eye, respectively. All diameters (anterior side cut, lamellar cut, and posterior side cut) were performed, 0.1 mm larger than the resulting diameter, thus overlapping each other. The donor cornea was placed into an artificial anterior chamber type Barron (Katena, Denville, USA) to achieve trephination from the epithelial side. Each laser procedure requires a disposable glass interface, which applanates the cornea completely during the laser procedure.

For laser trephination of the recipient's cornea, the eye was fixated by means of a vacuum suction ring. The glass cone interface was placed within the suction ring so that the cornea was completely applanated. We performed a complete penetrating laser trephination after which the corneal button was removed with forceps and a spatula under microscopic control. If necessary, a microscissor was used to complete the incision. The top hat profile was used in Fuchs dystrophy, whereas the mushroom profile was used in keratoconus patients (Figure 3).

2.5. Suturing. In all patients, a peripheral iridotomy was performed at the 12-o'clock position [16]. After temporary fixation of the donor button in the recipient bed with 8 interrupted sutures, a permanent wound closure was achieved by a 16-bite double-running diagonal cross-stitch suture (10–0 nylon) according to Hoffmann [17] (Figure 4). We attempted to suture as deep as 90% of the total corneal thickness. The eight cardinal sutures were placed at the site of orientation teeth with the excimer laser and at the site of the alignment incisions with the femtosecond laser as well as possible (Figure 5). In cases of wound gaping or graft override, additional interrupted sutures were used to ensure proper donor-host alignment at the end of surgery.

3. Results

Generally, the laser action time for trephination was much shorter for femtosecond compared to excimer laser trephination (Figure 6). The distribution of pachymetry values for the grafts is depicted in Figure 7. No intraoperative complications have been noticed. Incisions had to be completed with scissors in almost all eyes of groups I/II but only 2 cases in groups III/IV. Decentration happened in none of the eyes in groups I/II, but in 3/1 eyes in groups III/IV. No additional interrupted sutures were necessary for groups I/II, but in 4/1 cases in groups III/IV. Orientation markers were aligned in all cases of the excimer groups; in contrast, orientation markers were not totally aligned in 7/1 cases in groups III/IV. After removal of 8 cardinal sutures, graft override appeared in none of groups I/II/IV but in one case of group III. Moreover, gaping occurred in 0/1 eyes of groups I/II but in 2/1 cases in groups III/IV. Intraoperative positive pressure from vitreous has occurred in all groups as follows: 3/9 eyes in groups I/II and 8/11 in groups III/IV (Figure 8). In particular,

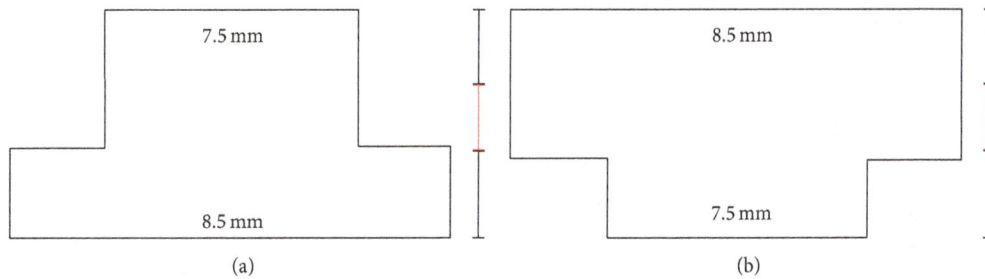

(a)   (b)

FIGURE 3: Different profiles of FLAK, upper and lower diameter are given in millimeters. Black and red bars indicate mean corneal thickness divided by 3 (meaning that the cornea was divided in anterior 2/3 and posterior 1/3). (a) Top hat profile used in Fuchs dystrophy enables a higher transplantation rate of corneal endothelial cells. (b) Mushroom profile used in keratoconus patients leads to less endothelial cell transplantation.

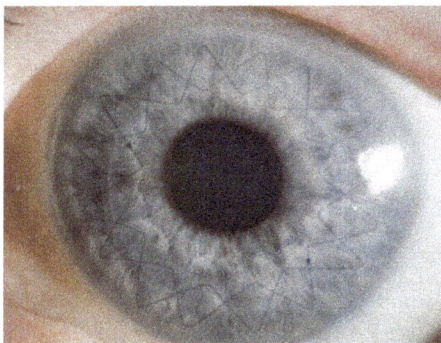

FIGURE 4: Corneal button sutured with double-running cross-stitch suture six weeks after excimer laser keratoplasty and 8 cardinal sutures for temporary fixation have been removed at the end of surgery.

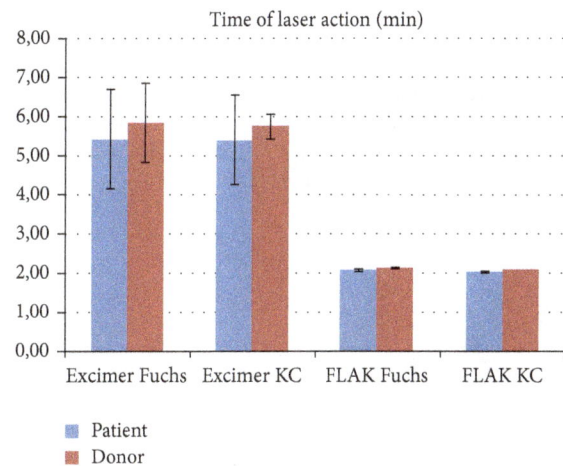

FIGURE 6: Time of laser action in minutes for all study groups separately for both patient and donor trephinations (Fuchs = Fuchs dystrophy, KC = keratoconus).

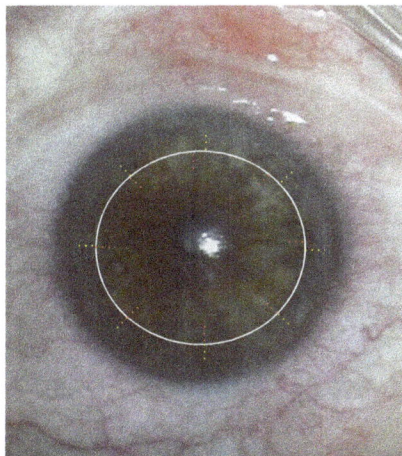

FIGURE 5: (Hypothetical diagram) different locations of radial incisions in donor and recipient (for better visualization, the red markings are in the donor and the yellow in recipient) after femtosecond laser trephination in keratoconus.

4. Discussion

Studies comparing an established corneal transplantation procedure with the new femtosecond laser technology that was introduced to clinical practice in 2006 were already carried out [18, 19]. In a recent publication, Birnbaum et al. have compared the results of 123 FLAK with conventional PKP in a randomized clinical study [18]. It has been revealed that despite the potential advantages of the femtosecond procedure it did not provide superior refractive results as compared to mechanical trephination. They found a topographic astigmatism after suture removal of about 6 diopters in the FLAK group.

A major advantage of femtosecond laser is the possibility to create different 3D profiles [18] (with the most widely spread ones being the top hat, mushroom, and zig-zag profile [13, 18]). It is considered mechanically stable [18]. Its stability is derived from the overlap, which is created by the side cut especially in the top hat configuration [20, 21]. Nevertheless, we found in our study that it was difficult to get it watertight without steps and gaps in comparison to the excimer laser keratoplasty. To avoid complications

positive vitreous pressure grade 2 appeared in 8 patients of the keratoconus FLAK group, but only in 1 patient of the Fuchs excimer laser group. An overview of the above given results is displaced in Figure 9.

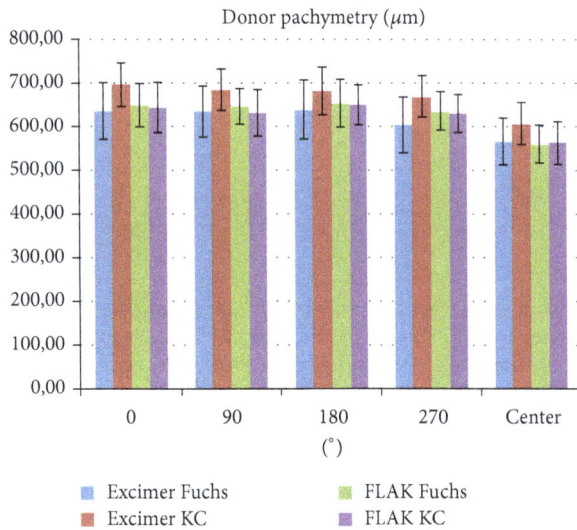

FIGURE 7: Distribution of pachymetry values for all study groups measured manually with ultrasound pachymetry at the center and in 4 midperipheral points at 0°, 90°, 180°, and 270° (KC = keratoconus, Fuchs = Fuchs endothelial dystrophy).

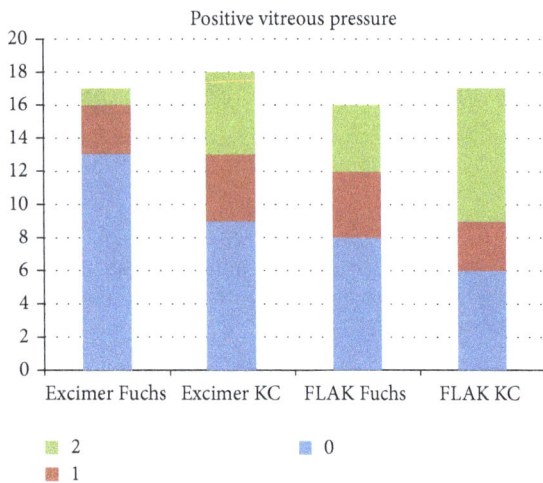

	Excimer	FLAK	
Fuchs		1	Graft decentration
KC		3	
Fuchs	1	1	Gaping
KC		2	
Fuchs			Anterior graft override
KC		1	
Fuchs	17	1	Not completely penetrated: patient
KC	18	1	
Fuchs		1	Additional interrupted sutures needed
KC		4	
Fuchs		1	Misalignment of incisions
KC		7	
Fuchs	2	4	Positive pressure from vitreous (grade 1)
KC	4	3	
Fuchs	1	4	Positive pressure from vitreous (grade 2)
KC	5	8	
	Excimer	FLAK	

FIGURE 9: Comparison of excimer versus femtosecond laser-assisted penetrating keratoplasty (FLAK): intraoperative results.

FIGURE 8: Positive pressure from vitreous (vis a tergo), depicted in three grades: 0 means no intraoperative pressure, 1 means iris prolapse till the level of the corneal incision, and 2 means iris prolapse beyond the level of the corneal incision.

recorded in earlier studies using the mushroom profile (e.g., infiltrates, steps, and ointment deposits), we successfully used an anterior part of the mushroom as thick as two-thirds of the mean of midperipheral donor and recipient thickness. This procedure may be recommended from our point of view.

The fact that FLAK created more gaps after the removal of the cardinal sutures resulted in the necessity to use more single interrupted sutures for correct donor-host adaptation. This was not due to a learning curve of the surgeon because a different cut profile was used in the FLAK group. Although, the mushroom profile has a relatively large diameter at the corneal surface, the wound apposition was less accurate. We have to admit that a suture depth of 90% can only be

intended and depends strongly on the experience of the surgeon. We further have to admit that there are no ideal geometrical settings for the mushroom profile. But a more likely explanation is that in keratoconus eyes the applanation done to the cone-shaped bulging cornea results in flattening. We believe that this extreme flattening effect leads to an alteration in the theoretically planned right angles of the anterior, posterior, and lamellar side cuts. Therefore, we got instead of right angles oblique angles and instead of a round trephination an oval- or pear-shaped trephination, which led to difficulty in fitting the properly cut donor button into the somehow distorted recipient bed. In particular, in keratoconus, orientation lines of donor and recipient tended not to match exactly (Figure 5). In such FLAK cases, an interrupted suturing technique might be more appropriate than a double-running suture.

It was obvious that the excimer laser needs more time to penetrate the cornea than the femtosecond laser. This is because the excimer laser digs from the surface a trench into the cornea while its energy is gradually absorbed [1]. On the other hand, the femtosecond laser creates cavitation bubbles at different depths of the cornea and thus an incision can be obtained faster [22]. We intended a complete perforation of the cornea during FLAK. If the femtosecond laser theatre is separated from the surgery room, it might be preferable to leave a stromal gap between 50 and 80 μm and to complete perforation in the surgery room. FLAK achieved an overwhelming number of cases with complete perforation of the cornea in comparison to the excimer PKP.

Another factor that must be considered here is the suturing technique. The double continuous running suture technique remains to be the suture of choice in FLAK [18]. In our study, the suturing was done down deep to the pre-Descemet's layer and not just at the level of the side cut of the profiled graft. In an ordinary PKP or Exc PKP, the suture is placed in the pre-Descemet's region of the donor cornea [23]. In Germany, the double-running cross-stitch suture according to Hoffmann is preferred over interrupted sutures, because it results in earlier visual rehabilitation and higher regularity of topography as long as the sutures are in place and a lower risk of suture loosening and need of suture replacement [17]. In case of corneal thinning, such as that in keratoconus, the suture may run through the anterior chamber at the recipient site.

One of the disadvantages of FLAK is that it generates a higher intraocular pressure than the Exc PKP. This was proved by direct intravitreal measurements [22, 24]. The sclera is inexpansible. Therefore, an increase in the volume of choroidal blood vessels produces disproportionate changes of intraocular volume and thus intraocular pressure. Moreover, it leads to major changes in the osmolarity of the vitreous. When the cornea is removed, the mechanical barrier to vitreous expansion is lost. In this situation, the iris-lens diaphragm is pushed forward (the so-called positive vitreous pressure or "vis a tergo"). In severe cases, it is impossible to maintain the anterior chamber and the cardinal sutures are difficult to place. Even the iris can be sutured to the corneal button thus leading to further difficulties. Moreover, a sudden increase in the intraocular pressure to values which are higher than the perfusion of the retinal vessels was recorded. However, this effect is only for a short time, due to the fast perforation of the cornea. Up to now, no central artery occlusion due to FLAK has been reported. By leaving a stromal gap and finishing the perforation in the surgery room, the suction ring can be removed earlier. This leads to reduction of pressure on the eye, thus enabling intraocular pressure reaching equilibrium and reducing positive vitreous pressure. Moreover, there are now also faster femtosecond laser platforms available which may help to further minimize this risk.

Decentration of corneal grafts in keratoconus patients with FLAK was more frequent than that in patients that were treated with excimer laser. Because of the flat applanation with the FLAK, it was more likely to obtain a decentered oval-shaped recipient incision. In contrast, in the excimer laser PKP, we have been using masks with orientation teeth which allow us to suture the first eight cardinal sutures with small risk of horizontal torsion because, according to the key-keyhole-principle, the orientation teeth in the donor fit exactly into the orientation notches of the recipient. Such a precise orientation is absent in the FLAK, since only radial markings are present. It became obvious that in the femtosecond laser trephined KC eyes these radial incision lines did not fit completely comparing donor and recipient. Therefore, the hypothesis that a better graft alignment can be achieved with FLAK cannot be confirmed with the geometrical settings in our study.

5. Conclusion

Intraoperative decentration, misalignment of the donor in the recipient bed, and need for additional interrupted sutures, as well as positive pressure from the vitreous, were more frequent when FLAK was performed.

Future comparative studies with a faster excimer laser platform and a concave femtosecond laser patient interface or even a "liquid interface" are needed to be carried out. These studies might show us less intraoperative complications regarding both techniques. The next step of our group is the presentation of best-spectacle corrected visual acuity, postoperative astigmatism, and regularity of topography after removal of all sutures in all eyes.

Conflict of Interests

The authors declare that there is no conflict of interests regarding the publication of this paper.

References

[1] B. Seitz, A. Langenbucher, and G. O. H. Naumann, "Perspektiven der Excimerlaser-Trepanation für die Keratoplastik," *Der Ophthalmologe*, vol. 108, no. 9, pp. 817–824, 2011.

[2] G. O. H. Naumann, B. Seitz, G. K. Lang, A. Langenbucher, and M. M. Kus, "193 nm excimer laser trephination in perforating keratoplasty. Report of 70 patients," *Klinische Monatsblätter für Augenheilkunde*, vol. 203, pp. 252–261, 1993.

[3] G. K. Lang, E. Schroeder, J. W. Koch, M. Yanoff, and G. O. H. Naumann, "Excimer laser keratoplasty. Part 1: basic concepts," *Ophthalmic Surgery*, vol. 20, no. 4, pp. 262–267, 1989.

[4] B. Seitz, A. Langenbucher, M. M. Kus, M. Küchle, and G. O. H. Naumann, "Nonmechanical corneal trephination with the excimer laser improves outcome after penetrating keratoplasty," *Ophthalmology*, vol. 106, no. 6, pp. 1156–1165, 1999.

[5] N. Szentmáry, A. Langenbucher, G. O. H. Naumann, and B. Seitz, "Intra-individual variability of penetrating keratoplasty outcome after excimer laser versus motorized corneal trephination," *Journal of Refractive Surgery*, vol. 22, no. 8, pp. 804–810, 2006.

[6] I. Bahar, I. Kaiserman, A. P. Lange et al., "Femtosecond laser versus manual dissection for top hat penetrating keratoplasty," *British Journal of Ophthalmology*, vol. 93, no. 1, pp. 73–78, 2009.

[7] I. Bahar, I. Kaiserman, P. McAllum, and D. Rootman, "Femtosecond laser-assisted penetrating keratoplasty: stability evaluation of different wound configurations," *Cornea*, vol. 27, no. 2, pp. 209–211, 2008.

[8] Y. Y. Y. Cheng, N. G. Tahzib, G. van Rij et al., "Femtosecond laser-assisted inverted mushroom keratoplasty," *Cornea*, vol. 27, no. 6, pp. 679–685, 2008.

[9] A. Ertan and G. Kamburoğlu, "Intacs implantation using a femtosecond laser for management of keratoconus: comparison of 306 cases in different stages," *Journal of Cataract and Refractive Surgery*, vol. 34, no. 9, pp. 1521–1526, 2008.

[10] M. Nubile, P. Carpineto, M. Lanzini et al., "Femtosecond laser arcuate keratotomy for the correction of high astigmatism after keratoplasty," *Ophthalmology*, vol. 116, no. 6, pp. 1083–1092, 2009.

[11] I. Ratkay-Traub, T. Juhasz, C. Horvath et al., "Ultra-short pulse (femtosecond) laser surgery: initial use in LASIK flap creation,"

Ophthalmology Clinics of North America, vol. 14, no. 2, pp. 347–355, 2001.

[12] F. Birnbaum, P. Maier, and T. Reinhard, "Perspectives of femtosecond laser-assisted keratoplasty," *Ophthalmologe*, vol. 108, no. 9, pp. 807–816, 2011.

[13] M. Farid, R. F. Steinert, R. N. Gaster, W. Chamberlain, and A. Lin, "Comparision of penetrating keratoplasty performed with the femtosecond laser zig-zag incision versus conventional blade trephination," *Ophthalmology*, vol. 116, no. 9, pp. 1638–1643, 2009.

[14] R. Shehadeh-Mashor, C. C. Chan, I. Bahar, A. Lichtinger, S. N. Yeung, and D. S. Rootman, "Comparison between femtosecond laser mushroom configuration and manual trephine straight-edge configuration deep anterior lamellar keratoplasty," *British Journal of Ophthalmology*, vol. 98, no. 1, pp. 35–39, 2014.

[15] R. M. Shtein, K. H. Kelley, D. C. Musch, A. Sugar, and S. I. Mian, "In vivo confocal microscopic evaluation of corneal wound healing after femtosecond laser-assisted keratoplasty," *Ophthalmic Surgery Lasers and Imaging*, vol. 43, no. 3, pp. 205–213, 2012.

[16] G. O. H. Naumann and H. Sautter, "Surgical procedures on the cornea," in *Surgical Ophthalmology*, F. C. Blodi, G. Mackensen, and H. Neubauer, Eds., pp. 433–497, Springer, Berlin, Germany, 1991.

[17] F. Hoffmann, "Suture technique for perforating keratoplasty," *Klinische Monatsblatter fur Augenheilkunde*, vol. 169, no. 5, pp. 584–590, 1976.

[18] F. Birnbaum, A. Wiggermann, P. C. Maier, D. Böhringer, and T. Reinhard, "Clinical results of 123 femtosecond laser-assisted penetrating keratoplasties," *Graefe's Archive for Clinical and Experimental Ophthalmology*, vol. 251, no. 1, pp. 95–103, 2013.

[19] E. Levinger, O. Trivizki, S. Levinger, and I. Kremer, "Outcome of 'mushroom' pattern femtosecond laser-assisted keratoplasty versus conventional penetrating keratoplasty in patients with keratoconus," *Cornea*, vol. 33, no. 5, pp. 481–485, 2014.

[20] M. Farid and R. F. Steinert, "Femtosecond laser-assisted corneal surgery," *Current Opinion in Ophthalmology*, vol. 21, no. 4, pp. 288–292, 2010.

[21] P. Maier, D. Böhringer, F. Birnbaum, and T. Reinhard, "Improved wound stability of top-hat profiled femtosecond laser-assisted penetrating keratoplasty in vitro," *Cornea*, vol. 31, no. 8, pp. 963–966, 2012.

[22] J. M. Vetter, M. Faust, A. Gericke, N. Pfeiffer, W. E. Weingärtner, and W. Sekundo, "Intraocular pressure measurements during flap preparation using 2 femtosecond lasers and 1 microkeratome in human donor eyes," *Journal of Cataract & Refractive Surgery*, vol. 38, no. 11, pp. 2011–2018, 2012.

[23] L. Buratto and E. Böhm, "The use of the femtosecond laser in penetrating keratoplasty," *The American Journal of Ophthalmology*, vol. 143, no. 5, pp. 737–742, 2007.

[24] K. Kamiya, H. Kobashi, K. Shimizu, A. Igarashi, and C. Boote, "Clinical outcomes of penetrating keratoplasty performed with the VisuMax femtosecond laser system and comparision with conventional penetrating keratoplasty," *PLoS ONE*, vol. 9, no. 8, Article ID e105464, 2014.

9

Evaluation of Intrastromal Riboflavin Concentration in Human Corneas after Three Corneal Cross-Linking Imbibition Procedures: A Pilot Study

Antonella Franch,[1] **Federica Birattari,**[1] **Gloria Dal Mas,**[1] **Zala Lužnik,**[2,3]
Mohit Parekh,[2] **Stefano Ferrari,**[2] **and Diego Ponzin**[2]

[1]*Department of Ophthalmology, SS Giovanni e Paolo Hospital, Sestiere Castello 6777, 30122 Venice, Italy*
[2]*Fondazione Banca degli Occhi del Veneto, c/o Padiglione G. Rama, Via Paccagnella 11, Zelarino, 30174 Venice, Italy*
[3]*Eye Hospital, University Medical Centre, Grablovičeva Ulica 46, 1525 Ljubljana, Slovenia*

Correspondence should be addressed to Antonella Franch; antofranch@hotmail.com

Academic Editor: Suphi Taneri

Purpose. To compare stromal riboflavin concentration after three corneal cross-linking (CXL) imbibition procedures: standard (EpiOff), transepithelial corneal (EpiOn), and iontophoresis-assisted technique (Ionto) using 0.1% hypotonic riboflavin phosphate. *Methods.* Randomized open-label pilot clinical study. Twelve corneas/12 patients with advanced keratoconus were randomly divided into 4 groups for CXL ($n = 3$). The corneas underwent imbibition with standard riboflavin EpiOff and with enhanced riboflavin solution (RICROLIN+) EpiOff, EpiOn, and iontophoresis techniques. Thereafter, deep anterior lamellar keratectomy procedure was performed and the obtained debrided corneal tissues were frozen. The maximal intrastromal riboflavin concentration was measured by high-performance liquid chromatography/mass spectrometry (mcg/dg). *Results.* The mean stromal concentration of riboflavin was 2.02 ± 0.72 mcg/dg in EpiOff group, 4.33 ± 0.12 mcg/g in EpiOff-RICROLIN+ group, 0.63 ± 0.21 mcg/dg in EpiOn-RICROLIN+ group, and 1.15 ± 0.27 mcg/dg in iontophoresis RICROLIN+ group. A 7-fold decrease in intrastromal riboflavin concentration was observed comparing EpiOn-RICROLIN+ and EpiOff-RICROLIN+ groups. *Conclusion.* The present pilot study indicates that both transepithelial CXL techniques in combination with hypotonic enhanced riboflavin formulation (RICROLIN+) were still inferior to the standard CXL technique; however, larger clinical studies to further validate the results are needed and in progress.

1. Introduction

Keratoconus (KC) is a progressive, degenerative, noninflammatory corneal thinning disease due to changes in organization and the structure of stromal corneal collagen fibers [1]. The disease usually manifests in the second decade of life with a relatively high prevalence in general population (1 in 1750 in white Europeans aged 10–44 years) [2]. In around 20% of keratoconic eyes, corneal transplantation is needed to restore vision [2].

In 2003, Wollensak with colleagues introduced the first available treatment option to halt the disease progression by chemically modifying the collagen fibers and increasing the corneal biomechanical strength and stability [3]. With the utilization of ultraviolet (UV) A light and riboflavin as a photosensitizer, they induced covalent cross-link bonds between collagen fibers [3]. Since then, numerous clinical studies and publications showed the efficacy and safety of corneal collagen cross-linking (CXL) technique in slowing down or halting KC progression. Currently, CXL has become a standard, low-invasive, and safe treatment option for progressive KC and several variations of the standard epithelium-off technique have been sought to avoid corneal epithelial debridement and thus increasing patients' safety and comfort [1]. However, when corneal epithelium is not removed, riboflavin penetration into the corneal stroma is decreased and lowers the efficacy of the procedure [4]. Thus, different strategies such as different riboflavin formulations that would enhance its penetration through intact epithelium, as well as prolongation of imbibition time, were used to overcome this issue. However, imbibition-time prolongation exposes corneas to excessive dehydration and thinning. Furthermore, deeper penetration of riboflavin can lead to increased corneal endothelium susceptibility to UVA toxicity [5].

To shorten the imbibition time, a new cross-linking technique was recently introduced using iontophoresis-assisted riboflavin administration (I-CXL). Due to riboflavin's small molecular weight, water solubility, and negative charge, it is a good candidate for iontophoresis [6]. Recently, the first preliminary results of up to 1 year postoperatively were reported indicating the efficacy of I-CXL in stabilizing the progression of CK [7]. Furthermore, a new hypoosmolar charged riboflavin solution (RICROLIN+; SOOFT Italia S.p.A., Montegiorgio, Italy) dextran-free that uses EDTA 0,1% and trometamol 0,05% as enhancers was introduced to optimize riboflavin stromal penetration by iontophoresis with fewer side effects [4, 5].

However, no comparative clinical studies on riboflavin penetration efficacy comparing transepithelial techniques to standard epithelium-off technique and the new riboflavin solution (RICROLIN+) were conducted to date.

Thus, the present pilot study aimed at determining differences in riboflavin concentration in the corneal stroma after three types of imbibition procedures (standard EpiOff, EpiOn, and iontophoresis-assisted administration) of 0.1% enhanced riboflavin solution were compared to a standard procedure in human corneas excised during deep anterior lamellar keratoplasty (DALK) was performed.

2. Materials and Methods

2.1. Pilot Study Design.
A randomized open-label pilot study was conducted at the ophthalmology department of the SS Giovanni e Paolo Hospital (Venice, Italy) between February and March 2014. Before enrollment, written informed consent was obtained from all patients in the clinical study. The aim of the pilot clinical trial was to compare the efficacy of riboflavin penetration into the corneal stroma using three corneal cross-linking imbibition techniques before replacing the anterior corneal tissue with a donor cornea using deep anterior lamellar keratoplasty due to advanced keratoconus.

The primary outcome measure was the maximum corneal stromal riboflavin concentration (mcg/dg).

2.2. Patient Selection.
Twelve patients (twelve corneas) with advanced keratoconus were selected for corneal cross-linking procedure before undergoing anterior lamellar keratoplasty (DALK).

The indication for DALK was defined after clinical and keratotopographical progression of keratoconus was identified.

Each patient had a pre- and postoperative standard ophthalmological examination, which included uncorrected distance visual acuity (UDVA), corrected distance visual acuity (CDVA), refractometry, corneal topography, pachymetry, endothelial cell count and confocal microscopy using, and slit-lamp biomicroscopy.

Only patients aged between 18 and 60 years were included in the study. The upper age limit was set at 60 years due to the nature of the disease [8]. Exclusion criteria included a corneal thickness less than 400 μm, corneal scarring, previous refractive or other corneal surgery, a history of chemical burns, severe infections, corneal stromal dystrophies, autoimmune disease, and wearing contact lens less than four weeks before enrollment.

2.3. Treatment.
Before DALK was performed, 12 eligible patients were randomized into four treatment groups: EpiOff group (gold standard or control group), EpiOff-RICROLIN+ group, EpiOn-RICROLIN+ group, and Ionto-RICROLIN+ group (Table 1).

EpiOff was designed as a control group (gold standard group) and included three eyes ($n = 3$). Riboflavin imbibition was performed according to a conventional collagen cross-linking protocol [9]. In short, after topical anesthetic instillation, the central corneal epithelium was removed to a diameter of 9 mm using a soft spatula. Standard riboflavin 0.1% eye drops (Ricrolin; SOOFT Italia S.p.A., Montegiorgio, Italy) were applied to the denuded cornea 1 drop every 1 to 2 minutes for 15 minutes. In EpiOff-RICROLIN+ group, after conventional corneal epithelium removal three corneas ($n = 3$) received RICROLIN+ (a hypotonic 0.1% riboflavin solution with enhancers dextran-free [including edetate sodium, tromethamine, bihydrate sodium phosphate monobasic, and bihydrate sodium phosphate bibasic]; SOOFT Italia S.p.A.) 1 drop every 1 to 2 minutes for 15 minutes. In EpiOn and Ionto groups, corneas received riboflavin imbibition via a transepithelial approach. In EpiOn-RICROLIN+ group, three corneas ($n = 3$) received RICROLIN+ for 30 minutes, 1 drop every 1 to 2 minutes. Although the enhancers in RICROLIN+ were designed to enable better riboflavin penetration into the corneal stroma through intact corneal epithelium, a longer imbibition time was used as reported in previous protocols [9]. Three corneas Ionto-RICROLIN+ group were soaked with RICROLIN+ using an iontophoresis system (IONTOFOR-CXL; SOOFT Italia S.p.A.) that was previously reported by Mastropasqua et al. [9]. For iontophoresis, two electrodes that are connected to a power generator are needed. One electrode (positive electrode) is placed on the patient's forehead, whereas the main negative electrode is contained in a rubber ring 10 mm in diameter, which is applied to the corneal surface and ensues constant riboflavin solution administration during the procedure. Iontophoresis is performed using a 1 mA/min intensity for 5 minute.

After riboflavin soaking, deep anterior lamellar keratoplasty (DALK) was started replacing 80% of the anterior portion of the diseased cornea with a healthy anterior corneal transplant.

Immediately after surgical removal of the anterior stromal tissue, slices from the EpiOff groups were frozen, while in the EpiOn and Ionto group the intact epithelium was

TABLE 1: Tested groups. Both EpiOff groups had a 15-minute imbibition with Ricrolin (standard) or RICROLIN+. The EpiOn group had a 30-minute imbibition and the Iontophoresis group had a 5-minute imbibition with RICROLIN+.

	EpiOff	EpiOff-RICROLIN+	EpiOn-RICROLIN+	Ionto-RICROLIN+
Number of corneas analyzed	2	3	3	3
Impregnation	Ricrolin	RICROLIN+	RICROLIN+	RICROLIN+
Impregnation time	15 min	15 min	30 min	5 min

TABLE 2: The mean intrastromal riboflavin concentration of each treatment group determined by HPLC/MS after three different imbibition techniques were used.

Treated group	EpiOff	EpiOff RICROLIN+	EpiOn RICROLIN+	Iontophoresis RICROLIN+
Mean (mcg/dg)	2.02	4.33	0.63	1.15
SD (mcg/dg)	0.72	0.12	0.21	0.27

HPLC/MS: high-performance liquid chromatography/mass spectrometry; SD: standard deviation.

removed before freezing to prevent the epithelial effect on the riboflavin concentration measurement.

2.4. Riboflavin Concentration Measurement. The concentration of riboflavin in each corneal stromal tissue sample was determined by high-performance liquid chromatography/ mass spectrometry (HPLC/MS) after homogenization (Ultra-turrax) and extraction in 50 : 50 (v/v) acetonitrile : water. The extracts were then centrifuged for 15 minutes at 10,000 rpm at 4°C. The sample extracts were diluted 100-fold with the initial mobile phase (10 : 90 100 mM ammonium formate buffer solution pH 3.2 : acetonitrile), and an aliquot of 5 μL was injected into the HPLC column (Kinetex C8, 50 × 2.1 mm, 2.6 μm). Samples were then analyzed using the Agilent 6410 Triple Quadruple Mass Spectrometer (Triple Quad MS) with an Electrospray Ionization (ESI) source (Agilent Technologies, USA). All data were acquired employing Agilent 6410 Quantitative Analysis version B.01.03 analyst data processing software. The calibration curve was obtained with a standard stock solution of riboflavin dissolved in 50 : 50 (v/v) acetonitrile : water to obtain an exact final concentration of 1 μg/mL. The target calibration range was 0.676–1.690 ng/mL (LOD was 0.676 ng/mL). The isocratic flow rate was set at 0.1 mL/min for the 3 min of duration of each assay. Riboflavin was ionized under positive ionization conditions. The predominant peak in the primary ESI spectra of riboflavin corresponds to the $[M-H-H_2O]^+$ ion at m/z 377, and a secondary peak was detected at m/z 243. Chromatograms were integrated and the calibration curves plotted as the peak area of riboflavin. The determination coefficient (r^2) was 0.999.

2.5. Statistical Analysis. The limitations of our pilot study include the small sample size, which disabled a reliable statistical analysis. Thus, the results are presented as the mean riboflavin concentration ± SD. Individual data are plotted in a scatter plot (Figure 1). The preliminary pilot results comparing the difference of riboflavin concentration in the four treatment groups were tested by the Kruskal-Wallis nonparametric test coupled with Dunn's multiple comparison test.

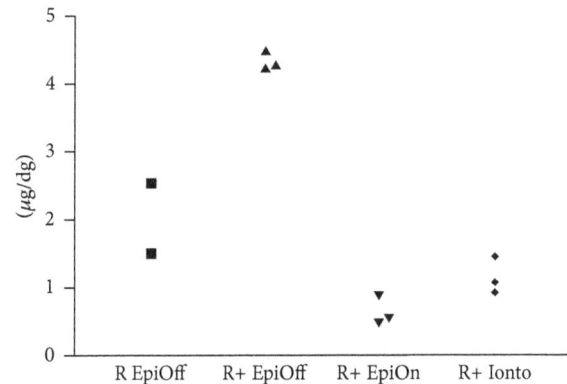

FIGURE 1: Scatter plot showing intrastromal riboflavin concentration (mcg/dg) per individual data in each group (Epi-Off, EpiOff-RICROLIN+, EpiOn-RICROLIN+, and iontophoresis RICROLIN+). The pilot study results confirm that iontophoresis-assisted riboflavin imbibition reaches higher riboflavin intrastromal concentrations compared to EpiOn technique, but still the efficacy of riboflavin imbibition is inferior to EpiOff standard technique.

3. Results and Discussion

3.1. Results. Recruitment for the pilot trial was completed after three months in 2013 with 12 eyes randomized into 4 treatment groups each containing 3 corneas, the Epi-Off, EpiOff-RICROLIN+, EpiOn-RICROLIN+, and Ionto-RICROLIN+ groups. The groups were balanced regarding donor age and preoperative corneal thickness values. However, one cornea of the EpiOff treatment group was lost for analysis because of technical problems.

Overall, the mean riboflavin concentration in the excised anterior corneal slices after riboflavin imbibition using these three CXL techniques is reported in Table 2.

The mean stromal concentration of riboflavin was 2.02 ± 0.72 mcg/dg (n = 2) in the EpiOff group (gold standard group), 4.33 ± 0.12 mcg/dg in the EpiOff-RICROLIN+ group, 0.63 ± 0.21 mcg/dg in the EpiOn-RICROLIN+ group, and 1.15 ± 0.27 mcg/dg in the iontophoresis RICROLIN+ group. The pilot study results confirm that iontophoresis-assisted riboflavin imbibition reaches higher riboflavin intrastromal concentrations compared to EpiOn technique, but still the efficacy of riboflavin imbibition is inferior to EpiOff standard technique.

However, due to the small pilot sample size and due to an unexpected high variability between the two samples treated with standard riboflavin and the EpiOff procedure, a reliable statistical analysis could not be performed, as higher numbers of patients are required.

Nevertheless, in the EpiOff-RICROLIN+ group a much better and consistent intrastromal riboflavin concentration was noticed. Furthermore, a 7-fold increase in intrastromal riboflavin concentration was observed comparing the EpiOff-RICROLIN+ group and the EpiOn-RICROLIN+ group (4.33 ± 0.12 mcg/dg and 0.63 ± 0.21 mcg/dg, resp.) (Figure 1). Thus, these pilot study results indicate that the increase in imbibition time (from 15 minutes to 30 minutes) could not overcome the decrease of riboflavin penetration due to intact epithelium. On the contrary, in the iontophoresis group the corneal epithelium-dependent inhibition of riboflavin penetration could be partially overcome with iontophoresis-assisted technique even though the imbibition time was reduced to 5 minute, if compared to the standard EpiOff group.

3.2. Discussion. After a decade of clinical and experimental studies, it is well known that sufficient concentration of riboflavin in corneal stroma is crucial to obtain a biomechanical effect of corneal CXL [4, 9]. Thus, since riboflavin cannot penetrate intact corneal epithelium due to its chemical properties, the central corneal epithelium is mechanically debrided in current standard CXL (EpiOff) techniques to allow sufficient riboflavin stromal imbibition [5]. However, epithelial removal causes various side effects, including intra- and postoperative pain as well as visual decline in the first three months after procedure. Furthermore, it can predispose patients to serious corneal infections and loss of corneal transparency due to abnormal corneal stromal scarring processes [5]. Thus, in recent years much effort has been put into the development of new efficient transepithelial riboflavin penetration techniques. Different strategies were studied to enhance transepithelial riboflavin penetration, such as increasing riboflavin imbibition time and new riboflavin solution formulations to facilitate its transepithelial penetration. For this reason, several enhancers were proposed, with Ricrolin TE (SOOFT, Montegiorgio, FM, Italy) formulation being the most studied one with no consensus regarding studied clinical effectiveness in comparison to the standard CXL technique [5]. Another strategy to enhance riboflavin penetration through intact corneal epithelium that was recently introduced is the iontophoresis technique [10]. This is a noninvasive technique, which enables the transfer of charged small molecules throughout the tissues by means of a low intensity electric field [11]. The rate at which the charged molecules can penetrate into the tissue can be additionally increased with changing the characteristics of the solution as was done in the case of riboflavin solution. A special hypotonic riboflavin solution formulation (RICROLIN+) was developed for iontophoretic drug delivery to optimize riboflavin imbibition through intact corneal epithelium. This

further enables shortening the treatment time as was recently shown in a 5-minute iontophoresis imbibition technique [9]. Moreover, a recent study by Mastropasqua et al. already compared the transepithelial (EpiOn and Ionto) techniques with the standard EpiOff technique for riboflavin stromal penetration, which showed a greater and deeper penetration rate of riboflavin when the iontophoresis-assisted transepithelial technique was used; however, the riboflavin concentrations were still lower than achieved with the standard EpiOff technique. Additionally, the study was done on human cadaver corneas not suitable for transplantation [9]. To date, no clinical comparative study evaluating these three CXL imbibition techniques was done on advanced keratoconus eyes.

Thus, in our recent pilot study we wanted to compare these three types of riboflavin imbibition procedures using a hypotonic 0.1% enhanced riboflavin solution formulation (RICROLIN+) with the standard CXL procedure in advanced keratoconic eyes immediately before deep anterior lamellar keratoplasty (DALK) was performed. Due to previous reports that showed no statistically significant differences in the intermediate and posterior corneal stromal riboflavin concentration among these 3 tested CXL techniques [4] and according to the fact that with DALK 80% of the diseased corneal tissue is removed, we could obtain enough corneal stromal material for further riboflavin concentration analysis using HPLC. Furthermore, to avoid the effect of the corneal epithelium in the transepithelial CXL group, the corneas were deepithelized before freezing. However, due to the small pilot sample size, the current pilot study is limited with reliable statistical analysis of the obtained results. Thus, although our preliminary pilot study data show no statistically significant difference in the mean stromal riboflavin concentration observed between the transepithelial techniques and the standard CXL technique, this might be due to an unexpected high variability between the two tested samples in the standard control group; therefore, the results were interpreted with caution and a larger number clinical study will be needed.

As expected, the lowest riboflavin penetration was observed in the passive EpiOn-RICROLIN+ and a slightly better permeability was observed in the iontophoresis group, reaching approximately 50% of the intrastromal concentration result of the standard EpiOff group. Importantly, the highest riboflavin concentrations were still found in the EpiOff group, with the pilot study results being similar to previously reported studies [4]. In fact, when we compare the EpiOn-RICROLIN+ group with the EpiOff-RICROLIN+ group, we observe a 7-fold decrease in intrastromal riboflavin concentration. These results demonstrate that also in our pilot study the increase in imbibition time (from 15 minutes to 30 minutes) could not overcome the barrier function of the intact corneal epithelium on riboflavin penetration, despite using the enhanced riboflavin solution formulation [4]. A recent study on rabbit eyes already showed that transepithelial riboflavin permeability was increased when using enhancers such as 0.01% benzalkonium chloride and 0.44% NaCl dextran-free; in our pilot study, we also demonstrated that with iontophoresis-assisted technique the results were better when compared to the EpiOn group but still inferior to the deepithelized CXL technique. The pilot study results might indicate that the corneal epithelium-dependent inhibition of riboflavin penetration might be at least partially successfully overcome with iontophoresis-assisted technique, if hypotonic enhanced riboflavin formulation was used, even though the imbibition time was reduced to 5 minutes. However, our encouraging pilot study results should be further evaluated in larger clinical studies that are already in progress.

Interestingly, we additionally observed a much better and consistent permeation in the EpiOff-RICROLIN+ group compared to the standard riboflavin group, indicating that further improvements (e.g., higher intrastromal riboflavin concentrations or shorter time treatments) could also be achieved in the EpiOff gold standard technique group.

4. Conclusions

In conclusion, the present pilot study indicates that both transepithelial CXL techniques in combination with hypotonic enhanced riboflavin formulation (RICROLIN+) were still inferior to the standard CXL technique. Furthermore, the highest riboflavin concentration was observed in the EpiOff-RICROLIN+ group, indicating that further improvements could also be achieved in the EpiOff gold standard technique group. Additionally, we demonstrated that prolongation of imbibition time yields an insufficient increase in the passive riboflavin penetration group (in the EpiOn group). On the contrary, if riboflavin is given by iontophoresis-assistance, a shortening of the imbibition time from 30 minutes to 5 minutes can be observed. Although, due to the small sample size, a reliable statistical analysis was not possible, these pilot study results are in accordance with previously reported data [4, 9] in human donor corneas. However, additional larger clinical studies are needed to further validate these results and the long-term efficacy of transepithelial CXL compared to the standard CXL protocol.

Conflict of Interests

The authors declare that there is no conflict of interests regarding the publication of this paper.

Acknowledgment

Zala Lužnik is the recipient of a Boehringer-Ingelheim travel grant.

References

[1] A. M. Sherif, "Accelerated versus conventional corneal collagen cross-linking in the treatment of mild keratoconus: a comparative study," *Clinical Ophthalmology*, vol. 8, pp. 1435–1440, 2014.

[2] D. M. Gore, A. J. Shortt, and B. D. Allan, "New clinical pathways for keratoconus," *Eye*, vol. 27, no. 3, pp. 329–339, 2013.

[3] G. Wollensak, E. Spörl, and T. Seiler, "Treatment of keratoconus by collagen cross linking," *Ophthalmologe*, vol. 100, no. 1, pp. 44–49, 2003.

[4] L. Mastropasqua, M. Lanzini, C. Curcio et al., "Structural modifications and tissue response after standard epi-off and iontophoretic corneal crosslinking with different irradiation procedures," *Investigative Ophthalmology & Visual Science*, vol. 55, no. 4, pp. 2526–2533, 2014.

[5] V. Soler, M. Cassagne, C. Laurent et al., "Iontophoresis transcorneal delivery technique for transepithelial corneal collagen crosslinking with riboflavin in a rabbit model," *Investigative Ophthalmology & Visual Science*, vol. 54, p. 4299, 2013.

[6] G. Bikbova and M. Bikbov, "Transepithelial corneal collagen cross-linking by iontophoresis of riboflavin," *Acta Ophthalmologica*, vol. 92, no. 1, pp. e30–e34, 2014.

[7] P. Vinciguerra, J. B. Randleman, V. Romano et al., "Transepithelial iontophoresis corneal collagen cross-linking for progressive keratoconus: initial clinical outcomes," *Journal of Refractive Surgery*, vol. 30, no. 11, pp. 746–753, 2014.

[8] A. J. Kanellopoulos and G. Asimellis, "Revisiting keratoconus diagnosis and progression classification based on evaluation of corneal asymmetry indices, derived from scheimpflug imaging in keratoconic and suspect cases," *Clinical Ophthalmology*, vol. 7, pp. 1539–1548, 2013.

[9] L. Mastropasqua, M. Nubile, R. Calienno et al., "Corneal cross-linking: intrastromal riboflavin concentration in iontophoresis-assisted imbibition versus traditional and transepithelial techniques," *American Journal of Ophthalmology*, vol. 157, no. 3, pp. 623.e1–630.e1, 2014.

[10] E. Eljarrat-Binstock and A. J. Domb, "Iontophoresis: a noninvasive ocular drug delivery," *Journal of Controlled Release*, vol. 110, no. 3, pp. 479–489, 2006.

[11] N. Dixit, V. Bali, S. Baboota, A. Ahuja, and J. Ali, "Iontophoresis—an approach for controlled drug delivery: a review," *Current Drug Delivery*, vol. 4, no. 1, pp. 1–10, 2007.

10

The Correlation Analysis between Corneal Biomechanical Properties and the Surgically Induced Corneal High-Order Aberrations after Small Incision Lenticule Extraction and Femtosecond Laser In Situ Keratomileusis

Wenjing Wu and Yan Wang

Tianjin Eye Hospital and Tianjin Eye Institute, Tianjin Ophthalmology and Visual Science Key Laboratory, Clinical College of Ophthalmology, Tianjin Medical University, No. 4, Gansu Road, Heping District, Tianjin 300020, China

Correspondence should be addressed to Yan Wang; wangyan7143@vip.sina.com

Academic Editor: Roberto Bellucci

Background. To investigate the correlation between corneal biomechanics and the surgically induced corneal high-order aberrations (HOAs) after small incision lenticule extraction (SMILE) and femtosecond laser in situ keratomileusis (FS-LASIK). *Methods.* A total of 150 right myopic eyes that underwent SMILE or FS-LASIK surgery were included in this retrospective study, 75 eyes in each group. The corneal hysteresis (CH) and the corneal resistance factor (CRF) with the corneal HOAs of the anterior, posterior, and total cornea were assessed preoperatively and three months postoperatively. Multivariate linear regression was applied to determine the correlations. *Results.* The preoperative CRF was significantly correlated with the induced 3rd–6th-order HOAs and spherical aberration of the anterior surface and the total cornea after SMILE and FS-LASIK surgeries ($P < 0.05$), postoperatively. The CRF was significantly correlated with the induced vertical coma of the anterior and posterior surfaces and the total cornea after SMILE surgery ($P < 0.05$). There was a significant correlation between the CRF and the induced posterior corneal horizontal coma after FS-LASIK surgery ($P = 0.013$). *Conclusions.* The corneal biomechanics affect the surgically induced corneal HOAs after SMILE and FS-LASIK surgery, which may be meaningful for screening the patients preoperatively and optimizing the visual qualities postoperatively.

1. Introduction

Currently, laser corneal refractive surgery has become an effective and safe method to correct myopia and astigmatism, especially by use of femtosecond laser in situ keratomileusis (FS-LASIK) and the advanced femtosecond laser small incision lenticule extraction (SMILE) [1, 2]. However, there remain a significant number of corneal high-order aberrations (HOAs) after surgery [3–5], leading to degraded visual qualities and subsequent patient dissatisfaction [6]. Many efforts have been made to investigate the resources of the induced aberrations [3, 4].

Recently, the preoperative corneal biomechanics were identified to play a significant role in the surgically induced astigmatism after cataract surgery [7]. The corneal biomechanics are also closely associated with the corneal HOAs in eyes after intracorneal ring segment implantation [8]. Hence,

we suppose that the surgically induced corneal HOAs after SMILE and FS-LASIK surgery may be influenced by the preoperative corneal biomechanics. However, to the best of our knowledge, little study has been done to quantitatively analyze the induced optical changes after SMILE and FS-LASIK surgery from the corneal biomechanical perspective.

Hence, this study was performed to investigate the possible relationships between corneal biomechanical parameters and the surgically induced corneal HOAs in myopic eyes after SMILE and FS-LASIK surgery. Considering these correlations may be important for optimizing the SMILE and FS-LASIK surgeries to achieve satisfactory visual qualities.

2. Materials and Methods

2.1. Subjects and Examinations. This study enrolled one hundred and fifty eyes of 150 myopic subjects, 75 right eyes

TABLE 1: The characteristics of the subjects in the SMILE and FS-LASIK groups.

Parameters	SMILE (n = 75 eyes) Mean ± SD (range)	FS-LASIK (n = 75 eyes) Mean ± SD (range)	P
Female/male	41/34	38/37	0.744
Age (years)	24.25 ± 5.38 (18 to 41)	24.28 ± 5.24 (18 to 42)	0.959
Sphere (D)	−5.12 ± 1.29 (−2.25 to −8.5)	−5.22 ± 1.76 (−1.50 to −10.50)	0.700
Cylinder (D)	−0.73 ± 0.70 (0 to −3.25)	−0.67 ± 0.52 (0 to −2.5)	0.507
MRSE (D)	−5.49 ± 1.35 (−2.75 to −8.875)	−5.56 ± 1.76 (−1.875 to −11.00)	0.808
CCT (μm)	547.69 ± 27.06 (503 to 620)	545.97 ± 27.71 (500 to 639)	0.701
Km (D)	43.08 ± 1.25 (40.5 to 46.4)	43.32 ± 1.22 (41.2 to 46.0)	0.221
IOP (mmHg)	15.80 ± 2.55 (10.1 to 20.1)	15.79 ± 2.78 (9.4 to 20.7)	0.988

MRSE: manifest refraction spherical equivalent, CCT: central corneal thickness, Km: mean corneal curvature, and IOP: intraocular pressure.

in the SMILE group and 75 right eyes in the FS-LASIK group. We retrospectively reviewed the clinical charts of patients who underwent SMILE or FS-LASIK surgery in our department. The inclusion criteria were as follows: subjects who had stable postoperative manifest refraction spherical equivalent (MRSE) within ±0.25 D, together with reliable corneal topographic evaluations and corneal biomechanical examinations preoperatively and 3 months postoperatively. Eyes with postoperative complications such as dry eye or steroid-induced high intraocular pressure were excluded as these complications may influence the corneal high-order aberrations [9, 10]. Seventy-five subjects (38 female/37 male) with the FS-LASIK surgery were included. Patients' age was 24.28 ± 5.24 years (mean ± SD); the range was 18 to 42 years. Spherical correction was −5.22 ± 1.76 D, ranging from −1.50 to −10.50 D, and the cylinder was −0.67±0.52 D, ranging from 0.00 to −2.50 D. Seventy-five subjects (41 female/34 male) who had myopic SMILE refractive surgery were matched for the patient age, sphere, and cylinder. The patients' age was 24.25 ± 5.38 years, ranging from 18 to 41 years. Myopic spherical corrections were −5.12 ± 1.29 D, ranging from −2.25 to −8.50 D. The cylinder was −0.73 ± 0.70 D, ranging from −0.00 to −3.25 D. Detailed clinical data are shown in Table 1. There were no statistically significant differences between the SMILE and FS-LASIK groups in the patients' gender, age, spherical diopter, cylindrical diopter, or MRSE preoperatively.

The research adhered to the tenets of the Declaration of Helsinki and received approval from the Institution Review Board of Tianjin Eye Hospital, Tianjin Medical University. Written informed consent was obtained from all participants after explanations of possible consequences.

Corneal wavefront aberrations were obtained using a rotating Scheimpflug Camera (Pentacam HR, Oculus, Wetzlar, Germany). The Pentacam HR has been used as a noninvasive and reproducible method for the measurement of corneal HOAs of the anterior and posterior surfaces and the total cornea [11, 12]. To avoid misleading effects, the corneas with preoperative scars were excluded from the study, and experienced ophthalmic technicians measured the corneal aberrations of the undilated eyes in low mesopic conditions. In this study, the wavefront aberrations of the anterior corneal surface, the posterior surface, and the total cornea, including the 3rd- to 6th-order HOAs, vertical coma, horizontal coma, and spherical aberration, were analyzed over 6.0 mm central corneal zone with the sign. The qualified readings preoperatively and at 3 months postoperatively were accepted for statistical analysis.

Patients underwent corneal biomechanical examinations through an Ocular Response Analyzer (ORA, Reichert Ophthalmic Instruments; Buffalo, NY, USA), which is the first instrument that could quantify the corneal biomechanical responses clinically [13]. This instrument used an air puff to deform the cornea and generate two principal corneal biomechanical parameters including the corneal hysteresis (CH) and the corneal resistance factor (CRF). CH represents the stiffness along the stromal lamellae; the CRF represents the overall mechanical resistance of the cornea, which is an indicator of the corneal elastic properties [13]. The ORA was used to obtain three or four consecutive measurements in each eye from every patient preoperatively and at 3 months postoperatively. The readings for the qualified examinations with the best waveform score were accepted for statistical analysis.

2.2. Surgical Technique. A single experienced surgeon (Yan Wang) performed all the SMILE and FS-LASIK surgeries. The surgical procedure was performed with topical anesthesia using 3 drops of oxybuprocaine hydrochloride (Benoxil, Santen, Inc., Osaka, Japan) applied 3 minutes before surgery. The same femtosecond laser system (VisuMax, Carl Zeiss Meditec AG, Germany) with a 500 kHz repetition rate was used for the SMILE procedure and the FS-LASIK procedure.

The SMILE procedure was performed with the VisuMax femtosecond laser system. The patient's eye was positioned under the interface cone, and the subject was asked to look at the blinking target light. The surgeon adjusted the position of the eye close to the interface cone. Once an appropriate centration (i.e., center of pupil) had been achieved, suction was applied [14–16]. Four cleavage planes were created, including two surfaces of the refractive lenticule, the vertical edge of the refractive lenticule, and a single side-cut incision peripherally of the cornea at the 12 o'clock position. The lenticule was separated from the stromal bed and removed with forceps through the small incision. The lenticule diameter was 6 mm. The optical zone diameter was equal to the lenticule diameter in patients with purely spherical refractive error. If the patient had astigmatism, the software added a transition zone to convert the oval lenticule into a circle. Therefore, the lenticule diameter was 6.0–6.1 mm, depending on the presence or absence of astigmatism [15, 17, 18]. The arc length of the small incision ranged from 2 to 5 mm. The target refraction was within ±0.25 D. The predicted depth of the anterior surface of the lenticule was 110 μm.

The VisuMax system was also used for flap creation in the FS-LASIK procedure; a 400 Hz Allegretto excimer laser system (WaveLight Laser Technologie AG, Germany) was used for stromal ablation with the wavefront-optimized ablation mode. The center of the ablation zone was aligned with the center of the pupil. After stromal ablation, the residual stromal bed was washed with the balanced salt solution, and the flap was repositioned. The target refraction was within ±0.25 D. The intended flap thickness was 100–110 μm with the flap diameters of 7.9–8.0 mm. The hinge of the corneal flap was in the nasal side. All eyes had ablations using an optical zone diameter of 6 mm surrounded by a transition zone of 1.0 mm.

2.3. Statistical Analysis. The normality of all data samples was checked with the Kolmogorov-Smirnov test. Differences between the preoperative and postoperative values were compared by the paired *t*-test; differences between SMILE and FS-LASIK were determined by two-tailed independent *t*-test.

Stepwise multivariate linear regression analysis was applied to investigate the determinants of corneal high-order aberrations, using criteria of probability-of-*F*-to-enter ≤ 0.050 and probability-of-*F*-to-remove ≥ 0.100. The dependent variable was the changes of the corneal HOAs of the anterior surface, the posterior surface, and the total cornea in SMILE and FS-LASIK, respectively. The explanatory variables include the preoperative CH and the CRF and the manifest refraction spherical equivalent (MRSE), the central corneal thickness (CCT), the intraocular pressure (IOP), and the mean corneal curvature. All regression analysis model assumptions were evaluated by analyzing the condition index in the collinearity diagnostics to exclude the collinearity among the explanatory variables. The Durbin-Watson value was also investigated to confirm the independence of the residual errors. If the condition index was larger than thirty, the last enrolled explanatory variable was excluded, and the other variables were included in the regression analysis. Only modes with the condition index larger than zero and less than thirty and the value of Durbin-Watson tests near two were included. A *P* value less than 0.05 was considered statistically significant. Statistical analysis was performed using SPSS statistical software (version 19.0, Chicago, USA).

3. Results

This study was comprised of seventy-five right eyes in the SMILE group and seventy-five right eyes in the FS-LASIK group. Detailed clinical data are shown in Table 1. Preoperatively, there were no statistically significant differences (*P* > 0.05, Student's *t*-test) between the two groups in the patients' gender, age, spherical diopter, cylindrical diopter, manifest refraction spherical equivalent (MRSE), central corneal thickness (CCT), mean corneal curvature, or intraocular pressure (IOP).

3.1. Corneal Biomechanics. Figure 1 illustrates that the corneal biomechanics significantly decreased after the SMILE (CH: *P* < 0.001, CRF: *P* < 0.001, paired *t*-test) and FS-LASIK (CH: *P* < 0.001, CRF: *P* < 0.001) surgeries. The postoperative CH and the CRF were significantly higher after SMILE than after FS-LASIK (*P* = 0.010, *P* = 0.019; Student's *t*-test, Figures 1(a) and 1(b)).

The CRF decreased 3.14 ± 1.06 mmHg while CH decreased 1.86 ± 1.13 mmHg after the SMILE surgery; the ratio of the CRF changes ((pre-CRF − post-CRF)/pre-CRF) was larger than the reduction ratio of CH (*P* = 0.001, Figure 1(c)) after the SMILE surgery. The CRF decreased 3.80 ± 1.53 mmHg while CH reduced 2.23 ± 1.33 mmHg after the FS-LASIK surgery. The ratio of the CRF changes after the FS-LASIK surgery was also larger than that of CH (*P* = 0.001, Figure 1(c)).

3.2. Corneal High-Order Aberrations (HOAs). The corneal HOAs of the anterior surface, the posterior surface, and the total cornea before and after SMILE and FS-LASIK are shown in Figure 2. The 3rd- to 6th-order HOAs and the spherical aberration of the anterior surface and the total cornea exhibit significant increases in both groups (*P* < 0.05).

There were significant differences between SMILE and FS-LASIK groups in the changes of corneal HOAs after surgeries (Figure 3). Specifically, the changes of the 3rd- to 6th-order HOAs, spherical aberration, and horizontal coma of the anterior surface and the total cornea were significantly lower after SMILE surgery than after FS-LASIK surgery (*P* < 0.05, Figure 3). The amounts of the induced vertical coma of the anterior surface and the total cornea were significantly higher after SMILE surgery (*P* = 0.042, *P* = 0.040, Figure 2), whereas the horizontal coma of the anterior cornea and the total cornea was significantly higher after FS-LASIK surgery than SMILE surgery. The induced posterior corneal horizontal coma was significantly lower after SMILE surgery (*P* < 0.001, Figure 3).

3.3. Multivariate Analysis of the Relations between Corneal Biomechanics and the Surgically Induced HOAs. The multivariable regression analyses of the surgically induced anterior corneal HOAs, posterior corneal HOAs, and total corneal HOAs are shown in Tables 2, 3, and 4, respectively. After both the SMILE and FS-LASIK procedures, the preoperative CRF showed significantly negative correlations with the induced 3rd- to 6th-order HOAs and the induced spherical aberration of the anterior surface (*P* < 0.01, Figure 4, Table 2) and the total cornea (*P* < 0.01, Figure 4, Table 4). The preoperative CRF also showed significant correlations with the induced vertical coma of the posterior cornea after the SMILE procedure (*P* = 0.024, Table 3, Figure 5). There was a significant correlation between the CRF and the induced horizontal coma of the posterior cornea after FS-LASIK surgery (*P* = 0.013, Table 3, Figure 5).

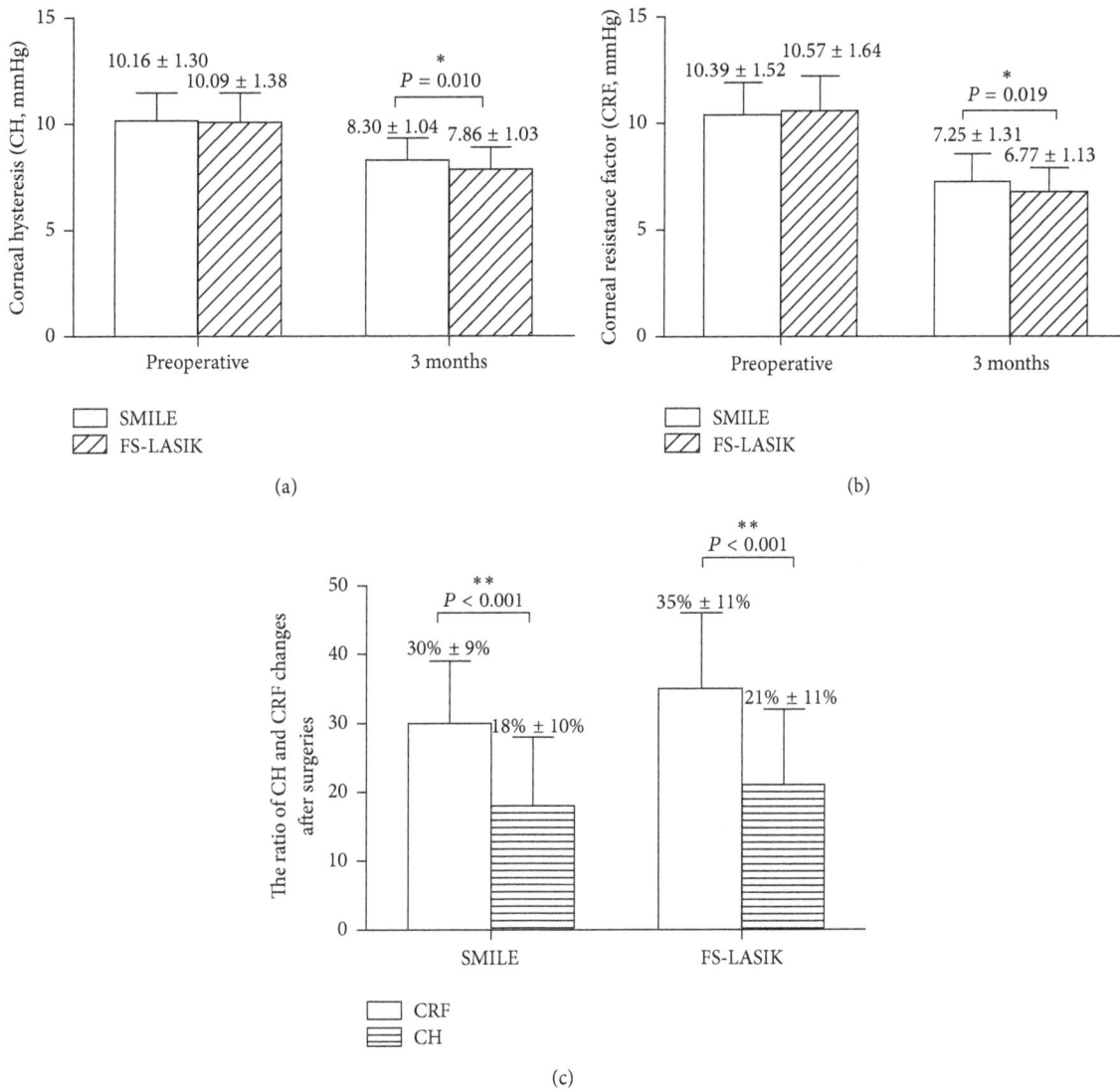

FIGURE 1: Comparison of the corneal hysteresis (CH) and the corneal resistance factor (CRF) between SMILE and FS-LASIK surgery (a, b); the ratio of CRF changes was significantly higher than that of CH after both the SMILE and the FS-LASIK surgeries (c). The ratio of CRF changes after surgery = ((preoperative CRF − postoperative CRF)/preoperative CRF), $^{**}P < 0.01$, $^{*}P < 0.05$.

TABLE 2: Stepwise multivariate linear regression analyses of factors that correlated with the alterations of the anterior corneal aberrations after SMILE and FS-LASIK.

Changes of anterior corneal HOAs	SMILE			Adjusted R^2	FS-LASIK			Adjusted R^2
	Priority	Beta	P		Priority	Beta	P	
3rd- to 6th-order HOAs	MRSE	−0.487	<0.001	0.303	MRSE	−0.755	<0.001	0.574
	CRF	−0.305	0.002		CRF	−0.210	0.007	
Spherical aberration	MRSE	−0.451	<0.001	0.279	MRSE	−0.701	<0.001	0.530
	CRF	−0.321	0.002		CRF	−0.299	<0.001	
Vertical coma	MRSE	0.332	0.003	0.135	MRSE	0.302	0.009	0.079
	CRF	0.229	0.037					
Horizontal coma	MRSE	0.237	0.040	0.043	MRSE	0.584	<0.001	0.332

HOAs: high-order aberrations, CRF: corneal resistance factor, MRSE: manifest refraction spherical equivalent, and beta: standardized coefficients.

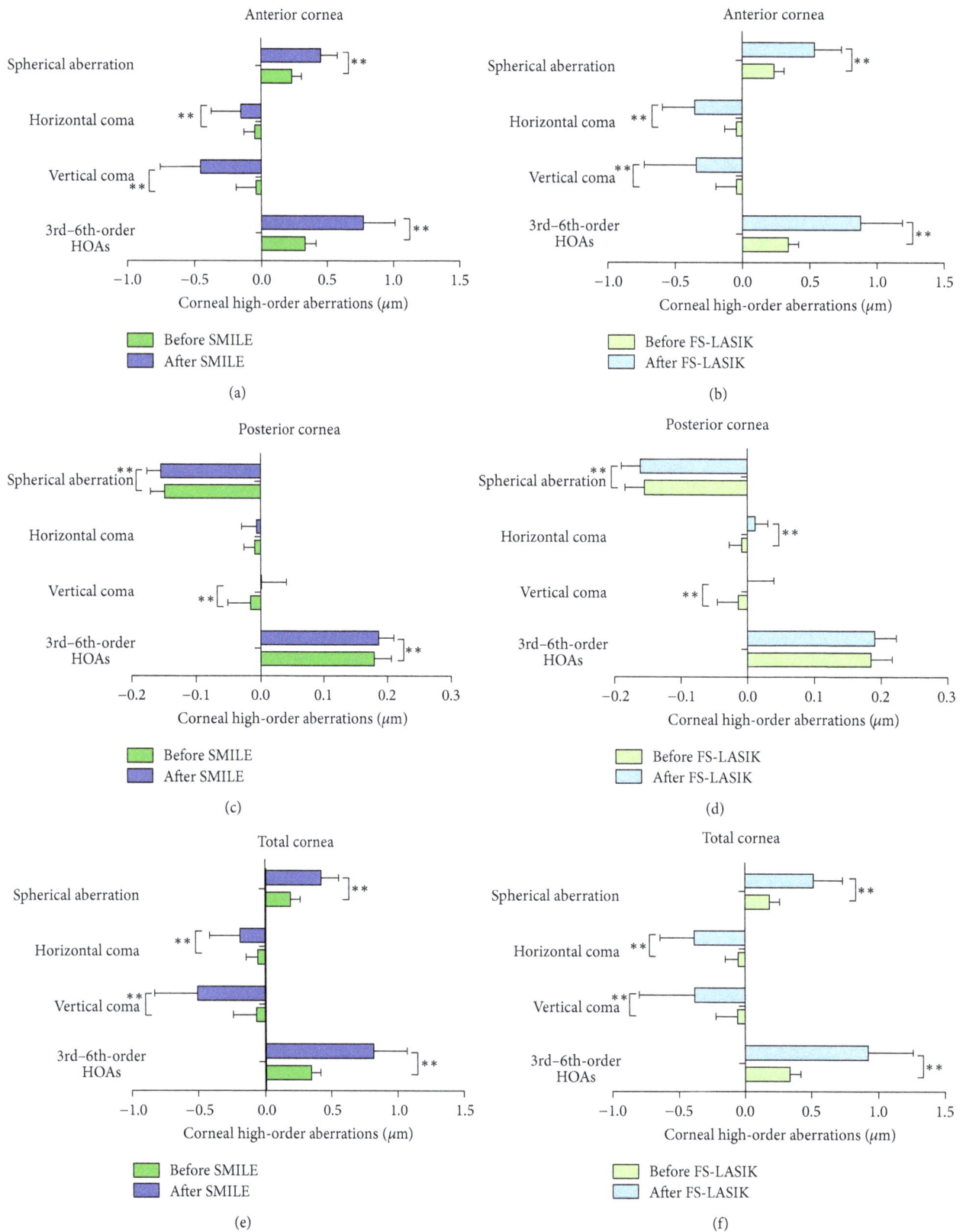

FIGURE 2: Comparison of the corneal HOAs of the anterior and posterior surfaces and the total cornea after SMILE and FS-LASIK surgeries. $^*P < 0.05$, $^{**}P < 0.01$. HOAs: high-order aberrations.

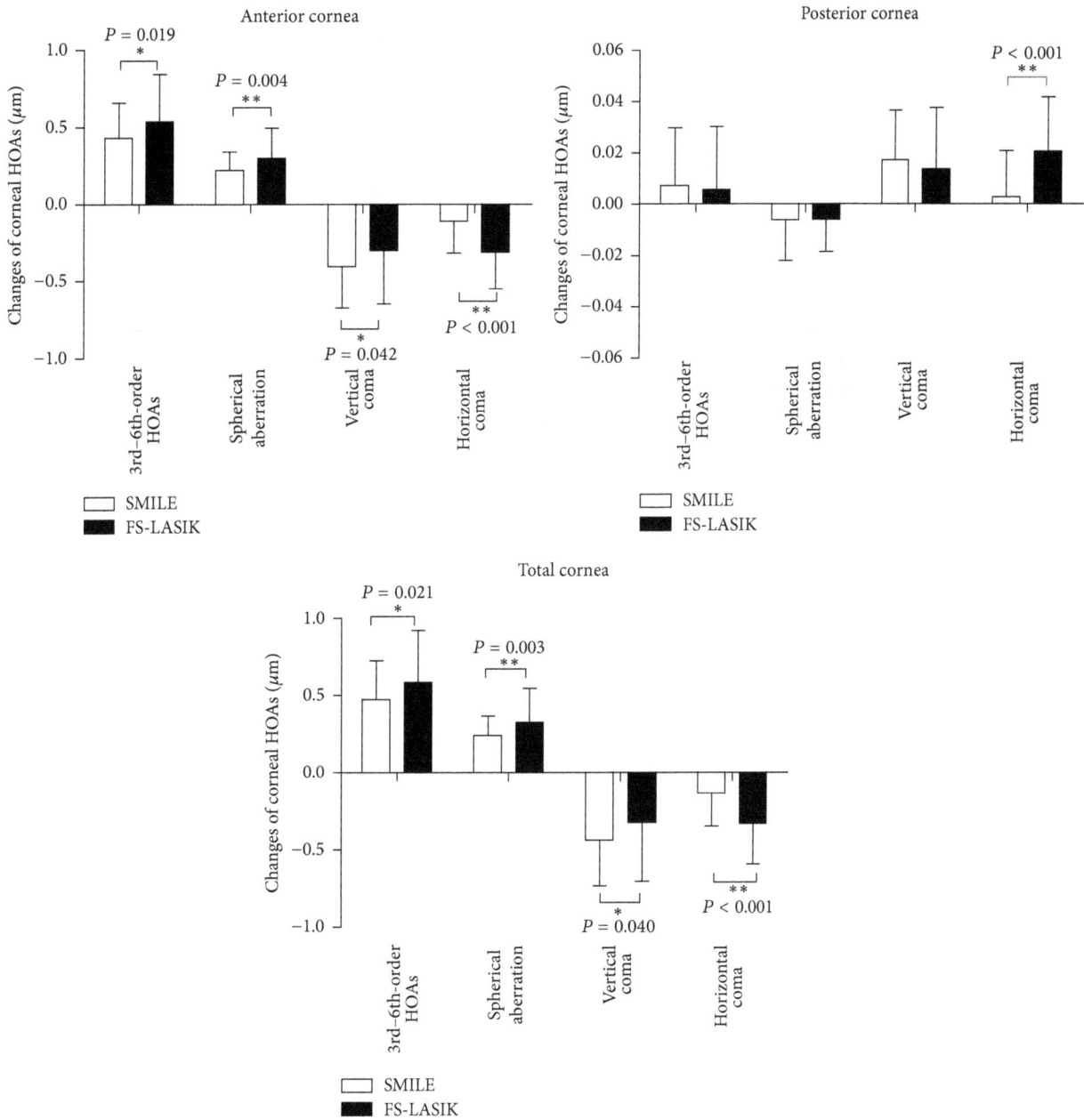

FIGURE 3: Comparison of the surgically induced corneal high-order aberrations (HOAs) of the anterior surface, the posterior surface, and the total cornea between SMILE and FS-LASIK. $^{*}P < 0.05$, $^{**}P < 0.01$. HOAs: high-order aberrations.

TABLE 3: Stepwise multivariate linear regression analyses of factors that correlated with the alterations of the posterior corneal aberrations after SMILE and FS-LASIK.

Changes of posterior corneal HOAs	SMILE			Adjusted R^2	FS-LASIK			Adjusted R^2
	Priority	Beta	P		Priority	Beta	P	
Vertical coma	CRF	−0.261	0.024	0.055				0.079
Horizontal coma					CRF	−0.280	0.013	0.107
					MRSE	−0.257	0.023	

HOAs: high-order aberrations, CRF: corneal resistance factor, MRSE: manifest refraction spherical equivalent, and beta: standardized coefficients.

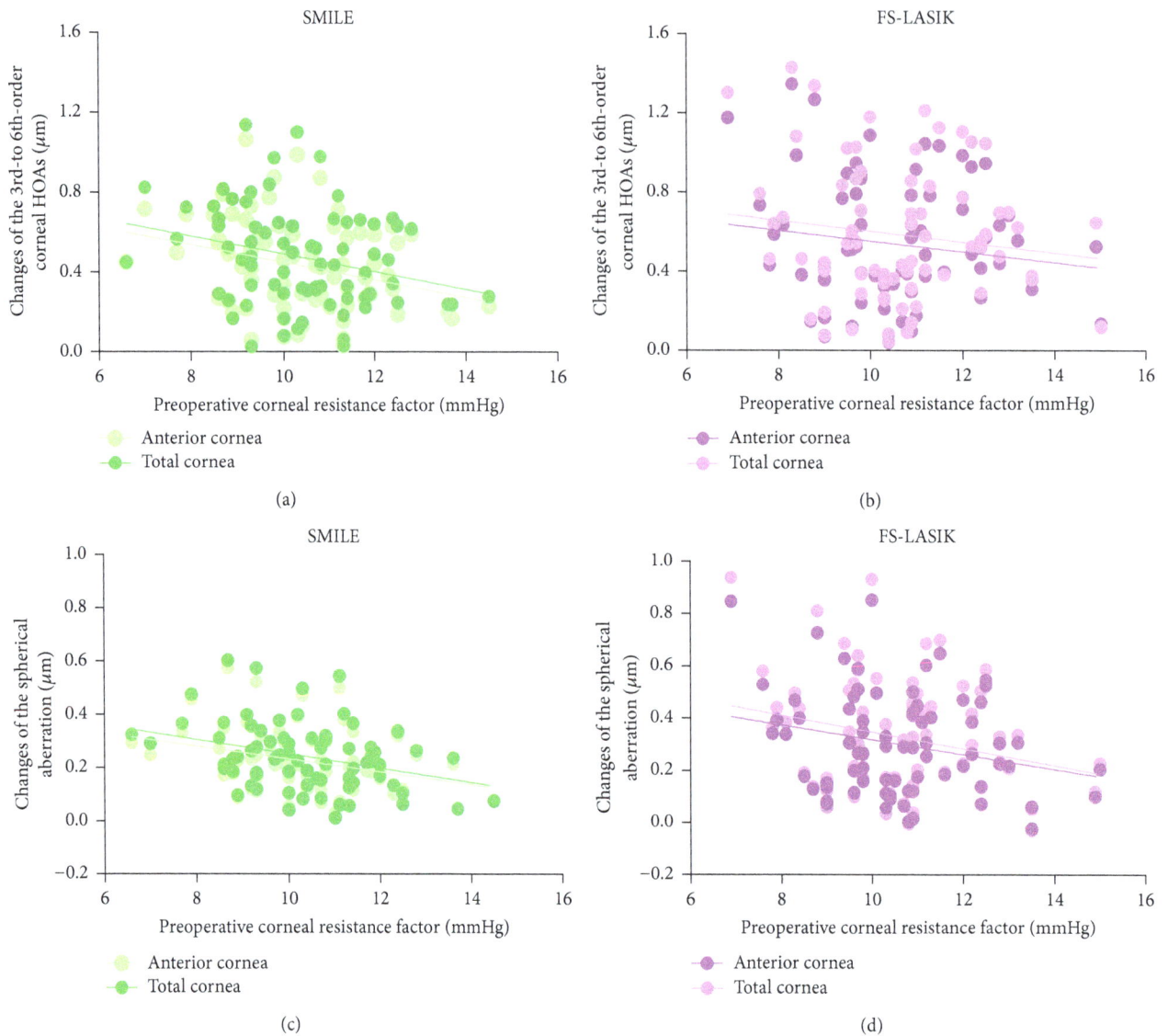

FIGURE 4: Scatter plots show the significant relations between the preoperative corneal resistance factor (CRF) and the changes in the corneal HOAs for the anterior cornea and the total cornea after SMILE and FS-LASIK surgeries.

TABLE 4: Stepwise multivariate linear regression analyses of factors that correlated with the alterations of the total corneal aberrations after SMILE and FS-LASIK.

Changes of total corneal HOAs	SMILE			Adjusted R^2	FS-LASIK			Adjusted R^2
	Priority	Beta	P		Priority	Beta	P	
3rd- to 6th-order HOAs	MRSE	−0.496	<0.001	0.298	MRSE	−0.760	<0.001	0.579
	CRF	−0.281	0.005		CRF	−0.200	0.010	
Spherical aberration	MRSE	−0.442	<0.001	0.280	MRSE	−0.697	<0.001	0.526
	CRF	−0.335	0.001		CRF	−0.302	<0.001	
Vertical coma	MRSE	0.338	0.003	0.136	MRSE	0.304	0.008	0.080
	CRF	0.223	0.043					
Horizontal coma	MRSE	0.289	0.012	0.084	MRSE	0.594	<0.001	0.344

HOAs: high-order aberrations, CRF: corneal resistance factor, MRSE: manifest refraction spherical equivalent, and beta: standardized coefficients.

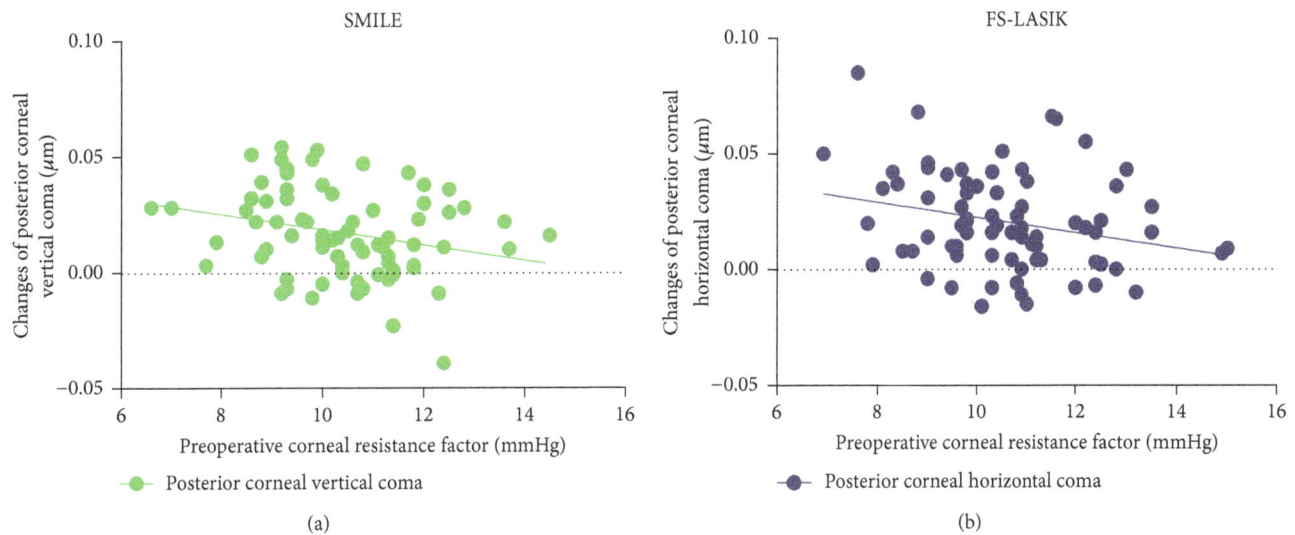

FIGURE 5: Scatter plots show the significant relations between the preoperative corneal resistance factor (CRF) and the changes of posterior corneal HOAs after SMILE and FS-LASIK surgeries.

4. Discussion

The present study aims to identify new factors influencing the corneal optical changes after corneal refractive surgeries through corneal biomechanical analysis. We provide evidence that the corneal biomechanics, especially the corneal resistance factor, were significantly correlated with the surgically induced corneal high-order aberrations (HOAs) after the SMILE and FS-LASIK procedures. To the best of our knowledge, this is the first study that investigates the correlations between the CH, the CRF, and the surgically induced corneal HOAs in myopic eyes after SMILE and FS-LASIK surgeries.

We found that the SMILE procedure was superior to the FS-LASIK surgery with respect to the corneal biomechanics. Reinstein et al. [19] and Roy et al. [20] also found better postoperative corneal biomechanics in the SMILE group through the mathematical analyses. Hence, high myopic subjects with lower corneal biomechanics preoperatively are suggested to undergo the SMILE surgery for better postoperative corneal biomechanics. Although some other studies found similar biomechanical results [18, 21] between SMILE and FS-LASIK surgery, the sample size is relative small (30 versus 30, 29 versus 35 eyes). Therefore, other randomized, prospective, contralateral studies with large sample sizes are still needed to confirm our results. Moreover, the present study also found that the CRF was more sensitive to the biomechanical changes after both the SMILE and FS-LASIK surgeries. Piñero et al. [22] also suggest that the CRF has more diagnostic ability than CH for the pathological changes occurring in keratoconic eyes that are characterized as disorganized corneal collagen and weakened corneal biomechanics. This may indicate that the CRF was more sensitive than CH to the optical changes after SMILE and FS-LASIK surgeries.

We also found that the SMILE procedure was superior to FS-LASIK with respect to the corneal high-order aberrations

(HOAs), which was in accordance with other studies [23, 24]. The optical advantages of the SMILE procedure may be associated with the flapless surgical technique [5]. These results may be important for those patients with larger pupil size or higher myopia [6, 25]. The SMILE procedure could be performed in these subjects to reduce the optical changes and improve their visual qualities. In addition, we also found the vertical coma was significantly increased after SMILE surgery, whereas the horizontal coma was significantly increased after FS-LASIK surgery. It might result from the superior incision along the vertical axis in SMILE procedure and the nasal-hinge flap in FS-LASIK surgery [5], which may cause imbalanced corneal healing responses and imbalanced optical changes along the axis. Although some studies demonstrated that decentrations [3, 4] play a role in the induction of coma after the SMILE surgery, other studies are still needed to investigate the resources of the vertical coma and horizontal coma to optimize the postoperative visual qualities.

The main finding in the present study is that the preoperative corneal biomechanical parameter CRF was independently correlated with the surgically induced corneal optical changes whatever the spherical equivalent was. These correlations indicated that the lower the CRF, the larger the induced corneal high-order aberrations after refractive surgeries. In other words, corneas with weaker mechanical and structural properties might be linked to more deformable corneal surfaces and larger optical changes of the cornea after surgeries. This might help explain why some subjects are more predisposed to poor visual qualities than others. In terms of correlations between corneal biomechanics and corneal aberrations, previous studies found that the corneal aberrations significantly increased in eyes that underwent radial keratectomy with reduced corneal biomechanical strengths [26, 27]. However, these studies did not investigate the correlations between the preoperative corneal biomechanics and the surgically induced corneal HOAs in eyes after surgery. Recently, Denoyer et al. demonstrated that the corneal biomechanical properties could influence the induced astigmatism in cataract surgery [7]. Piñero et al. also found that the corneal biomechanical properties were correlated with the corneal HOAs after intraocular ring segment implantation [8]. All of these findings demonstrate that the corneal biomechanical properties might be important factors associated with the corneal optical changes after surgeries. Our findings suggest that the clinical surgeons should pay more attention to the corneal biomechanical parameters preoperatively since patients with lower corneal structural properties may suffer from higher corneal HOAs, limiting the potential visual benefits of the SMILE and FS-LASIK surgeries. The corneal biomechanical characteristics might be included in the algorithm of corneal refractive surgeries to optimize the postoperative visual qualities of the SMILE and FS-LASIK surgeries.

There are some limitations in this study. Although this study enrolled 150 subjects, future studies with larger sample size would be needed to confirm our initial observations. Moreover, the present study investigated the correlations between corneal biomechanics and the surgically induced corneal HOAs in the advanced SMILE surgery and the established FS-LASIK surgery. Future studies may demonstrate the possible associations between corneal biomechanics and the surgically induced corneal HOAs in other corneal procedures.

In summary, the changes of corneal high-order aberrations after SMILE and FS-LASIK surgeries were associated with corneal biomechanical properties. Corneal biomechanics may be meaningful for screening patients preoperatively and optimizing the visual qualities postoperatively.

Conflict of Interests

The authors declare that there is no conflict of interests regarding the publication of this paper.

Acknowledgments

This study was supported by research grants from the National and Science Program Grant (no. 81470658), China, and the Tianjin Research Program of Application Foundation and Advanced Technology (14JCZDJC35900).

References

[1] W. Sekundo, K. S. Kunert, and M. Blum, "Small incision corneal refractive surgery using the small incision lenticule extraction (SMILE) procedure for the correction of myopia and myopic astigmatism: results of a 6 month prospective study," *British Journal of Ophthalmology*, vol. 95, no. 3, pp. 335–339, 2011.

[2] B. Pajic, I. Vastardis, B. Pajic-Eggspuehler, Z. Gatzioufas, and F. Hafezi, "Femtosecond laser versus mechanical microkeratome-assisted flap creation for lasik: a prospective, Randomized, Paired-eye study," *Clinical Ophthalmology*, vol. 8, pp. 1883–1889, 2014.

[3] M. Li, J. Zhao, H. Miao et al., "Mild decentration measured by a scheimpflug camera and its impact on visual quality following

[4] K. Kamiya, K. Umeda, A. Igarashi, W. Ando, and K. Shimizu, "Factors influencing the changes in coma-like aberrations after myopic laser in situ keratomileusis," *Current Eye Research*, vol. 36, no. 10, pp. 905–909, 2011.

[5] I. G. Pallikaris, G. D. Kymionis, S. I. Panagopoulou, C. S. Siganos, M. A. Theodorakis, and A. I. Pallikaris, "Induced optical aberrations following formation of a laser in situ keratomileusis flap," *Journal of Cataract and Refractive Surgery*, vol. 28, no. 10, pp. 1737–1741, 2002.

[6] C. Villa, R. Gutiérrez, J. R. Jiménez, and J. M. González-Méijome, "Night vision disturbances after successful LASIK surgery," *British Journal of Ophthalmology*, vol. 91, no. 8, pp. 1031–1037, 2007.

[7] A. Denoyer, X. Ricaud, C. Van Went, A. Labbé, and C. Baudouin, "Influence of corneal biomechanical properties on surgically induced astigmatism in cataract surgery," *Journal of Cataract & Refractive Surgery*, vol. 39, no. 8, pp. 1204–1210, 2013.

[8] D. P. Piñero, J. L. Alio, R. I. Barraquer, and R. Michael, "Corneal biomechanical changes after intracorneal ring segment implantation in Keratoconus," *Cornea*, vol. 31, no. 5, pp. 491–499, 2012.

[9] N. Deschamps, X. Ricaud, G. Rabut, A. Labbé, C. Baudouin, and A. Denoyer, "The impact of dry eye disease on visual performance while driving," *American Journal of Ophthalmology*, vol. 156, no. 1, pp. 184.e3–189.e3, 2013.

[10] J. Qu, F. Lu, J. Wu et al., "Wavefront aberration and its association with intraocular pressure and central corneal thickness in myopic eyes," *Journal of Cataract and Refractive Surgery*, vol. 33, no. 8, pp. 1447–1454, 2007.

[11] E. Juhasz, K. Kranitz, G. L. Sandor, A. Gyenes, G. Toth, and Z. Z. Nagy, "Wavefront properties of the anterior and posterior corneal surface after photorefractive keratectomy," *Cornea*, vol. 33, no. 2, pp. 172–176, 2014.

[12] S. Koh, N. Maeda, T. Nakagawa et al., "Characteristic higher-order aberrations of the anterior and posterior corneal surfaces in 3 corneal transplantation techniques," *The American Journal of Ophthalmology*, vol. 153, no. 2, pp. 284–290, 2012.

[13] A. Plakitsi, C. O'Donnell, M. A. Miranda, W. N. Charman, and H. Radhakrishnan, "Corneal biomechanical properties measured with the Ocular Response Analyser in a myopic population," *Ophthalmic and Physiological Optics*, vol. 31, no. 4, pp. 404–412, 2011.

[14] J. Zhang, Y. Wang, W. Wu, L. Xu, X. Li, and R. Dou, "Vector analysis of low to moderate astigmatism with small incision lenticule extraction (SMILE): results of a 1-year follow-up," *BMC Ophthalmology*, vol. 15, article 8, 2015.

[15] A. Ağca, A. Demirok, K. İ. Çankaya et al., "Comparison of visual acuity and higher-order aberrations after femtosecond lenticule extraction and small-incision lenticule extraction," *Contact Lens and Anterior Eye*, vol. 37, no. 4, pp. 292–296, 2014.

[16] F. Lin, Y. Xu, and Y. Yang, "Comparison of the visual results after SMILE and femtosecond laser-assisted LASIK for myopia," *Journal of Refractive Surgery*, vol. 30, no. 4, pp. 248–254, 2014.

[17] S. Wei and Y. Wang, "Comparison of corneal sensitivity between FS-LASIK and femtosecond lenticule extraction (ReLEx flex) or small-incision lenticule extraction (ReLEx smile) for myopic eyes," *Graefe's Archive for Clinical and Experimental Ophthalmology*, vol. 251, no. 6, pp. 1645–1654, 2013.

[18] A. Agca, E. B. Ozgurhan, A. Demirok et al., "Comparison of corneal hysteresis and corneal resistance factor after small

SMILE in the early learning curve," *Investigative Ophthalmology & Visual Science*, vol. 55, no. 6, pp. 3886–3892, 2014.

incision lenticule extraction and femtosecond laser-assisted LASIK: a prospective fellow eye study," *Contact Lens and Anterior Eye*, vol. 37, no. 2, pp. 77–80, 2014.

[19] D. Z. Reinstein, T. J. Archer, and J. B. Randleman, "Mathematical model to compare the relative tensile strength of the cornea after PRK, LASIK, and small incision lenticule extraction," *Journal of Refractive Surgery*, vol. 29, no. 7, pp. 454–460, 2013.

[20] A. S. Roy, W. J. Dupps Jr., and C. J. Roberts, "Comparison of biomechanical effects of small-incision lenticule extraction and laser *in situ* keratomileusis: finite-element analysis," *Journal of Cataract and Refractive Surgery*, vol. 40, no. 6, pp. 971–980, 2014.

[21] I. B. Pedersen, S. Bak-Nielsen, A. H. Vestergaard, A. Ivarsen, and J. Hjortdal, "Corneal biomechanical properties after LASIK, ReLEx flex, and ReLEx smile by Scheimpflug-based dynamic tonometry," *Graefe's Archive for Clinical and Experimental Ophthalmology*, vol. 252, no. 8, pp. 1329–1335, 2014.

[22] D. P. Piñero, J. L. Alio, R. I. Barraquer, R. Michael, and R. Jiménez, "Corneal biomechanics, refraction, and corneal aberrometry in keratoconus: an integrated study," *Investigative Ophthalmology and Visual Science*, vol. 51, no. 4, pp. 1948–1955, 2010.

[23] S. Ganesh and R. Gupta, "Comparison of visual and refractive outcomes following femtosecond laser—assisted LASIK with SMILE in patients with myopia or myopic astigmatism," *Journal of Refractive Surgery*, vol. 30, no. 9, pp. 590–596, 2014.

[24] A. Gyldenkerne, A. Ivarsen, and J. Ø. Hjortdal, "Comparison of corneal shape changes and aberrations induced by FS-LASIK and SMILE for myopia," *Journal of Refractive Surgery*, vol. 31, no. 4, pp. 223–229, 2015.

[25] T. Oshika, S. D. Klyce, R. A. Applegate, H. C. Howland, and M. A. El Danasoury, "Comparison of corneal wavefront aberrations after photorefractive keratectomy and laser *in situ* keratomileusis," *American Journal of Ophthalmology*, vol. 127, no. 1, pp. 1–7, 1999.

[26] M. R. Bryant, K. Szerenyi, H. Schmotzer, and P. J. McDonnell, "Corneal tensile strength in fully healed radial keratotomy wounds," *Investigative Ophthalmology and Visual Science*, vol. 35, no. 7, pp. 3022–3031, 1994.

[27] R. A. Applegate, G. Hilmantel, and H. C. Howland, "Corneal aberrations increase with the magnitude of radial keratotomy refractive correction," *Optometry and Vision Science*, vol. 73, no. 9, pp. 585–589, 1996.

11

Responses of the Ocular Anterior Segment and Refraction to 0.5% Tropicamide in Chinese School-Aged Children of Myopia, Emmetropia, and Hyperopia

Ying Yuan,[1,2] Zhengwei Zhang,[2] Jianfeng Zhu,[1] Xiangui He,[1] Ergang Du,[3] Kelimu Jiang,[2] Wenjing Zheng,[2] and Bilian Ke[2]

[1]Shanghai Eye Disease Prevention & Treatment Center, Shanghai 200040, China
[2]Department of Ophthalmology, Shanghai General Hospital, Shanghai Jiao Tong University School of Medicine, Shanghai 200080, China
[3]Chinese Medicine Hospital of Zhejiang Province, Hangzhou, Zhejiang 310006, China

Correspondence should be addressed to Bilian Ke; kebilian@126.com

Academic Editor: Terri L. Young

Purpose. To investigate the changes of anterior segment after cycloplegia and estimate the association of such changes with the changes of refraction in Chinese school-aged children of myopia, emmetropia, and hyperopia. *Methods.* 309 children were recruited and eligible subjects were assigned to three groups: hyperopia, emmetropia, or myopia. Cycloplegia was achieved with five cycles of 0.5% tropicamide. The Pentacam system was used to measure the parameters of interest before and after cycloplegia. *Results.* In the myopic group, the lenses were thinner and the lens position was significantly more posterior than that of the emmetropic and hyperopic groups in the cycloplegic status. The correlations between refraction and lens thickness (age adjusted; $r = 0.26$, $P < 0.01$), and lens position (age adjusted; $r = -0.31$, $P < 0.01$) were found. After cycloplegia, ACD and ACV significantly increased, while ACA significantly decreased. Changes in refraction, ACD, ACV, and ACA were significantly different among the three groups ($P < 0.05$, all). Changes of refraction were correlated with changes of ACD ($r = 0.41$, $P < 0.01$). *Conclusions.* Myopia presented thinner lenses and smaller changes of anterior segment and refraction after cycloplegia when compared to emmetropia and hyperopia. Changes of anterior chamber depth were correlated with refraction changes. This may contribute to a better understanding of the relationship between anterior segment and myopia.

1. Introduction

Myopia is a significant public health problem worldwide and is especially prominent in East Asian countries such as China and Singapore [1–6]. The incidence of myopia tends to increase in adolescence and is the main cause of low vision among the population [7]. The exact mechanism underlying development of myopia has not been well elucidated, but it is clear that the ocular refraction components including corneal, anterior segment, lens thickness (LT), vitreous chamber depth, and axial length are mismatched in myopia. The crystalline lens accounts for almost 20% of the eye's refracting power. During emmetropization of human eyes, the crystalline lens undergoes thinning and

flattening [8, 9]. However, the role of the lens in myopia onset and progression is still controversial. A longitudinal study from Singapore showed that changes in LT were biphasic in different refractive status [10]. Other studies with myopia models indicated that the role of the lens in refractive error development was nonexistent [11]. Moreover, the importance of lens position (LP), defined as anterior chamber depth (ACD) + LT/2, has rarely been investigated in myopes. Therefore, we conducted this cross-sectional study to investigate the association between LT, LP, and myopia.

Evaluation of the ocular anterior segment was essential in clinical ophthalmology. During accommodation, the LT and anterior lens curvature changed which would lead to a change in anterior segment structure. The role of anterior segment in myopia development has also come to the attention of researchers currently. Previous work reported that the anterior chamber angle (ACA) and ACD increased with myopia progression [12, 13]. Meanwhile, myopes usually showed insufficient accommodation or even accommodative lag [14, 15]. However, the effect of accommodation on the anterior segment of myopia remained unclear. So we investigated the relationship between change of anterior segment and change of refraction before and after cycloplegia here.

In this study, 0.5% tropicamide was used to relax accommodation and Pentacam was used to investigate the front corneal radius, back corneal radius, ACD, ACV, and ACA in myopia, emmetropia, and hyperopia before and after cycloplegia. Subjective refraction was also measured before and after application of tropicamide. Additionally, LT and LP after cycloplegia were measured to investigate the role of lens in myopia development. The results would shed more light on the relationship between anterior segment and myopia.

2. Materials and Methods

2.1. Subjects. Three hundred and nine children from one primary school in Chongming, Shanghai, China, were invited to participate in our study. Children with eye diseases and a history of ocular trauma and surgery or who could not cooperate during Pentacam measurements were excluded. The parameters of interest were measured bilaterally but only data from the right eyes were compared. This study was approved by the Human Research Committee of Shanghai General Hospital, Shanghai Jiao Tong University School of Medicine. We obtained informed written consent from at least one legal guardian, as well as verbal consent, from each child. The study's protocol conformed to the restrictions established by the Declaration of Helsinki.

2.2. Ocular Examination. All participants underwent a complete ophthalmic examination which included visual acuity, slit-lamp biomicroscopy, and the refraction of noncycloplegic and cycloplegic state. Best-corrected visual acuity was assessed monocularly with linear logMAR charts if the child had an uncorrected visual acuity higher than 0.0logMAR (i.e., vision > 0.0logMAR). A Haag-Streit slit-lamp (Koeniz, Switzerland) was used to examine the anterior segment. Five cycles of tropicamide (0.5%, one drop per cycle) were administered 5 minutes apart. About 30 minutes after application of the eye drops, children without pupillary light reflex were examined by an autorefractometer (RK-F1, Canon), which generated 5 valid readings of refraction, and the median value was used for analyses.

2.3. Pentacam Measurement. Anterior segment parameters were measured before and after application of tropicamide (determined by an absence of pupillary light reflex) with the Pentacam system. The Oculus Pentacam is a noninvasive evaluative test of ocular anterior segment topography using Scheimpflug photography. The mechanics of the system have been described in detail elsewhere [16]. Participants were seated comfortably and asked to keep their chin on

TABLE 1: Patient demographics and refractive status.

	Emmetropia	Hyperopia	Myopia
Pre-SE (D)	-0.30 ± 0.56	0.33 ± 1.05	-1.93 ± 1.21
Post-SE (D)	0.03 ± 0.25	1.16 ± 1.23	-1.85 ± 1.25
n	104 (37.01%)	58 (20.64%)	119 (42.35%)
Male/female	56/48	29/29	58/61
Age (y)	8.64 ± 1.53	8.12 ± 1.59	9.43 ± 1.32

SE: spherical equivalence.

the chinrest and forehead resting against the forehead strap. Every participant was instructed to keep both eyes open and to fixate on the black target in the center of the blue fixation beam when the instrument was in scan mode. The real-time image on the computer screen was adjusted manually by moving a joystick in the directions indicated on the screen. When the image met x-, y-, and z-plane alignment criteria, the scan was automatically commenced in an automatic release mode. Only scans registering as acceptable ("OK") on the instrument's "QS" (quality specification) output were used for analysis.

2.4. Definitions and Statistical Analysis. Spherical equivalence (SE) was calculated as the spherical power plus half-negative cylinder power. Emmetropia was defined as an SE between -0.5 D and $+0.5$ D after cycloplegia, myopia as an SE ≤ -0.5 D, and hyperopia as an SE $\geq +0.5$ D. The results were expressed as mean ± standard deviation. All statistical evaluations were performed using SAS version 9.2 (SAS Institute). Shapiro-Wilk test was used to assess normal distribution. Levene's test was used to test the variance homogeneity. Paired t-test, independent sample t-test, and one-way analysis of variance (ANOVA) with pairwise Bonferroni posttests were used to analyze the differences between variables. Wilcoxon signed ranks test and Kruskal-Wallis test were applied when the normality assumption and homogeneity of the variance assumption were violated. Pearson correlation coefficient was used to determine the association between refractive error and biometric parameters. $P < 0.05$ was considered statistically significant. All tests were two-tailed.

3. Results

Of the 309 participants examined, 281 children (90.94% of participants) aged 6–13 years (mean, 8.87 ± 1.54 years) were selected for analysis in this study, including 138 girls (49.11%) and 143 boys (50.89%) (Table 1). Twenty-eight children (9.96%) were excluded due to poor cooperation or low scan quality. No subject had a pupil response to light after the application of 5 drops of 0.5% tropicamide. All measurements of the anterior segment were normally distributed both before and after cycloplegia. The overall distributions of measurements before and after cycloplegia, as well changes between the two sessions, are detailed in Table 2.

3.1. Relationship between Crystalline Lens and Refractive Status. The mean LT and LP in the cycloplegic state were

TABLE 2: Anterior segment parameters before and after cycloplegia among refractive groups.

	Emmetropia	Hyperopia	Myopia
Pre-ACD (mm)	2.93 ± 0.23	2.81 ± 0.23[a]	3.12 ± 0.24[a,b]
Post-ACD (mm)	3.03 ± 0.22	2.99 ± 0.21	3.17 ± 0.23[a,b]
ΔACD	0.10 ± 0.08	0.18 ± 0.10[a]	0.06 ± 0.06[a,b]
P value	<0.01	<0.01	<0.01
Pre-ACV (mm³)	162.33 ± 22.82	153.90 ± 23.50[a]	178.86 ± 28.63[a,b]
Post-ACV (mm³)	174.38 ± 23.28	172.02 ± 23.60	185.10 ± 26.30[a,b]
ΔACV	12.05 ± 10.90	18.12 ± 14.97[a]	6.24 ± 13.23[a,b]
P value	<0.01	<0.01	<0.01
Pre-ACA (°)	36.94 ± 4.57	35.02 ± 4.86[a]	38.64 ± 5.15[a,b]
Post-ACA (°)	35.22 ± 7.86	35.87 ± 7.92	37.75 ± 7.66
ΔACA	−1.72 ± 7.38	0.85 ± 6.46[a]	−0.89 ± 6.51
P value	<0.05	0.321	0.138
Post-LT (mm)	3.43 ± 0.19	3.46 ± 0.19	3.31 ± 0.18[a,b]
Post-LP (mm)	4.75 ± 0.21	4.72 ± 0.20	4.83 ± 0.20[a,b]

ACD: anterior chamber depth, ACV: anterior chamber volume, ACA: anterior chamber angle, LT: lens thickness, LP: lens position, and Δ: difference between the pre- and postparameter.
[a]$P < 0.05$ compared with the emmetropia group.
[b]$P < 0.05$ compared with the hyperopia group.

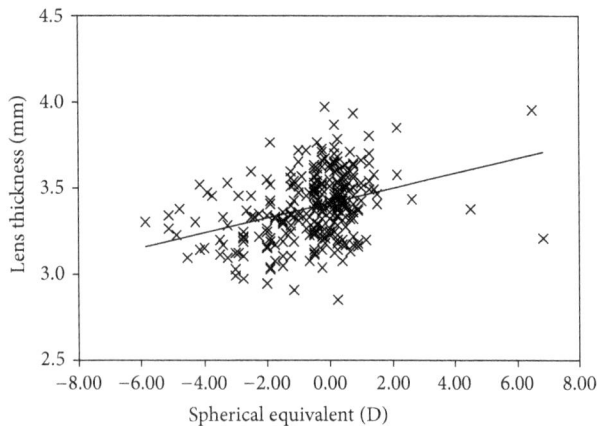

FIGURE 1: Association between lens thickness and refractive status in the cycloplegia.

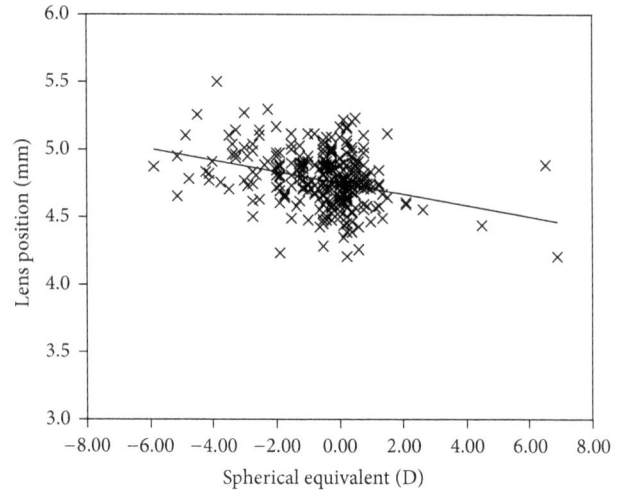

FIGURE 2: Association between lens position and refractive status in the cycloplegia.

significantly different among the myopic, emmetropic, and hyperopic groups ($P < 0.01$). A positive association was found between the LT and refractive status (age adjusted; $r = 0.26$, $P < 0.01$; Figure 1), while a negative association was noted between the LP and refractive error (age adjusted; $r = -0.31$, $P < 0.01$; Figure 2). The LT significantly decreased with increasing age, from age 6 to 13 years (SE adjusted; $r = -0.31$, $P < 0.01$). No significant difference was found in LT and LP between boys and girls. And there was no

significant difference in sex among the myopic, emmetropic, and hyperopic groups. We analyzed the difference in age among the three groups and found the age in the myopic group was different from the emmetropic and hyperopic groups.

3.2. Tropicamide-Induced Changes in Anterior Segment Parameters and Their Association with Refractive Status. After application of tropicamide, the values of ACD and ACV increased (both $P < 0.01$), while ACA decreased significantly ($P < 0.05$). The front and back corneal radius and corneal astigmatism were not significantly different from before cycloplegia ($P > 0.05$, resp.). A high correlation was found between ACD and ACV both before and after cycloplegia ($r = 0.81$, $P < 0.01$, and $r = 0.80$, $P < 0.01$, resp.).

Changes in the ACD (ΔACD) and volume (ΔACV) after cycloplegia were less pronounced in the myopes than those in the emmetropes or hyperopes ($P < 0.05$; Table 2). The change of ACA (ΔACA) was different among refractive groups ($P < 0.05$; Table 2). ΔACA of the myopic and emmetropic group had a decrement ($P = 0.14$, $P < 0.05$, resp.), while that of the hyperopic group had an increment ($P = 0.32$). There was no significant difference between genders for ΔACD, ΔACV, and ΔACA in any group (Table 3). No significant difference based on age was found for corneal radius, corneal astigmatism, ACD, ACV, and ACA.

3.3. Relationship between Changes in SE (ΔSE) and Changes in Anterior Segment. Cycloplegia with application of 0.5% tropicamide significantly changed the mean SE from −0.87 D to −0.54 D ($P < 0.01$; Table 1), which was statistically smaller in the myopic group (from −1.93 D to −1.85 D, ΔSE 0.08 ± 0.48 D) than in the emmetropic (from −0.30 D to 0.03 D, ΔSE 0.33 ± 0.53 D) and hyperopic (from −0.30 D to 1.16 D, ΔSE 0.86 ± 0.77 D) groups. However, changes of ACD per diopter in any group were not statistically significant, with myopes

TABLE 3: Difference in anterior segment parameters between genders among the three groups.

	ΔACD			ΔACV			ΔACA		
	Male	Female	P	Male	Female	P	Male	Female	P
Total	0.097 ± 0.008	0.097 ± 0.007	0.975	10.706 ± 14.336	10.986 ± 12.727	0.863	−0.996 ± 0.595	−0.676 ± 0.564	0.697
Emmetropia	0.101 ± 0.011	0.096 ± 0.011	0.718	11.232 ± 11.400	13.000 ± 10.910	0.412	−2.773 ± 1.003	−0.496 ± 1.025	0.117
Hyperopia	0.188 ± 0.017	0.169 ± 0.020	0.470	19.690 ± 16.935	16.552 ± 12.808	0.430	2.910 ± 1.316	−3.146 ± 0.945	<0.05
Myopia	0.047 ± 0.007	0.063 ± 0.008	0.127	5.707 ± 13.377	6.754 ± 13.179	0.668	−1.233 ± 0.791	−0.564 ± 0.893	0.577

ACD: anterior chamber depth, ACV: anterior chamber volume, ACA: anterior chamber angle, and Δ: difference between pre- and postparameter.

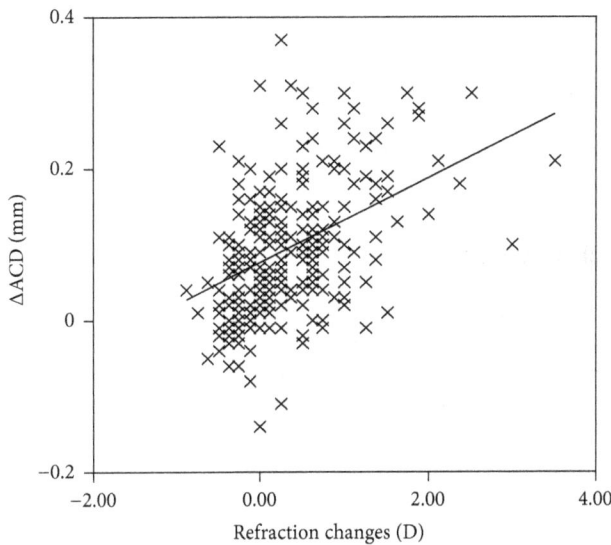

FIGURE 3: Association between the change of anterior chamber depth and the change of refraction.

presenting 0.16 ± 0.33 mm/D, emmetropes 0.21 ± 0.45 mm/D, and hyperopes 0.20 ± 0.62 mm/D. The association between ΔACD, ΔACV, and ΔSE was demonstrated by Pearson correlation. It was found that ΔSE was positively associated with ΔACD ($r = 0.41$, $P < 0.01$; Figure 3). The weaker association was found between ΔSE and ΔACV ($r = 0.22$, $P < 0.01$).

4. Discussion

In the current study, we evaluated the change of anterior segment and refraction and their associations due to cycloplegia in different refractive status. The finding indicated that ACD, ACV, and ACA changed significantly after cycloplegia. And ΔACD was correlated with refraction changes. Myopic children had smaller ΔACD, ΔACV, and ΔACA when compared to emmetropic and hyperopic children.

We found that lenses in the myopic group were significantly thinner than that in the emmetropic and hyperopic group, with LT 3.31 mm in myopes, 3.43 mm in emmetropes, and 3.46 mm in hyperopes. In human eyes, every diopter of reduced accommodation produces only a 0.06 mm decrease in lens thickness [17]. The 0.12 mm decreased in the LT in the myopia would result in an excess −2 D. This was consistent with the average refractive error −1.85 ± 1.25 D in the myopic

group. We further took advantage of the Emsley simplified eye model and relevant geometrical optics mechanism to probe the changes of LT as well as LP and their effect on the development of myopia. For eyes with thinner lenses, the focal length would increase due to the reduction lens refractive power. Additionally, the nodal point would have backward movement as LP changed. Both of them could lead to the image of objects located posteriorly to the retina. This can result in hyperopic defocus of retina and then increase the degree of myopia.

Animal experiments have proved that a concave lens could lead to myopia onset and development [18], which was consistent with the theory of hyperopic defocus. Lambert has found that removing the crystalline lens and implanting an intraocular lens in a neonatal monkey eye retarded its axial elongation [19]. This phenomenon may be caused by the relative static intraocular lens which cannot become thinner with age. Gradually, these eyes with such intraocular lenses produced myopic defocus. A longitudinal study in Chinese children revealed that newly developed myopia had slightly lower lens power than in children with persistent emmetropia, when they were still at emmetropic state [20]. Consequently, the crystalline lens could be an important contributor to myopia onset and development and may be a clue to the physician to observe refractive development. However, the children in our study, aged 6 to 13 years, had mild to moderate myopia. Further studies need to be conducted to investigate the role of the crystalline lens in myopia progression, including different degrees of myopia.

We found a significant increase in ACD as well as ACV after application of tropicamide in any group, which was consistent with the result of previous reports [21–23]. However, there was no significant difference in the front and back corneal radii before and after cycloplegia. In sum, the changes in ACD and ACV may be due to the decrease of LT which was caused by axial flattening and backward movement of the lens. Furthermore, a smaller increment in ACD was seen in the myopic group and a greater increment in the emmetropic and hyperopic groups in our study. It may be one of the optical structure basements to insufficient accommodation in myopia. When accommodation occurs, the refractive index of ocular increased due to the increase of LT and decrease of anterior segment. In myopia, it had a smaller change in anterior segment, which may lead to a less increased refractive power during accommodation.

In addition, after relaxing accommodation by tropicamide, the change of refraction was smaller in myopia compared to emmetropia and hyperopia. It was thought that the refraction change after cycloplegia was mainly associated with the decrease of lens power which was due to the decrease of the lens surfaces curvature, lens position, and lens thickness [24]. However, the accompanying changes in anterior chamber depth may also play a role in the refraction change after cycloplegia. In this study, we found a significant change of anterior segment after cycloplegia and found a positive correlation between ΔACD and ΔSE. The probability was significant, although the correlation coefficient was low. ΔACD caused by per diopter change in myopia is slightly smaller. It may prove that the insufficient accommodation in myopia is related to the anterior structure. This may be caused by the thickened ciliary muscle in myopia which had poor contractility and dilatability [25]. As the subjects had mostly mild to moderate myopia in our study, the function of ciliary muscle may not change significantly. A 0.19 mm ΔACD per diopter accommodation was found in our study. This was different from the result of previous studies, which measured the ocular dimensions at different accommodation stimuli [26]. It may be due to the fact that the actual accommodative responses were less than the stimuli especially in myopia.

We also found that ACA changed after cycloplegia and ΔACA differed in different refractive groups. ΔACA in the hyperopic group was a slight increment, whereas in the emmetropic and myopic groups there was a decrement (although the change in the myopic group was statistically insignificant). Contrary to our results, Tsai and associates [27] recently found that the ACA in myopes and emmetropes increased significantly after diagnostic cycloplegia using 1% tropicamide, as observed with the Pentacam system. The discrepancy between their results and ours can be explained by the following. Firstly, the concentrations of tropicamide were different (0.5% in our study and 1% in Tsai et al.'s study), which could cause cycloplegia and pupil dilation to different degrees and result in different changes in anterior lens displacement. Secondly, the baseline anterior segment parameters were different. Subjects in the Tsai et al. study had larger ACA before cycloplegia than ours. Therefore, the value of ΔACA may depend on both the anterior segment configurations at baseline and the response to tropicamide. However, the exact mechanism needs further investigation. Tsai et al. [27] also proved that there was no association between the change of intraocular pressure (IOP) and the change of ACA in school-aged children. So the importance of the change of ACA after cycloplegia in youths is different from that in elders. The relationships between ACA and refractive status and IOP are still not clear.

There were some limitations in this study. First, the pharmacological cycloplegia after application of 0.5% tropicamide may be incomplete. It was thought that good cycloplegia and dilation were achieved with atropine. But it took too long to reach maximum dilation and had more adverse effect [28]. In China, 0.5% tropicamide has been routinely used for refraction or dilated fundus examination in children. For this, the result of our study may be more helpful in clinical practice. Second, commercially available anterior segment measurement instruments could not image the posterior surface of the lens. Further study will be needed to investigate more ocular biometric parameters among more subjects.

In conclusion, children with myopia presented thinner and more posterior lenses, as well as smaller changes of anterior segment parameters and refraction after cycloplegia. The change of ACD was correlated with the change of refraction. This would help in better understanding the relationship between anterior segment and myopia.

Conflict of Interests

The authors declare that there is no conflict of interests regarding the publication of this paper.

Authors' Contribution

Ying Yuan and Zhengwei Zhang equally contributed to this paper.

Acknowledgments

Grant information: this work was supported by the National Natural Science Foundation of China (Grant no. 81200713), the Foundation of Interdisciplinary Research of "Medical and Engineering or Science" of Shanghai Jiao Tong University (Grant no. YG2011MS62), the Natural Science Foundation of Shanghai, China (Grant no. 09ZR1425400), the Hospital Training Plan of Medical Talent in 2012 (12RC06), and Shanghai Key Laboratory of Fundus Disease.

References

[1] M. He, W. Huang, Y. Zheng, L. Huang, and L. B. Ellwein, "Refractive error and visual impairment in school children in rural southern China," *Ophthalmology*, vol. 114, no. 2, pp. 374–482, 2007.

[2] M. He, J. Zeng, Y. Liu, J. Xu, G. P. Pokharel, and L. B. Ellwein, "Refractive error and visual impairment in urban children in southern China," *Investigative Ophthalmology and Visual Science*, vol. 45, no. 3, pp. 793–799, 2004.

[3] Y.-H. Guo, H.-Y. Lin, L. L. K. Lin, and C.-Y. Cheng, "Self-reported myopia in Taiwan: 2005 Taiwan National Health Interview Survey," *Eye*, vol. 26, no. 5, pp. 684–689, 2012.

[4] M. Dirani, Y.-H. Chan, G. Gazzard et al., "Prevalence of refractive error in Singaporean Chinese children: the strabismus, amblyopia, and refractive error in young Singaporean Children (STARS) study," *Investigative Ophthalmology & Visual Science*, vol. 51, no. 3, pp. 1348–1355, 2010.

[5] S. Vitale, R. D. Sperduto, and F. L. Ferris III, "Increased prevalence of myopia in the United States between 1971–1972 and 1999–2004," *Archives of Ophthalmology*, vol. 127, no. 12, pp. 1632–1639, 2009.

[6] C.-W. Pan, Y.-F. Zheng, A. R. Anuar et al., "Prevalence of refractive errors in a multiethnic Asian population: the Singapore epidemiology of eye disease study," *Investigative Ophthalmology and Visual Science*, vol. 54, no. 4, pp. 2590–2598, 2013.

[7] Q. S. You, L. J. Wu, J. L. Duan et al., "Prevalence of myopia in school children in greater Beijing: the Beijing Childhood Eye study," *Acta Ophthalmologica*, vol. 92, no. 5, pp. e398–e406, 2014.

[8] D. O. Mutti, K. Zadnik, R. E. Fusaro, N. E. Friedman, R. I. Sholtz, and A. J. Adams, "Optical and structural development of the crystalline lens in childhood," *Investigative Ophthalmology and Visual Science*, vol. 39, no. 1, pp. 120–133, 1998.

[9] K. Zadnik, D. O. Mutti, R. E. Fusaro, and A. J. Adams, "Longitudinal evidence of crystalline lens thinning in children," *Investigative Ophthalmology and Visual Science*, vol. 36, no. 8, pp. 1581–1587, 1995.

[10] H.-B. Wong, D. Machin, S.-B. Tan, T.-Y. Wong, and S.-M. Saw, "Ocular component growth curves among Singaporean children with different refractive error status," *Investigative Ophthalmology and Visual Science*, vol. 51, no. 3, pp. 1341–1347, 2010.

[11] J. G. Sivak, "The role of the lens in refractive development of the eye: animal models of ametropia," *Experimental Eye Research*, vol. 87, no. 1, pp. 3–8, 2008.

[12] B. Urban, M. Krętowska, M. Szumiński, and A. Bakunowicz-Łazarczyk, "Evaluation of anterior chamber depth measurements in emmetropic, hypermetropic and myopic eyes in children and adolescents using OCT Visante," *Klinika Oczna*, vol. 114, no. 1, pp. 18–21, 2012.

[13] L. Xu, W. F. Cao, Y. X. Wang, C. X. Chen, and J. B. Jonas, "Anterior chamber depth and chamber angle and their associations with ocular and general parameters: the Beijing Eye Study," *American Journal of Ophthalmology*, vol. 145, no. 5, pp. 929–936.e1, 2008.

[14] J. Gwiazda, F. Thorn, J. Bauer, and R. Held, "Myopic children show insufficient accommodative response to blur," *Investigative Ophthalmology and Visual Science*, vol. 34, no. 3, pp. 690–694, 1993.

[15] D. O. Mutti, G. L. Mitchell, J. R. Hayes et al., "Accommodative lag before and after the onset of myopia," *Investigative Ophthalmology & Visual Science*, vol. 47, no. 3, pp. 837–846, 2006.

[16] H. Shankar, D. Taranath, C. T. Santhirathelagan, and K. Pesudovs, "Repeatability of corneal first-surface wavefront aberrations measured with Pentacam corneal topography," *Journal of Cataract and Refractive Surgery*, vol. 34, no. 5, pp. 727–734, 2008.

[17] G. L. van der Heijde and J. Weber, "Accommodation used to determine ultrasound velocity in the human lens," *Optometry and Vision Science*, vol. 66, no. 12, pp. 830–833, 1989.

[18] E. L. Smith III, L.-F. Hung, B. Arumugam, and J. Huang, "Negative lens-induced myopia in infant monkeys: effects of high ambient lighting," *Investigative Ophthalmology and Visual Science*, vol. 54, no. 4, pp. 2959–2969, 2013.

[19] S. R. Lambert, A. Fernandes, C. Drews-Botsch, and M. Tigges, "Pseudophakia retards axial elongation in neonatal monkey eyes," *Investigative Ophthalmology and Visual Science*, vol. 37, no. 2, pp. 451–458, 1996.

[20] R. Iribarren, I. G. Morgan, Y. H. Chan, X. Lin, and S.-M. Saw, "Changes in lens power in Singapore Chinese children during refractive development," *Investigative Ophthalmology and Visual Science*, vol. 53, no. 9, pp. 5124–5130, 2012.

[21] L. Gao, X. Zhuo, A. K. H. Kwok, N. Yu, L. Ma, and J. Wang, "The change in ocular refractive components after cycloplegia in children," *Japanese Journal of Ophthalmology*, vol. 46, no. 3, pp. 293–298, 2002.

[22] M. Palamar, Z. Alkan, S. Egrilmez, and A. Yagci, "Influences of tropicamide on anterior segment parameters with Pentacam in healthy individuals," *Journal of Ocular Pharmacology and Therapeutics*, vol. 29, no. 3, pp. 349–352, 2013.

[23] J. Bhatia, "Effect of tropicamide and homatropine eye drops on a-scan parameters of the phakic normal eyes," *Oman Medical Journal*, vol. 26, no. 1, pp. 23–25, 2011.

[24] D. O. Mutti, K. Zadnik, S. Egashira, L. Kish, J. D. Twelker, and A. J. Adams, "The effect of cycloplegia on measurement of the ocular components," *Investigative Ophthalmology and Visual Science*, vol. 35, no. 2, pp. 515–527, 1994.

[25] S. Jeon, W. K. Lee, K. Lee, and N. J. Moon, "Diminished ciliary muscle movement on accommodation in myopia," *Experimental Eye Research*, vol. 105, pp. 9–14, 2012.

[26] Y. Sun, S. Fan, H. Zheng, C. Dai, Q. Ren, and C. Zhou, "Noninvasive imaging and measurement of accommodation using dual-channel SD-OCT," *Current Eye Research*, vol. 39, no. 6, pp. 611–619, 2014.

[27] I.-L. Tsai, C.-Y. Tsai, L.-L. Kuo, S.-W. Liou, S. Lin, and I.-J. Wang, "Transient changes of intraocular pressure and anterior segment configuration after diagnostic mydriasis with 1% tropicamide in children," *Clinical and Experimental Optometry*, vol. 95, no. 2, pp. 166–172, 2012.

[28] N. Loewen and J.-C. Barry, "The use of cycloplegic agents. Results of a 1999 survey of German-speaking centers for pediatric ophthalmology and strabology," *Strabismus*, vol. 8, no. 2, pp. 91–99, 2000.

12

Safety and Biocompatibility of a New High-Density Polyethylene-Based Spherical Integrated Porous Orbital Implant: An Experimental Study in Rabbits

Ivan Fernandez-Bueno,[1,2] Salvatore Di Lauro,[1,3] Ivan Alvarez,[4] Jose Carlos Lopez,[1] Maria Teresa Garcia-Gutierrez,[1] Itziar Fernandez,[1,5] Eva Larra,[4] and Jose Carlos Pastor[1,3]

[1]Instituto Universitario de Oftalmobiologia Aplicada (IOBA), University of Valladolid, 47011 Valladolid, Spain
[2]Centro en Red de Medicina Regenerativa y Terapia Celular de Castilla y Leon, Valladolid, Spain
[3]Department of Ophthalmology, Hospital Clinico Universitario, 47005 Valladolid, Spain
[4]AJL Ophthalmic S.A., 01510 Miñano, Spain
[5]Networking Research Center on Bioengineering, Biomaterials and Nanomedicine (CIBER-BBN), Valladolid, Spain

Correspondence should be addressed to Ivan Fernandez-Bueno; ifernandezb@ioba.med.uva.es

Academic Editor: Suphi Taneri

Purpose. To evaluate clinically and histologically the safety and biocompatibility of a new HDPE-based spherical porous orbital implants in rabbits. *Methods.* MEDPOR (Porex Surgical, Inc., Fairburn, GA, USA), OCULFIT I, and OCULFIT II (AJL Ophthalmic S.A., Vitoria, Spain) implants were implanted in eviscerated rabbis. Animals were randomly divided into 6 groups ($n = 4$ each) according to the 3 implant materials tested and 2 follow-up times of 90 or 180 days. Signs of regional pain and presence of eyelid swelling, conjunctival hyperemia, and amount of exudate were semiquantitatively evaluated. After animals sacrifice, the implants and surrounding ocular tissues were processed for histological staining and polarized light evaluation. Statistical study was performed by ANOVA and Kaplan-Meier analysis. *Results.* No statistically significant differences in regional pain, eyelid swelling, or conjunctival hyperemia were shown between implants and/or time points evaluated. However, amount of exudate differed, with OCULFIT I causing the smallest amount. No remarkable clinical complications were observed. Histological findings were similar in all three types of implants and agree with minor inflammatory response. *Conclusions.* OCULFIT ophthalmic tolerance and biocompatibility in rabbits were comparable to the clinically used MEDPOR. Clinical studies are needed to determine if OCULFIT is superior to the orbital implants commercially available.

1. Introduction

The first orbital implants were made of glass, plastic, cartilage, and silicone [1–4]. Although the motility of these implants proved to be excellent, the majority led to necrosis, infection, or exposure and was ultimately removed [5]. Hydroxyapatite and porous polyethylene were first introduced as new implant materials in the 1980s and in the 1990s, respectively [6, 7]. These porous implants have been successfully used for improving prosthetic motility and thus have provided a more natural and cosmetically pleasing look for anophthalmic patients [8].

At present, high-density polyethylene (HDPE) spherical implants, such as MEDPOR (Porex Surgical, Inc., Fairburn, GA, USA), are widely used for implantation into the resulting cavity of eviscerated or enucleated globes. HDPE implants are smooth and malleable, which make the implantation easier [7]. MEDPOR has pores greater than 150 μm, permitting the ingrowth of host vascular and soft tissue. This biointegration reduces the infection rates because it enables immune response to infection and allows delivery of systemically administered antibiotics [9, 10]. Nevertheless, the use of these materials is accompanied by some complications, such as

TABLE 1: Animal distribution and follow-up time for each orbital implant type.

Implants type	Number of animals (n)	Follow-up (days)
MEDPOR (Porex Surgical, Inc., Fairburn, GA, USA)	4	90
	4	180
OCULFIT I (AJL Ophthalmic S.A., Vitoria, Spain)	4	90
	4	180
OCULFIT II (AJL Ophthalmic S.A., Vitoria, Spain)	4	90
	4	180

blepharoptosis, eye discharge, implant exposure, conjunctival contracture and/or dehiscence, ectropion, and implant infection and/or extrusion [11]. To reduce complication rates, some changes in implant surface have been made, such as creating a smooth porous anterior surface that helps to reduce implant exposure (MEDPOR SST, Porex Surgical, Inc.) or giving a cone-shaped form to the implant (MEDPOR MCOI, Porex Surgical, Inc.). Although efforts have been made to reduce postoperative complications, reported rates of implant exposure still vary up to 34% [11–15], and it is necessary to remove the implant in up to 29% of the patients [7, 12, 16].

Because of the importance of anophthalmic implants to patients and because of the limitations described above of the existing implants, new materials and implant shape designs are currently under investigation. In this study, we used eviscerated rabbits to evaluate clinically and histologically the safety and biocompatibility of new HDPE-based spherical porous orbital implants (OCULFIT; AJL Ophthalmic S.A., Vitoria, Spain).

2. Materials and Methods

2.1. Experimental Animals. The use of animals in this study was in accordance with the recommendations of the Association for Research in Vision and Ophthalmology (ARVO) for the Use of Animals in Ophthalmic and Vision Research. It was approved by the Animal Research and Welfare Ethics Committee of the University of Valladolid (Spain) in agreement with European (Council Directive 2010/63/UE) and Spanish regulations (RD 53/2013). Twenty-four ($n = 24$) female rabbits (New Zealand White), weighing between 3.5 and 4.5 kg at implantation time, were used in this study. The animals had normal findings upon complete ophthalmic examinations consisting of slit-lamp biomicroscopy and indirect ophthalmoscopy. Animals were randomly divided into 6 groups ($n = 4$ each) according to 3 implant materials and 2 follow-up times per material (Table 1). HDPE spherical 12 mm diameter implants with smooth porous surface were used. The MEDPOR ($n = 8$; Porex Surgical, Inc.) is a clinically validated implant and served as the control. The OCULFIT I ($n = 8$; AJL Ophthalmic S.A.) is an HDPE-based implant, and the OCULFIT II ($n = 8$; AJL Ophthalmic S.A.) is a similar HDPE-based implant, but it is coated

with poly(ethylene glycol) diacrylate (PEGDA) hydrogel. The animals were followed up for 90 ($n = 12$) or 180 days ($n = 12$) after implantation. Animals housing was in accordance with the European regulation with free access to food and water during the experiment.

2.2. Surgical Technique. The surgical procedure was performed on the right eye of all rabbits. The animals were anesthetized by an intramuscular injection of ketamine (30 mg/kg; Imalgene 1000, Merial, Lyon, France) and xylazine (6 mg/kg; Rompún 2%, Bayer HealthCare, Kiel, Germany). Pinna and pedal reflexes were used to monitor the level of anesthesia. Prophylactic antibiotic treatment was established with benzylpenicillin procaine/benzathine (7 IU/kg; Shotapen LA, VIRBAC, Carros, France). Analgesia was applied by subcutaneous injection of butorphanol (0.1 mg/kg; Torbugesic Vet, Fort Dodge Animal Health, Fort Dodge, IA, USA). The periorbital area was cleansed by a solution of povidone iodine (5% Betadine; Meda Manufacturing, Bordeaux, France). Topical anesthesia was applied on the right eye prior to the surgical procedure (Colircusí Anestésico Doble; Alcon Cusí S.A., Barcelona, Spain). One milliliter of 1 : 200,000 epinephrine (1 mg/mL; B Braun Medical S.A., Barcelona, Spain) and 2% lidocaine (B Braun Medical S.A.) in phosphate-buffered saline (B Braun Medical S.A.) was given by a retrobulbar injection as a hemostatic agent and to minimize postoperative pain, respectively.

An eyelid speculum was placed to retract the eyelids prior to globe removal. A 360° conjunctival peritomy was performed, and Tenon's capsule was bluntly separated from the underlying sclera. A full-thickness incision around the corneal limbus of the right eye was made using a 15° blade knife (Alcon Laboratories, Inc., Fort Worth, TX, USA), and the entire cornea was removed. After separating the entire uvea from the scleral shell, all intraocular contents were completely removed using an Abadie curette (8 mm; Moria SA, Antony, France). The internal surface of the sclera was wiped with gauze soaked in 96% alcohol to denature any residual uveal pigment. To control hemorrhage, a disposable electrocautery pen (Bovie Medical Corporation, Clearwater, FL, USA) was used at the bleeding points of the scleral shell when necessary. Sclerotomy was performed by four relaxing radial scleral incisions between the rectus muscle insertions. Sterile intraocular 12 mm diameter implants were inserted, and the anterior sclera was closed with 5-0 polyglactin suture (Péters Surgical, Bobigny Cedex, France). The Tenon's capsule and the conjunctiva were closed with 6-0 polyglactin suture (Péters Surgical). Finally, ophthalmic tobramycin (Tobrex Ungüento; Alcon Cusí S.A.) was applied. Fentanyl sustained release patches (25 μg/h; Duragesic Matrix 25, Janssen-Cilag S.A., Madrid, Spain) were used postoperatively to maintain analgesia until 72 h [17, 18].

2.3. Clinical Evaluation. After surgery, clinical examinations were performed on days 1, 7, 15, 30, 45, 60, 90, 120, 150, and/or 180. Animals were not sedated for clinical evaluation. Signs of regional tenderness by palpation and presence of eyelid swelling, conjunctival hyperemia, and amount of exudate were evaluated in each rabbit according to Hackett and

McDonald irritation and inflammation scoring system [19]. The severity of these clinical signs was investigated and graded as none (0), mild (1), moderate (2), or severe (3) on each day of examination by the same ophthalmologist (SDL). Eye swelling and conjunctival hyperemia were assessed by slit-lamp biomicroscopy (Kowa SL-15; KowaOptimed Inc., CA, USA) in every follow-up time.

2.4. Histological Evaluation. The rabbits were anesthetized as previously described and then euthanized with intravenous injection of sodium pentobarbital (200 mg/kg; Dolethal, Vétoquinol, Cedex, France) at 90 or 180 days after implantation. A 5-0 polyglactin suture was placed at the central superior sclera to facilitate sample orientation during tissue processing. Then, the orbital content was exenerated.

The sockets were fixed for at least 24 hours in 10% formalin and then cut through the sagittal plane and processed in an automatic tissue processor (Leica ASP300; Leica Microsystems, Wetzlar, Germany). Two paraffin blocks from each socket were made. After that, multiple 3 μm thick microscope sections at different levels were obtained. Hematoxylin & eosin (HE; Merck KGaA, Darmstadt, Germany) and periodic acid of Schiff (PAS; Merck KGaA) stained slides were examined by standard light microscopy.

Evaluation of the overall inflammatory and tissue responses at the contact surface with the orbital implant was made by an experienced pathologist (JCL). All samples were also examined under polarized light.

2.5. Statistical Analysis. Statistical analysis of the clinical parameters was performed using R Statistical Software version 3.1.0 (Foundation for Statistical Computing, Vienna, Austria). The statistical significance level was set at 5%. Given the ordinal nature of clinical parameters, a Kruskal-Wallis one-way nonparametric analysis of variance (ANOVA) was used to compare median values of the three materials at each time point. Homogeneity of variance assumption was checked by the robust Brown-Forsythe Levene-type test using the group medians, implemented in R lawstat package [20]. Pairwise comparisons were performed by Mann-Whitney U tests with Bonferroni correction for multiple testing.

For each of the clinical parameters, the number of days until the value reached 0 (stabilization) was also evaluated. Kaplan-Meier survival analysis was applied to estimate the probability that the stabilization time exceeded time t. The log-rank test was used to compare the univariate stabilization times of the three implant types. The R survival package was used for this analysis [21].

3. Results

3.1. Clinical Evaluation. Clinical examinations were performed on days 1, 7, 15, 30, 45, 60, 90, 120, 150, and/or 180. Endpoint times were performed at 90 or 180 days after implantation. However, at 90 days after implantation, one animal in the MEDPOR group and one in the OCULFIT II group were lost to follow-up due to posterior paresis and subsequent ethical sacrifice. Their sockets were removed and submitted for histological processing and evaluation.

3.2. Clinical Parameter Follow-Up. There were no significant differences in regional tenderness, eyelid swelling, or conjunctival hyperemia among the different orbital implants and/or time points (Figures 1(a)–1(c)). However at 45 days after implantation, the exudate from eyes with OCULFIT II was significantly greater than that from eyes with OCULFIT I (p value: 0.0137) (Figure 1(d)). Comparison with MEDPOR was statistically significant at the 10% level (p values 0.0968 and 0.0644 for OCULFIT I and OCULFIT II, resp.), and differences in the amount of exudate were statistically different from 0 at 5% level. The amount of exudate in MEDPOR eyes was greater than OCULFIT I eyes (95% confidence interval [CI] MEDPOR, OCULFIT I: [0.04, 1.02]) and lower than OCULFIT II eyes (95% CI MEDPOR, OCULFIT II: [−1.69, −0.16]).

3.3. Time to Stabilization. For regional tenderness in all three groups, the average time for the rabbits to reach 0 (none) was 7 days (Figure 1(a)). There were no significant differences among the three survival curves (log-rank test: 1; p value: 0.612). For eye swelling in all three groups, the average time to reach 0 (none) edema was 11 days (Figure 1(b)). There were no significant differences among the three survival curves (log-rank test: 0; p value: 1). For conjunctival hyperemia, the average time to reach 0 (none) congestion was 15 days for the OCULFIT I group and 30 days for the MEDPOR and the OCULFIT II groups (Figure 1(c)). However, the differences among the three survival curves were not significant (log-rank test: 2.3; p value: 0.322). Exudate levels in none of the three groups became stabilized at 0 (none) during the 180-day follow-up (Figure 1(d)). At 90 days, 3 rabbits had 0 amount of exudate in the MEDPOR treated group, 4 in the OCULFIT I group, and only 2 in the OCULFIT II group. The probability of having exudate on day 90 was 0.571, 0.500, and 0.714, respectively, among the groups. There were no significant differences among the three survival curves (log-rank test: 1.1; p value: 0.585). At 180 days, the median exudate values were 0 in the MEDPOR group and 0.5 in the OCULFIT I and OCULFIT II groups. For the OCULFIT I group, the median exudate value remained unchanged at 0.5 from 60 days to the end of the experiment. For the OCULFIT II group, the median exudate value remained at 0.5 from 120 days. Neither OCULFIT group reached 0.

3.4. Histological Evaluation. After cutting the sclera with the implants in the sagittal plane, the inner implant materials were exposed. The MEDPOR implant appeared as an aggregate of small spherical granules of about 1 mm diameter (Figure 2(a)). In contrast, both OCULFIT inserts looked more compact and composed of multiple microgranules (Figure 2(b)). On gross examination, peripheral fibrovascularization from orbital tissue was also noted for all three implants.

Under polarized light, two types of birefringent materials were identified at 90 and 180 days (Figure 3). All three types of implant specimens appeared as birefringent intraocular solid material adjacent to the internal surface of the sclera (Figures 3(a) and 3(b)). Furthermore, another material composed of birefringent cylindrical units and consistent with

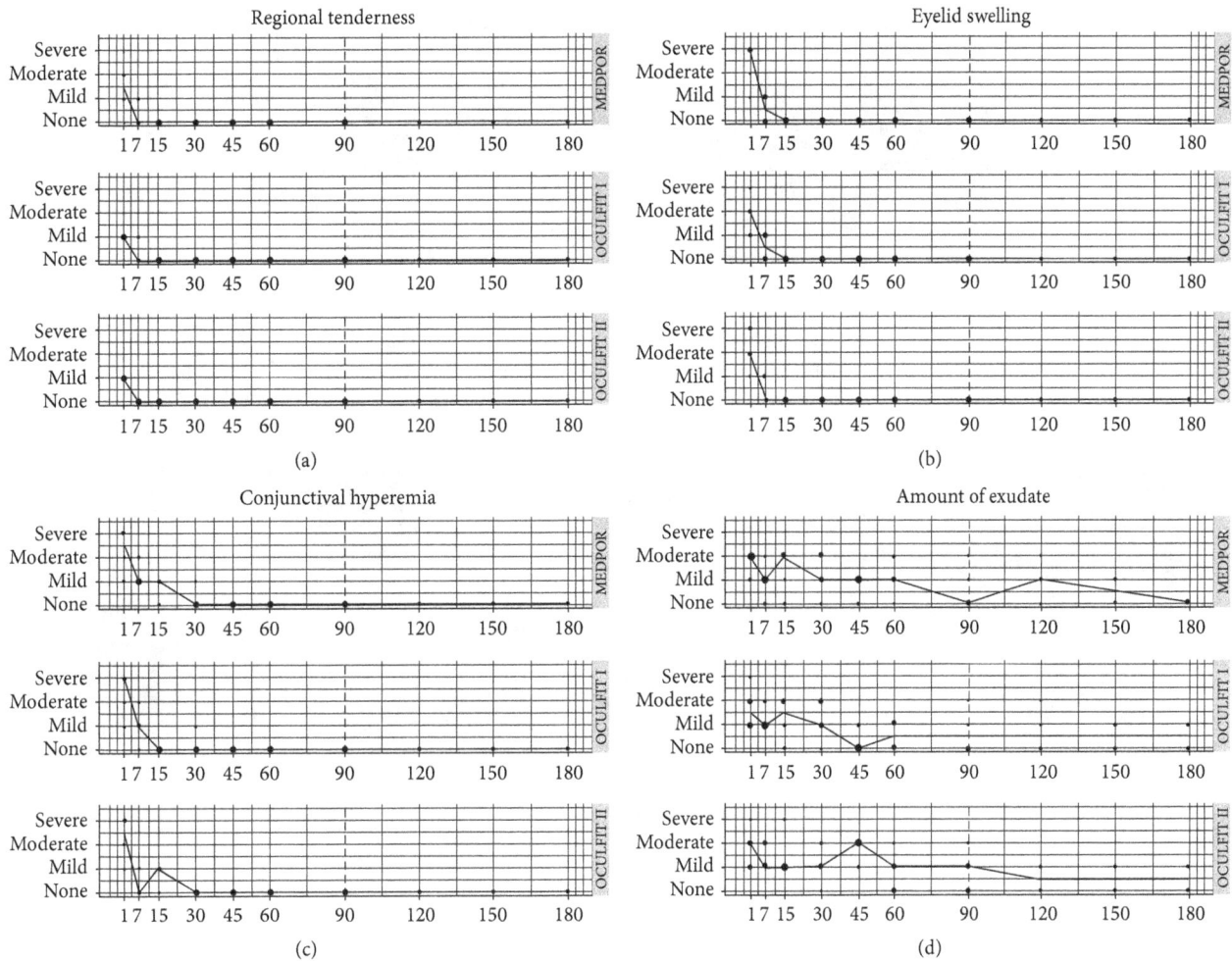

FIGURE 1: Clinical evaluation follow-up after orbital implantation. The severities of regional tenderness (a), eyelid swelling (b), conjunctival hyperemia (c), and amount of exudate (d) were recorded at each time point after insertion of the MEDPOR, OCULFIT I, and OCULFIT II implants. Clinical signs were graded as none, mild, moderate, or severe according to Hackett and McDonald scoring system [19]. Clinical examinations were performed on days 1, 7, 15, 30, 45, 60, 90, 120, 150, and 180 after implantation. Bubble sizes are proportional to the number of animals.

surgical suture was present in the peripheral adipose tissue (Figure 3(c)).

The main histological findings in HE and PAS stained slides were similar in all three types of implants evaluated at both time points. The most common changes included the presence of a loose granulation tissue with an associated foreign body giant cell reaction (Figures 4(a)–4(c)). Also, metaplastic changes (bone marrow metaplasia) were present in two MEDPOR samples (Figure 4(d)), and focal intraocular hemorrhage was present in two OCULFIT I samples (Figure 4(e)). Two OCULFIT II specimens (Figure 4(f)) had focal osseous metaplasia.

4. Discussion

The present study described the ophthalmic and histological evaluation of two new HDPE-based spherical integrated porous orbital implants (OCULFIT) in rabbits. Globe removal is a traumatic event for the patient. Cosmetic results are remarkably important to limit the postoperative psychological effects of the patient [22]. In this sense, there were remarkable advancements in orbital implant surgery during the latter part of the 20th century. Spherical integrated porous orbital implants have been widely used throughout the world [9]. However, postoperative complications and implant removal still occur [11–16] and new products have to be studied. Preclinical studies are necessary prior to clinically used approval. In this sense, the socket of rabbits after evisceration of the globe is a widely and currently used model to adequately test intraocular implants [23–25]. In this experimental study in rabbits, we found that, at 90 and 180 days, the tolerance and biocompatibility of the OCULFIT implants was as good as the MEDPOR, an implant in current clinical use.

OCULFIT implants are designed to be implanted into the socket after evisceration of the globes. Different biopolymers have been added to the HDPE to improve flexibility and hydrophilicity of the implants. OCULFIT orbital implants

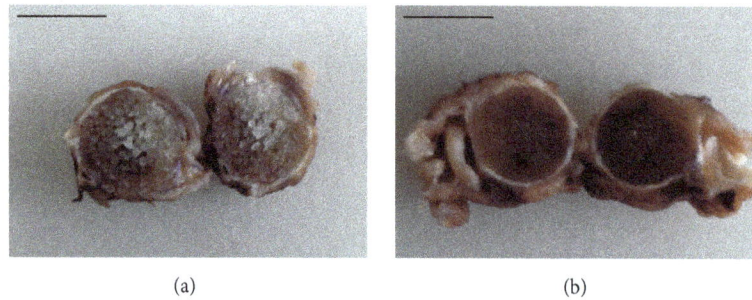

(a)   (b)

FIGURE 2: Macroscopic findings at 90 days after orbital implantation. After cutting the eyes through the sagittal plane, the MEDPOR implant (a) appeared as an aggregate of small spherical granules, while OCULFIT I (b), as well as OCULFIT II, was more compact and composed of multiple microgranules. Peripheral ingrowth of host vasculature and soft tissue was present in both materials. Scale bars: 12 mm.

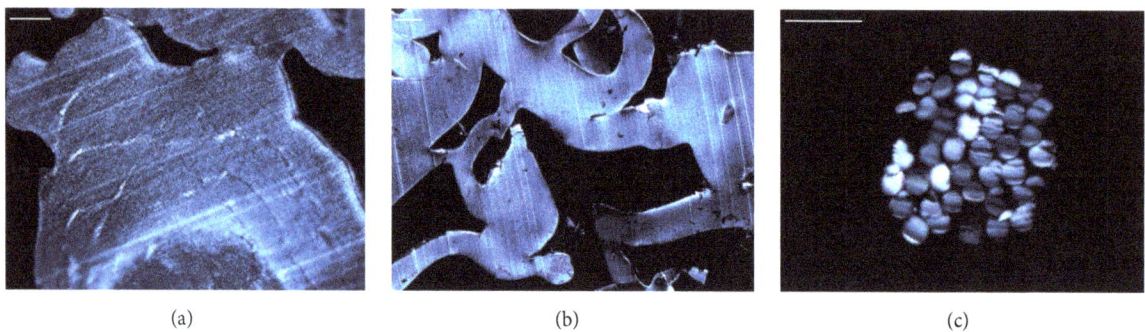

(a)   (b)   (c)

FIGURE 3: Histological evaluation under polarized light at 90 days after orbital implantation. Orbital implants MEDPOR, OCULFIT I, and OCULFIT II appeared as birefringent intraocular solid material adjacent to the internal surface of the sclera ((a), (b)). Birefringent cylindrical units were present in the peripheral adipose tissue (c). Scale bars: 20 μm ((a), MEDPOR; (c)) and 50 μm ((b), OCULFIT II).

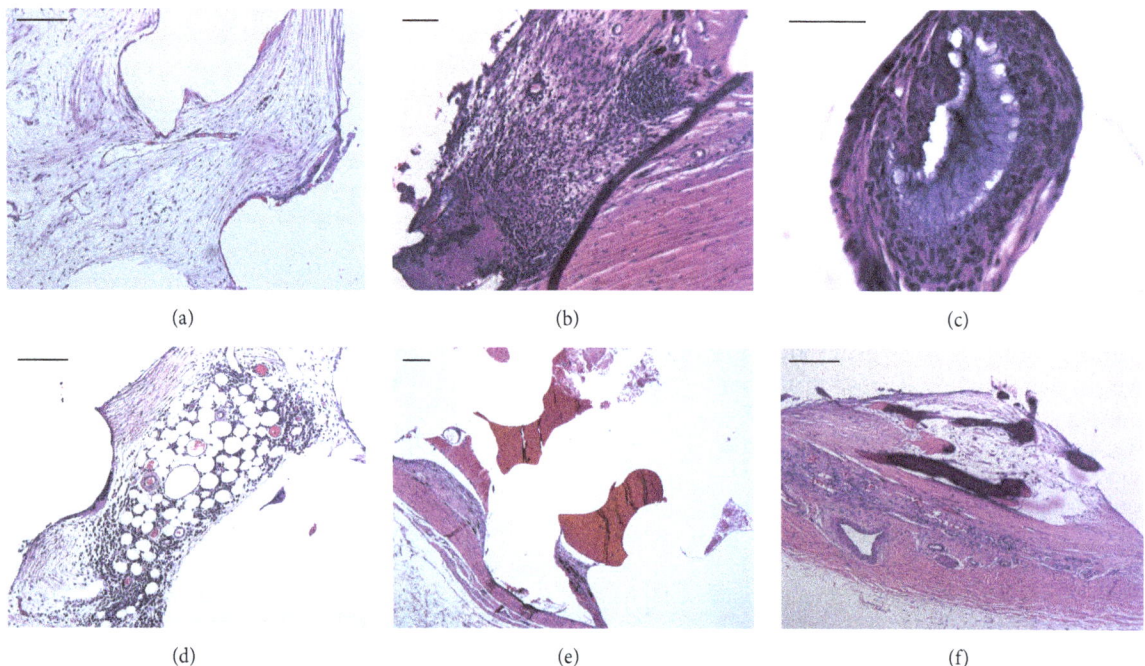

(a)   (b)   (c)

(d)   (e)   (f)

FIGURE 4: Histological findings in hematoxylin & eosin (HE) stained sections at 180 days after orbital implantation. Loose granulation tissue (a) with an associated foreign body giant cell reaction ((b), (c)) was commonly observed at 90 and 180 days after MEDPOR, OCULFIT I, and OCULFIT II implantation. Metaplastic changes (d), focal intraocular hemorrhage (e), and focal osseous metaplasia (f) were occasionally observed at 180 days after MEDPOR, OCULFIT I, and OCULFIT II implantation, respectively. Scale bars: 50 μm ((a), (d), MEDPOR; (e), OCULFIT I; (f), OCULFIT II) and 20 μm ((b), OCULFIT I; (c), OCULFIT II).

have an interconnected, opened porous structure that allows the ingrowth of host orbital vasculature and soft tissue, which integrates the implant with the host's body. The OCULFIT implants have a smooth anterior surface and a posterior porous surface that helps implant integration and minimizes their exposure. The difference between OCULFIT I and OCULFIT II is that the latter is covered with poly(ethylene glycol) diacrylate (PEGDA) hydrogel, which increases the hydrophilicity and theoretically reduces the integration time of the implants. In the experimental study presented here, both OCULFIT I and OCULFIT II were similar with respect to regional tenderness, eyelid swelling, and conjunctival hyperemia. However, the OCULFIT I caused small amount of exudate during the follow-up period; conjunctival hyperemia was stabilized 15 days before the OCULFIT II; and OCULFIT I had better results regarding the amount of exudate present.

MEDPOR, a polyporous form of polyethylene, is now widely used to compensate for the loss of volume in an anophthalmic socket after globe removal [8, 11]. In addition to its use in anophthalmic socket surgery, MEDPOR is commonly used in craniofacial reconstruction surgery. The porous character of MEDPOR enables fibrovascular proliferation of orbital tissue, reduces the risk of migration, exposure, and extrusion, and minimizes the risk of infection [9, 10]. MEDPOR has a hydrophobic and negatively charged surface that acts as a protective envelope to inhibit the adherence of bacteria and to reduce the postoperative infection rate [26]. This material is also nontoxic, nonallergenic, and highly biocompatible. MEDPOR is currently a very popular orbital implant material and [11], thus, an adequate, clinically validated control to test the tolerance and biocompatibility characteristics of the OCULFIT implants.

In our follow-up clinical evaluations, we found that the three implants tested were similar with respect to regional tenderness, eyelid swelling, and conjunctival hyperemia. However, OCULFIT I caused the smallest amount of exudate during the follow-up period, while MEDPOR induced more and OCULFIT II induced the most exudate. Conjunctival hyperemia was stabilized with OCULFIT I 15 days before the other two materials; and furthermore, it had considerably better results regarding the amount of exudate present. Although the amount of exudate did not become stabilized at 0 during either the 90 days or the 180 days of follow-up periods, the differences between the 0 and 0.5 median exudate values were not clinically relevant. In this case, OCULFIT I became stabilized at 60 days, OCULFIT II at 120 days, and MEDPOR at 180 days. However, there were no significant statistical differences in any case. The presence of continuous exudate during this study may be secondary to implant movement (rubbing) over the sclero-conjunctival surface, as previously described in human patients [22, 27], or remnant tear secretion due to nonremoval of the lacrimal glands. Exudate cultures to detect possible infectious origin were not performed in this study.

Macroscopic evaluation of the implant during tissue processing revealed differences between the MEDPOR and OCULFIT implants regarding the internal structure of the polyethylene granules. This finding may be due to manufacturing differences. However, we observed no differences in microscopic structure when the implants were viewed under polarized light. The birefringent cylindrical units found in the peripheral adipose tissue may correspond to surgical sutures that were used to close the scleral and conjunctival tissues and which did not absorb.

The histological findings were consistent with those previously observed in experimental rabbits [23–25] and in human patients where orbital inflammatory responses to integrated implants, characterized by a foreign body giant cell reaction, have been described [28, 29]. Host tissue growing into an implant does not turn off the foreign body response [7]. During the follow-up period, we found neither implant exposure nor infection clinical signs, which are the most serious complications associated with integrated orbital implants after globe removal [26]. We did find focal intraocular hemorrhage in two OCULFIT I samples. These may have been secondary to implant movement. Metaplastic modifications found in MEDPOR and OCULFIT II specimens were also previously described in anophthalmic sockets with an ocular implant [30].

5. Conclusions

In summary, OCULFIT ophthalmic tolerance and biocompatibility in rabbits were comparable to the clinically used MEDPOR orbital implant. Indeed, OCULFIT I had better experimental results. Although OCULFIT II implants induce more exudate in this animal study, the PEGDA hydrogel used to coat them may be loaded with growth factors that can be released in a controlled fashion to reduce the inflammatory response after implantation procedure. In this sense, OCULFIT II implants open a new opportunity to induce rapid integration with the recipient's tissues. Clinical studies are needed to determine conclusively if OCULFIT is superior to the orbital implants commercially available at present.

Conflict of Interests

Ivan Alvarez and Eva Larra are employees of AJL Ophthalmic S.A. All the other authors report no conflict of interests.

Acknowledgments

The authors would like to thank Ms. Nieves Fernandez (IOBA, Spain) for her technical assistance in the histological processing of tissue samples and Britt Bromberg, Ph.D., of Xenofile Editing, for his collaboration with the English version of the paper. This research has been the result of several projects supported by different grants from Gobierno del Pais Vasco (Gaitek IG-2010/0000113 and Etorgai IEI09-018) and Centro para el Desarrollo Tecnologico Industrial (CDTI) with collaboration of Ministerio de Economia y Competitividad (CENIT CEN-20091021). Ivan Fernandez-Bueno was supported by Centro en Red de Medicina Regenerativa y Terapia Celular de Castilla y Leon, Spain.

References

[1] A. Hornblass and B. J. Herschorn, "Double sphere orbital implantation in enucleation and evisceration," *Ophthalmic Plastic and Reconstructive Surgery*, vol. 1, no. 1, pp. 65–68, 1985.

[2] A. G. Tyers and J. R. O. Collin, "Baseball orbital implants: a review of 39 patients," *British Journal of Ophthalmology*, vol. 69, no. 6, pp. 438–442, 1985.

[3] H. A. Helms, H. E. Zeiger Jr., and A. Callahan, "Complications following enucleation and implantation of multiple glass spheres in the orbit," *Ophthalmic Plastic & Reconstructive Surgery*, vol. 3, no. 2, pp. 87–89, 1987.

[4] I. den Tonkelaar, H. E. Henkes, and G. K. van Leersum, "Herman Snellen (1834–1908) and Muller's 'reform-auge'. A short history of the artificial eye," *Documenta Ophthalmologica*, vol. 77, no. 4, pp. 349–354, 1991.

[5] W. J. Johnson, "The perfect socket: the ocularist's view," in *Principles and Practice of Ophthalmic Plastic and Reconstructive Surgery*, S. Bosniak, Ed., pp. 1127–1133, W.B. Saunders, Philadelphia, Pa, USA, 1996.

[6] A. C. Perry, "Integrated orbital implants.," *Advances in Ophthalmic Plastic and Reconstructive Surgery*, vol. 8, pp. 75–81, 1990.

[7] R. A. Goldberg, S. C. Dresner, R. A. Braslow, N. Kossovsky, and A. Legmann, "Animal model of porous polyethylene orbital implants," *Ophthalmic Plastic and Reconstructive Surgery*, vol. 10, no. 2, pp. 104–109, 1994.

[8] D. M. Moshfeghi, A. A. Moshfeghi, and P. T. Finger, "Enucleation," *Survey of Ophthalmology*, vol. 44, no. 4, pp. 277–301, 2000.

[9] A. Hornblass, B. S. Biesman, and J. A. Eviatar, "Current techniques of enucleation: a survey of 5,439 intraorbital implants and a review of the literature," *Ophthalmic Plastic & Reconstructive Surgery*, vol. 11, no. 2, pp. 77–88, 1995.

[10] S. Lee, N. Maronian, S. P. Most et al., "Porous high-density polyethylene for orbital reconstruction," *Archives of Otolaryngology—Head and Neck Surgery*, vol. 131, no. 5, pp. 446–450, 2005.

[11] S.-K. Jung, W.-K. Cho, J.-S. Paik, and S.-W. Yang, "Long-term surgical outcomes of porous polyethylene orbital implants: a review of 314 cases," *British Journal of Ophthalmology*, vol. 96, no. 4, pp. 494–498, 2012.

[12] P. L. Custer and K. M. Trinkaus, "Porous implant exposure: Incidence, management, and morbidity," *Ophthalmic Plastic and Reconstructive Surgery*, vol. 23, no. 1, pp. 1–7, 2007.

[13] D. Liu, "Evisceration techniques and implant extrusion rates: a retrospective review of two series and a survey of ASOPRS surgeons," *Ophthalmic Plastic and Reconstructive Surgery*, vol. 23, no. 1, pp. 16–21, 2007.

[14] C. L. Shields, Y. Uysal, B. P. Marr et al., "Experience with the polymer-coated hydroxyapatite implant after enucleation in 126 patients," *Ophthalmology*, vol. 114, no. 2, pp. 367–373, 2007.

[15] Z. Tabatabaee, M. Mazloumi, M. T. Rajabi et al., "Comparison of the exposure rate of wrapped hydroxyapatite (Bio-Eye) versus unwrapped porous polyethylene (Medpor) orbital implants in enucleated patients," *Ophthalmic Plastic & Reconstructive Surgery*, vol. 27, no. 2, pp. 114–118, 2011.

[16] J. Y. Chuo, P. J. Dolman, T. L. Ng, F. V. Buffam, and V. A. White, "Clinical and histopathologic review of 18 explanted porous polyethylene orbital implants," *Ophthalmology*, vol. 116, no. 2, pp. 349–354, 2009.

[17] P. L. Foley, A. L. Henderson, E. A. Bissonette, G. R. Wimer, and S. H. Feldman, "Evaluation of fentanyl transdermal patches in rabbits: blood concentrations and physiologic response," *Comparative Medicine*, vol. 51, no. 3, pp. 239–244, 2001.

[18] J. Liaw and Y.-C. Lin, "Evaluation of poly(ethylene oxide)-poly(propylene oxide)-poly(ethylene oxide) (PEO-PPO-PEO) gels as a release vehicle for percutaneous fentanyl," *Journal of Controlled Release*, vol. 68, no. 2, pp. 273–282, 2000.

[19] R. B. Hackett and T. O. McDonald, "Eye irritation," in *Advances in Modern Toxicology: Dermatoxicology*, F. Marzulli and H. Maibach, Eds., pp. 749–815, Hemisphere Publishing Corporation, Washington, DC, USA, 4th edition, 1991.

[20] J. L. Gastwirth, Y. R. Gel, W. L. W. Hui, V. Lyubchich, W. Miao, and K. Noguchi, *Lawstat: An R Package for Biostatistics, Public Policy, and Law. R Package Version 2.4.*, 2013.

[21] T. Therneau, "A Package for Survival Analysis in S. R package version 2.37-4," 2013.

[22] J.-S. Song, J. Oh, and S. H. Baek, "A survey of satisfaction in anophthalmic patients wearing ocular prosthesis," *Graefe's Archive for Clinical and Experimental Ophthalmology*, vol. 244, no. 3, pp. 330–335, 2006.

[23] D. Miyashita, F. Chahud, G. E. B. da Silva, V. B. de Albuquerque, D. M. Garcia, and A. A. V. E Cruz, "Tissue ingrowth into perforated polymethylmethacrylate orbital implants: an experimental study," *Ophthalmic Plastic and Reconstructive Surgery*, vol. 29, no. 3, pp. 160–163, 2013.

[24] K. Kalwerisky, L. Mihora, C. N. Czyz, J. A. Foster, and D. E. E. Holck, "Rate of vascularization and exposure of silicone-capped porous polyethylene spherical implants: an animal model," *Ophthalmic Plastic and Reconstructive Surgery*, vol. 29, no. 5, pp. 350–356, 2013.

[25] D. R. Jordan, S. Brownstein, M. Dorey, V. H. Yuen, and S. Gilberg, "Fibrovascularization of porous polyethylene (Medpor) orbital implant in a rabbit model," *Ophthalmic Plastic and Reconstructive Surgery*, vol. 20, no. 2, pp. 136–143, 2004.

[26] J.-R. You, J.-H. Seo, Y.-H. Kim, and W.-C. Choi, "Six cases of bacterial infection in porous orbital implants," *Japanese Journal of Ophthalmology*, vol. 47, no. 5, pp. 512–518, 2003.

[27] D. R. Jordan, S. Gilberg, and A. Bawazeer, "Coralline hydroxyapatite orbital implant (bio-eye): experience with 158 patients," *Ophthalmic Plastic and Reconstructive Surgery*, vol. 20, no. 1, pp. 69–74, 2004.

[28] M. Rosner, D. P. Edward, and M. O. M. Tso, "Foreign-body giant-cell reaction to the hydroxyapatite orbital implant," *Archives of Ophthalmology*, vol. 110, no. 2, pp. 173–174, 1992.

[29] W. R. Nunery, G. W. Heinz, J. M. Bonnin, R. T. Martin, and M. A. Cepela, "Exposure rate of hydroxyapatite spheres in the anophthalmic socket: histopathologic correlation and comparison with silicone sphere implants," *Ophthalmic Plastic and Reconstructive Surgery*, vol. 9, no. 2, pp. 96–104, 1993.

[30] J. H. Kim, M. J. Lee, H.-K. Choung et al., "Conjunctival cytologic features in anophthalmic patients wearing an ocular prosthesis," *Ophthalmic Plastic and Reconstructive Surgery*, vol. 24, no. 4, pp. 290–295, 2008.

13

Evaluation of the Effectiveness of Surgical Treatment of Malignant Glaucoma in Pseudophakic Eyes through Partial PPV with Establishment of Communication between the Anterior Chamber and the Vitreous Cavity

Marek Rękas,[1] Karolina Krix-Jachym,[1] and Tomasz Żarnowski[2]

[1]*Ophthalmology Department, Military Institute of Medicine, Szaserów Street 128, 04-141 Warsaw, Poland*
[2]*Department of Diagnostics and Microsurgery of Glaucoma, Medical University of Lublin, Chmielna Street 1, 20-079 Lublin, Poland*

Correspondence should be addressed to Marek Rękas; rekaspl@gmail.com

Academic Editor: Paolo Fogagnolo

Purpose. Determination of partial posterior vitrectomy (PPV) in the proposed modification for treatment of malignant glaucoma. *Methods.* The prospective, consecutive, single-center case series study involved patients in whom symptoms of malignant glaucoma occurred after combined cataract and glaucoma surgery or after glaucoma surgery in pseudophakic eye. When medical and laser treatment were not successful, partial PPV with establishment of communication between the anterior chamber and the vitreous cavity was performed. Efficacy measures were intraocular pressure (IOP) reduction, corrected distance visual acuity (CDVA), AND the number of antiglaucoma medications. Surgical success and occurring complications were also evaluated. *Results.* The study enrolled 20 eyes of 17 patients. Average IOP was reduced from 30.4 ± 14.2 (SD) mmHg to 14.6 ± 3.2 (SD) mmHg one year after surgery ($P < 0.00001$). A statistically significant reduction of the number of antiglaucoma medications was obtained from 3.3 ± 1.1 (SD) preoperatively to 1.2 ± 1.1 (SD) at the end of follow-up. Statistically significant improvement of CDVA was observed 3, 6, and 12 months after surgery. *Conclusions.* Partial PPV with establishment of communication between the anterior chamber and the vitreous cavity enables effective IOP control over a 12-month observation; however, in most cases, it is necessary to use antiglaucoma medications for IOP control.

1. Introduction

Surgical treatment of malignant glaucoma is based on interrupting the sequence of events lying at the foundation of its pathophysiological process. In the classical form of this complication, aqueous humor accumulates in the area of the vitreous cavity due to ciliary block, and, as a result of this, there is an increase in the vitreous pressure that is transferred to the structures of the anterior segment causing a forward movement of the lens-iris diaphragm [1]. Most often, malignant glaucoma develops quickly, within days after primary surgery with a clear cause-effect relationship with the performed procedure, although its occurrence can also be postponed [2–4]. Recurrences of malignant glaucoma are observed both after PPV that was initially effective and after conservative treatment [5–8]. It seems that the characteristic clinical picture of malignant glaucoma with recurrences is caused by the preservation of the primary mechanism that is found at the basis of aqueous humor accumulation in the posterior segment of the eye.

Observations resulting from the application of PPV for the treatment of malignant glaucoma in pseudophakic eyes make it possible to state that elimination of adhesion of the vitreous body, lens capsule, and its zonula to the plane of the iris, pupil, and iridectomy restores normal aqueous humor flow from the posterior to the anterior segment of the eye [6, 9]. While PPV unburdens the vitreous chamber and improves anatomical proportions in the anterior chamber, preservation of communication between the posterior and anterior segments of the eye is decisive to the stability of this procedure.

Surgical treatment in malignant glaucoma is usually applied when conservative and laser treatment do not have the intended effect [6, 9, 10]. On the other hand, the time that passes from diagnosis has an impact on the nature of complications and the effectiveness of surgical procedure. Certain authors stress that the greatest chance for permanent success of PPV in the case of malignant glaucoma is related to quick implementation of surgical treatment [11].

The goal of the study was to evaluate surgical treatment of malignant glaucoma in pseudophakic eyes by partial PPV extended by communication of the anterior chamber and vitreous cavity through removal of zonules and of the anterior and posterior capsule in the area of the iridectomy which was formed during primary glaucoma surgery.

2. Materials and Methods

2.1. Patients. The following treatment schedule was applied when symptoms of malignant glaucoma occurred: mannitol 2 g per kg intravenously once or twice a day, acetazolamide 250 mg *tid*, and locally: atropine 1% *qid*, Cosopt (dorzolamide hydrochloride-timolol maleate ophthalmic solution) *bid*, and 0.1% dexamethasone phosphate *tid*. The next step was laser treatment (capsulotomy through the iridectomy). These methods were of temporary effect in most cases. Sustainable improvement after medical and laser treatment was obtained in only 2 cases (9.1%). Regardless of using all available methods most of malignant glaucoma cases (20 eyes) needed to be treated surgically because of a weak effect of conservative treatment. The indication for surgical treatment was diagnosis of malignant glaucoma in eyes after cataract and glaucoma surgery or after glaucoma surgery in pseudophakic eyes based on symptoms such as progressive increase of IOP together with axial shallowing of the anterior chamber in the presence of a patent iridotomy, despite the application of conservative and laser treatment [6, 9, 10, 12, 13].

All patients required IOP reduction and restoration of anatomical relationships to prevent further progression of malignant glaucoma and its complications.

Exclusion criteria included suprachoroidal hemorrhage, pupillary block, hypotony progressing with shallowing of the anterior chamber or choroidal detachment, and inflammation in the anterior or posterior segment of the eyeball requiring conservative or surgical procedures of a different type.

Seventeen patients (20 eyes) with symptoms of malignant glaucoma occurring at various time after primary surgery were recruited into the study.

2.2. Preoperative Examination. During qualification, medical history concerning prior procedures and applied treatments was taken. During baseline examination, IOP, uncorrected distance visual acuity (UDVA), and corrected distance visual acuity (CDVA) were measured, the anterior segment was examined with consideration of anterior chamber depth, eye

fundus examination along with evaluation of c/d and measurement of central corneal thickness and axial length (AXL) was performed, and gonioscopic examination was conducted. The anterior and posterior segments were evaluated in terms of fulfillment of the inclusion criteria.

2.3. Surgical Technique. All surgeries were performed with retrobulbar anesthesia (2% xylocaine and 0.5% bupivacaine) by one surgeon (M.R.). The anterior chamber was opened (1.2 mm) at the 5:00 or 7:00 position depending on the eye that was being operated on. The anterior chamber was filled with viscoelastic (Viscoat, Alcon Laboratories, Inc.). A trocar was inserted into the vitreous cavity through the pars plana at a distance of 3.5 mm from the corneal limbus, and after that 25-gauge PPV was performed, which included removal of the anterior part of the vitreous body. After the vitreous chamber was unburdened, the anterior chamber was filled using Viscoat, adhesions around the present iridectomy, iris-lens adhesions, iridocorneal adhesions, and iris-capsule adhesions were released, and then the anterior chamber was opened in the projection of the iridectomy. A 25-gauge needle was inserted through this opening, puncturing the anterior and posterior capsule in the area of the iridectomy. There are few possible ways (through the anterior chamber or from behind) to clear the iridectomy and all of these methods can be used interchangeably. The iridectomy, posterior capsulotomy, and hyaloidotomy may be performed using a vitrectomy tip or using other surgical instruments. In this case series fragments of the circumferential capsule and zonula were removed with a 25-gauge vitrector, and communication was established between the anterior and posterior chamber and vitreous cavity.

During the surgery we pay particular attention to performing vitrectomy in properly wide range in case the vitreous remnants do not disturb the flow through iridotomy and at the end of surgery we avoid leaving the vitreous in the sclerotomies.

At the end of surgery, after the spontaneous deepening of anterior chamber was achieved, the site of the previously performed glaucoma surgery was revised, the anterior chamber was filled using Viscoat, and wounds in the corneal limbus were sealed, sometimes with the application of single Nylon 10/0 sutures.

2.4. Postoperative Protocol. Standard ophthalmological examination was performed on days 1 and 7 and 1, 3, 6, and 12 months after surgery. IOP, UDVA, and CDVA (Snellen chart and log MAR) were determined, and the anterior and posterior segments of the eye were examined. Postoperative course was analyzed, including the occurrence of complications and the number of applied antiglaucoma medications.

Complete surgical success was defined for two criteria: IOP $\leq$ 18 mmHg and IOP $\leq$ 21 mmHg without antiglaucoma medications, and satisfactory success was defined as IOP at these two levels without and with a maximum of two antiglaucoma medications. Ineffectiveness of the previous filtration procedure was identified when IOP $\geq$ 21 mmHg was stated or when it was necessary to use antiglaucoma medications [14].

Complications were qualified as "early" if they occurred in the first week after surgery; other complications were qualified as "late" complications. A postoperative IOP $\geq$ 21 mmHg was considered to be raised. Cystoid macular edema was stated based on deterioration of visual acuity and characteristic biomicroscopic image, and optical coherent tomography (OCT) was performed in order to confirm the diagnosis [15]. Other complications were identified based on clinical picture. A recurrence of malignant glaucoma was considered to be shallowing of the anterior chamber with accompanying progressive IOP increase after malignant glaucoma surgery. In the case of recurrence or suspected obstruction resulting from the formation of fibrin membranes in the area of iridectomy, unblocking of communication between the anterior and posterior segments was performed using Nd:YAG laser with energy 1–5 mJ.

2.5. Statistical Analysis.

Statistical analysis of the investigated variables was performed with the Shapiro-Wilk and paired Wilcoxon tests. Friedman ANOVA for matched groups and rank means and rank sums were also used for post hoc comparison. The Kaplan-Meier method was used to determine survival curves, and differences between them were tested by the log-rank test. A P value of 0.05 or less was considered significant. The calculations were performed with Statistica 10.0 PL.

3. Results

3.1. Demographic Data.

From January 2005 to March 2010 1689 eyes were treated with glaucoma surgery in single clinic (Military Institute of Medicine in Warsaw), 960 (56.8%) with penetrating surgery and 729 (43.2%) with nonpenetrating surgery. 1417 (83.9%) of conducted surgeries were combined with phacoemulsification, while 272 (16.1%) were antiglaucoma surgeries without phacoemulsification. The decision to perform a combined procedure depended on vision loss connected with cataract development, the number of antiglaucoma medications used, and the state of the glaucoma. Subtype of the glaucoma surgery was chosen individually for each patient.

In analyzed material malignant glaucoma occurred in 22 eyes (1.3%). Among patients with penetrating surgery, malignant glaucoma occurred in 2.3% of patients, whereas after nonpenetrating surgery this complication was not found ($P = 0.00004$). The statement was made that penetrating surgery is the risk factor of malignant glaucoma occurrence. The risk of malignant glaucoma after phacotrabeculectomy and phacoiridencleisis was equivalent ($P = 0.058$). When the frequency of malignant glaucoma after trabeculectomy and iridencleisis was compared, the difference was not statistically significant ($P = 0.416$). In the group of patients with malignant glaucoma 40.9% eyes underwent surgical treatment with the method of phacoiridencleisis, 22.7% phacotrabeculectomy, 18.2% iridencleisis, 13.6% trabeculectomy, and 4.5% seton valve implantation before this complication occurred. The phakic eyes with malignant glaucoma and malignant

TABLE 1: Patients' demographic data.

Demographic data	Mean (SD)	Me	Range
AXL	21.8 ± 0.8	21.9	19.9–23.8
IOL (D)	24.9 ± 2.4	24.5	22.0–32.0
CCT (μm)	539.5 ± 26.9	541.5	492.0–579.0
ACD (mm)	1.8 ± 0.6	2.0	0.5–2.3
c/d	0.8 ± 0.2	0.8	0.3–1.0
$CDVA_0$ (log MAR)	0.9 ± 0.7	0.7	0.1–2.3
IOP_0	30.4 ± 14.2	25.0	17.0–65.0

AXL: axial length; IOL: intraocular lens; CCT: central corneal thickness; ACD: anterior chamber depth; c/d: cup/disc ratio; $CDVA_0$: corrected distance visual acuity before surgery; IOP_0: intraocular pressure before surgery; SD: standard deviation; Me: median number.

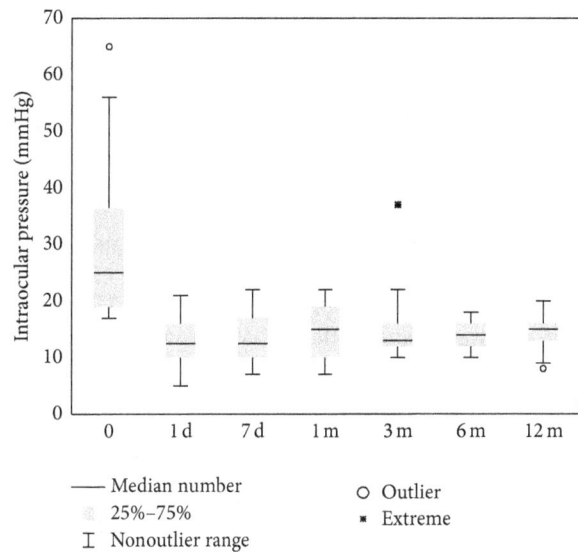

FIGURE 1: Median number, outlier, and extreme of intraocular pressure at specific time after surgery.

glaucoma cases after cataract surgery were not analyzed for the study purpose.

Twenty eyes of 17 patients (15 women, 2 men) with an average age of 62.9 ± 13.3 (SD) years (Me 64, range: 43–85 years) were recruited into the study. The mean time elapsed from primary glaucoma surgery was about two months but differed markedly equal to 61.4 ± 190.5 (SD) days (Me 2.5; from 1 to 840 days). The mean time of observation was 405 ± 366.1 (SD) days (Me 360; from 7 to 1440 days). Demographic data is presented in Table 1.

3.2. Intraocular Pressure Control.

During a 12-month observation period, significant variance of the IOP value was stated ($\chi^2_{ANOVA} = 38.73$; $P < 0.001$), which resulted from statistically significant IOP reduction on day 1 after surgery (rank means 3.72, rank sum 67.0, and $P < 0.05$) that was maintained until the end of observation ($\chi^2_{ANOVA} = 2.51$; $P = 0.77462$) (Figure 1, Table 2).

Preoperative mean IOP was 30.4 ± 14.2 (SD) mmHg and decreased during the first day, on average, by 49.3% (range: 11.8–80.8%) to 13.4 ± 4.4 (SD) mmHg (rank means 3.72, rank

TABLE 2: Mean values, median number, standard deviations, ranges of intraocular pressure, and number of medications at specific times after surgery.

Time	Intraocular pressure (mmHg)				Medications (n)			
	Mean (SD)	Me	Range	$P^\wedge$	Mean (SD)	Me	Range	P^*
Pre-op	30.4 ± 14.2	25	17–65		3.3 ± 1.1	3	1–5	
1st day	13.4 ± 4.4	12.5	5–21	<0.05	0.0 ± 0.0	0	—	0.000089
7th day	13.3 ± 4.4	12.5	7–22	<0.05	0.0 ± 0.2	0	0-1	0.000089
1st month	14.6 ± 4.6	15	7–22	<0.05	0.5 ± 1.0	0	0–3	0.000196
3rd month	15.2 ± 6.1	13	10–37	<0.05	0.7 ± 1.1	0	0–4	0.000196
6th month	14.4 ± 2.5	14	10–18	<0.05	0.9 ± 1.0	1	0–3	0.000982
12th month	14.6 ± 3.2	15	8–20	<0.05	1.2 ± 1.1	1	0–3	0.002218

SD: standard deviation; n: number of medications; Friedman ANOVA (χ^2_{ANOVA} = 38.73; P < 0.001); post hoc test (rank means, rank sum)$^\wedge$; Wilcoxon signed-rank test*; Me: median number.

sum 67.0, and P < 0.05). After 12 months of follow-up, mean IOP was 14.6 ± 3.2 (SD) mmHg and was reduced, on average, by 43.0% (range: 5.8–72.3%) relative to initial values (rank means 2.94, rank sum 53.0, and P < 0.05) (Table 2).

3.3. Medications. Fewer medications were used after surgery than before the procedure. The mean number of antiglaucoma medications applied preoperatively was 3.3 ± 1.1 (SD) (Me 3; range: 1–5), and, at the end of follow-up, this number was significantly reduced to 1.2 ± 1.1 (SD) (Me 1; range: 0–3) (Z = 3.059412, P = 0.002218) (Table 2).

3.4. Surgical Success. The complete success rate after 12 months of follow-up for the criteria 18 and 21 mmHg was, respectively, 46.0% and 49.0%, whereas the qualified success rate was, respectively, 76.2 and 85.7% (Figure 2). It should be noted that a large drop of the percentage of patients fulfilling the complete success criterion is observed after the operation, which is related to the necessity of applying antiglaucoma medications for the purpose of IOP control (Figure 2). In 94.4% of cases, IOP ≤ 18 mmHg was achieved after surgery, and a >30.0% reduction of its value relative to initial values was achieved in 72.2% of cases during the same observation period.

3.5. Corrected Distance Visual Acuity. The mean log MAR of CDVA changed from 0.9 ± 0.7 (SD) before surgery to 0.7 ± 0.6 (SD) on day 1 after surgery (rank means 0.50, rank sum 6.50, and P > 0.05); the CDVA after 12 months was 0.3 ± 0.5 (SD) (rank means 2.92, rank sum 38.0, and P < 0.05) (Table 3).

3.6. Complications. The following early complications were observed: raised IOP (5%), inflammatory exudate in the anterior chamber (5%), vitreous hemorrhage (10%), and posterior adhesions (5%). Progressive shallowing of the anterior chamber without increase of IOP was observed in the first week after surgery in 8 cases (40%). Among the late complications, fibrosis was observed in 3 eyes (15.0%), recurrence of malignant glaucoma in 3 eyes (15%), cystoid macular edema in 2 eyes (10%), and retinal detachment in 1 eye (5%).

TABLE 3: Mean values, median number, standard deviations, ranges of corrected distance visual acuity at specific times after surgery.

Time	Corrected distance visual acuity (log MAR)			
	Mean (SD)	Me	Range	P^*
Pre-op	0.9 ± 0.7	0.7	0.1–2.3	
1st day	0.7 ± 0.6	0.5	0–2.3	>0.05
7th day	0.7 ± 0.7	0.3	0–2.3	>0.05
1st month	0.5 ± 0.7	0.3	0–2.3	>0.05
3th month	0.3 ± 0.4	0.2	0–1.9	<0.05
6th month	0.3 ± 0.5	0.1	0–1.9	<0.05
12th month	0.3 ± 0.5	0.2	0–1.9	<0.05

SD-standard deviation; log MAR-*logarithm* of the *minimum angle of resolution*; Friedman ANOVA (χ^2_{ANOVA} = 35.19; P < 0.001)-post-hoc test (rank means, rank sum)*, Me-median number.

4. Discussion

Despite well-established methods of conservative treatment and laser procedures to treat malignant glaucoma, it is documented that surgical management to release entrapped aqueous fluid remains the most efficacious.

Until Chaundry and coworkers emphasized that establishing patent communication between the anterior chamber and vitreous cavity is the most important part of surgery in cases of malignant glaucoma, pars plana vitrectomy with or without lens extraction was applied to treat malignant glaucoma and was not successful in all cases [5, 6, 12, 16].

The surgical method presented here reflects contemporary views on how to treat malignant glaucoma. Evacuation of vitreous and aqueous humor from the vitreous cavity and establishment of communication with the anterior chamber help stop the vicious mechanism that eventually leads to increased IOP. In postoperative follow-up, it is important to maintain patency of newly created passages by using an Nd:YAG laser, as this helps diminish the number of recurrences. The data presented here clearly demonstrates the significant decrease of IOP on day 1 after surgery and at the end of follow-up. The efficacy of the surgery is further confirmed by the reduction of the number of antiglaucoma

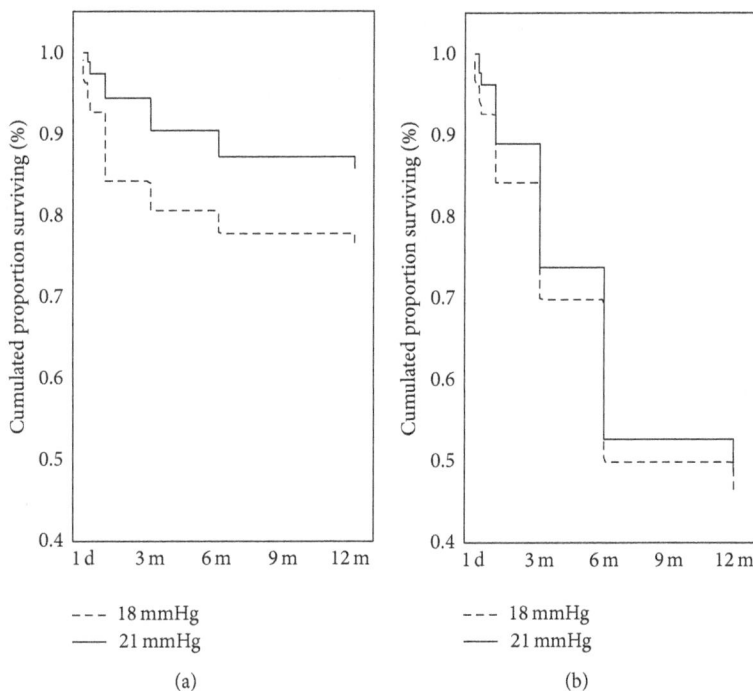

FIGURE 2: Cumulative surviving proportion (Kaplan-Meier) for success criterion of intraocular pressure less than or equal to 18 and 21 mmHg. (a) Qualified success rate (log-rank test; 2,004523, $P = 0.04501$); (b) complete success rate (log-rank test; 0.7002498, $P = 0.48377$).

medications from about 3 before surgery to about 1 after the operation.

The complete success rate in our whole group of patients for the two criteria of IOP reduction, the IOP ≤ 18 mmHg and IOP ≤ 21 mmHg criteria, was 46% and 45%, respectively, whereas the qualified success rate was 76.2% and 85.7%, respectively. It is noteworthy that there is a great difference between complete and qualified success rates. This is related to the fact that ant-glaucoma drops were frequently necessary to control IOP in our case series.

The most typical and difficult complication of malignant glaucoma surgery is the recurrence of malignant glaucoma. Tsai and coworkers described reoccurrence of symptoms in 33% of pseudophakic eyes treated with PPV and in 75% of phakic eyes after PPV [7]. Lois et al. did not observe recurrence of malignant glaucoma in 5 eyes treated surgically with zonulo-hyaloido-vitrectomy, but the follow-up was relatively short (1–9 months) [12]. Sharma and coworkers also did not note return of malignant glaucoma symptoms in their study, but the procedure of vitrectomy-phacoemulsification-vitrectomy was performed only in 4 eyes [17]. Debrouwere et al. compared percentage of recurrence after conventional vitrectomy (75%) and anterior vitrectomy with iridectomy and zonulectomy (66%), and they did not notice any after total PPV with iridectomy and zonulectomy [18]. In our study, 11 eyes (55%) exhibited isolated shallowing of the anterior chamber after surgical treatment of malignant glaucoma. In all cases, Nd-YAG capsulotomy was performed, and the laser beam was directed through a patent iridotomy/iridectomy or through the pupil. In eight eyes that did not show IOP

elevation, deepening of the anterior chamber was achieved. In three eyes with concomitant raised IOP, frank recurrence was regarded; however, only in one case reoperation was needed.

Failure of preceding glaucoma surgery was formerly described in the literature [5, 6, 9, 12]. In our study it was observed in 11 eyes (55%), and this made administration of antiglaucoma drops necessary.

At present, although new methods of treating malignant glaucoma are very promising, it is not possible to totally prevent complications. However, their occurrence can be limited by using new methods and making the decision to treat malignant glaucoma surgically as quickly as possible. Posterior pars plana vitrectomy with concomitant zonulectomy and capsulectomy seems to be efficacious as far as IOP control, post-op visual acuity, and reduction of medications are concerned. In general, it is plausible to perform it without delay before severe complications develop.

The study of malignant glaucoma has its limitations. Its pathomechanism is not fully understood, and the role of communication between the anterior chamber and posterior segment of the eye needs to be elucidated. The onset of malignant glaucoma differs, its frequency is low, and the application of various methods of treatment in groups of patients poses some ethical issues. It seems that further multicenter studies are needed to establish long-term success and optimal instrumentation in a larger group of patients.

5. Conclusions

Partial PPV with peripheral lens capsule excision communicating anterior chamber and vitreous cavity allows effective

IOP control in 12-month follow-up of 20 operated eyes, although in most cases there was a necessity of additional use of local antiglaucoma treatment in order to obtain the desired level of IOP after operation. In case of recurrences connected with occlusion of created tunnel between anterior chamber and vitreous cavity Nd-Yag laser may be used to restore communication between anterior and posterior segments of the eye. Such a management will usually result in complete resolution of the condition.

Ethical Approval

The study was approved by the appropriate ethics committee and was performed in accordance with the ethical standards laid down in the 1964 Declaration of Helsinki and its later amendments. Written informed consent was obtained from all patients before the procedure.

Disclaimer

The study sponsor had no involvement in design and conduct of the study; collection, management, analysis, and interpretation of the data; and preparation, review, or approval of the paper.

Conflict of Interests

The authors declare that there is no conflict of interests regarding the publication of this paper. The authors have no proprietary interest in any of the materials, products, or methods mentioned in this paper.

Acknowledgments

This paper was presented at 6th International Congress on Glaucoma Surgery ICGS 2012, Glasgow, UK, 13–15 September 2012. The study was supported with grant obtained from the Military Institute of Medicine (Grant no. 207).

References

[1] M. H. Luntz and M. Rosenblatt, "Malignant glaucoma," *Survey of Ophthalmology*, vol. 32, no. 2, pp. 73–93, 1987.

[2] R. Levene, "Malignant glaucoma: proposed definition and classification," in *Perspectives in Glaucoma. Transactions of the First Scientific Meeting of the American Glaukoma Society*, M. B. Shields, I. Pollack, and A. Kolker, Eds., pp. 243–350, Slack, Thorofare, NJ, USA, 1998.

[3] P. P. Ellis, "Malignant glaucoma occurring 16 years after successful filtering surgery," *Annals of Ophthalmology*, vol. 16, no. 2, pp. 177–179, 1984.

[4] S. Ruben, J. Tsai, and R. Hitchings, "Malignant glaucoma and its management," *British Journal of Ophthalmology*, vol. 81, no. 2, pp. 163–167, 1997.

[5] G. A. Byrnes, M. M. Leen, T. P. Wong, and W. E. Benson, "Vitrectomy for ciliary block (malignant) glaucoma," *Ophthalmology*, vol. 102, no. 9, pp. 1308–1311, 1995.

[6] J. W. Harbour, P. E. Rubsamen, and P. Palmberg, "Pars plana vitrectomy in the management of phakic and pseudophakic malignant glaucoma," *Archives of Ophthalmology*, vol. 114, no. 9, pp. 1073–1078, 1996.

[7] J. C. Tsai, K. A. Barton, M. H. Miller, P. T. Khaw, and R. A. Hitchings, "Surgical results in malignant glaucoma refractory to medical or laser therapy," *Eye*, vol. 11, no. 5, pp. 677–681, 1997.

[8] D. S. Greenfield, C. Tello, D. L. Budenz, J. M. Liebmann, and R. Ritch, "Aqueous misdirection after glaucoma drainage device implantation," *Ophthalmology*, vol. 106, no. 5, pp. 1035–1040, 1999.

[9] M. G. Lynch, R. H. Brown, R. G. Michels, I. P. Pollack, and W. J. Stark, "Surgical vitrectomy for pseudophakic malignant glaucoma," *American Journal of Ophthalmology*, vol. 102, no. 2, pp. 149–153, 1986.

[10] P. A. Chandler, R. J. Simmons, and W. M. Grant, "Malignant glaucoma. Medical and surgical treatment," *American Journal of Ophthalmology*, vol. 66, no. 3, pp. 495–502, 1968.

[11] A. S. Scott and V. H. Smith, "Retrolental decompression for malignant glaucoma," *British Journal of Ophthalmology*, vol. 45, pp. 654–661, 1961.

[12] N. Lois, D. Wong, and C. Groenewald, "New surgical approach in the management of pseudophakic malignant glaucoma," *Ophthalmology*, vol. 108, no. 4, pp. 780–783, 2001.

[13] M. M. K. Muqit and M. J. Menage, "Malignant glaucoma after phacoemulsification: treatment with diode laser cyclophotocoagulation," *Journal of Cataract and Refractive Surgery*, vol. 33, no. 1, pp. 130–132, 2007.

[14] L. De Jong, A. Lafuma, A.-S. Aguadé, and G. Berdeaux, "Five-year extension of a clinical trial comparing the EX-Press glaucoma filtration device and trabeculectomy in primary open-angle glaucoma," *Clinical Ophthalmology*, vol. 5, no. 1, pp. 527–533, 2011.

[15] R. Gallego-Pinazo, S. Martínez Castillo, R. Dolz-Marco, A. Lleó-Pérez, and M. Díaz-Llopis, "Analysis of prognostic factors by spectral-domain optical coherence tomography in pseudophakic cystoid macular oedema," *Archivos de la Sociedad Espanola de Oftalmologia*, vol. 87, no. 1, pp. 23–24, 2012.

[16] N. A. Chaudhry, H. W. Flynn Jr., T. G. Murray, D. Nicholson, and P. F. Palmberg, "Pars plana vitrectomy during cataract surgery for prevention of aqueous misdirection in high-risk fellow eyes," *The American Journal of Ophthalmology*, vol. 129, no. 3, pp. 387–388, 2000.

[17] A. Sharma, F. Sii, P. Shah, and G. R. Kirkby, "Vitrectomy-phacoemulsification-vitrectomy for the management of aqueous misdirection syndromes in phakic eyes," *Ophthalmology*, vol. 113, no. 11, pp. 1968–1973, 2006.

[18] V. Debrouwere, P. Stalmans, J. Van Calster, T. Spileers, T. Zeyen, and I. Stalmans, "Outcomes of different management options for malignant glaucoma: a retrospective study," *Graefe's Archive for Clinical and Experimental Ophthalmology*, vol. 250, no. 1, pp. 131–141, 2012.

14

Expression of HGF and c-Met Proteins in Human Keratoconus Corneas

Jingjing You,[1] Li Wen,[1] Athena Roufas,[1] Chris Hodge,[1,2] Gerard Sutton,[1,2,3] and Michele C. Madigan[1,4]

[1]*Save Sight Institute, Discipline of Clinical Ophthalmology, The University of Sydney, Sydney, NSW 2000, Australia*
[2]*Vision Eye Institute, Chatswood, NSW 2067, Australia*
[3]*Auckland University, Auckland 1010, New Zealand*
[4]*School of Optometry & Vision Science, UNSW, Kensington, NSW 2052, Australia*

Correspondence should be addressed to Jingjing You; jing.you@sydney.edu.au

Academic Editor: Neil Lagali

Keratoconus (KC) is a progressive degenerative inflammatory-related disease of the human cornea leading to decreased visual function. The pathogenesis of KC remains to be understood. Recent genetic studies indicate that gene variants of an inflammation-related molecule, hepatocyte growth factor (*HGF*), are associated with an increased susceptibility for developing KC. However HGF protein expression in KC has not been explored. In this initial study, we investigated late-stage KC and control corneas for the expression of HGF and its receptor mesenchymal-epithelial transition factor (c-Met/Met). KC buttons (~8 mm diameter) ($n = 10$) and whole control corneas ($n = 6$) were fixed in 10% formalin or 2% paraformaldehyde, paraffin embedded and sectioned. Sections were immunolabelled with HGF and c-Met antibodies, visualised using immunofluorescence, and examined with scanning laser confocal microscopy. Semiquantitative grading was used to compare HGF and c-Met immunostaining in KC and control corneas. Overall, KC corneas showed increased HGF and c-Met immunostaining compared to controls. KC corneal epithelium displayed heterogeneous moderate-to-strong immunoreactivity for HGF and c-Met, particularly in the basal epithelium adjacent to the cone area. Taken together with the recent genetic studies, our results further support a possible role for HGF/c-Met in the pathogenesis of KC.

1. Introduction

Keratoconus (KC) is the most common primary human degenerative corneal disease with a prevalence of around 1 in 2000 worldwide [1]. It is bilateral, asymmetric, and progressive, leading to corneal thinning and irregularity [2]. Onset primarily occurs in the 2nd decade of life and is associated with significant decreasing visual function [2] and morbidity [3]. KC is the main indication recorded for corneal grafts in Australia [4], and currently its progression can only be halted through surgical interventions including collagen cross-linking that stiffens the cornea using riboflavin and UVA [5]. More recently a surgical procedure was developed transplanting isolated Bowman's layer from donor corneas to KC eyes as a further late-stage intervention [6].

The histopathology of KC is well described and includes epithelial and stromal thinning within the apical cone region, breaks in the Bowman's layer, focal fibrosis, and anterior stromal keratocyte apoptosis [2, 7]. However the underlying pathogenesis of KC remains unclear. Recent evidence indicates a role for inflammation in the disease, with increased recruitment of inflammatory cells (e.g., macrophages, lymphocytes, and antigen presenting cells) [8] and inflammatory markers such as interleukin-1 (IL-1) and transforming growth factor-beta (TGF-β) [9] observed in KC corneal tissue sections. Increased expression of inflammatory markers such as interleukin-6 (IL-6), tumour necrosis factor alpha (TNF-α), and matrix metalloproteinase 9 (MMP-9) has also been found in tears collected from KC patients compared to controls [10]. Furthermore, a recent review examining the biochemical

TABLE 1: Characteristics of KC patients.

[a]KC	Gender	Age at diagnosis (yrs.)	Age at surgery (yrs.)	Contact lenses (Y or N)	History of allergy and/or atopy (Y or N)	[b]DALK (Y or N)
1	F	24	32	Y	N	N
2	F	23	30	N	Y asthma	Y
3	F	30	37	N	N	Y
4	M	27	32	N	Y atopy and asthma	N
5	M	25	32	N	N	Y
6	F	18	21	N	Y atopy and asthma	N
7	M	24	28	Y	N	N
8	M	24	43	Y	N	N
9	F	20	31	Y	N	N
10	F	32	38	Y	N	Y

[a]Grade 4 KC: severe; VA >6/7.5 with contact lens correction; severe corneal thinning and Munson's sign.
[b]DALK: deep anterior lamellar keratoplasty.

changes in KC proposed a "two-hit hypothesis" with a "genetic predisposition to the corneal disease and a second hit that may induce abnormalities of inflammatory components" [11].

Single nucleotide polymorphism (SNP) refers to a change in a single nucleotide within a DNA sequence and is the most common type of genetic variation observed in the human genome [12]. SNPs have been widely studied as genetic markers for human disease. Two parallel genome-wide association studies identifying potential SNPs associated with KC, using independent sample cohorts, reported a significant association between KC and the hepatocyte growth factor (HGF) gene, identifying two single nucleotide polymorphisms (SNPs; rs3735520 and rs17501108) in the promoter region [13]. Further, Burdon et al. (2011) also examined HGF protein abundance in the serum of controls correlating to the rs3735520 genotype and found a significant increase in HGF serum protein associated with the minor allele T [13].

HGF is a pleiotropic growth factor that activates the HGF/c-Met pathway after binding to its receptor, mesenchymal-epithelial transition factor (c-Met/Met). Once activated, downstream pathways such as mitogen-activated protein kinase (MAPK) cascades, PI3K-Akt axis or Janus kinase/signal transducers, and activators of transcription (JAK/STAT) pathways may be activated [14]. HGF has been implicated in several cellular roles within the cornea. For example, together with MMP-1, HGF is reported to initiate human corneal epithelial cell migration in vitro [15], and exogenous HGF has been found to promote the proliferation of both corneal epithelial and endothelial cells [16]. In injured rabbit corneas, Wilson et al. (1999) reported an obvious increase of HGF mRNA expression in keratocytes and c-Met mRNA expression in epithelial cells compared to unwounded corneas, suggesting that the HGF/c-Met pathway plays a role in corneal wound healing [17]. Studying bovine corneal wound healing in organ culture models, Carrington and Boulton (2005) showed that HGF delayed epithelial layer formation, together with increased differentiation of keratocytes

to myofibroblasts, compared with untreated and keratinocyte growth factor (KGF) treated corneas [18].

The expression of HGF and c-Met proteins in human KC corneas has not been investigated to date. One study has reported increased serum HGF expression for at least the minor allele of HGF SNP rs3735520, associated with increased potential for developing KC [13]. As a first step in assessing the role of HGF protein and its receptor (c-Met) in KC, we used corneal buttons from patients with severe KC and control human corneas to compare and examine the distribution and expression of these proteins.

2. Materials and Methods

KC corneal tissue buttons (Vision Eye Institute, Chatswood, NSW Australia) and donor corneas (Lions New South Wales (NSW) Eye Bank) were obtained with consent and approval from the Sydney Eye Hospital Human Research Ethics Committee (HREC 2013/1041). All procedures were in accordance with the Declaration of Helsinki. Informed consent was obtained from all participants prior to collection of KC buttons. Normal donor corneas were obtained from the Lions NSW Eye Bank following appropriate consent and HREC approval.

2.1. Corneal Specimens. Ten corneal buttons were collected from KC patients (age range from 18 to 32 years) undergoing corneal transplantation at Vision Eye Institute. All KC patients were diagnosed on the basis of clinical signs and corneal topography and were classified as KC grade 4 (most severe stage) (Table 1). Six normal donor corneas (age range 53 to 83 years) were obtained from the Lions NSW Eye Bank (Table 2).

KC corneal buttons (~8 mm diameter), with the cone apex location marked, were fixed in 10% neutral buffered formalin (NBF). Whole corneas were fixed in 2% paraformaldehyde/PBS (pH 7.4). All specimens were paraffin embedded and cut at 6 μm. Sections were collected on Super-Frost Plus

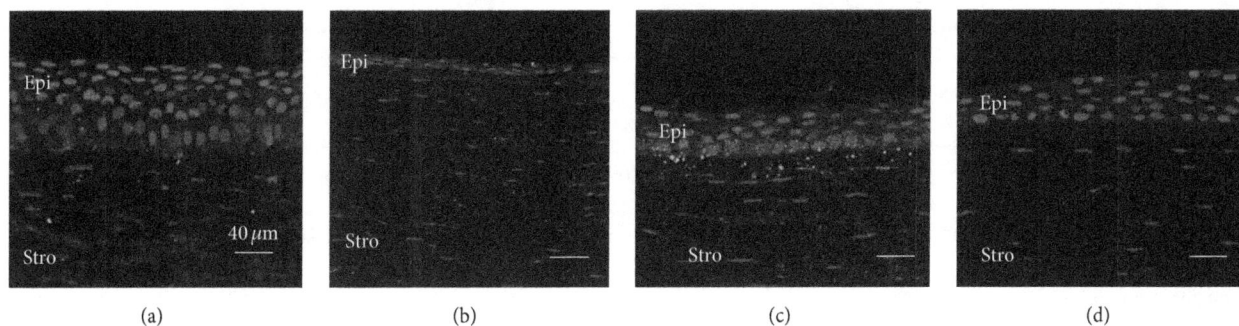

(a)   (b)   (c)   (d)

FIGURE 1: Representative images showing increased HGF expression in basal epithelial cells adjacent to the cone region in KC (a), compared to the relatively more uniform expression seen in all layers of control cornea epithelium at a similar location (c). Strong HGF stromal staining (keratocyte and extracellular matrix) is also observed in KC and control corneas (a to c). No immunostaining is apparent in the Ig negative control (d). *(a) Region adjacent to the cone in KC cornea, (b) cone region in KC cornea, (c) central region of control cornea, and (d) Ig negative control cornea. Epi: epithelium, Stro: stromal. Green: HGF; blue: nuclei.*

TABLE 2: Characteristics of control corneas.

Control	Gender	Age (yrs.)
1	M	67
2	F	53
3	F	64
4	F	67
5	M	83
6	M	63

slides (Menzel-Glaser, Saarbruckener, Germany) and dried before use.

2.2. Immunohistochemistry.

Sections were dewaxed and rehydrated through alcohols to water. For antigen retrieval, sections were incubated in 0.01 M citrate buffer (pH 6) at 85°C for 10 minutes, cooled to 40°C, and rinsed in Tris-buffered saline (TBS, pH 7.4) with 0.1% Tween-20 (TBST). Sections were incubated at room temperature (RT) in 5% bovine serum albumin (BSA) in TBST for 30 minutes, followed by incubation overnight at 4°C in HGF or c-Met primary antibodies, or appropriate negative controls (Mouse or Rabbit IgG) (Table 3). After overnight incubation, sections were washed in TBST and incubated in either goat anti-mouse Alexa Fluor 488 or donkey anti-rabbit Alexa Fluor 488.

For co-immunolabelling experiments, a separate series of slides were prepared and HGF visualised with Alexa Fluor 488 and c-Met visualised with Alexa Fluor 594, combined with nuclear Hoechst stain (Table 3).

Immunolabelling was repeated at least twice per specimen for each antibody, and appropriate Ig controls were included for each experiment. All slides were mounted in 20% glycerol/PBS, coverslipped, sealed with nail varnish, and viewed using a Zeiss LSM700 scanning laser confocal microscope and image software (Zen 2011, Carl Zeiss MicroImaging GHBH, Jena, Germany). Where more than one colour was to be detected, multichannel excitation bleed-through was minimized using fluorochromes with separated peak excitations. Emission bleed-through was minimized by multitracking, where signal crosstalk between neighbouring channels was corrected by performing a sequential image capture routine.

2.3. Semiquantitative Analysis for HGF and c-Met.

Semiquantitative grading of single-immunolabelled sections was used to assess the intensity and distribution of HGF and c-Met immunoreactivity in the corneal epithelium, stroma, and endothelium. Grading for KC buttons was made in the region adjacent to the cone (Adj) and for control corneas in a similar central corneal region. Immunolabelling of the thinned cone area of KC buttons was examined in each specimen but was not graded for comparison with controls because of the obviously altered morphology (only 1-2 epithelial layers present). The grading scale used was based on the intensity of the immunofluorescence (0 = no staining, 0.5 = very weak, 1 = weak, 2 = moderate, and 3 = strong) and the percentage (%) area immunolabelled (0 = 0%, 1 = 1% to 10%, 2 = 11% to 50%, and 3 > 50%) as described previously [19]. A final grade of 0 to 6 (intensity + % area immunolabelled) was then given for each specimen and this data is used to generate frequency histograms for HGF and c-Met immunostaining in KC and control specimens, respectively.

3. Results and Discussion

All KC corneas showed a thickened epithelium adjacent to the more central cone region (Figures 1(a) and 2(a)), compared to similar regions in the control corneas (Figures 1(c) and 2(c)), as we previously reported [19]. Only one to two layers of flattened epithelium were observed within the cone region (Figures 1(b) and 2(b)). Weak and more evenly distributed cytoplasmic immunostaining for HGF and c-Met was detected in the epithelium of control corneas (Figures 1(c) and 2(c)). In KC corneas, moderate-to-strong cytoplasmic immunostaining was seen within the basal and wing cell epithelial layers adjacent to the cone region (green fluorescence, Figures 1(a) and 2(a)). Only weak-to-moderate immunostaining of HGF and c-Met was detected in the KC cone region (Figures 1(b) and 2(b)).

Co-immunolabelling for HGF and c-Met showed that c-Met (red) was primarily localised in the epithelium of

TABLE 3: Primary antibodies and negative controls used for immunostaining.

Primary antibody	Company	Final concentration used
Mouse anti-human HGF	Santa Cruz Biotechnology, Inc. (Dallas, Texas, USA)	2 μg/mL
Rabbit anti-human c-Met	Santa Cruz Biotechnology, Inc.	0.4 μg/mL
Mouse anti-human IgG	Zymed Laboratories (Thermo Fisher Scientific, Waltham, Massachusetts, USA)	2 μg/mL
Rabbit anti-human IgG	Zymed Laboratories	0.4 μg/mL
Alexa Fluor 488 goat anti-mouse IgG	Molecular Probes (Life Technologies, Carlsbad, California, USA)	2 μg/mL
Alexa Fluor 488 donkey anti-rabbit IgG	Molecular Probes	2 μg/mL
Alexa Fluor 594 donkey anti-rabbit IgG	Molecular Probes	2 μg/mL
Hoechst	Molecular Probes	1 μg/mL

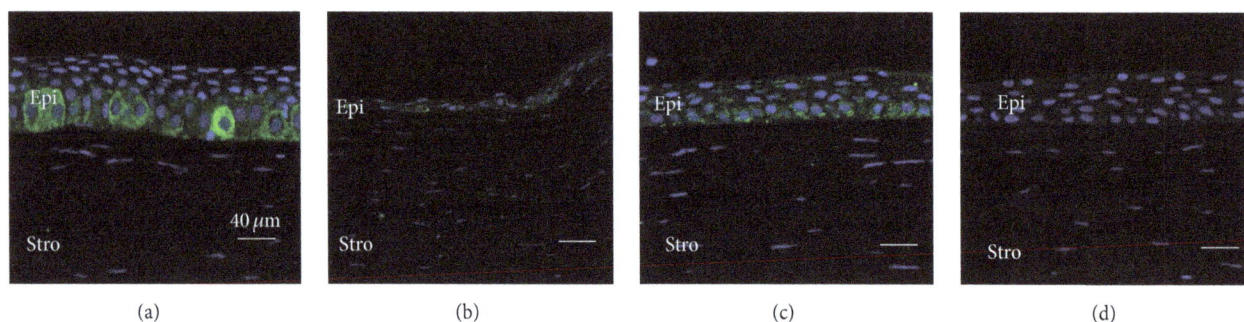

(a)   (b)   (c)   (d)

FIGURE 2: Representative images showing increased c-Met expression in basal epithelial cells adjacent to the cone region in KC (a), compared to the relatively more uniform expression seen in all layers of control cornea epithelium at a similar location (c). Weak c-Met staining is detected in the stroma in both KC and control corneas (a to c). No immunostaining is apparent in the Ig negative control (d). *(a) Region adjacent to the cone in KC cornea, (b) cone region in KC cornea, (c) central region of control cornea, and (d) Ig negative control. Epi: epithelium; Stro: stromal. Green: HGF; blue: nuclei.*

both control and KC corneas (Figure 3). HGF (green) was primarily localised within the stroma (both keratocytes and extracellular matrix) of control and KC corneas (Figure 3). Weak and relatively uniform immunostaining was observed in similar regions from control corneas for HGF and c-Met (Figure 3(a)). However, for KC corneas, increased HGF staining (green) was detected in the basal epithelium adjacent to the cone region and colocalised with increased c-Met staining (red) (Figure 3(d)). Limbal areas of control corneas showed slightly stronger stromal immunostaining of HGF compared to the central region of control corneas (Figure 3(b)).

Semiquantitative grading of HGF and c-Met immunostaining in KC samples was increased overall compared to the control corneas for similar regions, as indicated by the skewed distribution of the frequency histograms (Figures 4(a) and 4(b)). Overall, a greater proportion of KC corneas showed > grade 3 immunostaining for both HGF and c-met (KC: 70% and 90%, resp., *versus* control: 16% and 66% resp.) (Figures 4(a) and 4(b)).

Despite the importance of the HGF/c-Met pathway in regulating a number of key cellular activities, little is known about its potential role in normal or KC human corneas. As a first step to understand the possible role(s) of this pathway, we examined patterns of HGF and c-Met protein expression

in both control and KC corneas. Higher levels of HGF and c-Met immunostaining were detected in the basal epithelium adjacent to the KC cone, compared to the weaker and more uniform epithelial staining pattern seen in control corneas.

In control corneas, we found HGF expression was more intense in the stroma compared to the epithelium. This is consistent with previous studies showing low level *HGF* mRNA expression in the human corneal epithelium compared to keratocytes and endothelium [16, 20]. The surface of normal rabbit corneal epithelium was reported to show only low level HGF protein [21]. Our immunostaining experiments detected stronger c-Met (HGF receptor) staining in epithelium compared to keratocytes in control corneas. This is consistent with *c-Met* mRNA findings, which showed that human corneal epithelium, keratocytes, and endothelium all expressed *c-Met*, but with highest mRNA expression in epithelium [16, 20, 21]. These observations suggest that secreted keratocyte HGF may preferentially bind to the epithelium that expresses higher levels of c-Met (HGF receptor), compared to keratocytes that express low levels of c-Met, thus potentially regulating key epithelial cellular activities such as cell proliferation [22].

HGF is reported to be involved in two major processes, cell proliferation and migration, and inflammatory-related

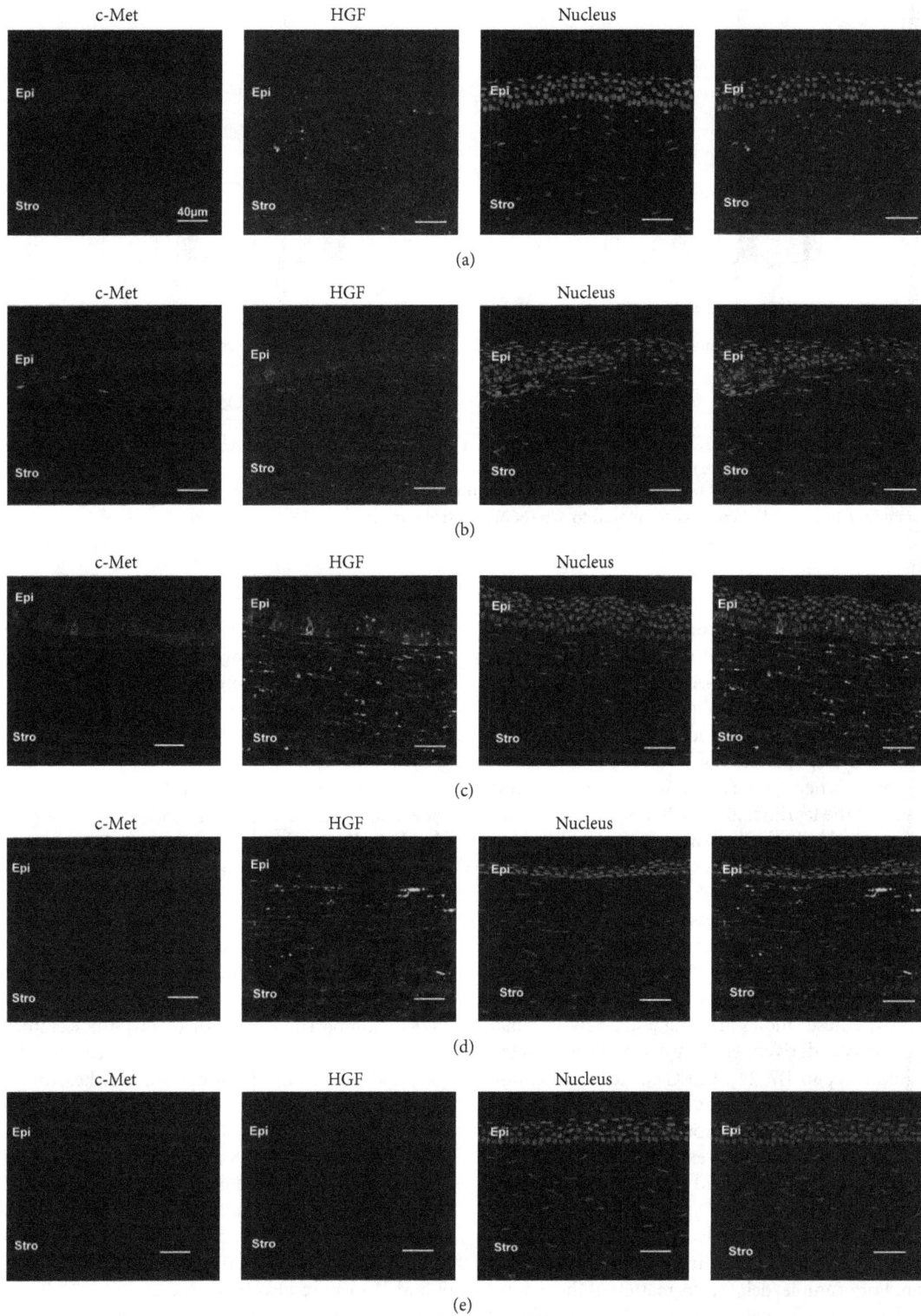

FIGURE 3: Representative images of central region of corneas with weak, uniform HGF (green), and c-Met (red) expression in all corneal layers (a). Patchy staining of HGF and c-Met is colocalised in the basal epithelium of both limbal regions (b) and adjacent to cone region of KC (c), with KC showing stronger staining than the limbal region. Strong HGF expression is seen within the stroma of both KC (c and d) and control corneas (a and b). (a) Central region of control cornea, (b) limbal region of control cornea, (c) region adjacent to the cone in KC cornea, (d) cone region in KC cornea, and (e) Ms and Rb Ig control.

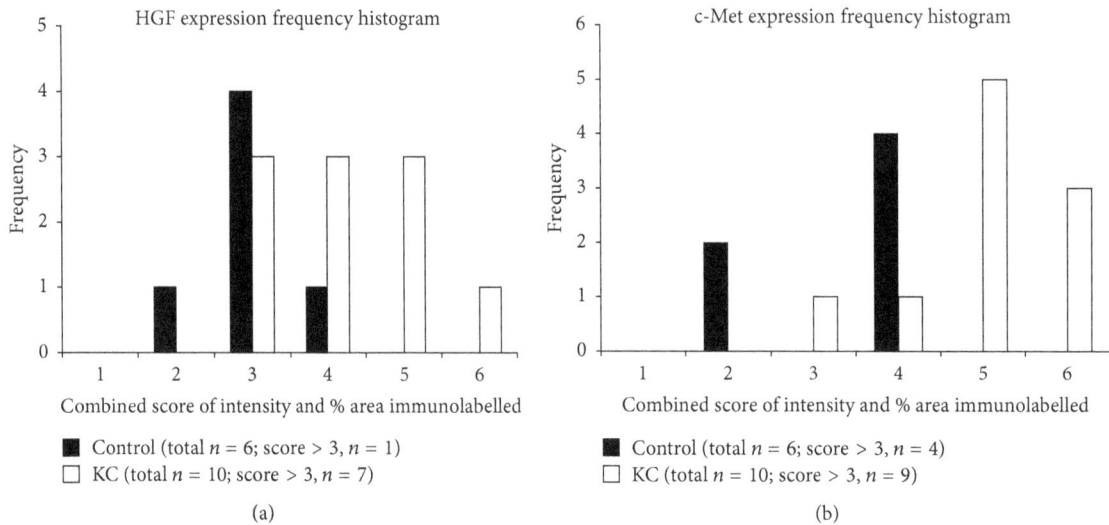

FIGURE 4: Frequency histograms for HGF (a) and c-Met (b) expression in KC and control corneas (combined score of staining intensity and % area coverage; range = 0 to 6). Note the right skewed distribution of HGF and c-Met immunostaining for KC corneas compared to controls. HGF staining had a combined score >3 in 7/10 (70%) KC corneas, compared to 1/6 (16%) control corneas. c-Met staining with a combined score >3 was seen in 9/10 (90%) KC corneas compared to 4/6 (66%) control corneas.

signalling cascades. HGF is a potent enhancer for corneal epithelial cell proliferation [16] and migration [23] *in vivo*, and increased *HGF* and *c-Met* mRNA expressions have been detected during corneal wound healing [16]. Increased HGF protein expression has been detected in the whole corneal epithelium, keratocytes, and tears of wounded compared to unwounded rabbit corneas [21]. *HGF* mRNA expression was also upregulated in the lacrimal gland when studying injured compared to unwounded rabbit corneas [17]. No difference in c-Met immunostaining was detected between wounded and unwounded rabbit corneas [21]. In secondary injured KC and control corneas, HGF expression in the stromal cells was reduced [24]. This was suggested to be most likely due to normal tissue repair pathways already being damaged or compromised, implying involvement of HGF in tissue regeneration [24]. These studies also suggested that lacrimal gland and keratocyte-derived HGF are closely associated with corneal tissue repair [17, 24]. In KC corneal epithelium, we observed increased HGF in the region adjacent to the cone, as well as increased c-Met; however it remains to be determined whether the increased expressions of HGF and c-Met observed are directly involved in KC pathogenesis or are secondary responses.

Poorly regulated and overexpressed HGF may be detrimental to tissues, related to the involvement of HGF in inflammation. For example, delayed formation of the epithelium layer and increased formation of stromal myofibroblasts have been detected during rabbit corneal wound healing, for corneas treated with recombinant HGF [18]. Applying recombinant HGF to corneas of mice with *Pseudomonas aeruginosa* keratitis also worsened the disease progression, with a significantly higher grade of corneal opacity and thinning compared to PBS-treated corneas [25]. *In vitro* treatment of corneal stromal keratocytes with proinflammatory

interleukin- (IL-) 1β increased *HGF* mRNA and protein production [26]. Elevated corneal HGF expression also enhanced proinflammatory cytokines and decreased anti-inflammatory cytokines in *Pseudomonas aeruginosa* keratitis in mice, most likely under the control of inflammatory cytokines and cell growth kinases [25].

KC has traditionally been described as a noninflammatory degenerative condition. However, emerging evidence clearly indicates that inflammation-related processes within the epithelium and stroma are involved in the pathogenesis of KC. Significant increases in proinflammatory molecules such as IL-6, IL-4, IL-5, IL-8, and IL-12 [27–29], MMP-1, MMP-3, MMP-7, and MMP-13 [28], and chemokine C-C motif ligand 5 (CCL5) [29] and significantly decreased levels of lactoferrin, serum albumin, and secreted IgA (sIgA) have been reported in KC compared to control tears [30]. Keratocytes in KC are reported to express more IL-1α receptors than controls [31], and one group has proposed that keratocyte apoptosis observed in KC may be induced by the binding of IL-1 receptors secondary to increased levels of IL-1 associated with epithelial trauma, for example, due to eye-rubbing [32]. Most recently, increased mRNA expression of *MMP-9* and its inducer proteins IL-6 and TNF-α were detected in KC corneal epithelium in an Indian cohort (>100 patients) compared to healthy controls ($n = 20$), and tear protein levels of MMP-9 and IL-6 were also increased in KC [33]. Treatment with topical cyclosporine A (an immunosuppressant) in a small group of KC patients ($n = 20$) reduced the tear levels of MMP-9 and appeared to halt the progression of KC, consistent with the involvement of inflammation in KC pathogenesis [33].

The link between *HGF* variants and KC susceptibility was first reported by Burdon et al., (2011) and then confirmed in an independent European cohort which replicated the association of SNP rs3735520 and detected a new *HGF* SNP rs2956540 [34]. In addition, an independent study of an Australian population of European descent ($n = 830$) focused on the *HGF* locus and detected a different SNP (rs4954218) significantly associated with KC [35]. The actual function of these *HGF* SNPs is unclear. However, a study of rs3735520 implicated a possible regulatory effect of this SNP for HGF protein expression in serum from KC patients [13]. As the SNPs identified to date are all located in the noncoding region of the gene (rs3735520, rs17501108, and rs1014091 in the upstream of *HGF* and rs2286194 in the intron between exon 8 and exon 9), it is likely that they will affect gene expression through mechanisms such as RNA splicing, transcription factor binding, and miRNA regulation [36]. Our results provide evidence of increased HGF protein in KC epithelium compared to control corneal epithelium; however the role of the reported HGF SNPs in the increased protein expression is unclear and will be further investigated.

4. Conclusion

Previous studies showed an independent, repeatable association between certain SNPs and *HGF* in KC [13, 34, 35]. The SNP variations detected were located in the noncoding region of *HGF* consistent with a role for these SNPs in the regulating HGF expression, and increased serum HGF expression associated with the minor SNP allele has been reported [37]. In the current study, we showed increased HGF protein expression within KC corneal epithelium. Taken together previous SNP studies, these observations indicate that the HGF/c-Met pathway may be involved in the pathogenesis of KC. Further studies investigating how the HGF/c-Met pathway may be altered in KC, including the associations between SNPs and protein expression and the role of inflammation requires further investigation. Studies on the downstream signalling pathways regulated by HGF/c-Met, such as MAPK cascades, the PI3K-Akt axis, and the JAK/STAT pathway may help to identify the potential role of this pathway in KC and in normal corneal homeostasis.

Conflict of Interests

The authors declare that they have no conflict of interests.

Acknowledgments

The authors thank the Medical School of Sydney University, Sydney Eye Hospital Foundation, and the Lions NSW Eye Bank for funding support. Michele C. Madigan is funded by the National Foundation for Medical Research & Innovation (NFMRI).

References

[1] Y. S. Rabinowitz, "Keratoconus," *Survey of Ophthalmology*, vol. 42, no. 4, pp. 297–319, 1998.

[2] C. N. J. Mcghee, "2008 Sir Norman McAlister gregg lecture: 150 years of practical observations on the conical cornea—what have we learned?" *Clinical and Experimental Ophthalmology*, vol. 37, no. 2, pp. 160–176, 2009.

[3] H. Wagner, J. T. Barr, and K. Zadnik, "Collaborative Longitudinal Evaluation of Keratoconus (CLEK) Study: methods and findings to date," *Contact Lens and Anterior Eye*, vol. 30, no. 4, pp. 223–232, 2007.

[4] K. A. Williams, M. T. Lowe, M. C. Keane et al., *The Australian Corneal Graft Registry 2012 Report*, Flinders University Press, Adelaide, Australia, 2012.

[5] G. R. Snibson, "Collagen cross-linking: a new treatment paradigm in corneal disease—a review," *Clinical and Experimental Ophthalmology*, vol. 38, no. 2, pp. 141–153, 2010.

[6] K. van Dijk, V. S. Liarakos, J. Parker et al., "Bowman layer transplantation to reduce and stabilize progressive, advanced keratoconus," *Ophthalmology*, vol. 122, no. 5, pp. 909–917, 2015.

[7] E. Sykakis, F. Carley, L. Irion, J. Denton, and M. C. Hillarby, "An in depth analysis of histopathological characteristics found in keratoconus," *Pathology*, vol. 44, no. 3, pp. 234–239, 2012.

[8] J. C. Fan Gaskin, I. P. Loh, C. N. McGhee, and T. Sherwin, "An immunohistochemical study of inflammatory cell changes and matrix remodeling with and without acute hydrops in keratoconus," *Investigative Opthalmology & Visual Science*, vol. 56, no. 10, pp. 5831–5837, 2015.

[9] L. Zhou, B. Y. J. T. Yue, S. S. Twining, J. Sugar, and R. S. Feder, "Expression of wound healing and stress-related proteins in keratoconus corneas," *Current Eye Research*, vol. 15, no. 11, pp. 1124–1131, 1996.

[10] I. Lema and J. A. Durán, "Inflammatory molecules in the tears of patients with keratoconus," *Ophthalmology*, vol. 112, no. 4, pp. 654–659, 2005.

[11] V. Galvis, T. Sherwin, A. Tello, J. Merayo, R. Barrera, and A. Acera, "Keratoconus: an inflammatory disorder?" *Eye*, vol. 29, no. 7, pp. 843–859, 2015.

[12] Y.-T. Huang, C.-J. Chang, and K.-M. Chao, "The extent of linkage disequilibrium and computational challenges of single nucleotide polymorphisms in genome-wide association studies," *Current Drug Metabolism*, vol. 12, no. 5, pp. 498–506, 2011.

[13] K. P. Burdon, S. Macgregor, Y. Bykhovskaya et al., "Association of polymorphisms in the hepatocyte growth factor gene promoter with keratoconus," *Investigative Ophthalmology & Visual Science*, vol. 52, no. 11, pp. 8514–8519, 2011.

[14] S. L. Organ and M. Tsao, "An overview of the c-MET signaling pathway," *Therapeutic Advances in Medical Oncology*, vol. 3, no. 1, supplement, pp. S7–S19, 2011.

[15] J. T. Daniels, G. A. Limb, U. Saarialho-Kere, G. Murphy, and P. T. Khaw, "Human corneal epithelial cells require MMP-1 for HGF-mediated migration on collagen I," *Investigative Ophthalmology and Visual Science*, vol. 44, no. 3, pp. 1048–1055, 2003.

[16] S. E. Wilson, J. W. Walker, E. L. Chwang, and Y.-G. He, "Hepatocyte growth factor, keratinocyte growth factor, their receptors, fibroblast growth factor receptor-2, and the cells of the cornea," *Investigative Ophthalmology and Visual Science*, vol. 34, no. 8, pp. 2544–2561, 1993.

[17] S. E. Wilson, Q. Liang, and W. J. Kim, "Lacrimal gland HGF, KGF, and EGF mRNA levels increase after corneal epithelial wounding," *Investigative Ophthalmology and Visual Science*, vol. 40, no. 10, pp. 2185–2190, 1999.

[18] L. M. Carrington and M. Boulton, "Hepatocyte growth factor and keratinocyte growth factor regulation of epithelial and stromal corneal wound healing," *Journal of Cataract and Refractive Surgery*, vol. 31, no. 2, pp. 412–423, 2005.

[19] J. You, L. Wen, A. Roufas, M. C. Madigan, and G. Sutton, "Expression of SFRP family proteins in human keratoconus corneas," *PLoS ONE*, vol. 8, no. 6, Article ID e66770, 2013.

[20] D.-Q. Li and S. C. G. Tseng, "Three patterns of cytokine expression potentially involved in epithelial-fibroblast interactions of human ocular surface," *Journal of Cellular Physiology*, vol. 163, no. 1, pp. 61–79, 1995.

[21] Q. Li, J. Weng, R. R. Mohan et al., "Hepatocyte growth factor and hepatocyte growth factor receptor in the lacrimal gland, tears, and cornea," *Investigative Ophthalmology and Visual Science*, vol. 37, no. 5, pp. 727–739, 1996.

[22] S. E. Wilson, Y.-G. He, J. Weng, J. D. Zieske, J. V. Jester, and G. S. Schultz, "Effect of epidermal growth factor, hepatocyte growth factor, and keratinocyte growth factor, on proliferation, motility and differentiation of human corneal epithelial cells," *Experimental Eye Research*, vol. 59, no. 6, pp. 665–678, 1994.

[23] J. K. Spix, E. Y. Chay, E. R. Block, and J. K. Klarlund, "Hepatocyte growth factor induces epithelial cell motility through transactivation of the epidermal growth factor receptor," *Experimental Cell Research*, vol. 313, no. 15, pp. 3319–3325, 2007.

[24] I. M. Cheung, C. N. McGhee, and T. Sherwin, "Deficient repair regulatory response to injury in keratoconic stromal cells," *Clinical and Experimental Optometry*, vol. 97, no. 3, pp. 234–239, 2014.

[25] X. Jiang, S. A. McClellan, R. Barrett, M. Foldenauer, and L. D. Hazlett, "HGF signaling impacts severity of *Pseudomonas aeruginosa* keratitis," *Investigative Ophthalmology and Visual Science*, vol. 55, no. 4, pp. 2180–2190, 2014.

[26] J. Weng, R. R. Mohan, Q. Li, and S. E. Wilson, "IL-1 upregulates keratinocyte growth factor and hepatocyte growth factor mRNA and protein production by cultured stromal fibroblast cells: interleukin-1β expression in the cornea," *Cornea*, vol. 16, no. 4, pp. 465–471, 1997.

[27] I. Lema, T. Sobrino, J. A. Durán, D. Brea, and E. Díez-Feijoo, "Subclinical keratoconus and inflammatory molecules from tears," *British Journal of Ophthalmology*, vol. 93, no. 6, pp. 820–824, 2009.

[28] S. A. Balasubramanian, S. Mohan, D. C. Pye, and M. D. P. Willcox, "Proteases, proteolysis and inflammatory molecules in the tears of people with keratoconus," *Acta Ophthalmologica*, vol. 90, no. 4, pp. e303–e309, 2012.

[29] A. S. Jun, L. Cope, C. Speck et al., "Subnormal cytokine profile in the tear fluid of keratoconus patients," *PLoS ONE*, vol. 6, Article ID e16437, 2011.

[30] S. A. Balasubramanian, D. C. Pye, and M. D. P. Willcox, "Levels of lactoferrin, secretory IgA and serum albumin in the tear film of people with keratoconus," *Experimental Eye Research*, vol. 96, no. 1, pp. 132–137, 2012.

[31] E. J. Fabre, J. Bureau, Y. Pouliquen, and G. Lorans, "Binding sites for human interleukin 1 α gamma interferon and tumor necrosis factor on cultured fibroblasts of normal cornea and keratoconus," *Current Eye Research*, vol. 10, no. 7, pp. 585–592, 1991.

[32] N. Efron and J. G. Hollingsworth, "New perspectives on keratoconus as revealed by corneal confocal microscopy," *Clinical and Experimental Optometry*, vol. 91, no. 1, pp. 34–55, 2008.

[33] R. Shetty, A. Ghosh, R. R. Lim et al., "Elevated expression of matrix metalloproteinase-9 and inflammatory cytokines in keratoconus patients is inhibited by cyclosporine A," *Investigative Ophthalmology and Visual Science*, vol. 56, no. 2, pp. 738–750, 2015.

[34] L. Dudakova, M. Palos, K. Jirsova et al., "Validation of rs2956540:G>C and rs3735520:G>A association with keratoconus in a population of European descent," *European Journal of Human Genetics*, vol. 23, no. 11, pp. 1581–1583, 2015.

[35] S. Sahebjada, M. Schache, A. J. Richardson, G. Snibson, M. Daniell, and P. N. Baird, "Association of the hepatocyte growth factor gene with Keratoconus in an Australian population," *PLoS ONE*, vol. 9, no. 1, Article ID e84067, 2014.

[36] Q. Huang, "Genetic study of complex diseases in the post-GWAS era," *Journal of Genetics and Genomics*, vol. 42, no. 3, pp. 87–98, 2015.

[37] K. P. Burdon, S. Macgregor, Y. Bykhovskaya et al., "Association of polymorphisms in the hepatocyte growth factor gene promoter with keratoconus," *Investigative Ophthalmology and Visual Science*, vol. 52, no. 11, pp. 8514–8519, 2011.

15

Characterization of Visual Symptomatology Associated with Refractive, Accommodative, and Binocular Anomalies

**Pilar Cacho-Martínez, Mario Cantó-Cerdán,
Stela Carbonell-Bonete, and Ángel García-Muñoz**

Departamento de Óptica, Farmacología y Anatomía, Universidad de Alicante, 03080 Alicante, Spain

Correspondence should be addressed to Pilar Cacho-Martínez; cacho@ua.es

Academic Editor: Edward Manche

Purpose. To characterize the symptomatology of refractive, accommodative, and nonstrabismic binocular dysfunctions and to assess the association between dysfunctions and symptoms. *Methods.* 175 randomised university students were examined. Subjects were given a subjective visual examination with accommodative and binocular tests, evaluating their symptomatology. Accommodative and binocular dysfunctions (AD, BD) were diagnosed according to the number of existing clinical signs: suspect AD or BD (one fundamental clinical sign), high suspect (one fundamental + 1 complementary clinical sign), and definite (one fundamental + 2 or more complementary clinical signs). A logistic regression was conducted in order to determine whether there was an association between dysfunctions and symptoms. *Results.* 78 subjects (44.6%) reported any kind of symptoms which were grouped into 18 categories, with "visual fatigue" being the most frequent (20% of the overall complaints). Logistic regression adjusted by the presence of an uncorrected refractive error showed no association between any grade of AD and symptoms. Subjects with BD had more likelihood of having symptoms than without dysfunction group (OR = 3.35), being greater when only definite BD were considered (OR = 8.79). *Conclusions.* An uncorrected refractive error is a confusion factor when considering AD symptomatology. For BD, the more the number of clinical signs used the greater the likelihood suffering symptoms.

1. Introduction

In order to maintain a clear single image when reading or doing near work, both accommodative and convergence systems must be adequate. If these mechanisms fail, leading to accommodative and/or vergence dysfunctions, subjects may complain of symptoms [1]. Several authors have reported that visual discomfort symptoms are prevalent among those subjects who have prolonged near work such as using a computer or reading [2–7] and complaints may include visual fatigue, headache, blurred vision, diplopia, loss of concentration when reading or doing near work, light sensitivity, or perceptual distortions involving letter movement and fading.

Scientific literature has revealed that accommodative and/or vergence anomalies are commonly found in clinical practice [1, 8–19] and may show different symptoms between patients [20, 21]. In this sense, several studies have focused on the measurement of visual discomfort symptoms in college students [2, 6, 22–24]. Several authors have related these dysfunctions to problems with reading or academic performance [25, 26]. Others [1, 27] have reported that these visual symptoms may have a negative effect on school performance or reading comprehension, even leading to avoidance of near work. It has also been shown [28] that children with more visual symptoms have lower academic achievement than those with fewer visual symptoms. And current clinical trials about convergence insufficiency have shown the improvement of academic behaviors [29] and the decrease in performance-related symptoms [30] after successful treatment.

In any case, although in the scientific literature we can see that the authors consider the presence of symptoms essential to diagnose accommodative and/or binocular anomalies [26, 31–42], it has been shown in a scoping review [43] considering articles since the last 30 years that there is no consensus as to which symptoms should be considered in the diagnosis of each of these anomalies. In this sense, few symptoms are specific to each entity and many of them overlap when considering an accommodative or binocular dysfunction, so that this information may influence clinical management as it is difficult to associate a particular dysfunction with a particular symptom. But also many of symptoms related to accommodative and binocular disorders may not be different from those related to other conditions as visual stress (or Meares-Irlen syndrome) [5, 44] or from those related to uncorrected refractive anomalies [45].

Under these premises, the aim of this study was to characterize the symptomatology of refractive, accommodative, and nonstrabismic binocular dysfunctions in a randomised sample of university students. A further aim was to assess the association between the various dysfunctions diagnosed and the symptoms reported by the patients.

2. Materials and Methods

This study is part of a larger research which intended to analyse the visual health of university students by means of analyzing the prevalence of accommodative and binocular dysfunctions of the university population of University of Alicante and to characterize their symptoms. This paper is related to the characterization of symptoms.

We conducted a prospective study of a population sample of university students from the University of Alicante, selected by means of simple random sampling of all students in all years of the degree courses taught at the University of Alicante. Simple random sampling was performed of the 26,326 students attending the University of Alicante at the time when the study was conducted. The randomization was done by the Computing Service of the University. Sample size was calculated by assuming an overall prevalence of accommodative and nonstrabismic binocular dysfunctions of 25% [11, 12, 18] with a confidence level of 95%, requiring a 5% for the proportion's estimation and a dropout rate of 20%, yielding a sample of 357 undergraduate and postgraduate students. As a requirement for obtaining data, students had to be aged between 18 and 35 years old. Establishing the upper age limit of 35 years was to avoid including prepresbyopic subjects in the study [46] who could bias the diagnosis of an accommodative and nonstrabismic binocular disorder.

Participants were initially contacted via an email informing them that they had been randomly selected from the university student population to participate in this research. Due to the low response rate yielded by this approach, it was decided to contact them by telephone to inform them of the study. Despite multiple attempts to contact students via email and telephone, there were 177 students who finally participated in the study, representing a response rate of 49.6%. There were a variety of reasons for nonresponse: 131 students did not respond either to emails or telephone calls, 6 lived elsewhere, 21 did not want to participate, and 20 students agreed to participate but did not attend their appointment.

This study was conducted in accordance with the Declaration of Helsinki, and the Ethics Committee of University of Alicante approved the study. All subjects gave their written informed consent once the nature of the study had been explained. All of the 177 students were given a visual examination, which besides a visual health examination and a refractive examination also included specific tests to determine the subject's accommodative and binocular status.

Visual examination consisted of the following procedures.

(i) *Sociodemographic Data.* Besides personal details, we also collected academic data such as number of hours of study per day and academic performance, this latter being calculated as the number of credits obtained divided by the number of credits studied in the last academic year.

(ii) *Clinical History.* Data were collected on the symptoms reported by the subjects. To this end, we did not use a questionnaire but we used the categories of symptoms described by García-Muñoz et al. [43] in a recent scoping review, in which they indicated the different types of symptoms which may be associated with accommodative and binocular dysfunction. We showed the list of 34 symptoms categories and patients were asked if they were suffering any type of these symptoms related to their vision. Several symptoms were fully explained to ensure understanding, for example, the symptom of "visual fatigue" (which refers specifically to symptoms described by patients such as tired eyes, eyestrain, or eye fatigue). Subjects were considered to present a visual symptomatology when they reported one or more symptoms. For the purpose of this analysis, a symptom was considered present when it was either the patients' main concern or if it occurred frequently, so that feeling the symptom once was not enough to render a positive answer.

(iii) *Refractive Examination.* This was performed by means of static retinoscopy and a subjective examination. The subjective examination was performed by means of monocular fogging method with crosscylinder followed by binocular balancing to a standard endpoint of maximum plus for best visual acuity. Once the maximum plus value for best visual acuity had been obtained, this result of the subjective examination was used as the baseline for all accommodative and binocular tests.

(iv) *Accommodative and Binocular Tests.* The following tests were performed. Phoria measurement was done with cover test. Unilateral and alternate cover test measurements [47–49] were done for distant and near vision while the subject was instructed to fixate on a single letter of 20/30 visual acuity. Using a prism bar, the deviation value was midway between the low and high neutral findings using an alternate cover test. Measurement of gradient AC/A ratio [50] was done using the cover test and −1.00 D lenses. We calculated AC/A ratio [50]. Monocular estimate method (MEM) dynamic retinoscopy [51] at 40 cm was done with the result of the subjective exam placed in a trial frame and using trial lenses. Monocular accommodative amplitude was measured by Donder's push-up method [52] using a single 20/30 Snellen line target in free space. The target was slowly moved towards the patient until reported blurring, and the distance from this point to the spectacle plane was then recorded in diopters. Monocular and binocular accommodative facility were measured following the procedure of Zellers et al. [53] at 40 cm and using ±2.00 D flipper lenses and the 20/30 letter line on Vectogram 9 (Bernell) which includes a suppression control for the binocular measurement. Monocular accommodative facility was measured in the same manner but without polarized glasses and with the nonviewing eye occluded. Both monocular and binocular accommodative facility were measured during one minute and the cycles per minute (cpm) were recorded, evaluating if the patient had difficulty in focusing with plus or minus lenses. Near point of convergence was measured in free space using an accommodative target of 20/30 visual acuity at 40 cm [54] and moving the target away from the subject at a speed of approximately 1 to 2 cm per second [55] until the break and recovery findings. Distance was calculated from the midsagittal plane of the patients' head to the nearest half centimeter. Positive and negative relative accommodations were measured with plus and minus, respectively, behind the phoropter, and using an accommodative target of 20/30 visual acuity at 40 cm [50] until sustained blur was detected. Positive and negative fusional vergences were determined at far and near vision with phoropter's Risley prism (with a smooth gradual increase in prism power) using an accommodative target of 20/30 visual acuity and performed according to the subject's type of heterophoria (for exophoria the positive fusional vergence was measured first and the negative fusional vergence was first performed for esophoria) [56, 57]. Vergence facility was measured in free space using an accommodative target of 20/30 visual acuity at 40 cm, with the prism combination of 3 Δ base-in/12 Δ base-out [58, 59] and evaluating if the patient had difficulty in fusing with the base-in or base-out prism. Determination of fusion was done by means of the 4-dot Worth test [50] and stereopsis was measured using graded circles of Randot SO-002 test [60] in free space.

Once all these tests had been performed, the results were analysed in order to determine the existence of refractive, accommodative, and/or binocular dysfunctions. In order to avoid bias, diagnosis of each dysfunction was completed by two authors different to the person who performed the visual examination, so that the persons who determined the diagnoses were masked to the symptoms.

The inclusion criteria for the study were applied to these initial data and consisted of having a visual acuity of 20/20 with the best correction, the absence strabismus or amblyopia, and any ocular or systemic disease that might affect the results. Two students presented an amblyopia and

strabismus so that the final number of subjects included in the study was 175, of whom 59 were male (33.7%) and 116 female (66.3%), with a mean age of 22.90 ± 3.96 years.

Patients were diagnosed with refractive dysfunction when a difference was detected between their habitual refraction and their subjective examination results obtained in this study. The clinical criteria applied to establish this difference were the following:

(i) A less negative subjective examination result than the habitual refraction; in other words, the patient was overcorrected for myopia (equal to or greater than 0.50 D).

(ii) Changes in the sphere or cylinder equal to or greater than 0.50 D, with which visual acuity was increased by at least one line with the new refraction.

Thus, subjects were classified into two refractive categories as follows:

(i) In subjects with an uncorrected refractive error, the patient used a prescription different to that indicated by the subjective examination, or the patient did not use a prescription but needed it.

(ii) In subjects without an uncorrected refractive error, the patient's habitual refraction was satisfactory.

Accommodative dysfunctions (AD) and binocular dysfunctions (BD) were diagnosed in accordance with the criteria described in the literature [42, 50]. However, since there is no enough scientific evidence to support the use of any given diagnostic criterion to accurately define each dysfunction [21], we decided to classify dysfunctions on the basis of the number of clinical signs associated with each dysfunction, classifying the signs that could be associated with each dysfunction as fundamental and complementary. The classification employed was as follows:

(i) Suspect AD or BD: one fundamental clinical sign.

(ii) High suspect AD or BD: one fundamental clinical sign + 1 complementary clinical sign.

(iii) Definite AD or BD: one fundamental clinical sign + 2 or more complementary clinical signs.

Table 1 gives the fundamental and complementary clinical signs used in this study to diagnose each accommodative and binocular dysfunction. For binocular conditions we used the classification made by Scheiman and Wick in which the calculated AC/A ratio is considered to diagnose a particular binocular condition. Following this classification high AC/A ratio conditions are convergence excess and divergence excess, low AC/A ratio includes convergence insufficiency and divergence insufficiency, and normal AC/A ratio conditions refer to fusional vergence dysfunction (also known as binocular instability [61]), basic esophoria, and basic exophoria. With these considerations, patients were grouped into different groups: patients with accommodative dysfunctions (AD), binocular dysfunctions (BD), and both accommodative and binocular anomalies (AD + BD).

TABLE 1: Clinical signs used in the study for diagnosing accommodative and binocular anomalies (AA: accommodative amplitude; MAF/BAF: monocular/binocular accommodative facility; MEM: monocular estimate method; PRA/NRA: positive/negative relative accommodation; PFV/NFV: positive/negative fusional vergence; NPC: near point of convergence; VF: vergence facility; Δ: prism diopters; D: diopters; cpm: cycles per minute; BO: base-out; BI: base-in).

Dysfunction	Fundamental sign	Complementary sign
Accommodative dysfunctions		
Accommodative insufficiency	Reduced AA: 2.00 D < minimum AA (15–0.25 × age)	MAF < 6 cpm with −2.00 D lenses BAF < 3 cpm with −2.00 D lenses MEM > 0.75 D PRA < 1.25 D
Accommodative excess	MAF < 6 cpm with +2.00 D lenses	PRA ≥ 3.50 D BAF < 6 cpm with +2.00 D lenses MEM < 0.25 D NRA < 1.50 D
Accommodative infacility	MAF < 6 cpm with ±2.00 D lenses	BAF < 3 cpm with ±2.00 D lenses PRA < 1.25 D NRA < 1.50 D
Binocular dysfunctions		
Convergence insufficiency	Significant exophoria at near vision (≥6 Δ), greater than far vision	PFV at near ≤ 11/14/3 Δ NPC ≥ 6 cm VF < 13,4 cpm with 12 Δ base-out prism BAF < 3 cpm with +2.00 D lenses MEM < 0.25 D NRA < 1.50 D
Convergence excess	Significant esophoria at near vision (≥1 Δ), greater than far vision	NFV at near ≤ 8/16/7 Δ VF < 13.4 cpm with 3 Δ base-in prism BAF < 3 cpm with −2.00 D lenses MEM > 0.75 D PRA < 1.25 D
Divergence excess	Significant exophoria at far vision (≥4 Δ), greater than near vision (the difference must be >5 Δ)	PFV at far ≤ 4/10/5 Δ PFV at near ≤ 11/14/3 Δ NPC ≥ 6 cm VF < 13,4 cpm with 12 Δ base-out prism BAF < 3 cpm with +2.00 D lenses MEM < 0.25 D NRA < 1.50 D
Basic esophoria	Significant esophoria at far and near vision of equal amount (deviations within 5 Δ of one another are considered equal)	NFV at far ≤ X/3/1 Δ and at near ≤ 8/16/7 Δ VF < 13.4 cpm with 3 Δ base-in prism BAF < 3 cpm with −2.00 D lenses MEM > 0.75 D PRA < 1.25 D

TABLE 1: Continued.

Dysfunction	Fundamental sign	Complementary sign
Basic exophoria	Significant exophoria at far and near vision of equal amount (deviations within 5 Δ of one another are considered equal)	PFV at far ≤ 4/10/5 Δ and at near ≤ 11/14/3 Δ NPC ≥ 6 cm VF < 13,4 cpm with 12 Δ base-out prism BAF < 3 cpm with +2.00 D lenses MEM < 0.25 D NRA < 1.50 D
Fusional vergence dysfunction	PFV and NFV reduced at far and near vision or VF < 13.4 cpm with both prisms of the combination used of 12 BO/3 BI	BAF < 3 cpm with ±2.00 D lenses PRA < 1.25 D and NRA < 1.50 D

Subjects who only presented an uncorrected refractive error were considered as the group of refractive dysfunction (RD).

And those subjects, who did not present any refractive, accommodative, or binocular dysfunction, were considered as the group named without dysfunction (WD).

2.1. Data Analysis. An analysis of the relationships between sociodemographic variables and the presence of symptoms was conducted using the samples as independent variables, using the chi-square test for categorical variables, the Mann-Whitney U test for continuous variables, and the Rho Spearman for correlation analysis. Significance level was 0.05 for all analysis.

Once the subjects had been classified according to the refractive, accommodative, or binocular dysfunction they presented, we analyzed their symptoms and the dysfunction diagnosed, conducting a logistic regression in order to determine whether there was an association between each dysfunction and the symptoms reported by the participants. This procedure yielded the raw odds ratio (OR). The presence of an uncorrected refractive error was considered a confounding variable, as it was associated with both the existence of symptoms and the presence of AD and BD ($p <$ 0.05). We thus determined the probability of having visual symptoms according to the dysfunctions diagnosed after having eliminated the effect that uncorrected refractive errors could have on this relationship and obtained an adjusted estimate of the association between the two variables by means of the adjusted odds ratio (OR).

Statistical analysis was performed using SPSS 20.0 for Windows.

3. Results

Of the 175 study participants, 61 subjects had some form of accommodative and/or binocular dysfunctions, 59 patients were classified as refractive dysfunction, and 55 subjects were grouped in the group without dysfunction. Furthermore, of the 61 subjects with some form of accommodative and/or

TABLE 2: Symptoms categories encountered in all subjects of the sample.

Symptoms	Number of complaints of patients	
	n	%
Visual fatigue	22	20.0
Headache	16	14.5
Dry or gritty eyes	14	12.7
Sore eyes	12	10.9
Blurred vision	11	10,0
Ocular pain	9	8.2
Red eye	7	6.4
Excessive sensitivity to light	6	5.5
Lack of concentration	2	1.8
Excessive blinking	2	1.8
Eye turn noticed	2	1.8
Difficulty in performing schoolwork	1	0.9
Words appearing to move or jump at near vision	1	0.9
Difficulty in focusing from one distance to another	1	0.9
Avoiding near task	1	0.9
Tearing	1	0.9
Pulling eyes	1	0.9
Feeling sleepy	1	0.9
Total	**110**	**100**

binocular anomalies, 33 of them also presented an uncorrected refractive error but they were classified as belonging to the accommodative or binocular dysfunction group.

Of the 175 subjects examined, 78 people (44.6%) reported having some kind of visual symptoms which were grouped into 18 different categories. Table 2 shows these categories encountered, together with the number of complaints reported by the patients.

TABLE 3: Symptoms related to subjects with refractive dysfunction and without dysfunction.

Dysfunction (n)	Number of patients with symptoms	Complaints	
		N	%
Without dysfunction (n = 55)	14	17	15.44
Visual fatigue		4	3.63
Headache		3	2.72
Ocular pain		3	2.72
Dry or gritty eyes		2	1.82
Blurred vision		1	0.91
Excessive sensitivity to light		1	0.91
Sore eyes		2	1.82
Red eye		1	0.91
Refractive dysfunction (n = 59)	27	43	39.08
Headache		9	8.18
Visual fatigue		7	6.36
Blurred vision		6	5.45
Dry or gritty eyes		5	4.55
Excessive sensitivity to light		3	2.72
Sore eyes		3	2.72
Ocular pain		2	1.82
Excessive blinking		2	1.82
Avoiding near task		1	0.91
Tearing		1	0.91
Lack of concentration		1	0.91
Difficulty in focusing from one distance to another		1	0.91
Pulling eyes		1	0.91
Feeling sleepy		1	0.91

An analysis of the sociodemographic data for the 175 university students revealed that there was no association between having symptoms (in general) and wearing contact lenses ($p = 0.44$), sex ($p = 0.17$), number of hours of study per day ($p = 0.068$), or students' academic performance ($p = 0.21$). When this analysis was done considering each type of symptoms isolated, there was only an association between the symptom of blurred vision and the number of hours per day ($p = 0.003$), so that patients with blurred vision studied more number of hours per day compared with patients without symptoms. Correlation analysis showed no correlation between the number of symptoms and the number of hours of study per day ($r = 0.13$, $p = 0.084$) or academic performance ($r = 0.13$, $p = 0.095$).

Tables 3, 4, 5, and 6 show the categories of symptoms detected in the different group of patients, without dysfunction, refractive, accommodative, and/or binocular dysfunctions.

Lastly, Table 7 shows the results of the logistic regression performed to determine the association between visual symptoms and the different dysfunctions diagnosed and gives the raw and adjusted OR for the presence of an uncorrected refractive error. This analysis was conducted for AD and BD dysfunctions both in general and according to the number of clinical signs present (suspect, high suspect, and definite).

Only relationships with a statistically significant raw or adjusted OR ($p < 0.05$) are shown.

4. Discussion

The results of this study of a university population selected by means of random sampling indicate the presence of different symptoms in subjects diagnosed with refractive, accommodative, and binocular dysfunctions. We found an association between visual symptomatology and binocular dysfunction, whereby the higher the number of clinical signs used to diagnose binocular dysfunction, the greater the likelihood of symptoms.

These findings, however, present some limitations. Despite being a randomised sample, our sample size was not large and this may have led to bias in the results. The AD and BD groups were sometimes small, which could lead to a statistical type II error; that is, no statistically significant differences appear when in fact they might exist in a larger sample. In addition to that, the small sample size makes it difficult to establish that this sample is representative of the whole university population. For that reason, results of this study only may be applied to the population analyzed and cannot be extrapolated to the general university population.

TABLE 4: Symptoms related to subjects with accommodative dysfunctions (AE: accommodative excess; AI: accommodative insufficiency).

Dysfunction (n)	Number of patients with symptoms	Complaints	
		N	%
Accommodative excess (n = 13)			
AE suspect (n = 1)	**1**	**1**	**0.91**
Red eye		1	0.91
AE high suspect (n = 7)	**3**	**5**	**4.55**
Dry or gritty eyes		2	1.82
Ocular pain		1	0.91
Sore eyes		1	0.91
Visual fatigue		1	0.91
AE definite (n = 5)	**4**	**4**	**3.63**
Red eye		1	0.91
Sore eyes		1	0.91
Visual fatigue		2	1.82
Accommodative insufficiency (n = 3)			
AI suspect (n = 3)	**2**	**5**	**4.55**
Blurred vision		1	0.91
Difficulty in performing schoolwork		1	0.91
Dry or gritty eyes		1	0.91
Visual fatigue		2	1.82
Accommodative infacility (n = 2)			
Accommodative infacility suspect (n = 3)	**1**	**1**	**0.91**
Sore eyes		1	0.91

Another important consideration when analyzing the results of this research is the diagnostic criteria we used which are different to other studies. Several authors have used different approaches for diagnosing an anomaly, from requiring patients to fail a test on two occasions [62] to use an algorithm to evaluate the degree of decompensated heterophoria [63, 64]. Scientific evidence has shown that there are different diagnostic criteria for these dysfunctions, showing that for several disorders some tests are more important than others [21]. This systematic review considering articles since the last 26 years [21] has shown for binocular conditions that the authors use different clinical criteria based on their own criteria, but there is a lack of studies which have evaluated the diagnostic accuracy (with data of predictive values, sensitivity and specificity, and ROC analysis) of clinical signs used for these anomalies. So the authors usually reach their diagnoses on the basis of the criteria they consider but without any explanation about why several clinical signs are used and others are not. In this sense, all authors consider for binocular disorders the measurement of the deviation, although other tests as NPC for convergence insufficiency are not used by all of them. The same happens with other binocular dysfunctions with large differences between authors although all of them agree with the measurement of the deviation. To date, there is only one study [42] which has evaluated the diagnostic validity for clinical signs associated with a high near exophoria, but it is necessary to explore more these data with greater samples and in other populations. For

this reason, we considered the phoria measurement as the fundamental clinical sign for all conditions.

For accommodative anomalies, diagnostic accuracy studies have shown that there is only certain evidence for several conditions. For accommodative insufficiency ROC analysis [26] has shown that the low accommodative amplitude is the test which has the potential discrimination ability for its diagnosis so we decided to use this clinical sign as the fundamental one. For accommodative excess the only study based on epidemiological criteria showed that a high positive relative accommodation (PRA) may be related to this anomaly [38]. However, this study had an important bias as the authors obtained the sensitivity values through the same tests previously used to diagnose the anomalies and without a ROC analysis. For this reason we decided not to use the PRA value as fundamental but only complementary. We used the fundamental clinical sign of failing monocular accommodative facility with plus lenses as this is the only monocular test which may be considered to be related to the accommodative system. The same was considered for accommodative infacility, being the test of failing monocular accommodative facility with plus and minus lenses, the fundamental clinical sign for its diagnosis.

As we can see, in the present study, we used this knowledge of scientific evidence to define which signs should be considered fundamental and which should be considered complementary. So, we created a specific methodology for classifying accommodative and binocular disorder. Some

TABLE 5: Symptoms related to subjects with binocular dysfunctions (CI: convergence insufficiency; CE: convergence excess; DE: divergence excess).

Dysfunction (*n*)	Number of patients with symptoms	Complaints	
		N	%
Convergence insufficiency (*n* = 17)			
CI suspect (*n* = 3)	2	3	**2.72**
Eye turn noticed		1	0.91
Headache		1	0.91
Visual fatigue		1	0.91
CI high suspect (*n* = 4)	2	4	**3.63**
Dry or gritty eyes		1	0.91
Ocular pain		1	0.91
Red eye		1	0.91
Sore eyes		1	0.91
CI definite (*n* = 10)	6	6	**5.45**
Excessive sensitivity to light		2	1.82
Dry or gritty eyes		1	0.1
Headache		1	0.91
Ocular pain		1	0.91
Visual fatigue		1	0.91
Convergence excess (*n* = 14)			
CE suspect (*n* = 2)	0	0	**0**
—			
CE high suspect (*n* = 6)	2	2	**1.82**
Blurred vision		1	0.91
Headache		1	0.91
CI definite (*n* = 6)	4	5	**4.55**
Blurred vision		2	1.82
Headache		1	0.91
Sore eyes		1	0.91
Visual fatigue		1	0.91
Divergence excess (*n* = 1)			
DE definite (*n* = 1)	1	1	**0.91**
Eye turn noticed		1	0.91
Basic exophoria (*n* = 1)			
Basic exophoria definite (*n* = 1)	1	2	**1.82**
Dry or gritty eyes		1	0.91
Sore eyes		1	0.91
Basic esophoria (*n* = 4)			
Basic esophoria high suspect (*n* = 2)	1	1	**0.91**
Visual fatigue		1	0.91
Basic esophoria definite (*n* = 2)	2	5	**4.55**
Lack of concentration		1	0.91
Ocular pain		1	0.91
Red eye		1	0.91
Sore eyes		1	0.91
Visual fatigue		1	0.91

TABLE 6: Symptoms related to subjects with both accommodative and binocular dysfunctions (CI: convergence insufficiency; CE: convergence insufficiency; AI: accommodative insufficiency; AE: accommodative excess; FVD: fusional vergence dysfunction).

Dysfunction (n)	Number of patients with symptoms	Complaints N	%
CI + AI (n = 2)			
CI definite + AI suspect (n = 2)	2	2	**1.82**
Dry or gritty eyes		1	0.91
Words appearing to move or jump at near vision		1	0.91
CI + AE (n = 2)			
CI suspect + AE high suspect (n = 1)	1	1	**0.91**
Red eye		1	0.91
CI definite + AE definite (n = 1)	0	0	**0**
—			
CE + AI (n = 1)			
CE high suspect + AI suspect (n = 1)	1	1	**0.91**
Red eye		1	0.91
FVD + AI (n = 1)			
FVD suspect + AI suspect (n = 1)	1	1	**0.91**
Visual fatigue		1	0.91

TABLE 7: Adjusted estimation of the association between visual symptomatology and all diagnosed dysfunctions including the different grades of dysfunctions according to the number of clinical signs used (RD: refractive dysfunction; AD: accommodative dysfunction; BD: binocular dysfunction; CI: confidence interval).

	Raw	CI 95%	p	OR Adjusted[†]	CI 95%	p
RD	2.47	1.12–5.47	0.026[*]	NA	NA	NA
AD suspect, high suspect, and definite	4.60	1.49–14.18	0.008[*]	2.34	0.55–9.97	0.249
AD high suspect and definite	3.91	1.15–13.23	0.029[*]	2.20	0.44–11.05	0.340
AD definite	11.71	1.21–113.81	0.034[*]	—	—	0.999
BD suspect, high suspect, and definite	3.84	1.58–9.35	0.003[*]	3.35	1.03–10.91	0.045[*]
BD high suspect and definite	4.28	1.69–10.85	0.002[*]	4.10	1.12–15.02	0.033[*]
BD definite	6.83	2.20–21.21	0.001[*]	8.79	1.59–48.65	0.013[*]
AD + BD	14.64	1.57–136.33	0.018[*]	8.79	0.84–91.49	0.069

[†]OR adjusted by an uncorrected refractive error.
[*]Significant association.

authors have performed similar classifications, diagnosing a disorder according to the number of clinical signs that the subject presented, mainly for convergence insufficiency [8, 36, 39, 40], but this is not the case for the other dysfunctions.

Results of this study reveal that there was no association between having symptoms and student's academic performance. Furthermore, students with more visual symptoms did not have lower academic achievement. These findings are different than those encountered by other authors who have shown a negative effect on school performance. Vaughn et al. [28] encountered that the higher the score in symptoms the poorer the academic performance in children. Shin et al. [1] found that children with both accommodative dysfunctions and a combination of accommodative and vergence dysfunctions had significantly lower academic scores. However they found that those patients with vergence dysfunctions alone had no relationship with academic achievement. In

addition to that, several clinical trials about the treatment of convergence insufficiency in children have shown the improvement of academic behaviours [29] and a significant decrease in performance-related symptoms (reading performance and attention) [30] after treatment. Comparisons are difficult to argue due to the different population examined (children versus adults) but in any case the only association we encountered was for blurred vision and the number of hours per day, showing that patients with blurred vision studied more number of hours per day compared with patients without symptoms. However it seems that in our university subjects the symptomatology does not affect their academic performance. In this sense, for university students, Grisham et al. [27] found an association between symptoms and reading performance. Comparisons are again difficult to discuss as they analyzed the reading performance considering a patient reading after one hour and two hours of near work, and in our study we have considered the academic performance as the number of credits obtained divided by the number of credits studied in the last academic year.

Interestingly, a closer analysis of the results reveals that numerous symptoms were associated with the different dysfunctions identified. We found 18 different categories of symptoms reported by the subjects, the most prevalent of which was "visual fatigue," mentioned in 20% of the reports.

It should also be noted that a quarter of people in the without dysfunction group (14 out of 55) presented symptoms similar to those with visual dysfunctions, such as visual fatigue, headache, or ocular pain. However, these subjects did not present any ocular or visual clinical sign which would explain this symptomatology. This finding suggests that some symptoms may be reported by patients and have no relationship with vision. In fact other authors have shown that several of these symptoms are related to other conditions as dry eye [3] and not only with a visual disorder. However as we did not test for these conditions as dry eye syndrome, we cannot explain any relationship.

As regards dysfunctions, we found that in all groups some patients presented clinical signs but did not report symptoms of any kind. This result is similar to that obtained in the study of Horwood et al. [65] which reports similar findings in a group of university students. In that study the authors used the CISS V-15 questionnaire. Although this survey was developed to monitor symptoms in persons with CI, Horwood et al. [65] used it as a screening tool to confirm the absence of significant visual symptoms. They encountered a strong mismatch between signs and symptoms. Particularly they demonstrated that symptoms often associated with convergence insufficiency (CI) are also common in young adults without clinical signs of CI and also that the majority of subjects with the clinical signs of CI had no symptoms.

Of particular interest is the fact that only the 46% (27 out of 59) of subjects with refractive dysfunction presented symptoms, even though most members of this group experienced an increase in visual acuity with the new correction. This finding suggests a deficit in the health education of these subjects, a possibility that should be taken into account by eye care professionals when conducting eye examinations. It is surprising that university students, who require greater visual demand than others, are not conscious of this visual health problem. However, it was the refractive dysfunction group which presented the highest number of symptoms, with 14 categories. Those most frequently reported were headache, visual fatigue, blurred vision, and dry or gritty eyes, symptoms typically associated with not wearing the proper correction. On the other hand, there were no complaints in the accommodative dysfunction group of difficulty in focusing from one distance to another or of headache, although in the literature such symptoms have been associated with these dysfunctions [43]. Furthermore, we did not find specific symptoms in the accommodative dysfunction or binocular dysfunction groups that were exclusively related to one dysfunction alone but rather observed that there were several categories common to both dysfunction groups, such as visual fatigue, blurred vision, or sore eyes. Therefore, one can conclude that the symptoms of visual problems are very similar in all refractive, accommodative, or binocular dysfunctions. This finding coincides with the results of the scoping review by García-Muñoz et al. [43], in which the authors found that most of the symptoms described in the scientific literature were related to both accommodative and binocular dysfunctions, although in that study the symptomatology of refractive dysfunctions was not determined.

Unadjusted associations between dysfunctions and symptoms were statistically significant in all dysfunction groups (refractive, accommodative, and binocular). The raw odds ratio indicated that those subjects with some kind of visual dysfunction were more likely to experience symptoms than those in the without dysfunction group.

However, when these associations were adjusted for the presence of an uncorrected refractive error, most of them ceased to be statistically significant, except for the group of binocular dysfunction. Particularly, for binocular dysfunctions, the odds ratio increased when high suspect and definite binocular dysfunction were considered. This implies that the more the clinical signs a subject presented, the greater the likelihood of experiencing symptoms. However this association does not mean that the more the clinical signs present the greater the frequency of symptoms as we did not examine the frequency of symptoms. In fact the study of Bade et al. [66] has shown that for children with convergence insufficiency there is no association between the severity of the clinical signs and their level of symptoms. For that reason future studies should show how this association encountered in our study may be modified if the frequency of symptoms is considered.

Our results indicate that an uncorrected refractive error contaminates the symptoms of visual dysfunction, fundamentally when an accommodative dysfunction is present. This should make us consider that when an accommodative anomaly is present and the patient has also an uncorrected refractive error, we cannot assure that patients' symptoms are due to the accommodative problem.

This influence of uncorrected refractive error suggests that when an accommodative or vergence dysfunction is detected, the refractive error should be corrected first before initiating a specific treatment to alleviate the patient's symptoms. This idea is consistent with the proposal made by Dwyer and Wick [67] who have suggested that correction of an uncorrected refractive error improves accommodative and binocular function. Nevertheless, it is unusual for studies of accommodative and binocular dysfunctions in adults to include details on how uncorrected refractive error has been managed and this may have led to research bias. Studies on prevalence of these conditions in adults [20] do not usually offer the prevalence rates about refractive dysfunctions. And even several authors exclude those subjects with refractive anomalies [11]. When considering diagnosis purposes [21] few studies refer to refractive anomalies [33, 34]. And for studies about treatment [68] only the clinical trials about convergence insufficiency [69–71] do detail the adequate prescription of refractive correction before the treatment. In future studies, researchers should consider the effect of an uncorrected refractive error on the prevalence, diagnosis, and treatment of accommodative and vergence dysfunctions to determine its influence in the management of these anomalies.

Conflict of Interests

The authors declare that there is no conflict of interests regarding the publication of this paper.

Acknowledgment

This work has been supported by "Vicerrectorado de Investigación, Desarrollo e Innovación" of the University of Alicante, Spain, GRE10-06.

References

[1] H. S. Shin, S. C. Park, and C. M. Park, "Relationship between accommodative and vergence dysfunctions and academic achievement for primary school children," *Ophthalmic and Physiological Optics*, vol. 29, no. 6, pp. 615–624, 2009.

[2] E. G. Conlon, W. J. Lovegrove, E. Chekaluk, and P. E. Pattison, "Measuring visual discomfort," *Visual Cognition*, vol. 6, no. 6, pp. 637–663, 1999.

[3] J. E. Sheedy, J. N. Hayes, and J. Engle, "Is all asthenopia the same?" *Optometry and Vision Science*, vol. 80, no. 11, pp. 732–739, 2003.

[4] R. G. Watten, "Reinvention of visual fatigue: accumulation of scientific knowledge or neglect of scientific history?" *Ophthalmic and Physiological Optics*, vol. 14, no. 4, pp. 428–432, 1994.

[5] B. J. W. Evans, "The need for optometric investigation in suspected Meares-Irlen syndrome or visual stress," *Ophthalmic and Physiological Optics*, vol. 25, no. 4, pp. 363–370, 2005.

[6] C. Chase, C. Tosha, E. Borsting, and W. H. Ridder, "Visual discomfort and objective measures of static accommodation," *Optometry and Vision Science*, vol. 86, no. 7, pp. 883–889, 2009.

[7] A. A. Yekta, T. Jenkins, and D. Pickwell, "The clinical assessment of binocular vision before and after a working day," *Ophthalmic and Physiological Optics*, vol. 7, no. 4, pp. 349–352, 1987.

[8] M. W. Rouse, E. Borsting, L. Hyman et al., "Frequency of convergence insufficiency among fifth and sixth graders. The Convergence Insufficiency and Reading Study (CIRS) group," *Optometry and Vision Science*, vol. 76, no. 9, pp. 643–649, 1999.

[9] E. Borsting, M. W. Rouse, P. N. Deland et al., "Association of symptoms and convergence and accommodative insufficiency in school-age children," *Optometry*, vol. 74, no. 1, pp. 25–34, 2003.

[10] J. E. Letourneau and S. Duci, "Prevalence of convergence insufficiency among elementary school children," *Canadian Journal of Optometry*, vol. 50, pp. 194–197, 1988.

[11] E. Porcar and A. Martinez-Palomera, "Prevalence of general binocular dysfunctions in a population of university students," *Optometry and Vision Science*, vol. 74, no. 2, pp. 111–113, 1997.

[12] F. Lara, P. Cacho-Martínez, Á. García-Muñoz, and R. Megías, "General binocular disorders: prevalence in a clinic population," *Ophthalmic and Physiological Optics*, vol. 21, no. 1, pp. 70–74, 2001.

[13] P. Dwyer, "The prevalence of vergence accommodation disorders in a school-age population," *Clinical & Experimental Optometry*, vol. 75, no. 1, pp. 10–18, 1992.

[14] S. Abdi and A. Rydberg, "Asthenopia in schoolchildren, orthoptic and ophthalmological findings and treatment," *Documenta Ophthalmologica*, vol. 111, no. 2, pp. 65–72, 2005.

[15] L. D. Pickwell, M. A. Viggars, and T. C. A. Jenkins, "Convergence insufficiency in a rural population," *Ophthalmic and Physiological Optics*, vol. 6, no. 3, pp. 339–341, 1986.

[16] M. Scheiman, M. Gallaway, R. Coulter et al., "Prevalence of vision and ocular disease conditions in a clinical pediatric population," *Journal of the American Optometric Association*, vol. 67, no. 4, pp. 193–202, 1996.

[17] M. W. Rouse, L. Hyman, M. Hussein, and H. Solan, "Frequency of convergence insufficiency in optometry clinic settings. Convergence Insufficiency and Reading Study (CIRS) Group," *Optometry and Vision Science*, vol. 75, no. 2, pp. 88–96, 1998.

[18] S. C. Hokoda, "General binocular dysfunctions in an urban optometry clinic," *Journal of the American Optometric Association*, vol. 56, no. 7, pp. 560–562, 1985.

[19] S. H. Hoseini-Yazdi, A. Yekta, H. Nouri, J. Heravian, H. Ostadimoghaddam, and M. Khabazkhoob, "Frequency of convergence and accommodative disorders in a clinical population of Mashhad, Iran," *Strabismus*, vol. 23, no. 1, pp. 22–29, 2015.

[20] P. Cacho-Martínez, Á. García-Muñoz, and M. T. Ruiz-Cantero, "Do we really know the prevalence of accomodative and nonstrabismic binocular dysfunctions?" *Journal of Optometry*, vol. 3, no. 4, pp. 185–197, 2010.

[21] P. Cacho-Martínez, Á. García-Muñoz, and M. T. Ruiz-Cantero, "Is there any evidence for the validity of diagnostic criteria used for accommodative and nonstrabismic binocular dysfunctions?" *Journal of Optometry*, vol. 7, no. 1, pp. 2–21, 2014.

[22] E. Borsting, C. H. Chase, and W. H. Ridder, "Measuring visual discomfort in college students," *Optometry and Vision Science*, vol. 84, no. 8, pp. 745–751, 2007.

[23] E. Borsting, C. Chase, C. Tosha, and W. H. Ridder, "Longitudinal study of visual discomfort symptoms in college students," *Optometry and Vision Science*, vol. 85, no. 10, pp. 992–998, 2008.

[24] S. A. Drew, E. Borsting, A. E. Escobar, C. Liu, E. Castellanos, and C. Chase, "Can chronic visual discomfort measures accurately predict acute symptoms?" *Optometry and Vision Science*, vol. 90, no. 10, pp. 1149–1155, 2013.

[25] H. D. Simons and J. D. Grisham, "Binocular anomalies and reading problems," *Journal of the American Optometric Association*, vol. 58, no. 7, pp. 578–587, 1987.

[26] B. Sterner, M. Gellerstedt, and A. Sjöström, "Accommodation and the relationship to subjective symptoms with near work for young school children," *Ophthalmic and Physiological Optics*, vol. 26, no. 2, pp. 148–155, 2006.

[27] J. D. Grisham, M. M. Sheppard, and W. U. Tran, "Visual symptoms and reading performance," *Optometry and Vision Science*, vol. 70, no. 5, pp. 384–391, 1993.

[28] W. Vaughn, W. C. Maples, and R. Hoenes, "The association between vision quality of life and academics as measured by the College of Optometrists in Vision Development Quality of Life questionnaire," *Optometry*, vol. 77, no. 3, pp. 116–123, 2006.

[29] E. Borsting, G. L. Mitchell, M. T. Kulp et al., "Improvement in academic behaviors after successful treatment of convergence insufficiency," *Optometry and Vision Science*, vol. 89, no. 1, pp. 12–18, 2012.

[30] C. Barnhardt, S. A. Cotter, G. L. Mitchell, M. Scheiman, and M. T. Kulp, "Symptoms in children with convergence insufficiency: before and after treatment," *Optometry and Vision Science*, vol. 89, no. 10, pp. 1512–1520, 2012.

[31] K. M. Daum, "Characteristics of exodeviations: I. A comparison of three classes," *American Journal of Optometry and Physiological Optics*, vol. 63, no. 4, pp. 237–243, 1986.

[32] M. Scheiman, M. Gallaway, and E. Ciner, "Divergence insufficiency: characteristics, diagnosis, and treatment," *American Journal of Optometry and Physiological Optics*, vol. 63, no. 6, pp. 425–431, 1986.

[33] G. A. Chrousos, J. F. O'Neill, B. D. Lueth, and M. M. Parks, "Accommodation deficiency in healthy young individuals," *Journal of Pediatric Ophthalmology and Strabismus*, vol. 25, no. 4, pp. 176–179, 1988.

[34] R. P. Rutstein, K. M. Daum, and J. F. Amos, "Accommodative spasm: a study of 17 cases," *Journal of the American Optometric Association*, vol. 59, no. 7, pp. 527–538, 1988.

[35] P. Dwyer, "Clinical criteria for vergence accommodation dysfunction," *Clinical & Experimental Optometry*, vol. 74, no. 4, pp. 112–119, 1991.

[36] E. Borsting, M. W. Rouse, and P. N. De Land, "Prospective comparison of convergence insufficiency and normal binocular children on CIRS symptom surveys," *Optometry and Vision Science*, vol. 76, no. 4, pp. 221–228, 1999.

[37] P. Cacho-Martínez, Á. García-Muñoz, F. Lara, and M. M. Seguí, "Diagnostic signs of accommodative insufficiency," *Optometry and Vision Science*, vol. 79, no. 9, pp. 614–620, 2002.

[38] Á. García, P. Cacho, and F. Lara, "Evaluating relative accommodations in general binocular dysfunctions," *Optometry and Vision Science*, vol. 79, no. 12, pp. 779–787, 2002.

[39] E. J. Borsting, M. W. Rouse, G. L. Mitchell et al., "Validity and reliability of the revised convergence insufficiency symptom survey in children aged 9 to 18 years," *Optometry and Vision Science*, vol. 80, no. 12, pp. 832–838, 2003.

[40] M. W. Rouse, E. J. Borsting, G. L. Mitchell et al., "Validity and reliability of the revised convergence insufficiency symptom survey in adults," *Ophthalmic and Physiological Optics*, vol. 24, no. 5, pp. 384–390, 2004.

[41] L. F. Marran, P. N. De Land, and A. L. Nguyen, "Accommodative insufficiency is the primary source of symptoms in children diagnosed with convergence insufficiency," *Optometry and Vision Science*, vol. 83, no. 5, pp. E281–E289, 2006.

[42] P. Cacho-Martínez, Á. García-Muñoz, and M. T. Ruiz-Cantero, "Diagnostic validity of clinical signs associated with a large exophoria at near," *Journal of Ophthalmology*, vol. 2013, Article ID 549435, 10 pages, 2013.

[43] Á. García-Muñoz, S. Carbonell-Bonete, and P. Cacho-Martínez, "Symptomatology associated with accommodative and binocular vision anomalies," *Journal of Optometry*, vol. 7, no. 4, pp. 178–192, 2014.

[44] L. Monger, A. Wilkins, and P. Allen, "Identifying visual stress during a routine eye examination," *Journal of Optometry*, vol. 8, no. 2, pp. 140–145, 2015.

[45] C. Haine, "The ophthalmic case historian," in *Borish's Clinical Refraction*, W. J. Benjamin, Ed., pp. 195–216, Butterworth-Heinemann, St. Louis, Mo, USA, 2006.

[46] G. E. Russell and B. Wick, "A prospective study of treatment of accommodative insufficiency," *Optometry and Vision Science*, vol. 70, no. 2, pp. 131–135, 1993.

[47] B. B. Rainey, T. L. Schroeder, D. A. Goss, and T. P. Grosvenor, "Reliability of and comparisons among three variations of the alternating cover test," *Ophthalmic and Physiological Optics*, vol. 18, no. 5, pp. 430–437, 1998.

[48] B. B. Rainey, T. L. Schroeder, D. A. Goss, and T. P. Grosvenor, "Inter-examiner repeatability of heterophoria tests," *Optometry and Vision Science*, vol. 75, no. 10, pp. 719–726, 1998.

[49] N. A. S. Barnard and W. D. Thomson, "A quantitative analysis of eye movements during the cover test—a preliminary report," *Ophthalmic and Physiological Optics*, vol. 15, no. 5, pp. 413–419, 1995.

[50] M. Scheiman and B. Wick, *Clinical Management of Binocular Vision: Heterophoric, Accommodative, and Eye Movement Disorders*, Lippincott Williams & Wilkins, Philadelphia, Pa, USA, 3rd edition, 2008.

[51] M. W. Rouse, R. London, and D. C. Allen, "An evaluation of the monocular estimate method of dynamic retinoscopy," *American Journal of Optometry and Physiological Optics*, vol. 59, no. 3, pp. 234–239, 1982.

[52] H. W. Hofstetter, "Useful age-amplitude formula," *Optometry and Vision Science*, vol. 38, pp. 42–45, 1950.

[53] J. A. Zellers, T. L. Alpert, and M. W. Rouse, "A review of the literature and a normative study of accommodative facility," *Journal of the American Optometric Association*, vol. 55, no. 1, pp. 31–37, 1984.

[54] M. Scheiman, M. Gallaway, K. A. Frantz et al., "Nearpoint of convergence: test procedure, target selection, and normative data," *Optometry and Vision Science*, vol. 80, no. 3, pp. 214–225, 2003.

[55] J. Siderov, S. C. Chiu, and S. J. Waugh, "Differences in the nearpoint of convergence with target type," *Ophthalmic and Physiological Optics*, vol. 21, no. 5, pp. 356–360, 2001.

[56] M. Rosenfield, K. J. Ciuffreda, E. Ong, and S. Super, "Vergence adaptation and the order of clinical vergence range testing," *Optometry and Vision Science*, vol. 72, no. 4, pp. 219–223, 1995.

[57] M. Rosenfield, "Prism adaptation: relevance in clinical practice," *Journal of Optometric Vision Development*, vol. 28, pp. 68–75, 1997.

[58] R. Gall, B. Wick, and H. Bedell, "Vergence facility: establishing clinical utility," *Optometry and Vision Science*, vol. 75, no. 10, pp. 731–742, 1998.

[59] R. Gall, B. Wick, and H. Bedell, "Vergence facility and target type," *Optometry and Vision Science*, vol. 75, no. 10, pp. 727–730, 1998.

[60] J. Saladin, "Phorometry and stereopsis," in *Borish's Clinical Refraction*, W. J. Benjamin, Ed., pp. 899–960, Butterworth-Heinemann, St. Louis, Mo, USA, 2006.

[61] B. J. W. Evans, *Pickwell's Binocular Vision Anomalies: Investigation and Treatment*, Elsevier Butterworth-Heineman, Edinburgh, Scotland, 5th edition, 2007.

[62] D. Stidwill, "Epidemiology of strabismus," *Ophthalmic and Physiological Optics*, vol. 17, no. 6, pp. 536–539, 1997.

[63] B. J. W. Evans, *Pickwell's Binocular Vision Anomalies: Investigation and Treatment*, Butterworth-Heinemann, Oxford, UK, 4th edition, 2002.

[64] M. Lambooij, M. Fortuin, W. Ijsselsteijn, B. Evans, and I. Heynderickx, "Measuring visual fatigue and visual discomfort associated with 3-D displays," *Journal of the Society for Information Display*, vol. 18, no. 11, pp. 931–943, 2010.

[65] A. M. Horwood, S. Toor, and P. M. Riddell, "Screening for convergence insufficiency using the CISS is not indicated in young adults," *British Journal of Ophthalmology*, vol. 98, no. 5, pp. 679–683, 2014.

[66] A. Bade, M. Boas, M. Gallaway et al., "Relationship between clinical signs and symptoms of convergence insufficiency," *Optometry and Vision Science*, vol. 90, no. 9, pp. 988–995, 2013.

[67] P. Dwyer and B. Wick, "The influence of refractive correction upon disorders of vergence and accommodation," *Optometry and Vision Science*, vol. 72, no. 4, pp. 224–232, 1995.

[68] P. Cacho-Martinez, A. Garcia-Muñoz, and M. T. Ruíz-Cantero, "Treatment of accommodative and nonstrabismic binocular dysfunctions: a systematic review," *Optometry*, vol. 80, no. 12, pp. 702–716, 2009.

[69] M. Scheiman, S. Cotter, M. Rouse et al., "Randomised clinical trial of the effectiveness of base-in prism reading glasses versus placebo reading glasses for symptomatic convergence insufficiency in children," *British Journal of Ophthalmology*, vol. 89, no. 10, pp. 1318–1323, 2005.

[70] M. Scheiman, G. L. Mitchell, S. Cotter et al., "A randomized clinical trial of treatments for convergence insufficiency in children," *Archives of Ophthalmology*, vol. 123, no. 1, pp. 14–24, 2005.

[71] M. Scheiman, G. L. Mitchell, S. Cotter et al., "A randomized clinical trial of vision therapy/orthoptics versus pencil pushups for the treatment of convergence insufficiency in young adults," *Optometry and Vision Science*, vol. 82, no. 7, pp. 583–593, 2005.

16

Inconsistencies Exist in National Estimates of Eye Care Services Utilization in the United States

Fernando A. Wilson,[1] Jim P. Stimpson,[2] and Yang Wang[1]

[1]College of Public Health, University of Nebraska Medical Center, 984350 Nebraska Medical Center, Omaha, NE 68198-4350, USA
[2]School of Public Health, City University of New York, 55 W. 125th Street, New York, NY 10027, USA

Correspondence should be addressed to Fernando A. Wilson; fernando.wilson@unmc.edu

Academic Editor: Antonio Benito

Background. There are limited research and substantial uncertainty about the level of eye care utilization in the United States. *Objectives.* Our study estimated eye care utilization using, to our knowledge, every known nationally representative, publicly available database with information on office-based optometry or ophthalmology services. *Research Design.* We analyzed the following national databases to estimate eye care utilization: the Medical Expenditure Panel Survey (MEPS), National Health Interview Survey (NHIS), Joint Canada/US Survey of Health (JCUSH), Behavioral Risk Factor Surveillance System (BRFSS), and the National Ambulatory Medical Care Survey (NAMCS). *Subjects.* US adults aged 18 and older. *Measures.* Self-reported utilization of eye care services. *Results.* The weighted number of adults seeing or talking with any eye doctor ranges from 87.9 million to 99.5 million, and the number of visits annually ranges from 72.9 million to 142.6 million. There were an estimated 17.2 million optometry visits and 55.8 million ophthalmology visits. *Conclusions.* The definitions and estimates of eye care services vary widely across national databases, leading to substantial differences in national estimates of eye care utilization.

1. Introduction

A recent report by the American Optometry Association (AOA) suggests that optometrists (OD) perform 88 million comprehensive eye exams annually, comprising 85% of all eye exams, compared to only 16 million (15%) exams performed by ophthalmologists (MD) [1]. These statistics have been widely cited in various reports on the eye care industry, and they have been used to demonstrate that most Americans rely on optometrists for their eye care needs [1–3]. However, the methodology used to generate these estimates is not available in the report, and there is significant uncertainty concerning the true number of eye care services that are being delivered in the US by optometrists, ophthalmologists, or other eye care professionals. To our knowledge, prior research examining the consistency and validity of current national estimates of eye care utilization across major publicly available healthcare databases does not exist. The uncertainty over utilization relative to the supply of eye care professionals—and thus uncertainty over whether the eye care needs of Americans

are being met—has important implications for the creation and funding of programs and policies that impact either utilization or supply in the eye care market. Our study estimates eye care utilization using every known nationally representative, publicly available database with information on office-based optometry or ophthalmology services.

2. Methods

To examine this issue, we analyzed the following publicly available databases: the Medical Expenditure Panel Survey (MEPS), National Health Interview Survey (NHIS), Joint Canada/US Survey of Health (JCUSH), and the National Ambulatory Medical Care Survey (NAMCS). To our knowledge, these databases contain all nationally representative data on office-based eye care utilization that are available to the public in the US. The NHIS is a national database collecting self-reported data on health and healthcare utilization and other measures using in-person interviews and is managed by the Centers for Disease Control and Prevention (CDC)

TABLE 1: Weighted number and percentage of adults aged 18 and older utilizing eye care services and weighted number of eye care visits in the United States stratified by nationally representative database.

	Weighted number of adults	Weighted number of visits	Weighted percent of adults visiting an eye care professional
Seeing or talking with any eye doctor in any setting in 12 months:			
2012 National Health Interview Survey (NHIS)[1]	87,850,196	N/A	38.0
2004 Joint Canada/US Survey of Health (JCUSH)[2]	99,472,902	142,634,037	48.3
Number of adults visiting an office-based optometrist in 12 months (ophthalmologists are excluded):			
2012 MEPS[3]	14,556,138	17,183,610	6.1
Number of adults visiting an office-based ophthalmologist in 12 months (optometrists are excluded):			
2012 MEPS[4]	30,434,241	55,756,866	12.8
2010 National Ambulatory Medical Care Survey (NAMCS)[5]	N/A	50,346,592	N/A
Having a dilated eye exam in 12 months:			
2008 NHIS[6]	89,335,468	N/A	40.4

[1] NHIS respondents were asked, "During the past 12 months, have you seen or talked to any of the following health care providers about your own health? ... An optometrist, ophthalmologist, or eye doctor (someone who prescribes eyeglasses)." Possible responses included "Yes," "No," "Refused," and "Don't know." This question was only asked to adults aged 18 and over.
[2] 2004 is the most recent survey year. JCUSH surveyed adults aged 18 and over by telephone. JCUSH respondents were asked, "In the past 12 months, how many times have you seen or talked with the following health care providers about your own health? ... An eye doctor including other people that prescribe lenses (such as an ophthalmologist or optometrist)?" Possible responses included a numerical response, "Refused," and "Don't know." Estimates in Table 2 were restricted to US residents only.
[3] MEPS respondents were asked about any medical events and corresponding medical care visits occurring in the prior 12 months. For each office-based medical care visit, respondents were also asked "What type of medical person did you talk to on {Visit Date}?" Possible responses included "optometrist" in addition to other specialties. In addition, MEPS supplements self-reported data on medical care utilization with surveys of respondents' medical providers (MD or DO). The Medical Provider component of MEPS provides detailed information on ophthalmology services.
[4] MEPS supplements self-reported data on medical care utilization with surveys of respondents' medical providers. The Medical Provider component of MEPS provides detailed information on ophthalmology services.
[5] 2010 is the most recent survey year. NAMCS is a national survey of office-based physicians who are nonfederally employed and engaged primarily in patient care activities.
[6] Respondents were asked, "When was the last time you had an eye exam in which the pupils were dilated? This would have made you temporarily sensitive to bright light." Possible responses included "Less than one month", "1–12 months", "13–24 months", "More than 2 years", "Never", "Refused", "Don't know".

[4]. The MEPS uses a subsample of NHIS respondents to provide detailed healthcare and other pieces of information for individuals and also includes a survey of respondents' medical providers [5]. The Agency for Healthcare Research and Quality (AHRQ) is responsible for administering the MEPS database. The JCUSH database is conducted by the CDC and Statistics Canada and consisted of random telephone surveys between November 2002 and March 2003 in both US and Canada [6]. JCUSH data are nationally representative for the US, providing information on eye care utilization. Finally, the NAMCS is a national database of physicians conducted by the CDC and provides clinical data on visits to ophthalmologists in the US [7].

In addition to the above databases, we also examined the Behavioral Risk Factor Surveillance System (BRFSS), which provides eye care utilization data restricted to adults aged 40 and over in a limited number of states [8]. We estimated the annual total number and percent of adults aged 18 years and older (40 years and older for BRFSS) who utilized eye care services and also the total number of eye care visits for databases providing these data. All analyses were weighted and adjusted for complex survey design using STATA 13 (College Station, TX).

3. Results

Table 1 shows a wide range of definitions and estimates of eye care services. MEPS differentiates between optometrists and ophthalmologists. The NHIS and JCUSH do not differentiate eye care professionals or their practice settings, and NAMCS only provides data on ophthalmologists. The weighted number of adults seeing or talking with any eye doctor ranges from 87.9 million for NHIS to 99.5 million for JCUSH. Total number of visits annually is 142.6 million from JCUSH. By comparison, MEPS results suggest that there are about 45 million adults visiting office-based optometrists and ophthalmologists annually, totaling 72.9 million visits. MEPS is the only database providing information on optometry specifically, and it indicates there are 14.6 million people utilizing optometry services annually in the US, resulting in 17.2 million visits. MEPS and NAMCS provide data on ophthalmology-only visits; MEPS estimates 55.8 million

TABLE 2: Weighted number and percentage of adults aged 40 and over utilizing eye care services in 11 states in 2008–2010, BRFSS[1].

	Weighted number	Weighted percent
Eyes examined by any doctor or eye care provider in 12 months[2]	10,703,480	62.4
Having a dilated eye exam in 12 months[3]	7,126,244	49.5

[1]States included Alabama, Indiana, Iowa, Connecticut, Missouri, New Mexico, North Carolina, Tennessee, Wyoming, Arkansas, and Georgia. Only the most recent data were used for each state within the study period 2008–10.

[2]Respondents were asked, "When was the last time you had your eyes examined by any doctor or eye care provider?" Possible responses included "Within the past month," "Within the past year," "Within the past 2 years," "2 or more years ago," "Never," "Refused," and "Don't know/Not sure."

[3]Respondents were asked, "When was the last time you had an eye exam in which the pupils were dilated? This would have made you temporarily sensitive to bright light." Possible responses included "Within the past month," "Within the past year," "Within the past 2 years," "2 or more years ago," "Never," "Refused," and "Don't know/Not sure."

TABLE 3: Total number of refractive eye exams performed annually in the US reported by AOA Excel and Jobson Medical Information LLC, 2012[1].

	Number
Number of refractive eye exams performed by optometrists only	88 million
Number of refractive eye exams performed by ophthalmologists only	16 million
Total annual exams	104 million

[1]AOA Excel and Jobson Medical Information LLC. The State of the Optometric Profession: 2013 (available at http://www.reviewob.com/Data/Sites/1/soop_070120134.pdf. Accessed February 19, 2015).

ophthalmology visits in 2012 compared to 50.3 million for NAMCS in 2010. NHIS indicated there were 89.3 million dilated eye exams performed in 2008—the most recent year available for this measure.

Table 2 provides BRFSS weighted estimates of eye exams performed annually. Unfortunately, BRFSS collected eye care data for only 11 states in the period 2008–10 and only for persons aged 40 and older. 62.4% of respondents in these states had their eyes examined by a doctor or eye care professional. This compares to a range of 45–55% for persons aged 40 and over in the NHIS and JCUSH databases (results not shown). The weighted percentage of respondents reporting a dilated eye exam (49.5%) is similar to the results reported in the 2008 NHIS (47.9%; not shown).

In contrast to the above analyses, Table 3 provides estimates reported by AOA Excel and Jobson Medical Information in "The State of the Optometric Profession: 2013." This report states that optometrists perform 88 million refractive eye exams annually. This statistic has been widely cited in various reports on the eye care industry. Unfortunately, we were not able to replicate or find information on the origin of this figure. It seems to be based on an analysis by Jobson's Practice Advancement Associates, but we could not find

details of this analysis or the source of data used. However, this estimate is high compared to results from the other databases on eye care utilization. For example, the NHIS—used in several studies on eye care—shows that there are about 88 million adults who "see or talk to" any eye doctor (optometrists, ophthalmologists, or other professionals) for any reason in a year.

Conversely, the AOA Excel/Jobson report's finding that there are only 16 million exams performed by ophthalmologists in 2012 seems low. The NAMCS—a national survey of medical providers—shows that there were 50.3 million ophthalmology visits annually among adults in 2010 (and 55.5 million visits among all age groups (not shown in Table 2)). Using ICD-9-CM procedure codes for eye examination (95.00–95.09), NAMCS data show that ophthalmologists performed 22.2 million exams for all age groups in 2010 (not shown in tables). 2010 was the most recent survey year for NAMCS and there were substantial missing values for the procedure codes, so the actual number of eye exams performed by ophthalmologists may be significantly higher today. 2012 MEPS data for ophthalmologists show that 31.5 million adults utilize ophthalmologists at least once in a year resulting in 55.8 million total visits, compared to 50.3 million visits from NAMCS.

The wide range of eye care utilization estimates is likely a function of the variance in question wording (see footnotes of Table 1), but it is also possible that there are differences in survey design and populations studied across the databases. Therefore, we compared utilization of office-based physicians and receipt of routine medical checkups for MEPS, NHIS, BRFSS, and NAMCS (Table 4). The difference between the lowest and highest number of people receiving medical checkups varied by about 4% across the databases. Similarly, there was a 1.5% difference in weighted number of visits between MEPS and NAMCS. These results suggest that variations in measurement of eye care service utilization are unlikely due to differences in survey design and instead are related to differences in measurement.

4. Discussion

We found that definitions and estimates of eye care services vary widely across databases, leading to substantial differences in national estimates of eye care utilization. Furthermore, only MEPS and the AOA report provide estimates on optometry services. However, the AOA estimate of optometry services may be high, and its estimate of ophthalmology services low, compared to other available databases. The methodology used to estimate these services was not provided and, thus, we cannot gauge the accuracy or limitations of their estimates. Interestingly, differences in national estimates of general physician-based medical care are relatively small across the databases.

Our study findings on the large differences in eye care utilization have wider implications for determining whether eye care professionals are currently meeting primary care needs in the US population or if there is an oversupply of professionals. One study suggests that one out of two adults aged 20 and over has eye sight problems—accounting

TABLE 4: A comparison of utilization of office-based physician services across databases in the US.

	Weighted number of adults	Weighted number of visits	Weighted percent of adults visiting a physician
Number of visits to an MD/DO in 12 months by adults (18 years or older):			
2012 MEPS	160,637,294	829,664,093	67.7
2010 NAMCS	N/A	817,302,463	N/A
Number of adults (18 years or older) who received a routine checkup by physician in 12 months:			
2012 NHIS	154,957,097	N/A	67.1
2012 BRFSS	161,513,385	N/A	67.7
2012 MEPS	154,480,018	N/A	67.5

for about 112.7 million Americans [8]. Our results suggest that the needs of persons with eye sight problems may be sufficiently met according to one survey (JCUSH) or that there may be underutilization of eye care services based on other surveys (MEPS/NAMCS). These estimates suggest that aggregate annual visits may range from 67.5 to 142.6 million in the US. The uncertainty over utilization relative to the supply of eye care professionals impacts decisions about the creation and funding of programs and policies that impact either utilization or supply of eye care services. It is likely that there will be increasing need for eye care services with the aging population in the US, but the empirical evidence is equivocal as to whether there is sufficient access to optometrists, ophthalmologists, and other professionals to meet the demand for services. The uncertainty highlighted in our study suggests a need for improved data collection efforts in eye care services, particularly the measurement of providers and services provided. An important priority of Health People 2020 is to decrease visual impairment in the US, and to help achieve this goal, an expert panel convened by the Centers for Disease Control and Prevention called for the establishment of a vision surveillance system [9–11]. Furthermore, the CDC recently issued a Funding Opportunity Announcement with the purpose of implementing a national vision surveillance system [12]. Existing data sources such as NHIS and BRFSS would be important components of this system, and the success of the surveillance system would require an effective assessment of eye care utilization [10–12]. However, our study emphasizes the importance of resolving uncertainties in estimates of eye care utilization across national surveys, thus providing a solid foundation for a vision surveillance system. Our research may also signal a need to examine inconsistencies in national estimates for other healthcare professions, particularly auxiliary or specialty services.

Conflict of Interests

The authors declare that there is no conflict of interests regarding the publication of this paper.

References

[1] AOA Excel and Jobson Medical Information LLC, *The State of the Optometric Profession: 2013*, 2015, http://www.reviewob.com/Data/Sites/1/soop_070120134.pdf.

[2] Harris Williams & Co, "Vision Industry Overview," 2015, http://www.harriswilliams.com/sites/default/files/content/hwco_hcls_vision_industry_updatev2.pdf.

[3] American Optometric Association, "AOA news," *President's Column*, vol. 52, no. 5, 2013, http://www.omagdigital.com/publication/?i=180556&p=6.

[4] Centers for Disease Control and Prevention, "About the National Health Interview Survey," 2015, http://www.cdc.gov/nchs/nhis/about_nhis.htm.

[5] Agency for Healthcare Research and Quality, "Medical Expenditure Panel Survey. Survey Background," 2015, http://meps.ahrq.gov/mepsweb/about_meps/survey_back.jsp.

[6] Centers for Disease Control and Prevention, "The Joint Canada/United States Survey of Health," 2015, http://www.cdc.gov/nchs/nhis/jcush.htm.

[7] Centers for Disease Control and Prevention, *Ambulatory Health Care Data*, 2015, http://www.cdc.gov/nchs/ahcd.htm.

[8] S. Vitale, L. Ellwein, M. F. Cotch, F. L. Ferris III, and R. Sperduto, "Prevalence of refractive error in the United States, 1999–2004," *Archives of Ophthalmology*, vol. 126, no. 8, pp. 1111–1119, 2008.

[9] Healthy People 2020, "Vision," 2015, http://www.healthypeople.gov/2020/topics-objectives/topic/vision/objectives?topicId=42.

[10] P. P. Lee, S. K. West, S. S. Block et al., "Surveillance of disparities in vision and eye health in the United States: an expert panel's opinions," *American Journal of Ophthalmology*, vol. 154, no. 6, supplement, pp. S3–S7, 2012.

[11] S. K. West and P. Lee, "Vision surveillance in the United States: has the time come?" *American Journal of Ophthalmology*, vol. 154, supplement 6, pp. S1–S2.e2, 2012.

[12] Centers for Disease Control and Prevention, "Establish a Vision and Eye Health Surveillance System for the Nation (RFA-DP-15-004)," 2015, http://www.cdc.gov/chronicdisease/about/foa/visioneyehealthsurveillance/index.htm.

17

Sulcus Fixation of Foldable Intraocular Lenses Guided by Ultrasound Biomicroscopy

Shasha Gao,[1] Tingyu Qin,[1] Shengnan Wang,[2] and Yong Lu[1]

[1]*Department of Ophthalmology, The First Affiliated Hospital of Zhengzhou University, Zhengzhou 450052, China*
[2]*Department of Ophthalmology, Beijing Ditan Hospital, Capital Medical University, Beijing, China*

Correspondence should be addressed to Yong Lu; lyong2002@126.com

Academic Editor: Lisa Toto

Background. To evaluate the clinical efficacy of suture fixation of foldable intraocular lens (IOL) in ciliary sulcus guided by ultrasound biomicroscopy (UBM). *Methods*. Thirty-five eyes of 32 cases needing suture fixation of foldable IOL in ciliary sulcus in our hospital were collected and divided into two groups: group A and group B. In group A, UBM was performed on 19 eyes of 17 cases before surgery to locate the projection position of ciliary sulcus in iris surface. In group B, the traditional sulcus fixation of IOL was performed on 16 eyes of 15 cases. The inserting position of needles, the haptics position of IOL and the IOL tilt, and decentration were observed by UBM examination 3 months after the surgery. Meanwhile, the vision and contrast sensitivity were analysed. *Results*. The differences in inserting position of the needle, the IOL tilt and decentration, the ratio of IOL haptics in sulcus, and uncorrected visual acuity were statistically significant ($P < 0.05$). The differences in best corrected visual acuity (BCVA) and contrast sensitivity were not statistically significant ($P > 0.05$). *Conclusions*. Sulcus fixation of foldable IOL aided by UBM can increase the accuracy of IOL haptics implanted into ciliary sulcus and reduce the IOL tilt and decentration.

1. Introduction

The sulcus suture fixation of the IOL was mentioned firstly by Girard [1] and Malbran et al. [2] and is widely used in the treatment of a defect of anterior or posterior capsule caused by contusion or penetration injury of the eyeball and complex surgeries. The application of a foldable IOL brings a small incision, few complications, a decrease of astigmatism, and quick recovery, significant advantages compared with a hard IOL [3]. However, because most scleral-sutured IOL procedures require that needles are placed behind the iris without direct visualization of the ciliary body, the possibility of asymmetric haptic location in the sulcus after intended sulcus implantation remains high [4].

Ultrasound biomicroscopy systems are suitable for imaging of virtually all anterior segment anatomy and pathology, including the cornea, iridocorneal angle, anterior chamber, iris, ciliary body, and lens. UBM is thus applicable for diagnostic imaging of corneal diseases, glaucoma, cysts, and tumors as well as lens implants. The ability of UBM to visualize the posterior chamber is useful for assessment of the position of the crystalline lens and lens implants which allows preoperative evaluation of the position of the sulcus before lens surgery, facilitating estimation of the postoperative intraocular lens position. In this study, we evaluated the clinical efficacy of sulcus suture fixation of the foldable IOL aided by UBM.

2. Patients and Methods

This study included 32 patients (35 eyes), 25 men and 7 women, who had transscleral fixation of foldable IOLs between 2012 and 2014. The mean age of the patients was 42 years with a range from 13 to 81. Eyes with infective ocular diseases, corneal diseases, severe iridocoloboma, abnormal pupil size and position, glaucoma, and retinal diseases were excluded to prevent the confounding effects in visual acuity. All patients gave their written informed consent prior to participation in the study.

The eyes were randomly divided into two groups according to the use of UBM examination. The UBM examination group (group A), including 17 cases (19 eyes), had UBM examination before sulcus fixation of foldable IOLs operation. The control group (group B), including 15 cases (16 eyes), had conventional sulcus fixation of foldable IOLs without UBM aiding. All the patients were followed up for 3 months after the surgery.

The method of sulcus location was as follows: first, the full UBM picture of the position where the haptic was intended to be sutured (usually at 2 o'clock and its corresponding 8 o'clock) was reviewed. A perpendicular line was drawn from the vertex of the ciliary sulcus (the cross point between iris back surface and ciliary body) to the scleral outside surface, and the length of this line which was the distance from the ciliary sulcus to the scleral outside surface was measured. Then, the line from the sulcus vertex to the back boundary of the corneal limbus at the scleral surface was drawn and measured. Last, the distance between the projecting position of the sulcus on the scleral surface and back boundary of corneal limbus at scleral surface was calculated according to the Pythagorean theorem (Figure 1).

For surgical methods, all surgeries were performed by the same surgeon under topical anesthesia and retrobulbar anesthesia. In group A, the needle was inserted and withdrawn at the projecting position of the sulcus on the scleral surface (2 o'clock and 8 o'clock) measured by UBM and the foldable IOL was implanted and sutured traditionally in the sulcus. In group B, the inserting and withdrawing positions of the needle were 1.5 mm away from the back boundary of the corneal limbus. The other surgical steps were the same as those in group A.

The UBM examination was performed on all patients 3 months after the surgery. The entire UBM image from 2 o'clock to 8 o'clock was determined. The scleral spur showed a high echo area like the olecranon in the UBM image and was the marker. The line between two olecranons of 2 o'clock and 8 o'clock was considered as the horizontal base line of the eyeball. For the IOL decentration, two perpendicular lines were drawn from both optical endpoints of the IOL to the base line and the distances between intersection points and the scleral spur were measured. The differences between these two distances were two times that of the IOL decentration (Figure 2). For the IOL tilt, a line parallel to the IOL optical endpoints connection through the left scleral spur on the UBM image was made and the angle between this line and the horizontal base line indicated the degree of IOL tilt (Figure 3).

3. Statistical Analysis

The Snellen preoperative and postoperative naked visual acuity (NVA) and the best corrected visual acuity (BCVA) were measured and converted into a logarithm of the minimum angle of resolution (logMAR) units for statistical analysis [5]. The contrast sensitivity at four different spatial frequencies (3, 6, 12, and 18 cycles per degree) was also measured by a CSV-1000E test lamp in a dark room and the logarithm of the result was analyzed statistically. The Wilcoxon matched pair test and Chi-square test were used for statistical analysis. A P value of less than 0.05 was considered statistically significant.

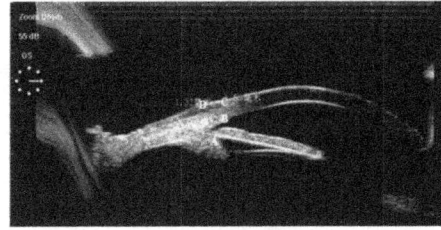

FIGURE 1: Location of sulcus by UBM before surgery (A = sulcus, B = scleral spur, C = back boundary of corneal limbus, and D = the projecting position of sulcus on the scleral surface).

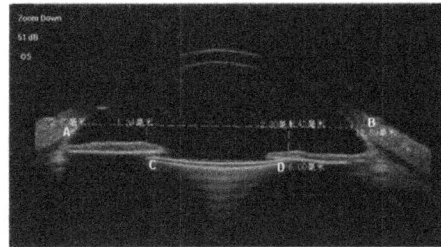

FIGURE 2: Measurement of IOL decentration (A, B = scleral spur, C, D = two optical endpoints of IOL).

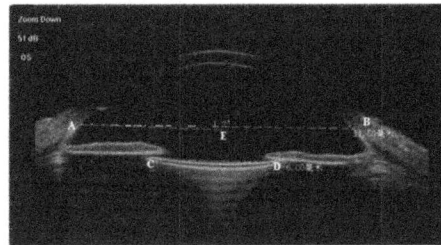

FIGURE 3: Measurement of IOL tilt (A, B = scleral spur, C, D = two optical endpoints of IOL, and line AE was the parallel line of line CD).

4. Results

4.1. The Age and Visual Acuity. The mean ages of group A and group B were 42.15 ± 22.03 and 44.27 ± 20.46 years, respectively, and the difference was not statically significant ($t = -0.28$, $P > 0.05$). The difference in preoperative and postoperative NVA and BCVA between the two groups was not statically significant. The difference in NVA between the two groups 3 months after surgery was statistically significant (Table 1).

4.2. The Needle Inserting and Withdrawing Position on the Scleral Surface. The needle insertion position at 2 o'clock in group A measured by UBM was 0.87 ± 0.17 mm away from the corneal limbus ranged from 0.607 mm to 1.21 mm and was different by 1.5 mm in group B ($t = -14.49$, $P < 0.001$). The needle withdrawing position at 8 o'clock in group A measured by UBM was 0.84 ± 0.18 mm away from the corneal limbus. It ranged from 0.600 mm to 1.19 mm which was different by 1.5 mm in group B ($t = -15.26$, $P < 0.001$).

TABLE 1: Comparison of VA between two groups (logMAR).

| | Preoperation | | Postoperation | |
	NVA	BCVA	NVA	BCVA
Group A	1.15 ± 0.25	0.27 ± 0.12	0.23 ± 0.11	0.14 ± 0.06
Group B	1.15 ± 0.27	0.29 ± 0.15	0.34 ± 0.15	0.15 ± 0.05
P value	0.81	0.78	0.03	0.7

VA = visual acuity, NVA = naked visual acuity.
BCVA = best corrected visual acuity.

TABLE 2: Haptic location 3 months after surgery.

	Both haptics in sulcus	One haptic in sulcus	No haptic in sulcus	P value
Group A	9	6	2	0.025
Group B	2	6	8	

4.3. The Haptic Position of IOL. Both haptics were in the sulcus in 9 eyes of group A (52.94%) and 2 eyes of group B. One haptic was in the sulcus in 6 eyes of group A and 6 eyes of group B. Neither of haptics was in the sulcus in 2 eyes of group A and 8 eyes of group B and the difference was statistically significant ($\chi^2 = 7.349$, $P = 0.025$) (Table 2).

4.4. IOL Tilt and Decentration. The mean IOL tilt was $2.83 \pm 1.10°$ in group A and $4.50 \pm 1.78°$ in group B and the difference was statistically significant ($t = -3.42$, $P = 0.002$). The mean IOL decentration was 0.28 ± 0.15 mm in group A and 0.49 ± 0.20 mm in group B and the difference was statistically significant ($t = -2.97$, $P = 0.005$).

4.5. The Contrast Sensitivity (CS). The sensitivity value for each spatial frequency showed no significant difference between the two groups at postoperative 3 months (Table 3).

5. Discussion

For correcting aphakia caused by different causes, implanting an IOL is the preferred method over glasses or contact lenses [6]. However, for the patients with inadequate capsular bag support, the transscleral sulcus fixation of the IOL is effective. Because of the blind nature of the surgical procedure, transscleral fixation also has disadvantages and blind manipulations make insertion of a needle through the ciliary sulcus more arduous.

The first practical UBM for imaging of the eye was developed by Pavlin et al. in the early 1990s [7]. UBM allows examination of the anterior segment of the eye which can show the ciliary sulcus clearly. In this study, we located the projection position of the ciliary sulcus in the iris surface by UBM and evaluated the clinical effects 3 months after the surgery. We found that the uncorrected visual acuity (UCVA) of patients in the UBM aided group was better than that in the control group, which is related to the suturing position. No statistically significant difference was found in BCVA between the two groups 3 months after the surgery. With the same measurement standard of the IOL, the difference in

TABLE 3: Contrast sensitivity 3 months after surgery.

	3 c/d	6 c/d	12 c/d	18 c/d
Group A	1.66 ± 0.14	1.73 ± 0.15	1.39 ± 0.20	0.74 ± 0.17
Group B	1.65 ± 0.15	1.72 ± 0.15	1.38 ± 0.19	0.73 ± 0.17
P value	0.47	0.94	0.81	0.83

suturing position between two groups caused the difference of the UCVA.

For the location of the ciliary sulcus, some scholars think that 1.5 mm posterior to the back boundary of limbus is the best position of fixing the IOL [8]. But UBM examination after surgery showed that the accuracy of locating the ciliary sulcus was not high [9]. In this study, the distance between the projecting position of the sulcus on the scleral surface and the back boundary of the corneal limbus was the inserting position of the needle. The difference in inserting position between the UBM aided group and the control group was statistically significant. UBM provides the personalized positioning of the ciliary sulcus which reduces the deviation of the surgical suture caused by anatomic differences.

The UBM appearance of haptics of the IOL was similar to the sclera which was characterized by high echoes during the UBM examination. The studies before showed that the rate of haptics in the sulcus was not high. Sewelam et al. [10] performed the UBM examination on patients who underwent the sulcus fixation of the IOL and found that only 55 percent of haptics were located in the sulcus. Alp et al. [9] evaluated the efficacy of a transillumination technique for the ciliary sulcus localization in transscleral fixations of posterior chamber intraocular lenses through UBM after the surgery and the rate of haptics in the sulcus was improved to 64 percent. In our study, the rate of haptics located in the sulcus in the control group was similar to that of the previous study, but the rate in the UBM examination group was obviously higher than that in the control group and the difference was statistically significant.

The IOL decentration and tilt are current research focuses and the position of the IOL can directly affect its optical performance [11]. Oshika et al. [12] reported that major tilting of an IOL caused a substantial amount of ocular coma-like aberration which may result in skewed distortion of the object image. Asymmetric fixation of IOL is the main cause for the presence of the IOL tilt or decentration. Now purkinje and scheimpflug imaging can detect the IOL tilt and decentration [11]. In addition, Loya et al. [4] reported the using of UBM to evaluate the IOL tilt and decentration. When the optic surface of the IOL was parallel to the horizontal baseline, the IOL had no tilt and when the difference between the two distances from both optical endpoints of the IOL to the base line was over 100 μm, the IOL was considered as decentration.

Contrast sensitivity measurements offer an objective measure of the quality of vision which is an important indicator for vision function [13]. The postoperative contrast sensitivity declined slightly compared with the preoperative one but there was no statistically significant difference between the two groups. The explanation might be due to the skilled operator. In both groups, the average IOL decentration and tilt were less than 0.5 mm and 5°, respectively, which caused little impact on the vision quality [14].

6. Conclusion

UBM guided sulcus fixation of foldable IOL increases the accuracy rate of haptics located in the sulcus and decreases the IOL decentration and tilt. The current study was limited by the short follow-up and small cases and the long term effect needs further investigation.

Conflict of Interests

All authors certify that they have no affiliations with or involvement in any organization or entity with any financial interests (such as honoraria, educational grants, participation in speakers' bureaus, membership, employment, consultancies, stock ownership, or other equity interest, and expert testimony or patent-licensing arrangements) or nonfinancial interest (such as personal or professional relationships, affiliations, knowledge, or beliefs) in the subject matter or materials discussed in this paper.

Acknowledgments

This study was supported by Research Funds for Ph.D. Programs of the First Affiliated Hospital of Zhengzhou University and by the Science and Technology Research Project of the Health Department of Henan Province (201403055 and 201303074). The authors wish to thank George Chin for helping them in preparing the paper and also want to thank the volunteers for participating in the study.

References

[1] L. J. Girard, "Pars plana phacoprosthesis (aphakic intraocular implant): a preliminary report," *Ophthalmic Surgery*, vol. 12, no. 1, pp. 19–22, 1981.

[2] E. S. Malbran, E. Malbran Jr., and I. Negri, "Lens guide suture for transport and fixation in secondary IOL implantation after intracapsular extraction," *International Ophthalmology*, vol. 9, no. 2-3, pp. 151–160, 1986.

[3] M. Taskapili, G. Gulkilik, M. S. Kocabora et al., "Comparison of sulcus implantation of single-piece hydrophilic foldable acrylic and polymethylmethacrylate intraocular lenses in eyes with posterior capsule tear during phacoemulsification surgery," *European Journal of Ophthalmology*, vol. 17, no. 4, pp. 595–600, 2007.

[4] N. Loya, H. Lichter, D. Barash, N. Goldenberg-Cohen, E. Strassmann, and D. Weinberger, "Posterior chamber intraocular lens implantation after capsular tear: ultrasound biomicroscopy evaluation," *Journal of Cataract and Refractive Surgery*, vol. 27, no. 9, pp. 1423–1427, 2001.

[5] S. D. Appel and R. L. Brilliant, "The low vision examination," in *Essentials of Low Vision Practice*, R. L. Brilliant, Ed., chapter 3, pp. 20–46, Butterworth-Heinemann, Boston, Mass, USA, 1999.

[6] T. Mutoh, Y. Matsumoto, and M. Chikuda, "Scleral fixation of foldable acrylic intraocular lenses in aphakic post-vitrectomy eyes," *Clinical Ophthalmology*, vol. 5, no. 1, pp. 17–21, 2011.

[7] C. J. Pavlin, K. Harasiewicz, M. D. Sherar, and F. S. Foster, "Clinical use of ultrasound biomicroscopy," *Ophthalmology*, vol. 98, no. 3, pp. 287–295, 1991.

[8] M. Monteiro, A. Marinho, S. Borges, L. Ribeiro, and C. Correia, "Evaluation of a new IOL scleral fixation technique without capsular support," *Journal Français d'Ophtalmologie*, vol. 29, no. 10, pp. 1110–1117, 2006.

[9] M. N. Alp, N. Buyuktortop, B. M. Hosal, G. Zilelioglu, and G. Kural, "Ultrasound biomicroscopic evaluation of the efficacy of a transillumination technique for ciliary sulcus localization in transscleral fixation of posterior chamber intraocular lenses," *Journal of Cataract and Refractive Surgery*, vol. 35, no. 2, pp. 291–296, 2009.

[10] A. Sewelam, A. M. Ismail, and H. El Serogy, "Ultrasound biomicroscopy of haptic position after transscleral fixation of posterior chamber intraocular lenses," *Journal of Cataract and Refractive Surgery*, vol. 27, no. 9, pp. 1418–1422, 2001.

[11] P. Rosales, A. De Castro, I. Jiménez-Alfaro, and S. Marcos, "Intraocular lens alignment from Purkinje and Scheimpflug imaging," *Clinical and Experimental Optometry*, vol. 93, no. 6, pp. 400–408, 2010.

[12] T. Oshika, G. Sugita, K. Miyata et al., "Influence of tilt and decentration of scleral-sutured intraocular lens on ocular higher-order wavefront aberration," *British Journal of Ophthalmology*, vol. 91, no. 2, pp. 185–188, 2007.

[13] R. Bellucci, "Multifocal intraocular lenses," *Current Opinion in Ophthalmology*, vol. 16, no. 1, pp. 33–37, 2005.

[14] F. Taketani, T. Matuura, E. Yukawa, and Y. Hara, "Influence of intraocular lens tilt and decentration on wavefront aberrations," *Journal of Cataract and Refractive Surgery*, vol. 30, no. 10, pp. 2158–2162, 2004.

18

The Prevalence and Distribution of Vitreoretinal Interface Abnormalities among Urban Community Population in China

Lei Liu,[1] **Song Yue,**[1] **Jingyang Wu,**[1] **Jiahua Zhang,**[1] **Jie Lian,**[2]
Desheng Huang,[3] **Weiping Teng,**[4] **and Lei Chen**[1,4]

[1]*Department of Ophthalmology, The First Affiliated Hospital of China Medical University, Shenyang 110001, China*
[2]*Department of Healthcenter, Fengyutan Community, Shenyang 110064, China*
[3]*Department of Epidemiology, School of Public Health, China Medical University, Shenyang 110122, China*
[4]*Key Laboratory of Endocrine Diseases in Liaoning Province, The First Hospital of China Medical University, Shenyang 110001, China*

Correspondence should be addressed to Lei Chen; leichen0501@163.com

Academic Editor: Takaaki Hayashi

The aim of this research was to identify the prevalence and distribution of vitreoretinal interface abnormalities (VIAs) among urban community population in Shenyang, China. According to the WHO criteria, a cross-sectional study was carried out among 304 Type 2 diabetes (T2D) patients and 304 people without diabetes as control over 45 years old. The presence of VIAs was determined by standardized grading of macular optical coherence tomography (Optovue OCT; Optovue, Inc., Fremont, CA) scans and two-field fundus photographs in at least one eye. For both men and women, high prevalence of VIAs (70.79%) was observed among over 65-years-old T2D patients. Prevalence of VIAs was observed to be high among T2D patients in all age groups compared to normal subjects. Prevalence of VIAs increased with age in all subjects. Prevalence of components of VIAs was epiretinal membrane (ERM) 11.43%, posterior vitreous detachment (PVD) 17.76%, vitreomacular traction syndrome (VMT) 5.67%, macular cysts/macular edema (MC/ME) 4.61%, full-thickness macular hole (FTMH) 0.82%, and partial thickness macular hole (PTMH) 0.74% in any eye, respectively. ERM and MC/ME were more prevalent in T2D in both males and females. The results highlight the need for early detection using OCT and approaches for the prevention of VIAs of diabetes in urban community.

1. Introduction

With the rapid development of economy, changes in lifestyle, and increasing intensification of old aging, the prevalence of diabetes was significantly rising, and the health impacts on human life became more and more serious in China [1]. According to the previous report, there were about 98.4 million people who had diabetes in 2013 and this number is predicted to be 142.7 million by 2035 in China [2]. Under this tendency, diabetic complications would be more prevalent. So we must pay more attention to prevention of various diabetic complications including diabetic eye diseases. One of the common complications of ocular in diabetes was vitreoretinal interface abnormalities (VIAs) [3]. VIAs include epiretinal membrane (ERM), vitreomacular traction (VMT), macular cysts or macular edema (MC/ME), partial thickness macular hole (PTMH), full-thickness macular hole (FTMH),

and posterior vitreous detachment (PVD) [4]. PTMH and FTMH always result in visual impairment and/or blindness. In early stage, most of the VIAs were asymptomatic [5]. Therefore, early detection and screening are most important. To date, there is no research on the prevalence of VIAs in Chinese population with diabetes. This community-based, cross-sectional survey was carried out to assess the gender differences in the prevalence of VIAs among Type 2 diabetes (T2D) and normal subjects in a Chinese urban community.

2. Methods

2.1. Study Population. Fengyutan health care center is a prevention model within Liaoning Diabetic Eye Center. It provides health service for more than 80,000 residents living in five communities (including Yutan, Yonghuan, Taoyuan,

TABLE 1: Definition for VIAs.

	Signs on OCT Scan	Representative
ERM	Which is characterized by hyperreflectivity of the membrane with corrugation on the surface of the internal membrane.	Figure 2(a)
Vitreomacular traction	Which was defined by the fact that the posterior hyaloid had detached from the retina but remained adhered to the retina in at least one location.	Figure 2(b)
Macular cysts	Which were defined as one or more cavities with well-defined margins within the retina that were often within low reflection.	Figure 2(c)
FTMHs	Which were considered as having hole in fovea including FTMH (steep, wide, foveal contours) and PTMH (lamellar).	Figure 2(d)
PVD	Which was defined by the fact that the posterior vitreous had detached from the retina without any adhesion.	Figure 2(e)

VIAs: vitreoretinal interface abnormalities.

Qingnian, and Zhongxin community) in Fengyutan Subdistrict, Shenyang, China. According to WHO criteria, T2D was diagnosed by general doctors and recorded in health files. Some details about this study had been reported previously [6]. Totally, 304 T2D residents and 304 normal subjects (control group) aged over 45 years who lived in Fengyutan community more than one year were selected from urban and suburb districts according to randomized resident health files. All of the selected subjects attended this study. The control group was matched for age and gender with diabetes.

2.2. Data Collection. Questionnaire including name, duration of diabetes, or hypertension was used to collect data. Peripheral venous blood sample was extracted over 8 h fasting. Laboratory examination including fasting plasma glucose (FPG), glycosylated hemoglobin (HbA$_1$c), triglyceride (TG), and total cholesterol (TC) concentration was tested in Fengyutan health care center. Participants were seated in a darkened room. Macular scans were photographed using optical coherence tomography (Optovue OCT; Optovue, Inc., Fremont, CA). Two 45-degree nonmydriatic digital camera (Type CR6-45NM, Canon Inc., Japan) photographic fields, centered at the optic disc and macular fovea, were taken from both eyes. All images including OCT and fundus were graded in a masked manner by two ophthalmologists at the Liaoning Diabetic Eye Center separately, who were well-trained to evaluate retinal photographs and OCT images according to standardized protocols and who were masked to subjects' characteristics. If the grades were inconsistent, the other ophthalmologist would give the final decision. There were 25 subjects that could not get a clear retinal or OCT image because of lens or cornea opacity. They accepted mydriasis with tropicamide 1% (Santen Pharmaceutical Co., Ltd., Shiga, Japan) before 15 minutes of dark adaptation and binocular indirect ophthalmoscope by two ophthalmologists who reviewed retinal or OCT images. VIAs were assessed according to a standardized protocol.

Definition for VIAs was shown in Table 1.

2.3. Ethics Committee. The Medical Ethics Committee of the First Affiliated Hospital of China Medical University approved the research protocol of this study and all subjects

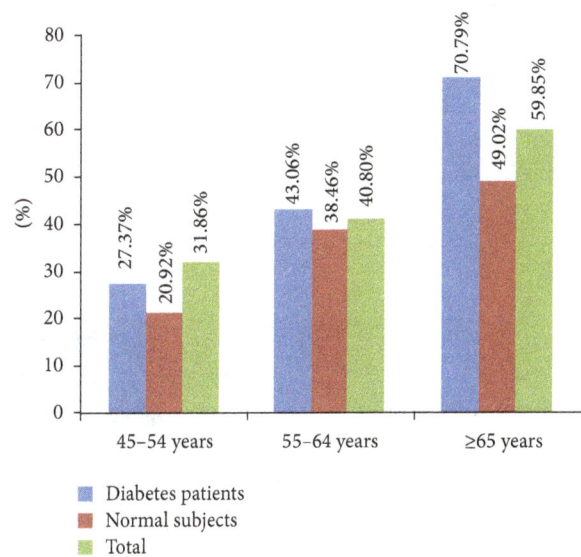

FIGURE 1: The prevalence of vitreoretinal interface abnormalities in different age groups.

gave informed written consent, according to the Declaration of Helsinki.

2.4. Statistical Analysis. Statistical analysis was carried out using a statistical software package (SPSS version 20.0, Chicago, IL). Descriptive statistics for continuous variables were determined as the mean ± standard deviation (SD). Otherwise, ratios and percentages for categorical variables were computed. The prevalence estimates were calculated. Chi-square test was used to determine the differences of VIAs prevalence between age groups. A P value <0.05 was considered to indicate statistical significance.

3. Results

According to Figure 1, the high prevalence of VIAs (70.79%) was observed among over 65-year-old T2D patients. Prevalence of VIAs was observed to be high among T2D patients in all age groups compared to normal subjects. The prevalence of VIAs was increased with age in all subjects. Both in males and

TABLE 2: Characteristics for all subjects.

	All participants	Type 2 diabetes patients	Normal subjects	P value*
Age, n (%)	608	304 (50.00)	304 (50.00)	
45–54 years	193 (31.74)	95 (31.25)	98 (32.24)	
55–64 years	212 (34.87)	108 (35.52)	104 (34.21)	0.93
≥65 years	203 (33.39)	101 (33.22)	102 (33.55)	
Sex, n (%)				
Females	340 (55.92)	172 (56.58)	168 (55.26)	
Males	268 (44.08)	132 (43.42)	136 (44.74)	0.74
Duration of DM, n (%)				
<5 years	125 (41.12)	125 (41.12)	N/A	
6–15 years	101 (33.22)	101 (33.22)	N/A	N/A
≥16 years	78 (25.66)	78 (25.66)	N/A	
Hypertension, n (%)				
Absent	270 (30.87)	125 (41.12)	145 (47.69)	
Present	338 (69.13)	179 (58.88)	159 (52.30)	0.10
FPG, mmol/L, mean ± SD	7.96 ± 2.43	9.23 ± 3.47	5.25 ± 1.08	<0.01
TG, mmol/L, mean ± SD	1.87 ± 0.45	1.99 ± 0.53	1.82 ± 0.34	<0.01
TC, mmol/L, mean ± SD	5.28 ± 1.68	5.79 ± 1.20	4.98 ± 1.45	<0.01
HbA_1c, %	7.88 ± 1.05	10.11 ± 1.76	5.78 ± 0.83	<0.01

Fasting plasma glucose (FPG); glycosylated hemoglobin (HbA_1c); triglyceride (TG); total cholesterol (TC).
*P value showed difference between Type 2 diabetes patients and normal control groups.

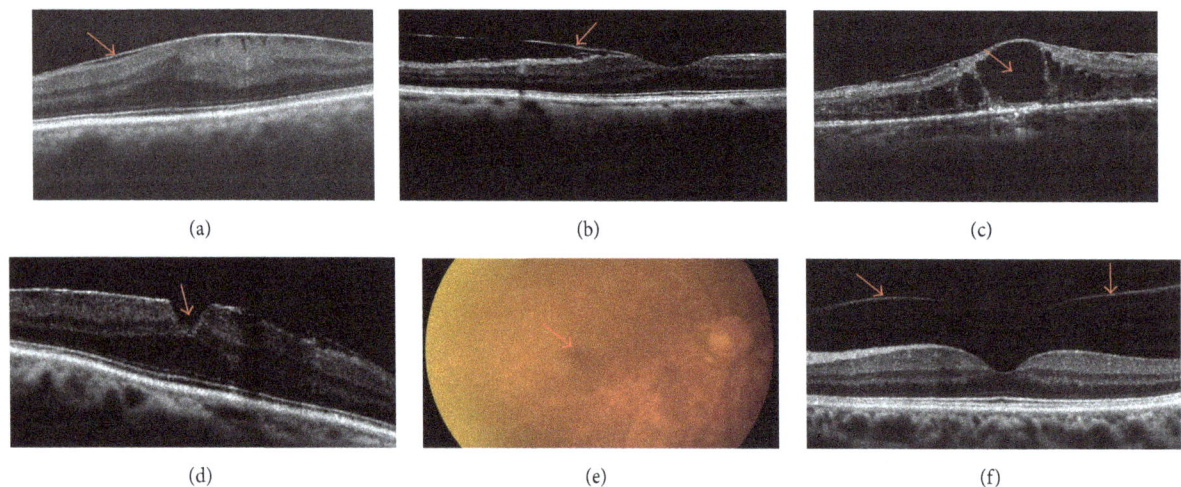

FIGURE 2: (a) Representative epiretinal membrane (ERM) image; (b) vitreomacular traction syndrome (VMT) image; (c) representative macular cysts/macular edema (MC/ME); (d) representative full-thickness macular hole (FTMH) image and representative partial thickness macular hole (PTMH) image; (e) representative posterior vitreous detachment (PVD) image. The red arrows indicate abnormities of fundus diseases.

in females, prevalence of components of VIAs was epiretinal membrane (ERM) 11.43%, posterior vitreous detachment (PVD) 17.76%, vitreomacular traction syndrome (VMT) 5.67%, macular cysts/macular edema (MC/ME) 4.61%, full-thickness macular hole (FTMH) 0.82%, and partial thickness macular hole (PTMH) 0.74% in any eye, respectively.

By comparison, no statistical difference was found in age, gender, and hypertension history between T2D patients and normal subjects (Table 2). We have found significant difference among two groups in FPG, TG, TC, and HbA_1c levels.

In males, the prevalence of ERM (19.31%), FTMH (1.10%), VMT (9.47%), and MC/ME (9.30%) was higher in T2D patients compared with normal subjects ($P = 0.001$). There was no significant statistical difference in the prevalence of ERM and MC/ME among three age groups both in T2D patients and in normal subjects groups. However, there was a significant association between the prevalence of PVD and

TABLE 3: The prevalence of VIAs within males in this study (number of eyes or %).

| Variables | Type 2 diabetes patients | | | | | Normal subjects | | | | | |
	45–54 years (n = 74)	55–64 years (n = 104)	≥65 years (n = 86)	P value*	Total (n = 264)	45–54 years (n = 98)	55–64 years (n = 94)	≥65 years (n = 80)	P value#	Total (n = 272)	P value†
ERM	15 (20.3)	17 (16.3)	19 (22.09)	0.58	51 (19.31)	5 (5.10)	11 (11.70)	10 (12.5)	0.16	26 (9.56)	0.001
PTMH	0	1 (0.96)	2 (2.32)		3 (1.10)	1 (1.02)	0	1 (1.25)		2 (0.73)	0.62
FTMH	1 (1.35)	1 (0.96)	1 (1.16)		3 (1.10)	0	0	1 (1.25)		1 (0.38)	0.03
VMT	4 (5.41)	6 (5.77)	15 (17.44)	0.008	25 (9.47)	3 (3.06)	3 (3.19)	6 (7.5)	0.27	12 (4.41)	0.03
MC/ME	3 (4.05)	6 (5.77)	8 (9.30)	0.37	17 (6.44)	1 (1.02)	2 (2.12)	4 (5.00)	0.23	7 (2.57)	0.03
PVD	10 (13.51)	28 (26.92)	37 (43.02)	<0.01	75 (28.4)	13 (13.27)	37 (39.36)	40 (50.00)	<0.01	90 (33.09)	0.24
VIAs	33 (44.59)	59 (56.73)	82 (95.35)	<0.01	174 (65.9)	23 (23.47)	53 (56.38)	62 (77.5)	<0.01	138 (50.74)	<0.01

Epiretinal membrane without schisis (ERM); macular cysts/macular edema (MC/ME); partial thickness macular hole (PTMH); full-thickness macular hole (FTMH); posterior vitreous detachment (PVD); vitreomacular traction syndrome (VMT).
*Difference analysis between three age groups in Type 2 diabetes patients.
#Difference analysis between three age groups in normal subjects.
†Difference analysis between Type 2 diabetes patients and normal subjects groups.

TABLE 4: The prevalence of VIAs within females in this study (number of eyes or %).

| Variables | Type 2 diabetes patients | | | | | Normal subjects (number of eyes) | | | | | |
	45–54 years (n = 116)	55–64 years (n = 112)	≥65 years (n = 116)	P value*	Total (n = 344)	45–54 years (n = 98)	55–64 years (n = 114)	≥65 years (n = 124)	P value#	Total (n = 336)	P value†
ERM	5 (4.31)	15 (13.39)	25 (21.55)	<0.01	45 (13.08)	7 (7.14)	9 (7.89)	11 (8.87)	0.89	27 (8.03)	0.03
PTMH	1 (0.86)	1 (0.89)	1 (0.86)		3 (0.87)	0	0	1 (0.81)		1 (0.29)	0.63
FTMH	1 (0.86)	0	2 (1.72)		3 (0.87)	0	2 (1.75)	1 (0.81)		3 (0.89)	0.73
VMT	4 (3.44)	6 (5.36)	9 (7.76)	0.35	19 (5.52)	3 (3.06)	4 (3.51)	6 (4.84)	0.76	13 (3.87)	0.31
MC/ME	3 (2.58)	5 (4.46)	14 (12.07)	<0.01	22 (6.39)	0	3 (2.63)	7 (5.65)		10 (2.98)	0.03
PVD	5 (4.31)	7 (6.25)	10 (8.62)	0.40	22 (6.39)	8 (8.16)	9 (7.89)	12 (9.68)	0.87	29 (8.63)	0.26
VIAs	19 (16.38)	34 (30.35)	61 (52.59)	<0.01	114 (33.14)	18 (18.37)	27 (23.68)	38 (30.64)	<0.01	83 (24.70)	<0.01

Epiretinal membrane without schisis (ERM); macular cysts/macular edema (MC/ME); partial thickness macular hole (PTMH); full-thickness macular hole (FTMH); posterior vitreous detachment (PVD); vitreomacular traction syndrome (VMT).
*Difference analysis between three age groups in Type 2 diabetes patients.
#Difference analysis between three age groups in normal subjects.
†Difference analysis between Type 2 diabetes patients and normal subjects groups.

age increasing both in normal subjects and in T2D patients. The prevalence of VMT was increased with age in T2D patients groups (Table 3).

In females, the prevalence of VIAs including ERM (13.08%) and MC/ME (6.39%) was higher in T2D patients compared with normal subjects. The prevalence of ERM and MC/ME was increased with age in T2D patients groups. There was no significant statistical difference in the prevalence of VMT and PVD among three age groups both in T2D patients and in normal subjects groups. In addition, there was no significant statistical difference in the prevalence of PTMH, FTMH, VMT, and PVD between normal subjects and T2D patients. The results were shown in Table 4. The prevalence of VIAs within all subjects in this study was shown in Table 5.

4. Discussion

To the best of our knowledge, this is the first study about prevalence of VIAs in subjects within Chinese urban residents. Strength of this research is the rate of gradable quality images. There were only 3.5% of images which were unreadable, with 96.5% of participants having gradable photographs at least in one eye. There were 70.79% diabetes patients over 65 years old with VIAs. That is to say, the possibility for diabetes with older age may be much higher compared with normal subjects. Not surprisingly, increasing age was significantly associated with VIAs. This has been reported by some other studies in the past [4, 7, 8].

Previous study reported that persons with diabetes were more likely to have ERM than persons without diabetes. It was consistent with our results. In many population-based studies, diabetes was a significant risk factor for ERM [9, 10].

Snead et al. [11] report the overall prevalence of PVD to be 57% in normal subjects. In addition, the prevalence of PVD in T2D was 63.3% [12]. The previous prevalence rates of PVD were higher compared with our results. This may be because of different checking methods (we did not use B-ultrasound) and different population. The prevalence of PVD in our study subjects was higher in males than that in females both in diabetes patients and in normal subjects. However, Khalatbari et al. reported that there was no

TABLE 5: The prevalence of VIAs within all subjects in this study (number of eyes or %).

Variables	Type 2 diabetes patients					Normal subjects					
	45–54 years (n = 190)	55–64 years (n = 216)	≥65 years (n = 202)	P value*	Total (n = 608)	45–54 years (n = 196)	55–64 years (n = 208)	≥65 years (n = 204)	P value#	Total (n = 608)	P value†
ERM	20 (10.52)	32 (14.81)	44 (21.78)	<0.01	96 (13.95)	12 (6.12)	20 (9.62)	21 (10.29)	0.28	53 (8.72)	<0.01
PTMH	1 (0.52)	2 (0.93)	3 (1.48)	0.62	6 (0.87)	1 (0.51)	—	2 (0.98)	—	3 (0.49)	0.31
FTMH	2 (1.05)	1 (0.46)	3 (1.48)	0.56	6 (0.87)	—	2 (0.86)	2 (0.98)	—	4 (0.66)	0.52
VMT	8 (4.21)	12 (5.56)	24 (11.88)	<0.01	44 (6.39)	6 (3.06)	7 (3.36)	12 (5.88)	0.29	25 (4.11)	0.02
MC/ME	6 (3.15)	11 (5.09)	22 (10.89)	<0.01	39 (5.66)	1 (0.51)	5 (24.04)	11 (5.39)	0.01	17 (2.79)	<0.01
PVD	15 (7.89)	35 (16.20)	47 (23.26)	<0.01	97 (14.09)	21 (10.71)	46 (22.12)	52 (25.49)	<0.01	119 (19.57)	0.09
VIAs	52 (27.37)	93 (43.06)	143 (70.79)	<0.01	288 (41.86)	41 (20.92)	80 (38.46)	100 (49.02)	<0.01	221 (36.35)	<0.01

Epiretinal membrane without schisis (ERM); macular cysts/macular edema (MC/ME); partial thickness macular hole (PTMH); full-thickness macular hole (FTMH); posterior vitreous detachment (PVD); vitreomacular traction syndrome (VMT).

*Difference analysis between three age groups in Type 2 diabetes patients.

#Difference analysis between three age-groups in normal subjects.

†Difference analysis between Type 2 diabetes patients and normal subjects groups.

significant discrepancy in the rates of posterior ocular disease according to different sex [13].

To date, there is no related report on the discrepancy of VMT prevalence in different age groups between males and females. From Table 5, we can conclude that VMT in all DM was increased with age. It was in accordance with the prevalence of VMT in male DM. However, this tendency was not seen in female DM patients. It may be due to gender differences. But further observational studies are needed to draw a conclusion in different ethnicity or area.

In our study, we did not investigate the prevalence of macular cysts and macular edema (MC/ME), respectively. Previous study reported that the overall weighted prevalence of ME was 3.8% in US diabetes and there was no difference in the prevalence of ME by age or sex [14]. This was similar to our results.

There were some limitations in our study. As a cross-sectional study, we only evaluated the prevalence for VIAs. The causality between VIAs and diabetes could in the future be explored using a prospective study design. In addition, the risk factors for VIAs were not analyzed in this study. Thirdly, because it was carried out in community, we only used OCT and fundus camera to detect abnormalities.

In summary, in this study, we investigated the prevalence of VIAs in diabetes and in normal subjects and analyzed the discrepancy within sex. There is the need for early detection using OCT and fundus camera approaches for the prevention of VIAs in China urban community.

Conflict of Interests

The authors declare that there is no conflict of interests regarding the publication of this paper.

Authors' Contribution

Lei Liu and Song Yue contributed to the work equally and should be regarded as co-first authors.

Acknowledgments

This study was supported by the National Natural Science Foundation of China (81300783); Liaoning Science and Technology Project (2009225005); Liaoning Department of Health Medical Peak of Construction Project (2010016); Important Platform of Science and Technology for the University in Liaoning Province (16010).

References

[1] H. Hu, M. Sawhney, L. Shi et al., "A systematic review of the direct economic burden of type 2 diabetes in china," *Diabetes Therapy*, vol. 6, no. 1, pp. 7–16, 2015.

[2] L. Guariguata, D. R. Whiting, I. Hambleton, J. Beagley, U. Linnenkamp, and J. E. Shaw, "Global estimates of diabetes prevalence for 2013 and projections for 2035," *Diabetes Research and Clinical Practice*, vol. 103, no. 2, pp. 137–149, 2014.

[3] A. Ophir, M. R. Martinez, P. Mosqueda, and A. Trevino, "Vitreous traction and epiretinal membranes in diabetic macular oedema using spectral-domain optical coherence tomography," *Eye*, vol. 24, no. 10, pp. 1545–1553, 2010.

[4] C. E. Myers, B. E. K. Klein, S. M. Meuer et al., "Retinal thickness measured by spectral-domain optical coherence tomography in eyes without retinal abnormalities: the Beaver Dam Eye Study," *American Journal of Ophthalmology*, vol. 159, no. 3, pp. 445–456, 2015.

[5] G. Ripandelli, T. Rossi, F. Scarinci, C. Scassa, V. Parisi, and M. Stirpe, "Macular vitreoretinal interface abnormalities in highly myopic eyes with posterior staphyloma: 5-year follow-up," *Retina*, vol. 32, no. 8, pp. 1531–1538, 2012.

[6] L. Liu, J. Geng, J. Wu et al., "Prevalence of ocular fundus pathology with type 2 diabetes in a Chinese urban community as assessed by telescreening," *BMJ Open*, vol. 3, no. 12, Article ID e004146, 2013.

[7] E. Hatef, A. Fotouhi, H. Hashemi, K. Mohammad, and K. H. Jalali, "Prevalence of retinal diseases and their pattern in Tehran: the Tehran eye study," *Retina*, vol. 28, no. 5, pp. 755–762, 2008.

[8] P. K. Nirmalan, J. Katz, A. L. Robin et al., "Prevalence of vitreoretinal disorders in a rural population of southern India: the

Aravind Comprehensive Eye Study," *Archives of Ophthalmology*, vol. 122, no. 4, pp. 581–586, 2004.

[9] K. Z. Aung, G. Makeyeva, M. K. Adams et al., "The prevalence and risk factors of epiretinal membranes: the Melbourne collaborative cohort study," *Retina*, vol. 33, no. 5, pp. 1026–1034, 2013.

[10] R. Kawasaki, J. J. Wang, H. Sato et al., "Prevalence and associations of epiretinal membranes in an adult Japanese population: the Funagata study," *Eye*, vol. 23, no. 5, pp. 1045–1051, 2009.

[11] M. P. Snead, D. R. J. Snead, A. S. Mahmood, and J. D. Scott, "Vitreous detachment and the posterior hyaloid membrane: a clinicopathological study," *Eye*, vol. 8, no. 2, pp. 204–209, 1994.

[12] L. Gella, R. Raman, V. Kulothungan, and T. Sharma, "Prevalence of posterior vitreous detachment in the population with type II diabetes mellitus and its effect on diabetic retinopathy: Sankara Nethralaya Diabetic Retinopathy Epidemiology and Molecular Genetic Study SN-DREAMS report no. 23," *Japanese Journal of Ophthalmology*, vol. 56, no. 3, pp. 262–267, 2012.

[13] D. Khalatbari, S. Stinnett, R. M. McCallum, and G. J. Jaffe, "Demographic-related variations in posterior segment ocular sarcoidosis," *Ophthalmology*, vol. 111, no. 2, pp. 357–362, 2004.

[14] R. Varma, N. M. Bressler, Q. V. Doan et al., "Prevalence of and risk factors for diabetic macular edema in the United States," *JAMA Ophthalmology*, vol. 132, no. 11, pp. 1334–1340, 2014.

19

Sublethal Photothermal Stimulation with a Micropulse Laser Induces Heat Shock Protein Expression in ARPE-19 Cells

Keiji Inagaki,[1,2] Takuya Shuo,[3] Kanae Katakura,[3] Nobuyuki Ebihara,[4] Akira Murakami,[2] and Kishiko Ohkoshi[1]

[1]Department of Ophthalmology, St. Luke's International Hospital, 9-1 Akashi-cho, Chuo-ku, Tokyo 104-8560, Japan
[2]Department of Ophthalmology, Juntendo University Graduate School of Medicine, Hongo 2-1-1, Bunkyo-ku, Tokyo 113-8421, Japan
[3]Institute for Medical Innovation, St. Luke's International University, 10-1 Akashi-cho, Chuo-ku, Tokyo 104-8560, Japan
[4]Department of Ophthalmology, Juntendo University Urayasu Hospital, 1-1 Tomioka 2-chome, Urayasu-shi, Chiba 279-0021, Japan

Correspondence should be addressed to Keiji Inagaki; inakei@luke.ac.jp

Academic Editor: Terri L. Young

Purpose/Aim of the Study. Subthreshold micropulse diode laser photocoagulation is an effective treatment for macular edema. The molecular mechanisms underlying treatment success are poorly understood. Therefore, we investigated the effects of sublethal laser energy doses on a single layer of densely cultured ARPE-19 cells as a model of the human retinal pigment epithelium (RPE). *Materials and Methods.* A single layer of densely cultured human ARPE-19 cells was perpendicularly irradiated with a micropulse diode laser. Nonirradiated cells served as controls. Sublethal laser energy was applied to form a photocoagulation-like area in the cultured cell layers. Hsp70 expression was evaluated using quantitative polymerase chain reaction and immunocytochemistry. *Results.* Photocoagulation-like areas were successfully created in cultured ARPE-19 cell layers using sublethal laser energy with our laser irradiation system. Hsp70 mRNA expression in cell layers was induced within 30 min of laser irradiation, peaking at 3 h after irradiation. This increase was dependent on the number of laser pulses. Hsp70 upregulation was not observed in untreated cell layers. Immunostaining indicated that Hsp70 expression occurred concentrically around laser irradiation sites and persisted for 24 h following irradiation. *Conclusion.* Sublethal photothermal stimulation with a micropulse laser may facilitate Hsp70 expression in the RPE without inducing cellular damage.

1. Introduction

Laser photocoagulation is widely used for treating various retinal diseases, including diabetic retinopathy [1], branch retinal vein occlusion [2], and central serous retinopathy [3]. Unfortunately, conventional laser treatments are destructive procedures used to create whole-layer damage to retinal tissue. Such invasive treatments are not suitable for macular diseases, including macular edema, because laser scars generally grow larger and create permanent scotomas. Laser scar enlargement, subretinal fibrosis, and subretinal neovascular membranes have been reported as serious complications of laser treatment [4–8].

Micropulse lasers were invented to reduce laser-induced burns that can occur with conventional laser treatment [9].

Lasers in the micropulse mode exert pulses of short laser applications, thereby diminishing the heat generated at the target site [10]. In fact, retinal coagulation scars are not visible upon fundoscopic examination, autofluorescent imaging, or optical coherence tomography [11, 12] when the eyes are treated with a subthreshold micropulse laser. Many studies have shown the clinical efficacy of this treatment [10, 13–17]; however, few studies have investigated the molecular mechanisms responsible for fluid absorption from retinal tissue [18]. Although thermal stimulation of the retinal pigment epithelium (RPE) is thought to be the key trigger for fluid absorption from an edematous retina, the molecular mechanisms of this process are not yet understood. Notably, Lavinsky et al. found slight morphological changes following laser irradiation with a low-energy output in Dutch-belted rabbits [19]. These changes were reversible (i.e., they did not cause permanent damage) when photocoagulation spots (visible burns) were barely visible on the retinal surface. These data suggested that biological cascades within the RPE may contribute to the therapeutic effects of sublethal photocoagulation during the treatment of macular edema.

Heat shock protein (Hsp) family members, which act as chaperone proteins, aid in refolding denatured proteins and are protective against apoptosis and inflammation [20–24]. In particular, elevated expression of Hsp is known to occur with increases in temperature. Upregulation of Hsp70 expression induced by laser irradiation is thought to play an important role in the improvement of macular edema [25]. Intriguingly, nondamaging laser irradiation induces Hsp70 expression within the RPE of hemizygous C57BL/6 mice [26], whereas low-energy laser irradiation induces RPE cell death in Dutch-belted rabbits [19]. Unfortunately, whether sublethal laser energy induces Hsp70 expression in human retinal tissue is still unknown.

In this study, as a first step towards understanding the molecular mechanisms through which micropulse laser application affects retinal tissue, we constructed a laser irradiation system to directly expose cultured human retinal pigment epithelial ARPE-19 cell layers to a sublethal dose of laser energy. The expression of Hsp70 at both the mRNA and protein levels was examined over time.

2. Materials and Methods

2.1. Cell Culture. The ARPE-19 immortal human RPE cell line [27] at passage 19 (ATCC CRL-2303, Lot number: 60279299) was purchased from American Type Culture Collection (Manassas, VA, USA), and all experiments were performed using the cells at passages 22 through 26. Cells were maintained in Dulbecco's modified Eagle's medium: Nutrient Mixture F-12 (DMEM/F-12, Gibco, Life Technologies, Carlsbad, CA, USA) supplemented with 10% fetal bovine serum (One Shot FBS; Gibco, Life Technologies) and 1% penicillin-streptomycin (Pen Strep; Gibco, Life Technologies) at 37°C in a 5% CO_2 incubator. Cell culture media were replaced 2-3 times a week. For laser applications, 3×10^5 cells were seeded on the glass bottoms (12 mm in diameter) of 35 cm² glass-bottomed culture dishes (Asahi Techno Glass, Tokyo, Japan) and left to stand for 30 min. Two milliliters of DMEM/F-12 was then added, and media were replaced on the fourth day of culture. Fully confluent cells were used in experiments on the eighth day of culture.

2.2. Laser Application. Diode lasers are primarily used for targeting of RPE cells in photocoagulation treatment in the clinical setting. Therefore, we constructed an experimental system that made it possible to irradiate a fully confluent layer of cultured cells. In order to directly irradiate cultured cell layers with a laser, as is performed in the clinical setting, a slit-lamp adapter for an 810 nm diode laser (Oculight SL; Iris Medical, Mountain View, CA, USA) was placed on top of a slit-lamp system created by cutting a slit-lamp microscope barrel (900 BM; Haag-Streit Diagnostics, Bern, Switzerland) and vertically fixing it onto a culture dish. After laser irradiation, cells were inspected with a confocal microscope (TCS

SP8; Leica Microsystems, Mannheim, Germany) equipped with a life cell imaging chamber (Stage Top Incubator; Tokai Hit, Shizuoka, Japan) and/or a phase-contrast microscope (DMI3000B; Leica Microsystems). Measurements of photocoagulated areas were performed using an image analyzer (LAS 4.2; Leica Microsystems) and Image J 1.47 public domain software (National Institutes of Health, Bethesda, MD, USA).

2.3. Cell Viability Assay. A LIVE/DEAD cell imaging kit (Molecular Probe, Life Technologies) was used to visualize live and dead cells after laser irradiation. The LIVE/DEAD reagent, composed of calcein-AM and ethidium homodimer-1, was directly added to conditioned media on cultured cells after laser irradiation and incubated for 15 min at 25°C. To discriminate between live and dead cells, the RPE cell layer was inspected with a confocal microscope with the appropriate filters in place. Live cells were able to hydrolyze calcein-AM and were therefore stained green, while dead cells were permeable to ethidium homodimer-1 and were therefore stained red.

2.4. Quantitative Reverse Transcription Polymerase Chain Reaction (qRT-PCR). All RNA isolation experiments were performed using a PureLink RNA Mini Kit with DNase (Ambion, Life Technologies) according to the manufacturer's instructions. First-strand cDNA was synthesized from 200 ng of total RNA using a High Capacity RNA-to-cDNA Kit (Applied Biosystems, Life Technologies). For quantification of *Hsp70* mRNA, one-twentieth of the above-mentioned cDNA was analyzed using TaqMan Fast Advanced Master Mix (Applied Biosystems, Life Technologies) and Taq-Man Gene Expression Assay probe-primer sets for *HSPA1A* (Hs00359163_s1; Applied Biosystems, Life Technologies). The level of *Hsp70* mRNA was determined by the $2^{-\Delta\Delta CT}$ method [28] using *GAPDH* (Hs02758991_g1, Applied Biosystems, Life Technologies) as an internal control.

2.5. Immunocytochemistry. Cells were fixed with 4% paraformaldehyde (Thermo Fischer Scientific, Waltham, MA, USA) and permeabilized using 0.1% Triton X-100. Cells were treated with Image-iT FX signal enhancer (Molecular Probe, Life Technologies), blocked in 10% normal goat serum (Molecular Probe, Life Technologies), and incubated with an anti-Hsp70 antibody (3A3; Abcam, Cambridge, UK) or anti-GAPDH antibody (loading control; Abcam). These primary antibodies were visualized with Alexa Fluor 488 Goat Anti-Mouse IgG antibody (Molecular Probe, Life Technologies), which served as a secondary antibody. Samples were counterstained with SlowFade Gold Antifade Mountant with 4′,6-diamidino-2-phenylindole (DAPI; Molecular Probe, Life Technologies). Immunofluorescent images of cells were captured with a confocal microscope, as described above.

2.6. Statistical Analyses. Student's *t*-tests and Mann-Whitney *U* tests were used to test mean differences for statistical significance. Statistical calculations were performed using SPSS software (SPSS, Inc., Chicago, IL, USA). Each experiment was conducted more than three times. Differences with *p* values of less than 0.05 were considered statistically significant.

3. Results

3.1. Laser Irradiation System for Cultured Cell Layers. Cells were irradiated on glass-bottomed dishes via a dichroic mirror and a perpendicular laser (Figures 1(a) and 1(b)). In order to uniformly expose the cell layer to laser energy, the culture dish was plated on black paper. Several methods of spreading black paper under culture dishes when performing laser irradiation in ARPE-19 cells have been previously reported [29, 30]. Additionally, culture media without phenol red were used to avoid blocking of the emitted diode laser light. The culture dish was placed on a mechanical stage so that the dish could be moved into the proper laser irradiation position in a flat X-Y plane. The stage was moved in 0.1 mm steps, and the cell layer was accurately irradiated with the laser in equal intervals. The position of the laser irradiation site was indicated by a red light pointing in the direction of the X- or Y-axis. The position along the Z-axis was then determined using the focal point of the laser. The focal point was defined as the position in which the laser aiming beam was most clearly projected onto the surface of the black paper.

When a cell layer was irradiated with a conventional continuous-wave mode laser, the laser irradiation site and its periphery gradually changed into a coagulation-like form. The formation of sparse annular intercellular spaces around the laser irradiation site was also observed in bright-field images obtained with a confocal microscope 2 h after laser irradiation (Figure 1(c) and Supplementary Material 1 in Supplementary Material available online at http://dx.doi.org/10.1155/2015/729792). These cell groups in the bright-field images remained viable, as indicated by green fluorescence staining with calcein-AM, an indicator of cell survival. In contrast, the laser irradiation site and nearby cells were dead, as indicated by red fluorescence staining with ethidium homodimer-1, an indicator of cell death (Figure 1(d)).

3.2. Morphological Changes in Cultured Cell Layers after Sublethal Micropulse Laser Irradiation. A laser provides intermittent irradiation in the micropulse mode, with the percentage of irradiation time set at a fixed number. This number is known as the duty cycle. In the micropulse mode, the duty cycle is 15%, with the laser irradiating for 0.3 ms during each 2.0 ms period. When the total micropulse laser exposure duration was 1000 ms, the duty cycle was repeated 500 times (Figure 2(a)).

Figure 2(b) shows phase-contrast images of irradiation sites 2 h after micropulse laser irradiation was performed with the following laser settings: duty cycle of 15%, laser exposure duration between 500 and 1000 ms, and laser power between 600 and 800 mW. Laser irradiation was performed at 1 mm intervals along the X- and Y-axes on each cell layer. Laser exposure duration was shortened with each 1 mm position change along the X-axis, but laser power remained constant. Laser power was decreased with each 1 mm position change along the Y-axis, but laser exposure duration remained constant. When the laser power was fixed at 800 mW, the coagulation area gradually decreased as the laser exposure time was shortened (1000 to 500 ms: 184 ± 8.8 to $81 \pm 13.5\,\mu m^2$). However, coagulation-like lesions were

no longer visible with phase-contrast microscopy when the laser power was 600 mW and the laser exposure duration was 600 ms. Coagulation area was significantly correlated with laser exposure duration. Additionally, coagulation area proportionally increased with laser power within the range examined (Spearman's correlation coefficient: $r > 0.8$, $p < 0.05$, Figure 2(c)).

Based on the observed changes in micropulse laser irradiation lesions in a cultured cell layer (Figure 2(b)), the optimal, reproducible sublethal laser settings were determined to be a laser exposure duration of 1000 ms, a duty cycle of 15%, and a laser power of 600 mW. Bright-field images, captured with a confocal microscope, revealed that cell morphology changed in sublethal photothermal stimulation sites where intercellular spaces were sparse (Figure 2(d)). However, almost all cells within sublethal photothermal stimulation sites were alive, even 24 h after micropulse laser irradiation (Figure 2(d)). Additionally, the coagulation-like area was significantly smaller for lesions created in the micropulse mode than for those created in the continuous-wave mode under the same energy conditions (Mann-Whitney U test: $p < 0.001$, Figures 2(e) and 2(f)).

3.3. Hsp Expression in Cultured Cell Layers following Sublethal Laser Irradiation. To investigate whether sublethal photocoagulation induced Hsp expression, which is important in reducing macular edema, we used qRT-PCR to examine the expression levels of *HSPA1A* mRNA, which encodes Hsp70 protein, in a cultured cell layer irradiated with a sublethal irradiation dose using a micropulse laser (Figure 2(d)). Cells were examined until 24 h after irradiation from each of the 81 irradiation positions in the X-Y plane. In the pretreated irradiation group, maximum *HSPA1A* mRNA expression was observed 3 h after photothermal stimulation. The expression of *Hsp70* mRNA was only slightly increased over baseline, even 24 h after irradiation (Figure 3(a)). Because the clinical efficacy of macular edema treatment has been shown to be better with high-density micropulse laser irradiation than with standard laser treatment [16], we also examined the effects of varying the number of laser irradiation lesions on *HSPA1A* mRNA levels by changing the spacing of laser irradiation lesions on the cultured cell layer, which resulted in an increase in the number of lesions from 81 to 477. As expected, a significant increase in *HSPA1A* mRNA expression was observed 3 h after irradiation in cell layers with a higher number of lesions (Figure 3(b)).

Actual Hsp70 protein levels in cultured cell layers were also examined after sublethal laser irradiation using immunocytochemistry with an anti-Hsp70 antibody (Figure 3(c)). Hsp70 immunofluorescent signals were present in concentric areas around laser irradiation sites. However, GAPDH, used as an endogenous control for qRT-PCR analyses of *HSPA1A* mRNA, was uniformly present throughout the cultured cell layer. The presence of cells within laser irradiation sites was confirmed with DAPI counterstaining. Even 24 h after photothermal stimulation, Hsp70 immunostaining persisted at laser irradiation sites.

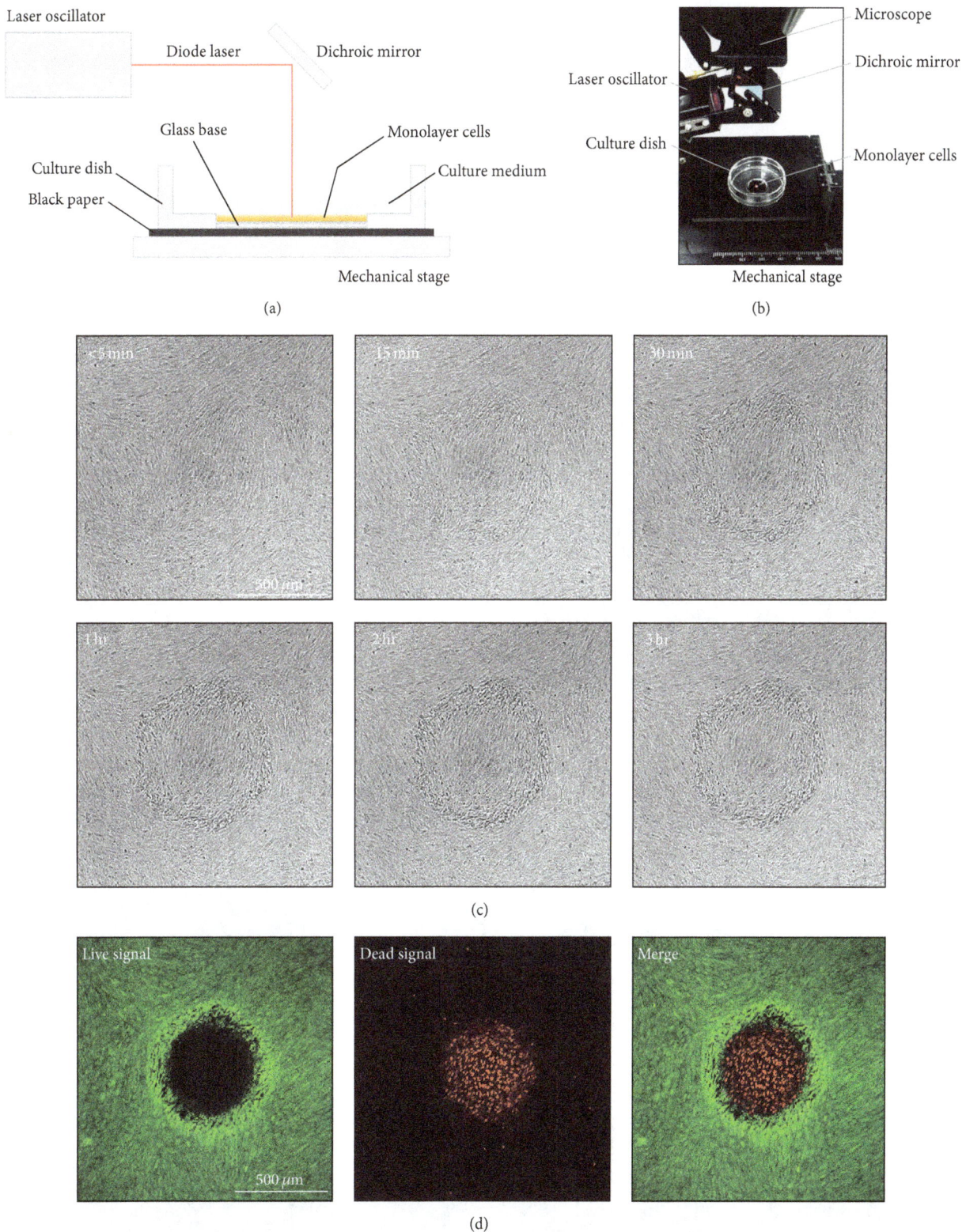

FIGURE 1: Experimental setup for laser irradiation of cultured cell layers. (a, b) A diode laser beam passed through a dichroic mirror to perpendicularly irradiate a full confluent cultured cell layer on a glass-based dish. To avoid blocking diode laser light, a phenol-red-free culture medium was used. (c) Confocal microscopy bright-field images of the irradiated cell layer. Spots were made using the continuous-wave mode with a power of 250 mW, duration of 500 ms, and spot size of 200 μm. The white dotted circle indicates the laser irradiation site. A video is also available (see Supplementary Material 1). (d) Two hours after laser irradiation (using the laser settings described in (c)), cell viability was assessed using LIVE/DEAD cell imaging reagents. Live cells were stained green, and dead cells were stained red. Fluorescent images were captured with confocal microscopy (projected images). Cells within the laser spot were dead, but cell groups forming the sparse annular intercellular spaces observed in the bright-field images were alive.

Laser irradiation mode: micropulse, 15% duty cycle
Laser ON time: 0.3 ms

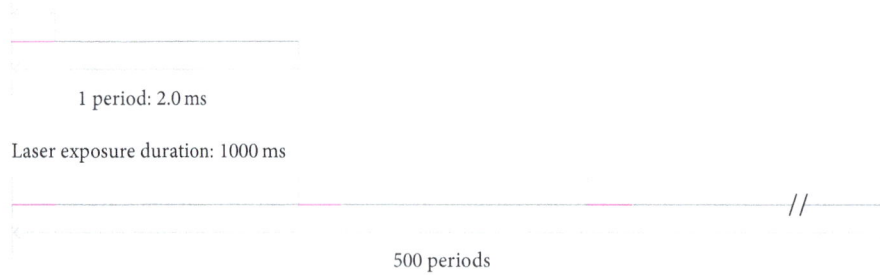

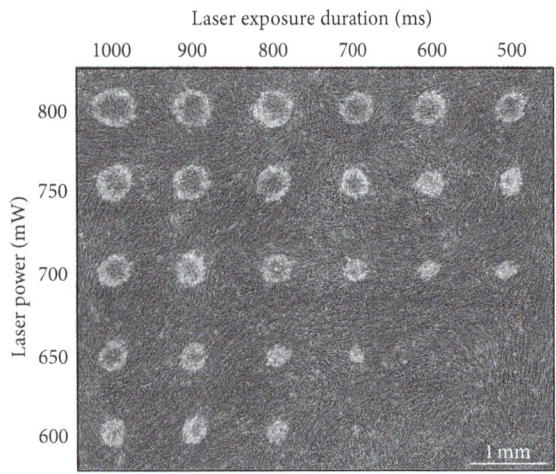

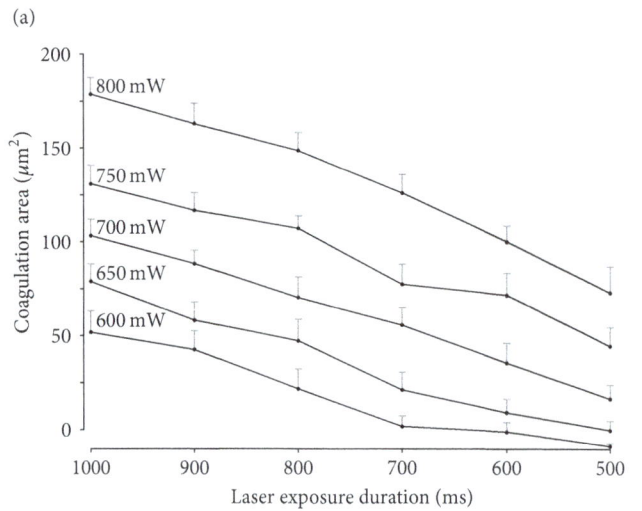

1 period: 2.0 ms

Laser exposure duration: 1000 ms

//

500 periods

(a)

(b)

(c)

After laser irradiation: 2 hr

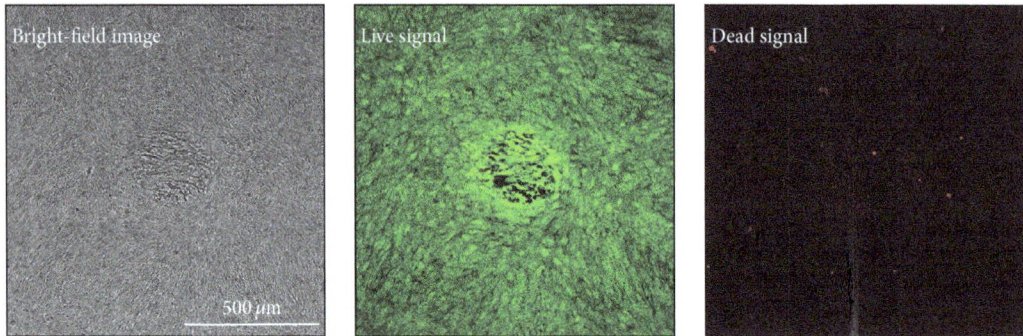

After laser irradiation: 24 hr

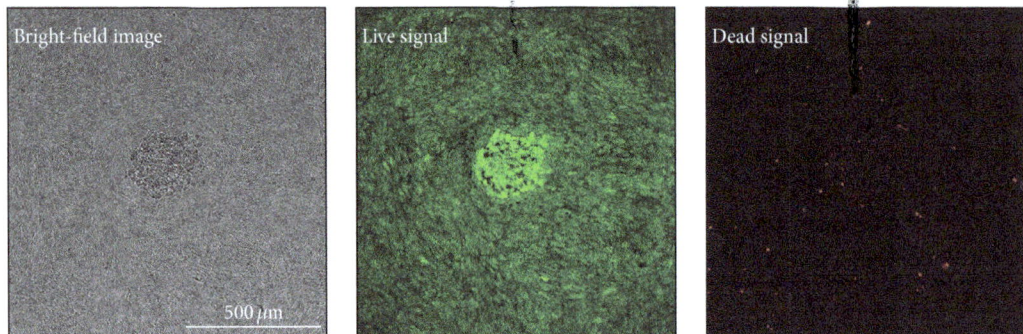

(d)

FIGURE 2: Continued.

Laser irradiation mode:	Micropulse, 15% duty cycle	Continuous-wave
Total laser energy (mJ):	90	90
Laser power (mW):	600	600
Laser exposure duration (ms):	1000	150

(e)

(f)

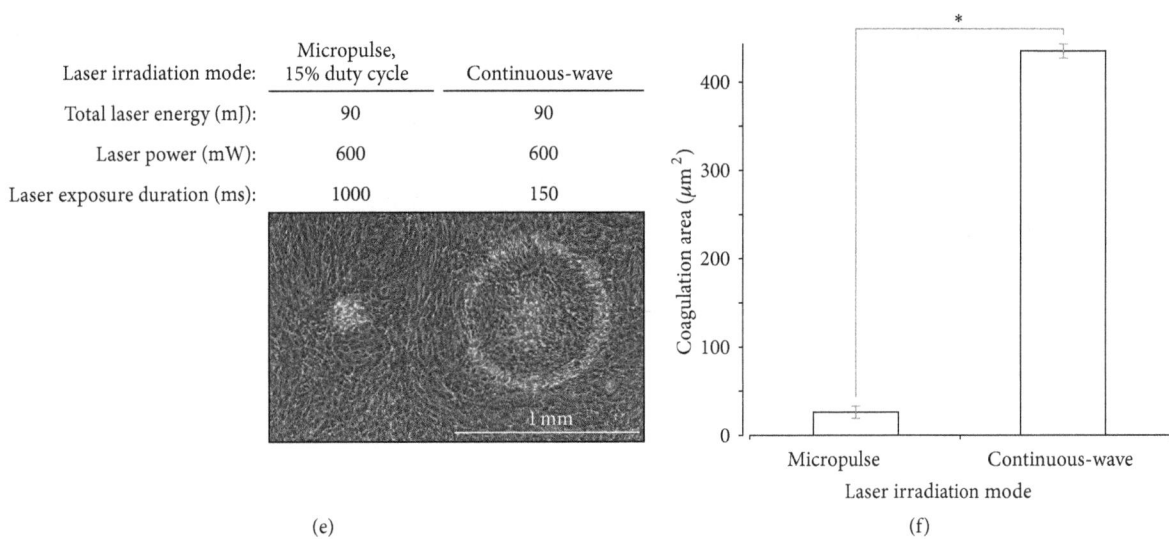

FIGURE 2: Establishment of laser parameters for sublethal photothermal stimulation on a cultured cell layer using micropulse-mode laser irradiation. (a) A micropulse-mode laser emits short, intermittent pulses of laser energy. At a 15% duty cycle, the laser was on for 0.3 ms during each 2.0 ms period. When the total laser exposure duration was 1000 ms, the laser cycle was repeated 500 times. (b) Representative phase-contrast microscopy images taken 2 h after laser irradiation with a micropulse laser. The laser had a 15% duty cycle and was set to various laser powers (600–800 mW) and laser exposure durations (500–1000 ms). Multiple spots were made on a single one-cell layer culture plate 1 mm apart in both the X and Y directions. The duration was varied along the X-axis, and power was varied along the Y-axis. The laser spot size remained constant at 200 μm. (c) Areas of morphological change are shown in (b), as measured with NIH Image J software. Data represent the mean ± standard error of 10 independent experiments. Both laser exposure duration and laser power were significantly correlated with coagulation area (Spearman's correlation coefficient: $r > 0.8$, $p < 0.05$). (d) Representative bright-field (left panels) and fluorescent (center and right panels) images around laser irradiation sites, as captured with confocal microscopy, at the indicated times following laser irradiation. Sublethal photothermal stimulation was performed with the following laser settings: 15% duty cycle, 1000 ms laser exposure duration, and 600 mW laser power. Note that no dead cell signals (red fluorescence) were observed within the 24 h following laser irradiation. (e) Representative phase-contrast microscopy images 2 h after laser irradiation of single-cell layers with a laser in the micropulse (left) and continuous-wave (right) modes. The total laser irradiation energy was 90 mJ in both cases. (f) Mean coagulation area of spots made with a laser in the micropulse and continuous-wave modes shown in (e). Error bars represent one standard error ($n = 12$). The asterisk (∗) indicates a statistically significant difference between means (Mann-Whitney U tests, $p < 0.01$).

4. Discussion

In this study, we established a system in which one layer of densely cultured cells could be irradiated with a diode laser. We successfully and repeatedly created coagulation-like lesions without inducing cell death. Moreover, we confirmed that sublethal micropulse photothermal stimulation induced Hsp70 expression in a cultured layer of ARPE-19 cells.

Previous reports in the literature have shown that the size of coagulation lesions created using a continuous-wave laser is dependent on laser duration and power in Dutch-belted rabbits [31, 32]. Our in vitro study results are consistent with this and revealed that this is also true for coagulation-like lesions made with a micropulse laser (Figures 2(b) and 2(c) and Supplementary Material 2). Using the same amount of energy, more tissue damage occurred in lesions created with a continuous-wave laser than in those created with a micropulse laser (Figures 2(e) and 2(f)). It is thought that micropulse lasers cause less damage than continuous-wave lasers because the pulses of very short, intermittent energy may allow for heat dissipation within tissue. This would reduce tissue temperature elevation during laser application.

Although numerous clinical studies have shown the efficacy of subthreshold micropulse laser treatments, the laser settings (i.e., laser power and pulse duration) used in these studies have not been consistent [10, 13–17]. Moreover, the optimal laser energy for subthreshold laser treatments has not yet been established, and surgeons often use continuous-wave laser modes for titrating laser settings [16, 17, 33]. Our study revealed that laser thermal damage caused by continuous-wave and micropulse laser modes differed (Figures 2(e) and 2(f)). Our results also suggested that laser power and exposure time titrations for the treatment of retinal disease should be performed using subthreshold micropulse photocoagulation and not continuous-wave laser photocoagulation.

Sublethal micropulse photothermal stimulation sites had cellular groups with sparse intercellular spaces that did not have any dead cells, even 24 h after laser irradiation, as determined using cell viability assays (Figure 2(d)). We presumed that these intercellular spaces represented the loss of cell-to-cell adhesion in the RPE layer, which may contribute to a dysfunctional blood retinal barrier in vivo, directly increasing fluid and molecule movement between the retina and choroidal tissues. Restoring the blood retinal barrier

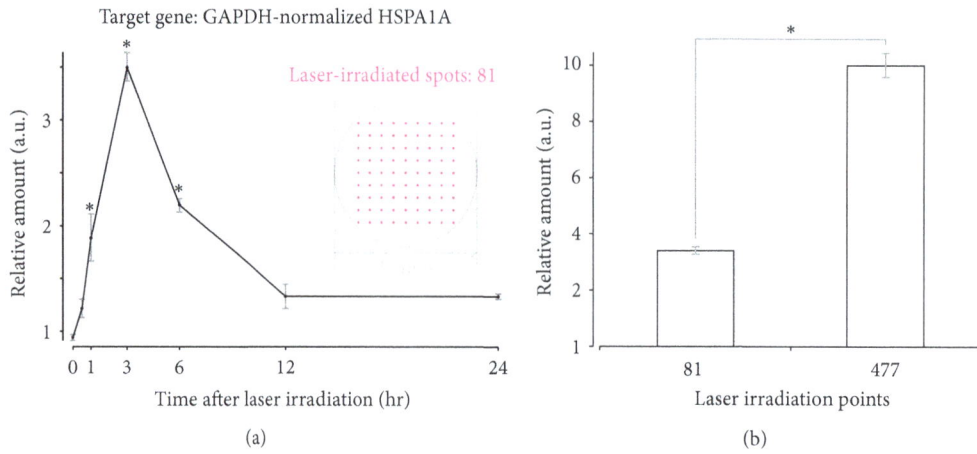

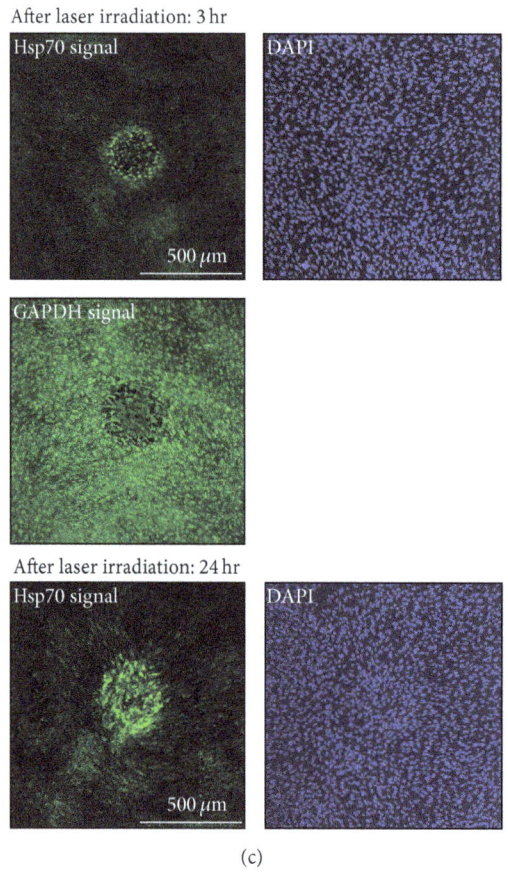

FIGURE 3: Changes in the expression of heat shock protein 70 (Hsp70) in cultured cell layers after sublethal photothermal stimulation. (a–c) Micropulse-mode laser irradiation sessions of cells on the glass-based dish were made using the following laser settings: 1000 ms exposure duration and 600 mW laser power. (a) Sublethal laser irradiation led to a transient upregulation of *HSPA1A* mRNA, which encodes the Hsp70 protein. At the indicated time points, total RNA was extracted, and *HSPA1A* mRNA levels were assessed using real-time quantitative reverse transcription polymerase chain reaction (qRT-PCR). *GAPDH* mRNA was used as an internal control. The data presented in the figure were normalized to the amount of *HSPA1A* mRNA in nonirradiated samples. Data represent mean values of three independent experiments. Error bars represent one standard deviation. The asterisk (∗) indicates statistical significance ($p < 0.05$), as determined using Student's t-tests. A schematic of the 81 laser irradiation spots on the cultured cell layer is shown in the insert. (b) Three hours following laser irradiation, *HSPA1A* mRNA upregulation was higher when 477 laser irradiation spots were made than when 81 spots were made. The asterisk (∗) indicates a statistically significant difference between means ($n = 3$, Student's t-test, $p < 0.001$). (c) Upregulation of Hsp70 protein at laser irradiation sites 3 h (upper and middle panels) and 24 h (lower panel) after sublethal photothermal stimulation. Cell layers were immunostained with the indicated antibodies and counterstained with 4′,6-diamidino-2-phenylindole (DAPI). Fluorescent images were captured with a confocal microscope (projected images). Immunofluorescent signals representing Hsp70 expression were detected around laser irradiation sites 24 h after laser irradiation (lower left).

with photothermal stimulation may lead to improvements in macular edema. Future research on proteins related to RPE cell adhesion and RPE tight junctions (e.g., occludin, claudin, and zonula occludens-1) is needed in RPE cell layers.

Several studies have shown that heated tissue remaining viable after conventional continuous-wave laser treatment undergoes a stress response, which includes production of beneficial intracellular biological factors (e.g., PEDF, TSP-1, SDF1, and Hsp) with antiangiogenic and restorative functions [25, 30, 34]. Because Hsp may block the activity of apoptotic and inflammatory pathways that cause cellular damage [20–24], upregulation of Hsp70 expression induced by laser irradiation is thought to be important for reducing macular edema following clinical laser therapy [25, 26]. In the current study, sublethal micropulse photothermal stimulation was shown to induce upregulation of Hsp70, the major Hsp in mammalian cells. Moreover, expression of *Hsp70* mRNA, quantified by real-time qRT-PCR, was temporarily upregulated in preconditioned cultured cell layers for 12 h following laser irradiation. This change was not observed in the untreated control group. Immunostaining indicated that expression of Hsp70 proteins in cultured cell layers occurred concentrically around laser-irradiated sites. Additionally, Hsp70 protein production persisted for 24 h after sublethal laser irradiation. This study is the first to report Hsp70 expression and upregulation in cultured cells following sublethal micropulse laser energy application.

The beneficial effects of subthreshold micropulse photocoagulation for diabetic macular edema are not observed immediately in the clinical setting but begin to become evident 3 months following therapy [10, 13–17]. Therefore, sublethal micropulse photothermal stimulation that induces Hsp70 upregulation may facilitate RPE remodeling and contribute to improvements in macular edema.

Our study had several limitations. First, we examined a monolayer of cultured cells, which may not have the same vertical heat conduction properties as an intact eye. Secondly, ARPE-19 cells exhibit some characteristics and features that are different from those of human RPE cells. Therefore, the laser irradiation system developed and used in this study should be further examined in ARPE-19 cells and in human RPE cells derived from retinal tissue and induced pluripotent stem cells.

5. Conclusions

In conclusion, while the therapeutic mechanism underlying the efficacy of micropulse laser therapy has not yet been determined, our data showed that Hsp70 may be a trigger for improving RPE health and function. Moreover, Hsp70 may be used as a biological marker to determine therapeutic laser levels for subthreshold micropulse photocoagulation. In addition, testing laser irradiation systems in a cultured layer of human RPE cells is advantageous because changes in cell morphology, molecular composition, cellular transcriptomes, and cellular proteomes after sublethal photothermal stimulation can be precisely assessed using live imaging microscopy, DNA microarrays, and mass spectrometry techniques.

Conflict of Interests

The authors declare that there is no conflict of interests regarding the publication of this paper.

Authors' Contribution

Keiji Inagaki and Takuya Shuo contributed equally to this work.

Acknowledgments

The authors are grateful to Emeritus Professor Tatsuro Irimura for helpful advice, and they wish to thank Hisashi Takahashi with the Toyohara Ophthalmic Instrument Company, Ltd. (Tokyo, Japan), for making the laser application system and for technical support.

References

[1] Early Treatment of Diabetic Retinopathy Study Research Group, "Photocoagulation for diabetic macular edema: early treatment diabetic retinopathy study report number 1," *Archives of Ophthalmology*, vol. 103, no. 12, pp. 1796–1806, 1985.

[2] The Branch Vein Occlusion Study Group, "Argon laser photocoagulation for macular edema in branch retinal vein occlusion," *American Journal of Ophthalmology*, vol. 98, pp. 271–282, 1984.

[3] J. W. Lim, S. W. Kang, Y.-T. Kim, S. E. Chung, and S. W. Lee, "Comparative study of patients with central serous chorioretinopathy undergoing focal laser photocoagulation or photodynamic therapy," *British Journal of Ophthalmology*, vol. 95, no. 4, pp. 514–517, 2011.

[4] H. Schatz, D. Madeira, H. R. McDonald, and R. N. Johnson, "Progressive enlargement of laser scars following grid laser photocoagulation for diffuse diabetic macular edema," *Archives of Ophthalmology*, vol. 109, no. 11, pp. 1549–1551, 1991.

[5] D. R. Guyer, D. J. D'Amico, and C. W. Smith, "Subretinal fibrosis after laser photocoagulation for diabetic macular edema," *American Journal of Ophthalmology*, vol. 113, no. 6, pp. 652–656, 1992.

[6] B. K. Rutledge, I. H. L. Wallow, and G. L. Poulsen, "Sub-pigment epithelial membranes after photocoagulation for diabetic macular edema," *Archives of Ophthalmology*, vol. 111, no. 5, pp. 608–613, 1993.

[7] M. P. Varley, E. Frank, and E. W. Purnell, "Subretinal neovascularization after focal argon laser for diabetic macular edema," *Ophthalmology*, vol. 95, no. 5, pp. 567–573, 1988.

[8] E. Midena, T. Segato, G. Bottin, S. Piermarocchi, and I. Fregona, "The effect on the macular function of laser photocoagulation for diabetic macular edema," *Graefe's Archive for Clinical and Experimental Ophthalmology*, vol. 230, no. 2, pp. 162–165, 1992.

[9] T. R. Friberg and E. C. Karatza, "Treatment of macular disease using a micropulsed and continuous wave 810 nm diode laser," *Ophthalmology*, vol. 104, no. 12, pp. 2030–2038, 1997.

[10] J. K. Luttrull, C. Sramek, D. Palanker, C. J. Spink, and D. C. Musch, "Long-term safety, high-resolution imaging, and tissue temperature modeling of subvisible diode micropulse photocoagulation for retinovascular macular edema," *Retina*, vol. 32, no. 2, pp. 375–386, 2012.

[11] K. Inagaki, K. Ohkoshi, and S. Ohde, "Spectral-domain optical coherence tomography imaging of retinal changes after conventional multicolor laser, subthreshold micropulse diode laser, or pattern scanning laser therapy in Japanese with macular edema," *Retina*, vol. 32, no. 8, pp. 1592–1600, 2012.

[12] K. Ohkoshi, E. Tsuiki, T. Kitaoka, and T. Yamaguchi, "Visualization of subthreshold micropulse diode laser photocoagulation by scanning laser ophthalmoscopy in the retro mode," *American Journal of Ophthalmology*, vol. 150, no. 6, pp. 856–862, 2010.

[13] M. L. Laursen, F. Moeller, B. Sander, and A. K. Sjoelie, "Subthreshold micropulse diode laser treatment in diabetic macular oedema," *British Journal of Ophthalmology*, vol. 88, no. 9, pp. 1173–1179, 2004.

[14] J. K. Luttrull, D. C. Musch, and M. A. Mainster, "Subthreshold diode micropulse photocoagulation for the treatment of clinically significant diabetic macular oedema," *British Journal of Ophthalmology*, vol. 89, no. 1, pp. 74–80, 2005.

[15] J. Figueira, J. Khan, S. Nunes et al., "Prospective randomised controlled trial comparing sub-threshold micropulse diode laser photocoagulation and conventional green laser for clinically significant diabetic macular oedema," *British Journal of Ophthalmology*, vol. 93, no. 10, pp. 1341–1344, 2009.

[16] D. Lavinsky, J. A. Cardillo, L. A. S. Melo Jr., A. Dare, M. E. Farah, and R. Belfort Jr., "Randomized clinical trial evaluating mET-DRS versus normal or high-density micropulse photocoagulation for diabetic macular edema," *Investigative Ophthalmology & Visual Science*, vol. 52, no. 7, pp. 4314–4323, 2011.

[17] K. Ohkoshi and T. Yamaguchi, "Subthreshold micropulse diode laser photocoagulation for diabetic macular edema in Japanese patients," *American Journal of Ophthalmology*, vol. 149, no. 1, pp. 133.e1–139.e1, 2010.

[18] A. K. Yu, K. D. Merrill, S. N. Truong, K. M. Forward, L. S. Morse, and D. G. Telander, "The comparative histologic effects of subthreshold 532- and 810 nm diode micropulse laser on the retina," *Investigative Ophthalmology and Visual Science*, vol. 54, no. 3, pp. 2216–2224, 2013.

[19] D. Lavinsky, C. Sramek, J. Wang et al., "Subvisible retinal laser therapy: titration algorithm and tissue response," *Retina*, vol. 34, no. 1, pp. 87–97, 2014.

[20] J. T. Beckham, G. J. Wilmink, M. A. Mackanos et al., "Role of HSP70 in cellular thermotolerance," *Lasers in Surgery and Medicine*, vol. 40, no. 10, pp. 704–715, 2008.

[21] S. Du, Q. Zhang, S. Zhang, L. Wang, and J. Lian, "Heat shock protein 70 expression induced by diode laser irradiation on choroid-retinal endothelial cells in vitro," *Molecular Vision*, vol. 18, pp. 2380–2387, 2012.

[22] D. Lanneau, A. de Thonel, S. Maurel, C. Didelot, and C. Garrido, "Apoptosis versus cell differentiation: role of heat shock proteins HSP90, HSP70 and HSP27," *Prion*, vol. 1, no. 1, pp. 53–60, 2007.

[23] M. N. Rylander, Y. Feng, J. Bass, and K. R. Diller, "Thermally induced injury and heat-shock protein expression in cells and tissues," *Annals of the New York Academy of Sciences*, vol. 1066, pp. 222–242, 2005.

[24] C. Sőti, E. Nagy, Z. Giricz, L. Vígh, P. Csermely, and P. Ferdinandy, "Heat shock proteins as emerging therapeutic targets," *British Journal of Pharmacology*, vol. 146, no. 6, pp. 769–780, 2005.

[25] M. A. Yenari, J. Liu, Z. Zheng, Z. S. Vexler, J. E. Lee, and R. G. Giffard, "Antiapoptotic and anti-inflammatory mechanisms of heat-shock protein protection," *Annals of the New York Academy of Sciences*, vol. 1053, pp. 74–83, 2005.

[26] C. Sramek, M. Mackanos, R. Spitler et al., "Non-damaging retinal phototherapy: dynamic range of heat shock protein expression," *Investigative Ophthalmology & Visual Science*, vol. 52, no. 3, pp. 1780–1787, 2011.

[27] K. C. Dunn, A. E. Aotaki-Keen, F. R. Putkey, and L. M. Hjelmeland, "ARPE-19, a human retinal pigment epithelial cell line with differentiated properties," *Experimental Eye Research*, vol. 62, no. 2, pp. 155–169, 1996.

[28] K. J. Livak and T. D. Schmittgen, "Analysis of relative gene expression data using real-time quantitative PCR and the $2^{-\Delta\Delta C_T}$ method," *Methods*, vol. 25, no. 4, pp. 402–408, 2001.

[29] P. Tababat-Khani, L. M. Berglund, C.-D. Agardh, M. F. Gomez, and E. Agardh, "Photocoagulation of human retinal pigment epithelial cells in vitro: evaluation of necrosis, apoptosis, cell migration, cell proliferation and expression of tissue repairing and cytoprotective genes," *PLoS ONE*, vol. 8, no. 8, Article ID e70465, 2013.

[30] N. Ogata, A. Ando, M. Uyama, and M. Matsumura, "Expression of cytokines and transcription factors in photocoagulated human retinal pigment epithelial cells," *Graefe's Archive for Clinical and Experimental Ophthalmology*, vol. 239, no. 2, pp. 87–95, 2001.

[31] A. Jain, M. S. Blumenkranz, Y. Paulus et al., "Effect of pulse duration on size and character of the lesion in retinal photocoagulation," *Archives of Ophthalmology*, vol. 126, no. 1, pp. 78–85, 2008.

[32] Y. M. Paulus, A. Jain, R. F. Gariano et al., "Healing of retinal photocoagulation lesions," *Investigative Ophthalmology & Visual Science*, vol. 49, no. 12, pp. 5540–5545, 2008.

[33] K. Inagaki, A. Iseda, and K. Ohkoshi, "Subthreshold micropulse diode laser photocoagulation combined with direct photocoagulation for diabetic macular edema in Japanese patients," *Nippon Ganka Gakkai zasshi*, vol. 116, no. 6, pp. 568–574, 2012.

[34] N. Binz, C. E. Graham, K. Simpson et al., "Long-term effect of therapeutic laser photocoagulation on gene expression in the eye," *The FASEB Journal*, vol. 20, no. 2, pp. 383–385, 2006.

20

Epigenetic Regulation of Werner Syndrome Gene in Age-Related Cataract

Xi Zhu, Guowei Zhang, Lihua Kang, and Huaijin Guan

Eye Institute, Affiliated Hospital of Nantong University, Nantong, Jiangsu 226001, China

Correspondence should be addressed to Huaijin Guan; gtnantongeye@gmail.com

Academic Editor: Jun Zhang

Purpose. To examine the promoter methylation and histone modification of WRN (Werner syndrome gene), a DNA repair gene, and their relationship with the gene expression in age-related cataract (ARC) lens. *Methods.* We collected the lenses after cataract surgery from 117 ARC patients and 39 age-matched non-ARC. WRN expression, DNA methylation and histone modification around the CpG island were assessed. The methylation status of Human-lens-epithelium cell (HLEB-3) was chemically altered to observe the relationship between methylation and expression of WRN. *Results.* The WRN expression was significantly decreased in the ARC anterior lens capsules comparing with the control. The CpG island of WRN promoter in the ARC anterior lens capsules displayed hypermethylation comparing with the controls. The WRN promoter was almost fully methylated in the cortex of ARC and control lens. Acetylated H3 was lower while methylated H3-K9 was higher in ARC anterior lens capsules than that of the controls. The expression of WRN in HLEB-3 increased after demethylation of the cells. *Conclusions.* A hypermethylation in WRN promoter and altered histone modification in anterior lens capsules might contribute to the ARC mechanism. The data suggest an association of altered DNA repair capability in lens with ARC pathogenesis.

1. Introduction

Age-related cataract (ARC) is one of the dominant causes of visual impairment in the elderly [1]. The disease can be classified as cortical, nuclear, and posterior subcapsular according to the location of the opacity within the lens [2]. ARC is a complex disease with multiple genetic and environmental risk components, including UV light, sun exposure, vitamin C deficiency, and hypertension [3], but its etiology is not fully understood [4, 5].

Oxidative stress has long been recognized as an important mediator of pathophysiology in lens epithelial cells (LECs) and also plays a vital role in the pathogenesis of cataract [6–8]. Recent studies have reported the association between reactive oxygen species- (ROS-) induced DNA damage of LECs and the development of cataract [8–10]. In our previous studies, we have also found that oxidative DNA damage marker, 8-oxoG, was significantly increased in ARC group compared with control group [11, 12]. Oxidative DNA lesions are repaired by nucleotide excision repair, double-strand break (DSB) repair, and base excision repair [13, 14]. The

WRN gene plays an important role in aging [15] and is known to function in repair of damaged DNA, particularly in repairing double-strand breaks [16]. The WRN protein belongs to RecQ family and has 1432 amino acids possessing both $3' \rightarrow 5'$ DNA helicase and $3' \rightarrow 5'$ DNA exonuclease activities. These biochemical functions are known to have roles in DNA replication, repair of DNA damage, gene transcription, and telomere maintenance [17]. WRN disruption causes Werner's syndrome (WS), an autosomal recessive segmental progeroid syndrome that results in accelerated aging and affects multiple organs and tissues [17]. Most WS patients develop bilateral ocular cataract when they are 20 years old and beyond [18, 19]. Previously, we reported that polymorphisms and copy number variations of WRN are associated with ARC [20, 21].

Epigenetics pertains to heritable alterations in gene expression that do not involve modification of the underlying genomic DNA sequence [22]. DNA methylation and histone modifications (including methylation, acetylation, sumoylation, and phosphorylation) are the major epigenetic mechanisms for gene expression [23]. Hypermethylation of

TABLE 1: Demographic information of study participants.

	Control	ARC
N	39	117
Age (mean ± SD)	69.66 ± 4.51	70.38 ± 7.72
Female N (%)	21 (54.8)	70 (60.1)
Male N (%)	18 (45.2)	47 (39.9)
Cortical N (%)	0	39 (33.3)
Nuclear N (%)	0	39 (33.3)
PSC N (%)	0	39 (33.3)

promoter CpG islands and histone H3 methylated at lysine 9 have been linked to heterochromatin and gene silencing, whereas histone H3 acetylated is enriched in euchromatic domains and correlates with active gene expressions [24–26]. DNA methylation is a critical regulator of gene expression in the eye and is necessary for the proper development and postmitotic survival of retinal neurons [27]. Aberrant methylation patterns have been associated with age-related macular degeneration, cataract, pterygium, and retinoblastoma [28–32]. Changes in histone modifications have also been observed in experimental models of diabetic retinopathy and glaucoma [22]. A decreased expression of WRN is related to aberrant DNA hypermethylation in various tumors; epigenetic inactivation of this gene may be a biomarker for selection of drugs for the treatment of cancer [33–37].

In this study, we investigated WRN expression in anterior lens capsules and lens cortex of ARC and age-matched controls and analyzed the correlation between epigenetic modification and expression profiles of WRN gene to explore the possible effect of epigenetics on the development of ARC.

2. Materials and Methods

2.1. Study Participants. The research followed the tenets of the Declaration of Helsinki. All participants signed the informed consent forms. The study was approved by the Ethics Committee of Affiliated Hospital of Nantong University.

We enrolled 117 ARC patients that consisted of three subgroups: age-related cortical cataract (ARC-C), age-related nuclear cataract (ARC-N), and age-related posterior subcapsular cataract (ARC-P). The criteria for ARC group included (1) opaque ocular lenses, (2) ≥50 years of age, and (3) $C \geq 4$, $N \geq 4$, and $P \geq 4$ according to the lens opacity classification system III (LOCSIII) [38] and excluded (1) complicated cataract due to high myopia, uveitis, ocular trauma, or other known causes and (2) hypertension, diabetes, or other systemic diseases. We enrolled 39 patients with vitreoretinal diseases who received transparent lens extraction as control group. The criteria for the control included (1) transparent ocular lenses and (2) ≥50 years of age and excluded (1) other major eye diseases such as glaucoma, myopia, diabetic retinopathy, and uveitis and (2) hypertension, diabetes, or other systemic diseases. The demographic information for all participants was listed in Table 1.

2.2. Anterior Lens Capsules and Lens Cortex Preparation. Anterior lens capsules that included lens epithelium (LE) and peripheral cortex were obtained through small incision extra capsular cataract surgery. The tissue was dissected and rapidly frozen in liquid nitrogen and then stored at −80°C for protein, RNA, and genomic DNA extraction.

2.3. RNA Isolation and cDNA Preparation. Total RNA from anterior lens capsules and lens cortex was isolated from the frozen tissues using TRIzol reagent (Invitrogen, Carlsbad, CA), and cDNAs were synthesized using PrimeScript RT reagent Kit (TaKaRa, Dalian, China).

2.4. Quantification of WRN mRNA. TaqMan gene expression assay probe (Applied Biosystems, Foster City, CA) was used for WRN mRNA quantification (Applied Biosystems assay ID: Hs01087915_m1). The results were normalized against the expression of housekeeping gene GAPDH from the same sample. RT-PCR was performed using ABI 7500 real time PCR system (Applied Biosystems, Foster City, CA). The fold change of WRN expression was determined using the comparative CT ($2^{-\Delta\Delta CT}$) method.

2.5. Western Blot Assay. The protein of anterior lens capsules and lens cortex was extracted in lysis buffer (1 M Tris-HCl at pH 7.5, 1% Triton X-100, 1% Nonidet p-40, 10% SDS, 0.5% sodium deoxycholate, 0.5 M EDTA, 10 mg/mL leupeptin, 10 mg/mL aprotinin, and 1 mM phenylmethylsulfonyl fluoride). Proteins were size-fractionated by sodium dodecyl sulfate-polyacrylamide gel electrophoresis and transferred onto polyvinylidene difluoride filter membranes (Millipore, Bedford, MA). Nonspecific protein binding to the membrane was blocked with blocking buffer (5% nonfat milk, 200 mM NaCl, 50 mM Tris, and 0.05% Tween 20). The blocked membrane was then incubated with mouse anti-human-WRN (1:800; Abcam, Cambridge, UK) and anti-GAPDH (1:1000; Santa Cruz, CA, USA) at 4°C for 18 h. The membrane was washed three times with TBST (20 mM Tris, 500 mM NaCl, and 0.1% Tween 20) for 5 min each time, followed by incubating with an alkaline phosphatase-conjugated goat anti-mouse IgG antibody (1:2000; Santa Cruz, CA, USA) for 2 h. Detection was performed using an ECL chemiluminescence kit (Pierce, Rockford, IL) and the signal was exposed to an X-ray film that was scanned using Image Quant software (Molecular Dynamics, Sunnyvale, CA, USA).

2.6. DNA Methylation Detection. DNA sequence of WRN from the NCBI genome database was used for the bioinformatic analysis. Transcription start site (TSS) of the gene was predicted by the online database (http://dbtss.hgc.jp/). CpG islands of WRN were predicted by using online software (http://www.urogene.org/methprimer/).

Genomic DNA from the frozen tissues and HLEB-3 was isolated by phenol/chloroform and ethanol extraction. Two micrograms of genomic DNA was treated with sodium bisulfite using the EpiTect Bisulfite Kit (Qiagen, Inc., Frederick, MD). EpiTect Control DNA (Qiagen, Inc.) was used as the positive controls in all experiments.

The bisulfite-sequencing PCR (BSP) primer was designed by web-based Meth Primer software (http://www.urogene.org/methprimer/) to cover a CpG island near WRN. The primers used for region 1 were 5′-TTATTTTGAAAGAAG-TTTTTTTTTGG-3′ (forward) and 5′-AAACAAACTATT-ATCCTCCCAACAC-3′ (reverse). The primers used for region 2 were 5′-TTTTTTGTGTTGGGAGGATAATAGT-3′ (forward) and 5′-AACAAAAAACAAAACTCCAAA-AAAA-3′ (reverse). The primers used for region 3 were 5′-AGGTCTCCAGCCGGCGGGCACTCA-3′ (forward) and 5′-TGAGGGGAAGAGGGGGTC-3′ (reverse). The primers used for region 4 were 5′-TTTAGTGTATTTTTTGAT-TGAAGTT-3′ (forward) and 5′-CTAAACAACTAAAAT-CCTACATCCC-3′ (reverse). The PCR products were gel-extracted and cloned into the pMD-20-T vector (Takara, Japan). Plasmid-transformed bacteria DH5a were grown for 14 h and the plasmid DNA was isolated. At least 10 clones were chosen for sequence analysis. The degree of methylation was presented as mC/CpG.

2.7. Chromatin Immunoprecipitation (ChIP) Assay. Chromatin immunoprecipitation (ChIP) assay was performed using Tissue Acetyl-Histone H3 ChIP kit and Tri-Methyl-Histone H3K9 ChIP kit (Epigentek, Farmingdale, NY, USA) according to the manufacturer's instructions. Briefly, the anterior lens capsules and cortex were cross-linked with 1% formaldehyde for 8 min and then homogenized. The homogenate was sonicated for 4 pulses of 15 sec each at level 2 using the microtip probe of a Branson Digital Sonifier (Model 450, Branson Ultrasonics Corporation, Connecticut, USA), followed by a 40 sec interval on ice between each pulse, to generate fragments of genomic DNA ranging from 200 to 800 bp in length. For the ChIP assays, equal amounts of treated chromatin were added to microwells containing immobilized antibody for the targeted protein or a negative control normal mouse IgG antibody. In addition, a small portion of treated chromatin, which was equal to 5% of the extracted genomic DNA, was used as the Input DNA to calculate the enrichment of the leptin promoter DNA after immunoprecipitation of the targeted proteins. After incubation for 90 min at 65°C to reverse the cross-links and elute the DNA, Fast-Spin columns were used for DNA purification. The primers for WRN promoter were 5′-CCGCCGCCTGACTTCGGACACC-3′ (forward) and 5′-TCGCACTCCCGCTGCACCCCAC-3′ (reverse).

2.8. Cell Culture and Demethylation Treatment. To test the relationship between the methylation and the expression of the WRN, an in vitro study of demethylation was performed. Human lens epithelium cell line (HLEB-3) was obtained from American Type Culture Collection (ATCC; Rockville, MD) and cultured in Eagle's minimum essential medium (Invitrogen-GIBCO, Carlsbad, CA) with 10% fetal bovine serum at 37°C in a humidified 5% CO_2 atmosphere. After reaching 80–90% confluency, the cells were demethylated by incubation in medium containing 3 mM of 5-aza-2-deoxy-cytidine (5-aza-dC) (Sigma, CA, USA) for 72 h. Whole cell protein extracts of HLEB-3 were isolated for Western blotting.

2.9. Statistical Analysis. One-way ANOVA analysis was used to determine the difference in averages between the four groups. P value <0.05 was considered statistically significant. Statistical analyses were performed with SPSS software (SPSS 17.0; SPSS, Inc., Chicago, IL).

3. Results

3.1. Expression of WRN in Anterior Lens Capsules and Lens Cortex. RT-PCR analysis was performed to investigate WRN mRNA content in anterior lens capsules and context of the ARC and the controls. Lower WRN mRNA (Figure 1(a)) expression in anterior lens capsules was detected in all three subtypes of ARC cases compared with the controls (P < 0.01).

To confirm the change of WRN in protein level between ARC and controls, Western blot analysis was performed. As shown in Figure 1(b), the expression pattern of WRN protein in anterior lens capsules was lower in all three subtypes of ARC cases compared with the controls (P < 0.01). However, WRN was undetected in lens cortex in both the ARC cases and the controls (data not shown).

3.2. Methylation Status of WRN. To analyze the relationship between methylation status and expression of WRN, we detected the methylation rate of WRN promoter in the DNA extracted from the anterior lens capsules and cortex of ARC and control group using BSP. Bioinformatic analysis indicated four CpG islands in the promoter of WRN (Figure 2(a)) (R1: −1287 to −1133, R2: −875 to −620, R3: −209 to 164, and R4: 173 to 324, relative to the TSS). Figures 2(b) and 2(c) showed a representative result of bisulfite genomic sequencing of the R3 fragment. Each row stands for a single plasmid clone, and each circle represents a CpG site. The unmethylated and methylated CpGs were represented by unfilled and filled cycles, respectively. As shown in Figure 2(b), the methylation rate of all three subtypes of ARC was higher than that of the control group at region 3 of WRN promoter. As shown in Figure 2(c), the methylation rate of lens cortex at region 3 was almost 100% in both ARC group and control group. The methylation rates at regions 1, 2, and 4 in WRN promoter were almost 100% in both ARC group and control group (data not shown).

3.3. Histone Modifications around the CpG Islands of the WRN Gene in ARC. In general, hypermethylation of H3-K9 exhibits the silencing of gene expression, whereas acetylation of H3 is associated with activation of gene expression. We performed ChIP to analyze the correlation between the histone modification and the expression profiles of WRN gene. ChIP analysis depicted that acetylated H3 levels were lower in all three subtypes of ARC than the control in anterior lens capsules while methylated H3-K9 was increased in all three subtypes of ARC (Figure 3). The histone modification of cortex was undetectable (data not shown).

3.4. Methylation Status and Protein Expression of WRN in HLEB-3 after Treatment with 5-Aza-dC. To test the relationship between the methylation and the expression of the WRN, an in vitro study of demethylation was performed. 5-Aza-dC

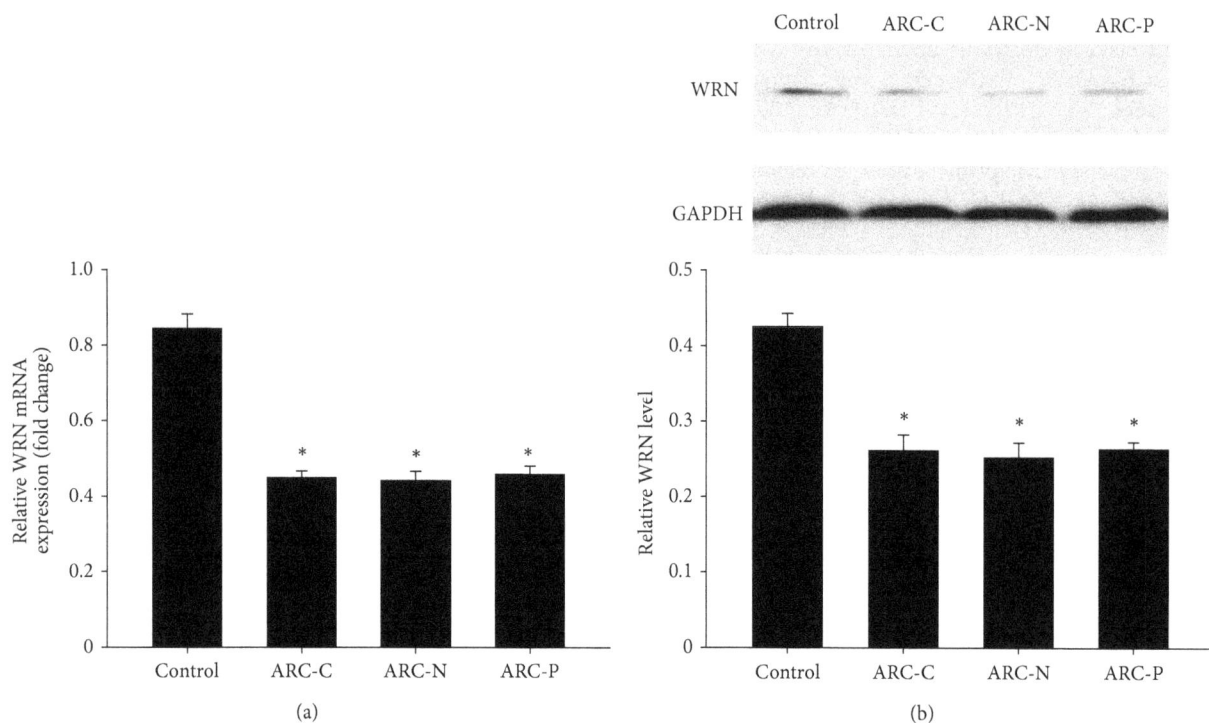

FIGURE 1: Relative expression of mRNA and protein levels of WRN in anterior lens capsules of control and ARC. (a) RT-PCR analysis of the expression of WRN in control ($n = 20$) and ARC-C ($n = 20$), ARC-N ($n = 20$), and ARC-P ($n = 20$). Values represent mean ± SD. $^*P < 0.01$. (b) WRN protein levels in control ($n = 9$) and ARC-C ($n = 9$), ARC-N ($n = 9$), and ARC-P ($n = 9$) anterior lens capsules were detected using Western blotting. Relative WRN protein level to GAPDH is presented as mean ± SD. $^*P < 0.01$.

is a DNA methyltransferase inhibitor which is used to inhibit DNA methylation. As shown in Figure 4(a), after treatment with 5-aza-dC, the methylation rate of WRN promoter in HLEB-3 was decreased in comparison with the untreated control. In contrast, the protein expression of WRN in HLEB-3 after treatment with 5-aza-dC was increased in comparison with the untreated control (Figure 4(b)).

4. Discussion

Although the pathophysiology of ARC is far from being clearly understood, it is well accepted that oxidative stress plays an important role in the disease pathogenesis. When reactive oxygen species (ROS) production exceeds the capacity of its removal by various mechanisms, they may cause oxidative damage to DNA [6–10]. In a normal physiologic condition, most oxidative DNA lesions are rapidly repaired by base excision repair (BER), nucleotide excision repair (NER), and double-strand break repair (DSBR) pathways [13, 14]. WRN is a protein functioning in the DSBR pathway and is also required for cellular DNA replication and mismatch repair [33]. Both mRNA and protein expression of WRN are downregulated in anterior lens capsules in ARC, implying a reduced DNA repair capability in the ARC lens from all included subtypes. The results have provided an additional evidence of DNA repair mechanism in ARC development by using patients' lens tissue.

We demonstrated that WRN undergoes epigenetic alterations in ARC lens tissue from all included subtypes and

this alteration is associated with the mRNA and protein expression of the gene. The treatment with a demethylating agent restored the WRN expression in HLEB-3. The results linked the epigenetic changes with the target gene expression and are consistent with the current knowledge on the effect of epigenetic modification on human genome.

It is of interest that the ARC-associated epigenetic changes of WRN gene only occur in anterior lens capsules but not in lens cortex in which both ARC cases and control had an undetectable or very weak expression of WRN and a very high degree of WRN methylation. Lens cortex is made up of lens fibers which are differentiated from LECs. The results suggest that the strategies to intervene epigenetic alteration in ARC should aim at anterior lens capsules.

We analyzed methylation status at four regions of WRN promoter in both ARC and control groups; only region 3 showed significant changes between the cases and the controls. This sequence-specific change is reasonable because this region contains the most abundant CpG islands among the four selected regions and spans the translation starting site.

5. Conclusions

Overall, our study found that aberrant epigenetic methylation in WRN DNA and the associated histone linked to low expression of WRN and lens opacity. This is the first report to show a relationship between the epigenetic modification of WRN gene and ARC by directly studying the lens tissue from human subjects. This study provided a deeper insight

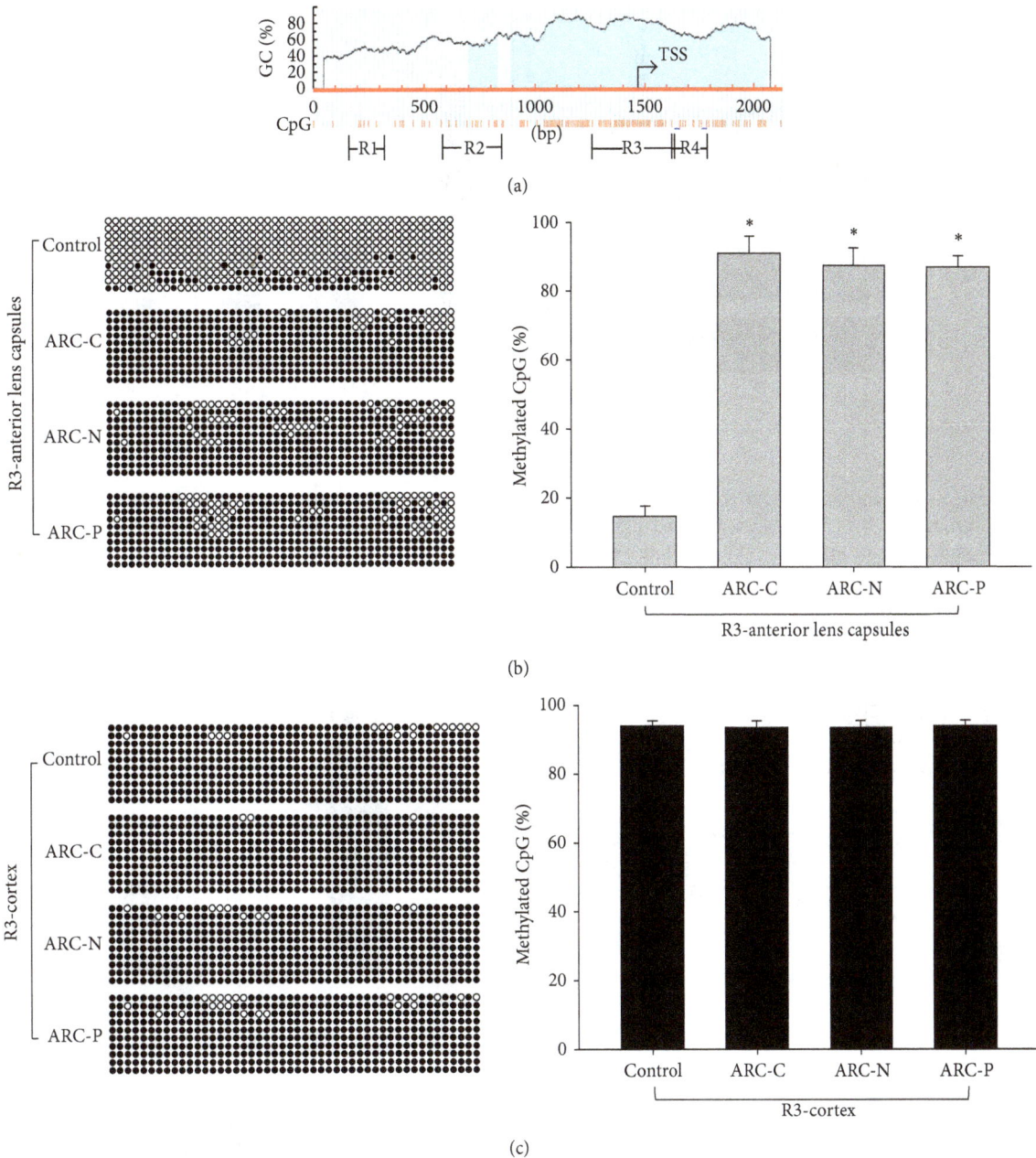

(a)

(b)

(c)

FIGURE 2: Methylation status at region 3 in WRN promoter in anterior lens capsules and cortex of control and ARC. (a) The positions of CpG islands within WRN promoter. In the following panels, each row of circles represents a single clone. Open and close circles represent unmethylated and methylated CpG sites, respectively. (b) Methylation status of region 3 in WRN promoter in anterior lens capsules of control ($n = 20$) and ARC-C ($n = 20$), ARC-N ($n = 20$), and ARC-P ($n = 20$). The ARC group displayed hypermethylation compared to the control group. $^*P < 0.01$. (c) Methylation status of region 3 in WRN promoter in lens cortex of control and ARC lens. There were no significant statistical differences between the ARC group and the control group. $P > 0.05$.

on the DNA repair mechanism in the pathogenesis of ARC, and the knowledge can be used to identify novel options for the prevention and therapy for ARC.

Disclaimer

The authors are responsible for the content and writing of the paper.

Conflict of Interests

The authors declare no conflict of interests.

Acknowledgments

This study was supported by the National Natural Science Foundation of China (no. 81270987 and no. 81070718), the 333

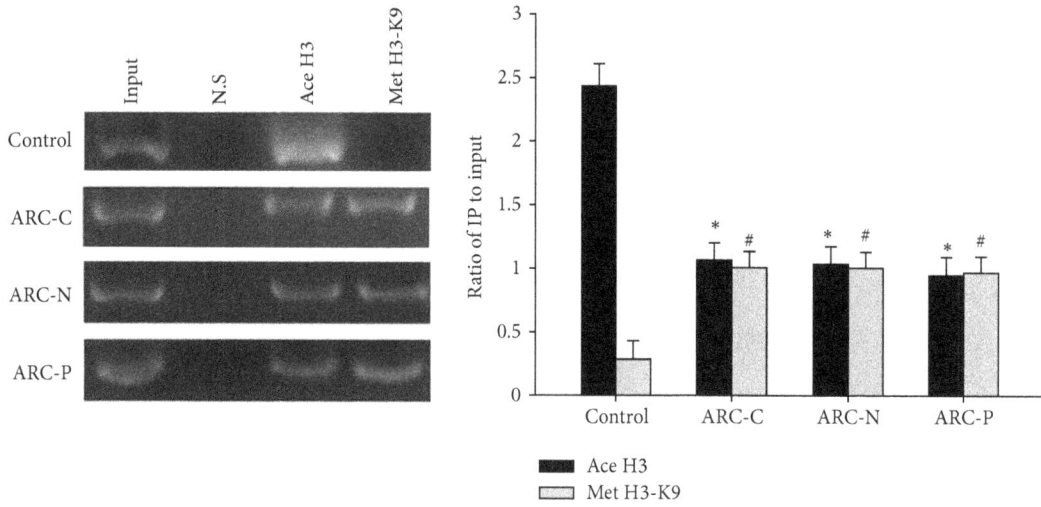

FIGURE 3: Histone modifications of the WRN promoter in anterior lens capsules of control and ARC. In anterior lens capsules, compared with the control group ($n = 10$), ChIP analysis revealed that acetylated H3 levels were lower in ARC-C ($n = 10$), ARC-N ($n = 10$), and ARC-P ($n = 10$). At the same time, methylated H3-K9 was increased. $^*P < 0.01$.

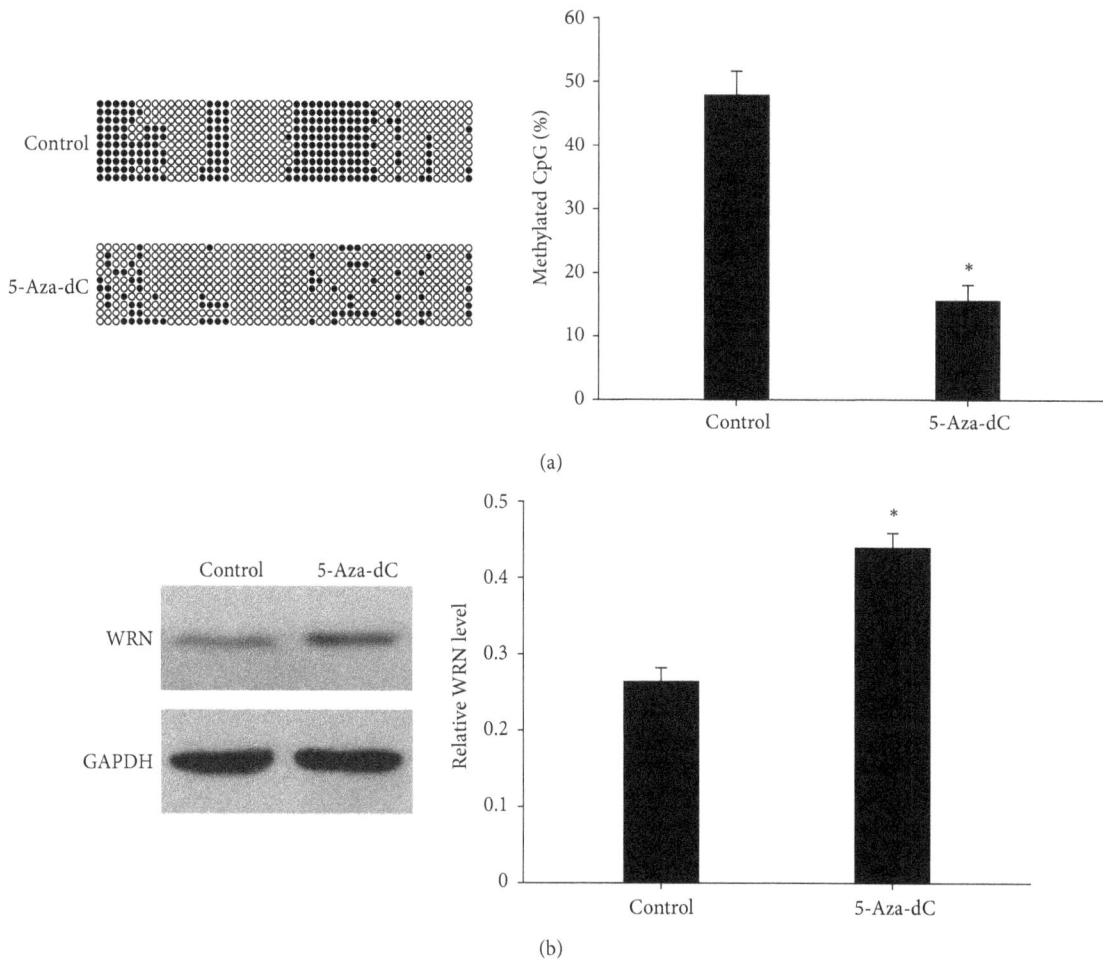

(a)

(b)

FIGURE 4: Relative methylation status and expression of protein levels of WRN in HLEB-3 after treatment with 5-aza-dC. In the following panels, each row of circles represents a single clone. Open and close circles represent unmethylated and methylated CpG sites, respectively. (a) After treatment with 5-aza-dC, the methylation rate of WRN in HLEB-3 was decreased. (b) Protein expression of WRN in the untreated control cells and in cells after treatment with 5-aza-dC. Relative WRN protein level to GAPDH is presented as mean ± SD. $^*P < 0.01$.

Project of Jiangsu Province, China (no. BRA2010173), and the Ordinary University Graduate Student Research Innovation project of Jiangsu Province, China (no. 03050487).

References

[1] B. Thylefors, "A global initiative for the elimination of avoidable blindness," *The American Journal of Ophthalmology*, vol. 125, no. 1, pp. 90–93, 1998.

[2] B. E. K. Klein, R. Klein, and K. L. P. Linton, "Prevalence of age-related lens opacities in a population: the Beaver Dam Eye Study," *Ophthalmology*, vol. 99, no. 4, pp. 546–552, 1992.

[3] J. Zuercher, J. Neidhardt, I. Magyar et al., "Alterations of the 5′untranslated region of *SLC16A12* lead to age-related cataract," *Investigative Ophthalmology & Visual Science*, vol. 51, no. 7, pp. 3354–3361, 2010.

[4] A. Shiels and J. F. Hejtmancik, "Genetic origins of cataract," *Archives of Ophthalmology*, vol. 125, no. 2, pp. 165–173, 2007.

[5] C. J. Hammond, H. Snieder, T. D. Spector, and C. E. Gilbert, "Genetic and environmental factors in age-related nuclear cataracts in monozygotic and dizygotic twins," *The New England Journal of Medicine*, vol. 342, no. 24, pp. 1786–1790, 2000.

[6] S. Ottonello, C. Foroni, A. Carta, S. Petrucco, and G. Maraini, "Oxidative stress and age-related cataract," *Ophthalmologica*, vol. 214, no. 1, pp. 78–85, 2000.

[7] O. Ates, H. H. Alp, I. Kocer, O. Baykal, and I. A. Salman, "Oxidative DNA damage in patients with cataract," *Acta Ophthalmologica*, vol. 88, no. 8, pp. 891–895, 2010.

[8] R. J. W. Truscott, "Age-related nuclear cataract—oxidation is the key," *Experimental Eye Research*, vol. 80, no. 5, pp. 709–725, 2005.

[9] W. Pendergrass, P. Penn, D. Possin, and N. Wolf, "Accumulation of DNA, nuclear and mitochondrial debris, and ROS at sites of age-related cortical cataract in mice," *Investigative Ophthalmology and Visual Science*, vol. 46, no. 12, pp. 4661–4670, 2005.

[10] Y. Zhang, L. Zhang, L. Zhang, J. Bai, H. Y. Ge, and P. Liu, "Expression changes in DNA repair enzymes and mitochondrial DNA damage in aging rat lens," *Molecular Vision*, vol. 16, pp. 1754–1763, 2010.

[11] L. Kang, W. Zhao, G. Zhang, and H. Guan, "Acetylated 8-oxoguanine DNA glycosylase 1 and its relationship with p300 and SIRT1 in lens epithelium cells from age-related cataract," *Experimental Eye Research*, 2015.

[12] B. Xu, L. Kang, G. Zhang et al., "The changes of 8-OHdG, hOGG1, APE1 and Pol beta in lenses of patients with age-related cataract," *Current Eye Research*, vol. 40, no. 4, pp. 378–385, 2015.

[13] R. D. Wood, M. Mitchell, J. Sgouros, and T. Lindahl, "Human DNA repair genes," *Science*, vol. 291, no. 5507, pp. 1284–1289, 2001.

[14] D. M. Wilson III, T. M. Sofinowski, and D. R. McNeill, "Repair mechanisms for oxidative DNA damage," *Frontiers in Bioscience*, vol. 8, pp. D963–D981, 2003.

[15] D. K. Singh, B. Ahn, and V. A. Bohr, "Roles of RECQ helicases in recombination based DNA repair, genomic stability and aging," *Biogerontology*, vol. 10, no. 3, pp. 235–252, 2009.

[16] H. Yan, J. McCane, T. Toczylowski, and C. Y. Chen, "Analysis of the Xenopus Werner syndrome protein in DNA double-strand break repair," *The Journal of Cell Biology*, vol. 171, no. 2, pp. 217–227, 2005.

[17] J. Gee, Q. X. Ding, and J. N. Keller, "Analysis of Werner's expression within the brain and primary neuronal culture," *Brain Research*, vol. 940, no. 1-2, pp. 44–48, 2002.

[18] L. H. Camacho, A. Mora-Bowen, R. Munden, W. R. Smythe, and N. G. Ordoñez, "Malignant mesothelioma: natural history, pathologic features and future therapies," *American Journal of Medicine*, vol. 120, no. 7, pp. E7–E9, 2007.

[19] M. Goto, "Hierarchical deterioration of body systems in Werner's syndrome: implications for normal ageing," *Mechanisms of Ageing and Development*, vol. 98, no. 3, pp. 239–254, 1997.

[20] S. Su, Y. Yao, R. R. Zhu et al., "The associations between single nucleotide polymorphisms of DNA repair genes, DNA damage, and age-related cataract: Jiangsu eye study," *Investigative Ophthalmology and Visual Science*, vol. 54, no. 2, pp. 1201–1207, 2013.

[21] J. Jiang, J. Zhou, Y. Yao et al., "Copy number variations of DNA repair genes and the age-related cataract: jiangsu eye study," *Investigative Ophthalmology & Visual Science*, vol. 54, no. 2, pp. 932–938, 2013.

[22] M. M. Liu, C. C. Chan, and J. S. Tuo, "Epigenetics in ocular diseases," *Current Genomics*, vol. 14, no. 3, pp. 166–172, 2013.

[23] T. Jenuwein and C. D. Allis, "Translating the histone code," *Science*, vol. 293, no. 5532, pp. 1074–1080, 2001.

[24] J. C. Rice and B. W. Futscher, "Transcriptional repression of BRCA1 by aberrant cytosine methylation, histone hypoacetylation and chromatin condensation of the BRCA1 promoter," *Nucleic Acids Research*, vol. 28, no. 17, pp. 3233–3239, 2000.

[25] J. A. Fahrner, S. Eguchi, J. G. Herman, and S. B. Baylin, "Dependence of histone modifications and gene expression on DNA hypermethylation in cancer," *Cancer Research*, vol. 62, no. 24, pp. 7213–7218, 2002.

[26] S. Fujii, R. Z. Luo, J. Yuan et al., "Reactivation of the silenced and imprinted alleles of ARHI is associated with increased histone H3 acetylation and decreased histone H3 lysine 9 methylation," *Human Molecular Genetics*, vol. 12, no. 15, pp. 1791–1800, 2003.

[27] I. O. Nasonkin, K. Lazo, D. Hambright, M. Brooks, R. Fariss, and A. Swaroop, "Distinct nuclear localization patterns of DNA methyltransferases in developing and mature mammalian retina," *The Journal of Comparative Neurology*, vol. 519, no. 10, pp. 1914–1930, 2011.

[28] Y. Wang, F. Li, G. Zhang, L. Kang, B. Qin, and H. Guan, "Altered DNA methylation and expression profiles of 8-oxoguanine DNA glycosylase 1 in lens tissue from age-related cataract patients," *Current Eye Research*, 2014.

[29] M. Gemenetzi and A. J. Lotery, "The role of epigenetics in age-related macular degeneration," *Eye*, vol. 28, no. 12, pp. 1407–1417, 2014.

[30] M. Beta, S. Chitipothu, V. Khetan, J. Biswas, and S. Krishnakumar, "Hypermethylation of adenomatosis polyposis coli-2 and its tumor suppressor role in retinoblastoma," *Current Eye Research*, pp. 1–10, 2014.

[31] R. A. Kowluru, J. M. Santos, and M. Mishra, "Epigenetic modifications and diabetic retinopathy," *BioMed Research International*, vol. 2013, Article ID 635284, 9 pages, 2013.

[32] L. Wei, B. Liu, J. Tuo et al., "Hypomethylation of the IL17RC promoter associates with age-related macular degeneration," *Cell Reports*, vol. 2, no. 5, pp. 1151–1158, 2012.

[33] R. Agrelo, W. H. Cheng, F. Setien et al., "Epigenetic inactivation of the premature aging Werner syndrome gene in human cancer," *Proceedings of the National Academy of Sciences of the United States of America*, vol. 103, no. 23, pp. 8822–8827, 2006.

[34] K. Futami, M. Takagi, A. Shimamoto, M. Sugimoto, and Y. Furuichi, "Increased chemotherapeutic activity of camptothecin in cancer cells by siRNA-induced silencing of WRN

helicase," *Biological and Pharmaceutical Bulletin*, vol. 30, no. 10, pp. 1958–1961, 2007.

[35] K. Masuda, K. Banno, M. Yanokura et al., "Association of epigenetic inactivation of the WRN gene with anticancer drug sensitivity in cervical cancer cells," *Oncology Reports*, vol. 28, no. 4, pp. 1146–1152, 2012.

[36] L. Wang, L. Xie, J. Wang, J. Shen, and B. Liu, "Correlation between the methylation of SULF2 and WRN promoter and the irinotecan chemosensitivity in gastric cancer," *BMC Gastroenterology*, vol. 13, no. 1, article 173, 2013.

[37] G. Supic, R. Kozomara, M. Brankovic-Magic, N. Jovic, and Z. Magic, "Gene hypermethylation in tumor tissue of advanced oral squamous cell carcinoma patients," *Oral Oncology*, vol. 45, no. 12, pp. 1051–1057, 2009.

[38] L. T. Chylack Jr., J. K. Wolfe, D. M. Singer et al., "The lens opacities classification system III," *Archives of Ophthalmology*, vol. 111, no. 6, pp. 831–836, 1993.

21

New Eye Cleansing Product Improves Makeup-Related Ocular Problems

Masako Okura,[1,2] Motoko Kawashima,[3] Mikiyuki Katagiri,[1] Takuji Shirasawa,[1] and Kazuo Tsubota[3]

[1]*Department of Aging Control Medicine, Juntendo University Graduate School of Medicine,*
 3-1-3 Hongo, Bunkyo-ku, Tokyo 113-8431, Japan
[2]*Eye Clinic Tenjin, 2-11-1 Tenjin, Chuo-ku, Fukuoka 8100001, Japan*
[3]*Department of Ophthalmology, Keio University School of Medicine, 35 Shinanomachi, Shinjuku-ku, Tokyo 1608582, Japan*

Correspondence should be addressed to Kazuo Tsubota; tsubota@z3.keio.jp

Academic Editor: Flavio Mantelli

Purpose. This study evaluated the effects of using a newly developed eye cleansing formulation (Eye Shampoo) to cleanse the eyelids for 4 weeks in a parallel-group comparative study in women with chronic eye discomfort caused by heavy use of eye makeup and poor eye hygiene habits. *Methods.* Twenty women participants who met the inclusion criteria were randomly allocated to 2 groups comprising 10 participants each. The participants were asked to use either artificial tears alone or artificial tears in conjunction with Eye Shampoo for 4 weeks. The participants answered the questionnaire again and were reexamined, and changes in symptoms within each group and variations of symptoms between the two groups were statistically analyzed. *Results.* In the group using only artificial tears, improvements in subjective symptoms but not in ophthalmologic examination results were found. In the group using Eye Shampoo together with artificial tears, significant improvements were observed in the subjective symptoms, meibomian orifice obstruction, meibum secretion, tear breakup time, and superficial punctate keratopathy. *Conclusion.* In patients with chronic eye discomfort thought to be caused by heavy eye makeup, maintaining eyelid hygiene using Eye Shampoo caused a marked improvement in meibomian gland blockage and dry eye symptoms.

1. Introduction

In recent years, a large number of cosmetics for the eye have become popular among young women. A large number of patients have reported various symptoms resulting from the use of such cosmetic products including oil-based makeup removers. These products also appear to increase the risk of meibomian gland dysfunction (MGD) in young people.

Eyelid hygiene has been reported to be an effective technique for managing MGD [1–3]. Several lid scrubs including OCuSOFT (OCuSOFT Corp., Rosenberg, Texas) are available commercially, and reports of their effectiveness have been published [3–7]. A hypoallergenic makeup removal product that can also be used for treatment of MGD was recently developed in Japan. This product, Eye Shampoo (MediProduct Co., Ltd., Tokyo, Japan), is a nonirritating eye cleansing formulation with a pH of 7.4,

an osmolarity of 300 mOsm/L, and ingredients with anti-inflammatory (dipotassium glycyrrhizate) and moisturizing (sodium hyaluronate) properties (Figure 1(a)).

In this study, we investigated the effectiveness of eyelid hygiene using Eye Shampoo for young women who routinely wore heavy makeup.

2. Methods

2.1. Subjects. Thirty women between 20 and 40 years of age were recruited. They currently use all the following makeup tools: foundation, eyelash makeup tools such as mascara, false eyelashes and eyelash extensions, eye shadow, eyeliner with inside liner, and eye makeup remover. Inclusion criteria included subjective symptoms of chronic eye discomfort and meibomian gland blockage. Individuals were excluded if they had currently undergoing treatment of ocular

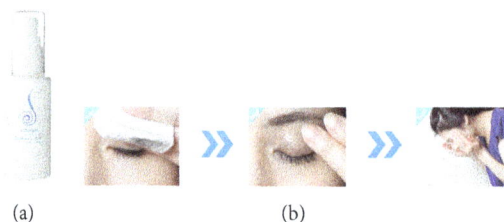

FIGURE 1: Lid hygiene technique. (a) Eye Shampoo (http://www.eyeshampoo.com/). (b) Lid cleansing using Eye Shampoo.

TABLE 1: Participants' demographic characteristics.

	Eye Shampoo group	Control group
N	10	10
Age (range), years	26.5 (21–33)	29.7 (20–39)
Contact lens use (yes : no)	8 : 2	7 : 3

surface diseases including blepharitis, dry eye disease, and Sjögren syndrome. Of the 30 women recruited, 29 gave informed consent to participate in the study. Each participant underwent screening for eligibility, received written and oral information about the study, and provided written consent to participate. Each also completed a background survey with questions including contact lens wear, history of laser in situ keratomileusis, eye-washing habits, history of chalazion, and use of eye drops. Screening examinations of the 29 volunteers were conducted, and 20 study participants who met the criteria were selected (mean age ± range, 28.1 ± 5.7 years) (Table 1).

This study followed the tenets of the Declaration of Helsinki, and the protocol was approved prospectively by the Shirasawa Clinical Research Center Ethical Review Board, Gunma, Japan.

2.2. Experimental Protocols. After consistency in ages and primary endpoints had been ensured, the patients were randomly allocated to either the control group, using only artificial tears ($n = 10$), or the Eye Shampoo group, using Eye Shampoo in conjunction with artificial tears ($n = 10$). Test products were sent by mail to the participants of each group and were used for 4 weeks, after which the examinations were repeated. Participants were allowed to use artificial tears up to 6 times per day.

The participants answered a study questionnaire and underwent eyelid margin and ocular surface examinations, including tear breakup time (BUT) and fluorescein staining score. Bacterial cultures were taken from the lid margin. They were also instructed to self-record their lid hygiene performing status and any adverse events in a study diary throughout the intervention period. Primary outcomes included subjective symptoms, meibomian orifice obstruction, and meibum secretion evaluated by compression.

2.3. Eyelid Hygiene Using Eye Shampoo. Study participants in the Eye Shampoo group used eye makeup remover and face-washing soap after awakening and before going to bed.

TABLE 2: Ocular symptoms questionnaire. Data were obtained before and 4 weeks after intervention.

	None	Mild	Moderate	Severe
Eye discomfort (feeling vague discomfort in eyes)	☐	☐	☐	☐
Feeling of dryness	☐	☐	☐	☐
Foreign body sensation	☐	☐	☐	☐
Bleary eyes	☐	☐	☐	☐
Gritty feeling	☐	☐	☐	☐
Burning sensation	☐	☐	☐	☐
Sore eyes	☐	☐	☐	☐
Hot	☐	☐	☐	☐
Eye discharge (gum in eyes)	☐	☐	☐	☐
Stringy mucus	☐	☐	☐	☐
Blurriness	☐	☐	☐	☐
Eyestrain	☐	☐	☐	☐
Eye pain	☐	☐	☐	☐
Lacrimation (excessive watering of the eye)	☐	☐	☐	☐
Itchiness	☐	☐	☐	☐
Red eye	☐	☐	☐	☐
Heaviness	☐	☐	☐	☐
Extra sensitivity to light	☐	☐	☐	☐
Excessive frequent eye blinking (frequent blinks)	☐	☐	☐	☐

They were asked to add Eye Shampoo to this hygiene regimen by pumping the Eye Shampoo onto the hand or a piece of cotton, gently spreading it around the eyes, lightly massaging it to remove any impurities at the root of the eyelashes, and washing it away (Figure 1(b)). They were allowed to use a cotton swab if they were still concerned about impurities. They were asked to place a drop of artificial tears in each eye after the eye-washing procedure. Participants in the control group followed the same hygiene regimen with the exception of the Eye Shampoo.

2.4. Subjective Symptom Questionnaire. The participants were asked to answer questions regarding 15 symptoms (Table 2). Responses of "none," "mild," "moderate," and "severe" were scored from 0 to 3, respectively. The totals were calculated and compared among the 15 symptoms.

TABLE 3: Comparison of symptoms, orifice obstruction, and decreased meibum secretion between the groups.

Group/task	Baseline	4 weeks		Variation	
	Mean ± SD	Mean ± SD	P (versus baseline)	Mean ± SD	P (between-group)
Subjective symptoms					
Control group	12.6 ± 4.8	9.3 ± 6.7	0.034*	−3.3 ± 4.0	0.005**
Eye Shampoo group	12.4 ± 5.8	1.7 ± 2.2	0.005**	−10.7 ± 6.3	
Orifice obstruction					
Control group	1.9 ± 0.3	1.9 ± 0.3	1.000	0.0 ± 0.0	0.001**
Eye Shampoo group	2.0 ± 0.0	0.7 ± 0.8	0.009**	−1.3 ± 0.8	
Decreased meibomian secretion					
Control group	1.9 ± 0.3	1.9 ± 0.3	1.000	0.0 ± 0.0	0.002**
Eye Shampoo group	2.0 ± 0.0	0.8 ± 0.9	0.014*	−1.2 ± 0.9	

*$P < 0.05$, **$P < 0.01$.

2.5. Eyelid Margin and Ocular Surface Examinations. Meibomian orifice obstruction and decreased meibum secretion were classified into 3 stages, scored as 0, 1, or 2. Decreased meibum secretion was evaluated with a 2-second duration of extrusion of the glands of the upper eyelid using the thumb. Meibomian gland orifice abnormalities (telangiectasia, displacement of the mucocutaneous junction, and eyelid margin abnormalities), BUT, superficial punctate keratopathy (SPK), eyelid culture, strip meniscometry, and measurement of eyelash length were also evaluated. Meibomian gland orifice abnormalities and SPK were classified into 3 stages, scored as 0, 1, or 2. Numerical values were indicated using mean ± standard deviation.

2.6. Statistical Analysis. Measurements for strip meniscometry, BUT, and eyelash length were analyzed using the t-test. For the parameters evaluated using three or four grades, intragroup comparisons were carried out and analyzed using the Wilcoxon signed rank test. Variations in the intergroup comparisons were evaluated with the Mann-Whitney U test. Significance was assumed to be $P < 0.05$.

3. Results

All participants completed the study, and results from all were included in the analysis. The lowest use rate among the participants was 62%.

3.1. Subjective Symptoms. Both groups exhibited significant improvement in subjective symptoms (control group, $P = 0.034$; Eye Shampoo group, $P = 0.005$) (Table 3, Figure 2). In the intergroup comparison of variations, scores in the Eye Shampoo group were significantly higher than those in the control group ($P = 0.005$) (Figure 3).

3.2. Eyelid Margin Examination. The Eye Shampoo group exhibited significant improvement in meibomian orifice obstruction scores ($P = 0.009$); scores were also higher in the Eye Shampoo group than in the control group ($P = 0.001$) (Figure 4). The Eye Shampoo group showed significant improvement in meibum secretion scores as well ($P = 0.002$)

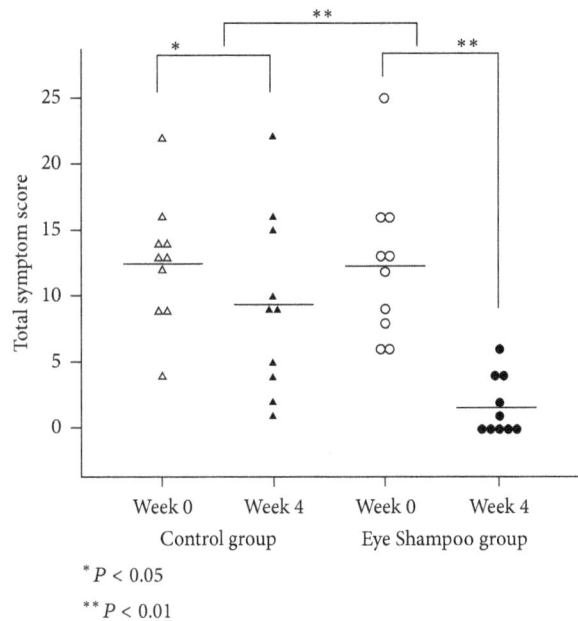

*$P < 0.05$
**$P < 0.01$

FIGURE 2: Subjective symptom scores for the two groups.

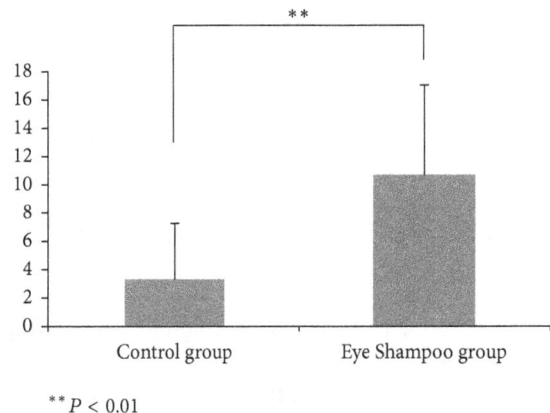

**$P < 0.01$

FIGURE 3: Variation in subjective symptom scores between the two groups.

TABLE 4: Comparison of strip meniscometry, tear film breakup time (BUT), and superficial punctate keratopathy (SPK) between the groups. SD, standard deviation.

Group/task	Baseline	4 weeks		Variation	
	Mean ± SD	Mean ± SD	P (versus baseline)	Mean ± SD	P (between-group)
Strip meniscometry (R)					
Control group	5.3 ± 3.6	5.1 ± 3.8	0.900	−0.2 ± 4.9	0.210
Eye Shampoo group	3.9 ± 2.0	5.8 ± 1.9	0.002**	1.9 ± 1.4	
Strip meniscometry (L)					
Control group	5.2 ± 3.8	5.6 ± 4.0	0.790	0.4 ± 4.6	0.283
Eye Shampoo group	4.1 ± 2.2	6.3 ± 3.3	0.014**	2.2 ± 2.3	
BUT (R)					
Control group	3.7 ± 1.1	3.2 ± 1.4	0.096	−0.5 ± 0.8	0.002**
Eye Shampoo group	3.7 ± 1.3	4.7 ± 1.6	0.008*	1.0 ± 0.9	
BUT (L)					
Control group	3.7 ± 1.1	3.3 ± 1.4	0.168	−0.4 ± 0.8	0.002**
Eye Shampoo group	3.7 ± 1.3	4.6 ± 1.4	0.004**	0.9 ± 0.7	
SPK					
Control group	0.7 ± 0.5	0.9 ± 0.3	0.157	0.2 ± 0.4	0.007**
Eye Shampoo group	0.6 ± 0.7	0.1 ± 0.3	0.025*	−0.5 ± 0.5	

*$P < 0.05$, **$P < 0.01$.

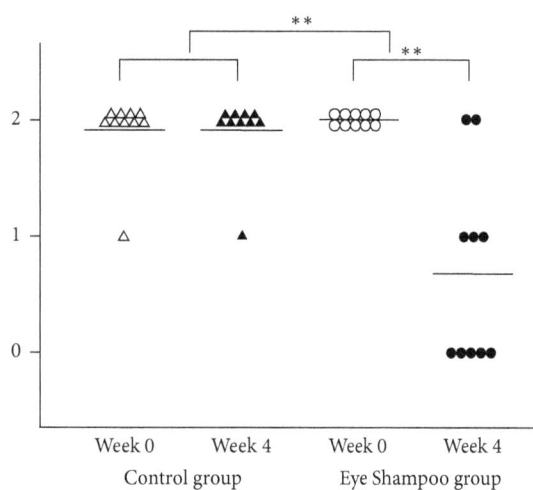

FIGURE 4: Meibomian gland orifice obstruction in the two groups. 0, absent; 1, slight; 2, prominent.

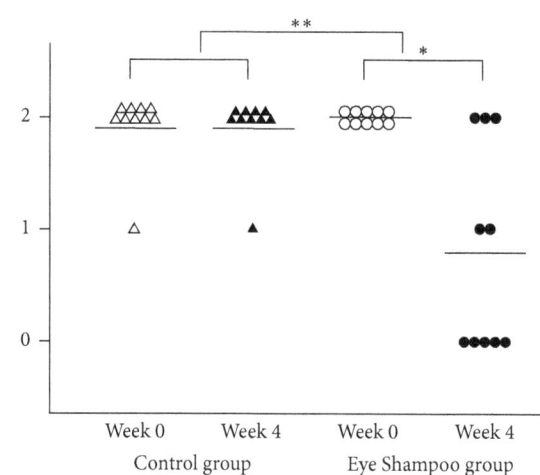

FIGURE 5: Meibum secretion in the two groups, evaluated by pressing the middle of the upper eyelid with a thumb. 0, expression with mild pressure; 1, expression with moderate pressure; 2, no expression with moderate pressure.

(Table 3, Figure 5). Abnormal findings around the orifices (vascular engorgement, anterior or posterior replacement, and irregular eyelid margin) were not significantly different in either group. Two images (Figures 6 and 7) show marked effects seen in the Eye Shampoo group, and one image (Figure 8) shows a typical presentation in the control group.

3.3. Ocular Surface Examination. No significant variation of BUT was recognized within the control group. However, BUT was significantly extended within the Eye Shampoo group and was also significantly higher in the Eye Shampoo group than in the control group (right eye: intragroup, $P = 0.008$; intergroup, $P = 0.002$; left eye: intragroup, $P = 0.004$;

intergroup, $P = 0.002$). No change in SPK was observed within the control group. However, both intragroup and intergroup variations in SPK were significantly higher in the Eye Shampoo group (intragroup, $P = 0.025$; intergroup, $P = 0.007$) (Table 4).

3.4. Other Examinations. There was no significant difference in strip meniscometry scores between the groups. However, in the intragroup comparisons, scores within the Eye Shampoo group were significantly improved after intervention (right eye, $P = 0.002$; left eye, $P = 0.014$).

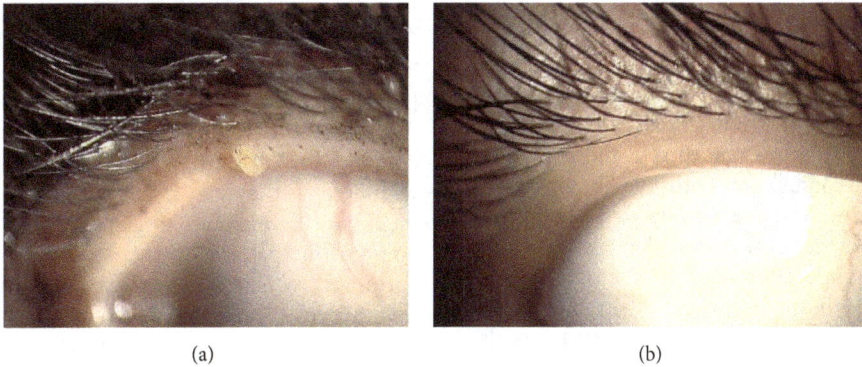

FIGURE 6: Plugging in the upper eyelid, with improvement after 4 weeks of intervention. (a) Week 0, with mascara and glue adhering to the eyelashes. (b) Week 4, after using artificial tears and Eye Shampoo.

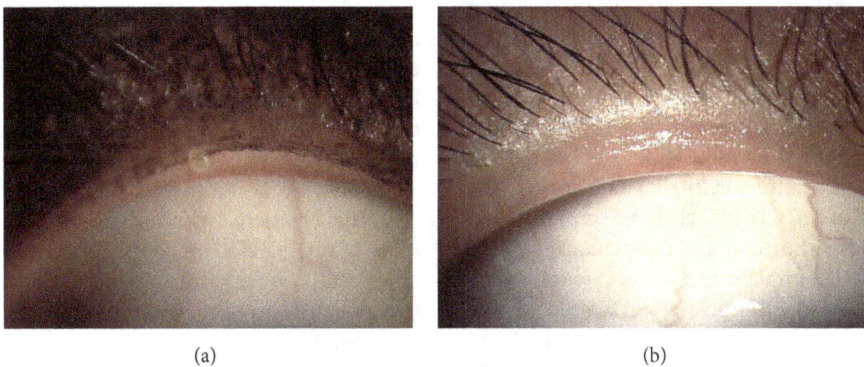

FIGURE 7: Tapioca sign in the upper eyelid, with improvement after 4 weeks of intervention. (a) Week 0, adhering to eyeliner inside eyelid margin. (b) Week 4, after using artificial tears and Eye Shampoo.

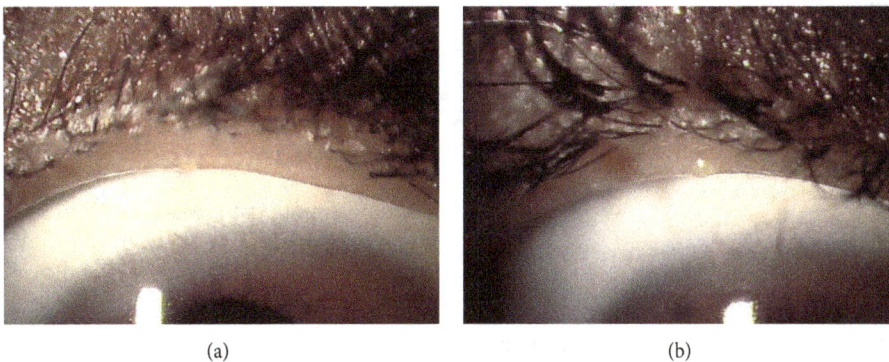

FIGURE 8: Tapioca sign in the upper eyelid, with no improvement after 4 weeks; eyelash extensions are present in both images. (a) Week 0. (b) Week 4, after using artificial tears.

Before intervention, resident microbiota was detected by bacterial culture in 3 participants in each of the two groups. After 4 weeks, however, resident microbiota was detected in 3 participants in the control group but in no participants in the Eye Shampoo group.

A questionnaire regarding subjective symptoms was administered to the participants at the conclusion of the study. We asked participants if they had become aware of "stinging," "blurred by oil," "feeling pain," "experiencing itchiness," and other symptoms after using eye makeup removers.

Eight participants in the control group responded with "blurred by oil," 2 responded with "stinging," and 1 responded with "foreign body sensation." In the Eye Shampoo group, no participants reported symptoms of "blurriness," "stinging," "itchiness," and so forth. However, 3 participants responded with "felt refreshed" and others responded favorably with comments such as "felt safe and was able to completely remove make up," "did not feel any stinging even though I scrubbed," and "knew that I had missed spots even after washing my face."

4. Discussion

Our results indicate that eyelid hygiene using Eye Shampoo markedly improved objective ocular surface findings, symptoms of dry eye, and chronic eye discomfort thought to be caused by the heavy use of eye makeup. In the group that used artificial tears in conjunction with Eye Shampoo, significant differences from the control group were observed in subjective symptoms, orifice obstruction, decreased meibum secretion by pressure application, and the examinations for BUT and SPK. A significant improvement in the volume of pooled tears (measured by strip meniscometry) was also noted in the Eye Shampoo group.

In the case of obstructive MGD, tear film abnormalities such as a decreased lipid layer thickness are directly caused by a decrease in meibum secretion. It has been reported that the tear film may become unstable because of the thinning of the lipid layer, which is reflected by short BUT. It has also been reported that the tear film in the lower cornea breaks up easily, and in that area, a corresponding corneal epithelium disorder may be observed [8]. The treatment goal is to improve abnormalities observable with a slit lamp, such as the short BUT and the resulting epithelial damage [9]. The site of decreased tear film stability is likely to be contaminated with eye makeup, thereby shortening BUT and causing SPK. In this study, we found that implementation of eyelid hygiene using Eye Shampoo helped minimize areas missed by eye makeup removal and kept the eyelid clean. This, in turn, led to reduction in obstruction, improvement of meibum secretion measured by pressure application, stabilization of tear film, improvement in subjective symptoms, increase in BUT, and improvement in SPK. It is also possible that this led to improved strip meniscometry measurements of the volume of pooled tears in the tear meniscus.

In the present study, no adverse events were reported and good results were obtained using Eye Shampoo. Moreover, no participants reported irritation using Eye Shampoo, an advantage of continuing lid hygiene. In addition, participants reported that Eye Shampoo was easily available and that they felt that their eyelashes were healthier. These suggest that continued use of Eye Shampoo could have additional favorable effects on the eyelashes; however, there are issues to be addressed, including no sample size calculation at the start of the study, the small sample size, and the fact that only young adults were included. Further investigation is warranted.

In recent years, "eye appeal makeup" has become popular among young people in Japan, and some have presented with dry eye symptoms due to obstructed meibomian glands at a young age. The most likely cause is an eye makeup technique called "inside liner," which is eyeliner that is applied to the eyelid margins over the meibomian glands so that the eyes will appear to be larger. Another cause may be that eyeliner, eye shadow, mascara, and foundation become mixed with sweat and tears over time, and the meibomian glands may become obstructed by the oils in the eye makeup. A thin, oily film mixed with pigments may cover the base of the eyelashes over the meibomian glands. Eye makeup may also migrate to the ocular surface through blinking or using eye drops [10, 11].

Kawakita et al. reported that the ocular surface migration rate (96%) and contamination scores of makeup applied to the base of the eyelashes increased when eye drops were also used [13]. We have encountered cases in which gel-like eyeliner that flaked off created a foreign body that remained in the conjunctiva. Furthermore, eyelash extensions must be used with care, as they may cause the area around the eyelashes, including the meibomian glands, to become contaminated. Some of the patients in this study presented with artificial entropion, which occurred as false eyelashes pressed the natural eyelashes down. Moreover, it appears that eyelid glue used to create a fold not only accelerates tear evaporation as it obstructs closure of the eyelid but also affects meibomian gland secretion. Blinking induces the meibomian glands to produce tears slowly from the eyelid margins. Lacrimal flow associated with blinking, which has been likened to pleated drapes [12], may thereby be affected. We have observed cases in which eyelid glue became twisted and entangled in the eyelashes over time, producing a dandruff-like appearance. It may be necessary to differentiate this presentation from that of Demodex [13–15], which, incidentally, we suspected in one of our study participants, although we did not detect Demodex upon examination with a speculum.

With cosmetics contaminating the eyes, tear film stability is further decreased, likely generating a vicious cycle. Our results suggest that, by regularly implementing eyelid hygiene, the symptoms of MGD could be improved relatively easily when eye makeup obstructs the meibomian glands in young people. There has been a recent tendency to overwork the eyes from a young age with eye makeup and other products. In this regard, implementation of daily eyelid hygiene to keep the eyelids clean could slow the aging of the eyes.

In conclusion, eyelid hygiene is an effective management technique for meibomian gland and ocular surface health.

Conflict of Interests

Kazuo Tsubota and Masako Okura received a financial support from MediProduct Co., Ltd., Tokyo, Japan. The other authors declare that there is no conflict of interests regarding the publication of this paper.

Acknowledgment

This study was supported by MediProduct Co., Ltd., Tokyo, Japan. The funders had no role in study design, data collection and analysis, publication decisions, or paper preparation.

References

[1] J. R. Paugh, L. L. Knapp, J. R. Martinson, and M. M. Hom, "Meibomian therapy in problematic contact lens wear," *Optometry and Vision Science*, vol. 67, no. 11, pp. 803–806, 1990.

[2] J. M. Romero, S. A. Biser, H. D. Perry et al., "Conservative treatment of meibomian gland dysfunction," *Eye and Contact Lens*, vol. 30, no. 1, pp. 14–19, 2004.

[3] J. E. Key, "A comparative study of eyelid cleaning regimens in chronic blepharitis," *The CLAO Journal*, vol. 22, no. 3, pp. 209–212, 1996.

[4] R. W. Bowman, J. M. Dougherty, and J. P. McCulley, "Chronic blepharitis and dry eyes," *International Ophthalmology Clinics*, vol. 27, no. 1, pp. 27–35, 1987.

[5] J. R. Wittpenn, "Eye scrub: simplifying the management of blepharitis," *Journal of Ophthalmic Nursing & Technology*, vol. 14, pp. 25–28, 1995.

[6] E. Goto and J. Shimazaki, "Meibomian gland dysfunction and its treatment," *Atarashii Ganka*, vol. 14, no. 11, pp. 1613–1621, 1997.

[7] J. M. Romero, S. A. Biser, H. D. Perry et al., "Conservative treatment of meibomian gland dysfunction," *Eye & Contact Lens*, vol. 30, no. 1, pp. 14–19, 2004.

[8] S. Den, "Diagnosis and treatment of meibomian gland dysfunction," *Atarashii Ganka*, vol. 25, no. 12, pp. 1655–1659, 2008.

[9] N. Yokoi and K. Tsubota, "Core mechanism of dry eye: hypothesis based on tear film instability," *Atarashii Ganka*, vol. 29, no. 3, pp. 291–297, 2012.

[10] T. Goto, X. Zheng, L. Gibbon, and Y. Ohashi, "Cosmetic product migration onto the ocular surface: exacerbation of migration after eyedrop instillation," *Cornea*, vol. 29, no. 4, pp. 400–403, 2010.

[11] A. Malik and C. Claoué, "Transport and interaction of cosmetic product material within the ocular surface: beauty and the beastly symptoms of toxic tears," *Contact Lens & Anterior Eye*, vol. 35, no. 6, pp. 247–259, 2012.

[12] N. Yokoi and G. A. Georgi, "Evaluation of meibomian gland function from the clinical aspect," *Atarashii Ganka*, vol. 28, no. 8, pp. 1073–1079, 2001.

[13] T. Kawakita, M. Kawashima, O. Ibrahim, D. Murato, and K. Tsubota, "Demodex-related marginal blepharitis in Japan," *Nippon Ganka Gakkai Zasshi*, vol. 114, no. 12, pp. 1025–1029, 2010.

[14] T. Kojima, R. Ishida, E. A. Sato et al., "In vivo evaluation of ocular demodicosis using laser scanning confocal microscopy," *Investigative Ophthalmology & Visual Science*, vol. 52, no. 1, pp. 565–569, 2011.

[15] S. H. Lee, Y. S. Chun, J. H. Kim, E. S. Kim, and J. C. Kim, "The relationship between demodex and ocular discomfort," *Investigative Ophthalmology & Visual Science*, vol. 51, no. 6, pp. 2906–2911, 2010.

22

Effect of Flat Cornea on Visual Outcome after LASIK

Engy Mohamed Mostafa

Ophthalmology Department, Sohag University, Naser City, Sohag 82524, Egypt

Correspondence should be addressed to Engy Mohamed Mostafa; engymostafa@yahoo.com

Academic Editor: Edward Manche

Purpose. To evaluate the effect of preoperative and postoperative keratometry on the refractive outcome after laser in situ keratomileusis (LASIK) for moderate and high myopia. *Methods.* Records of 812 eyes (420 patients) with myopia ≥ -6 D who had LASIK at Sohag Laser Center, Egypt, from January 2010 to November 2013, were retrospectively analyzed. Main outcome measures were postoperative corrected distance visual acuity (CDVA), postoperative spherical equivalence, and postoperative Q factor. *Results.* LASIK was performed in 812 eyes (mean age 21.8 ± 5.2 years). Patients were grouped according to the degree of preoperative myopia into three groups: Group 1, -6 to -7.9 D; Group 2, -8 to -9.9 D; and Group 3, -10 to -12 D. The refractive outcome among the different myopia groups was stratified by pre- and postoperative keratometry. A trend toward greater undercorrection was noted in eyes with preoperative keratometry <43.5 D compared with those with steeper keratometry >46 D in all myopia groups. The undercorrection was also noted in postoperative keratometry groups <35 D. *Conclusions.* Preoperative and postoperative keratometry appeared to influence the refractive outcome especially in high myopic eyes.

1. Introduction

The principal theory of laser refractive surgery is that the optical power of the eye can be changed by modifying the corneal curvature [1]. Laser in situ keratomileusis (LASIK) is performed to correct myopia and myopic astigmatism by ablating the corneal tissue and flattening the central anterior corneal curvature. The subsequent increase in the corneal radius lowers the dioptric power of the cornea and allows accurate correction of myopic defects [2].

Although laser in situ keratomileusis (LASIK) has been shown to be safe and effective for the treatment of myopia [3, 4], greater outcome variability has been reported in eyes with higher degrees of myopia [5].

Many factors have been investigated to find what influences the predictability of LASIK including patient age [6], optical zone diameter [6], epithelial hyperplasia [7], and preoperative keratometry (K) [5].

The question of whether the preoperative K power influences outcomes in myopic patients has been studied somewhat in patients undergoing photorefractive keratometry (PRK) procedures and more in hyperopic LASIK [8], and the findings are contradictory. Therefore, we tried to deduct the effect of both pre- and postoperative keratometry on moderate to high myopic patients undergoing LASIK since the literature is unclear regarding their influence.

2. Patients and Methods

The case records of 812 consecutive eyes of 420 patients with moderate and high myopia ≥ -6 D were retrospectively analyzed. LASIK was done at Sohag Laser Center, Egypt, from January 2010 to November 2013. Data obtained from the case records included patient age, spherical equivalent (SE) refraction (pre- and postoperative), corrected distance visual acuity (CDVA) (pre- and postoperative), and keratometry (pre- and postoperative) and details of intraoperative complications. Follow-up was repeated at 3 and 6 months postoperatively. Exclusion criteria were (1) eyes with spherical equivalence > -12 D, (2) eyes with follow-up of less than 6 months, (3) eyes with intraoperative complications, (4) eyes with preoperative CDVA <0.3, (5) eyes that needed undercorrection due to thin corneas not permitting total correction, and (6) eyes with previous ocular surgeries. Rabinowitz criteria [9–11] were applied meticulously to screen for keratoconus and exclude risk factors.

TABLE 1: Demographics of all eyes and the three groups stratified by degree of myopia.

Myopia group (D)	Patient age (years) (mean ± SD)	Number of eyes	Preoperative SE (D) (mean ± SD)	Preoperative keratometry (D) (Mean ± SD)	Postoperative SE (mean ± SD)	Postoperative keratometry (D) (mean ± SD)
All eyes	21.8 ± 5.2	812	−8.5 ± 3.2	42.3 ± 4.1	−0.13 ± 1.1	36.36 ± 3.8
−6 to −7.9 D	22.8 ± 8.1	370	−7.2 ± 0.4	44.2 ± 1.7	0 ± 1.1	36.9 ± 4.5
−8 to −9.9 D	21.1 ± 6.9	289	−9.1 ± 0.2	45.2 ± 1.9	−0.1 ± 1.4	36.2 ± 2
−10 to −12 D	21.5 ± 7.2	153	−11.00 ± 0.5	44.9 ± 1.4	−0.3 ± 1.00	36 ± 3.3

SE: spherical equivalence; D: Diopter.

TABLE 2: Postoperative CDVA stratified by preoperative keratometry.

Myopia group (D)	Postoperative CDVA (log MAR) Mean ± SD			t-test comparing eyes with Preop K <42 D and >46 D	ANOVA comparing 3 groups with different Preop K
	Preop K <42 D (number of eyes)	Preop K = 42 to 45.9 D (number of eyes)	Preop K >46 D (number of eyes)		
−6 to −7.9 D	0.0 ± 0.11 (109)	0.0 ± 0.12 (119)	0.0 ± 0.16 (142)	0.21	0.657
−8 to −9.9 D	0.05 ± 0.15 (66)	0.0 ± 0.13 (114)	0.11 ± 0.2 (109)	0.032*	0.27
−10 to −12 D	0.12 ± 0.29 (28)	0.18 ± 0.29 (58)	0.18 ± 0.4 (67)	0.015*	0.04*

CDVA: corrected distance visual acuity; Preop: preoperative; K: keratometry; ANOVA: analysis of variance.

Corneal keratometry (K) was measured in the flat and steep axes using a Scheimpflug topography system (Sirius, CSO, Italy). Pre- and postoperative average K = (K flat + K steep)/2. Change in K (ΔK) was calculated as preoperative minus postoperative average K. Visual acuity was recorded using logMAR.

3. LASIK Procedure

One refractive eye surgeon (EM) operated on the patients using the same nomogram for all treatments. The minimum residual stromal bed was planned to be 280 μm with emmetropia being the goal in all cases. Superior hinged lamellar flaps were created with a Moria M2 microkeratome using a 90 μm single use head and 9.0 mm ring. Laser ablation was performed using the VISX Star S4 IR, creating a 6.5 mm optical zone with 8.0 mm blend zone with centration over the center of the pupil. Following noncustomized ablation, the flap was replaced and the patients then received fluoroquinolone QID for 7 days and prednisolone acetate 1% drops QID for 7 days and then tapering over 3 weeks. Our final outcomes were compared at the 6-month follow-up.

For the purpose of analysis, patients were divided into three groups based on the degree of preoperative myopia: Group 1, −6 D to −7.9 D; Group 2, −8 to −9.9 D; and Group 3, −10 to −12 D. The reported refractive values correspond to spectacle plane. The refractive outcome among the different myopic groups was further stratified by pre- and postoperative keratometry. The study was approved by the ethical committee of Sohag Faculty of Medicine.

Statistical analysis was performed using the SPSS program. Means were compared using the unpaired t-test (2-tailed), while nonparametric data were analyzed using the chi-square test. Trends in data were tested using an analysis

of variance, and the relationship between preoperative keratometry and postoperative refraction was studied by linear regression.

4. Results

The demographics of the 420 patients (155 men, 265 women) and the three groups which are stratified according to the degree of preoperative myopia are reported in Table 1. No statistically significant difference existed between the 3 myopic matched cohort groups in mean age (P = 0.26).

4.1. Preoperative Keratometry. The data was further stratified according to the mean preoperative keratometry (K) power into 3 subdivisions: (1) K < 42 D, (2) K = 42–45.9 D, and (3) K > 46 D. There was a statistically significant difference in postoperative spherical equivalence in both groups, 2 and 3, when the corneal power was less than 42 D and more than 46 D (P = 0.032 and P = 0.015, resp.) (Figure 1(a)) and the same applies to the corrected distance visual acuity (Table 2). In patients with similar preoperative myopia, greater undercorrection was noted in eyes with preoperative keratometry <42 D. Although this was seen in all myopia subgroups, the difference was greatest in those with higher preoperative myopia (SE of −10.0 to −12 D) (P = 0.015).

4.2. Postoperative Keratometry. In Table 3, the postoperative corneal powers were divided into three subdivisions: (1) K < 35 D, (2) K = 35–38.9 D, and (3) K > 39 D. There was a statistically significant difference in postoperative spherical equivalence and corrected distance visual acuity in all groups of myopia when the corneal power was less than 35 D and more than 38 D. In patients

TABLE 3: Postoperative CDVA stratified by postoperative keratometry.

Myopia group (D)	Postoperative CDVA Mean ± SD			t-test comparing eyes with Postop K <35 D and >39 D	ANOVA comparing 3 groups with different Postop K
	Postop K <35 D	Postop K = 35–38.9 D	Postop K >39 D		
−6 to −7.9 D	0.0 ± 0.6	0.0 ± 0.6	0.0 ± 0.5	0.05*	0.42
−8 to −9.9 D	0.1 ± 1.2	0.1 ± 1	0.0 ± 1.1	0.033*	0.47
−10 to −12 D	0.13 ± 1.3	0.1 ± 1.2	0.1 ± 1.2	0.02*	0.15

CDVA: corrected distance visual acuity; Postop: postoperative; K: keratometry; ANOVA: analysis of variance.

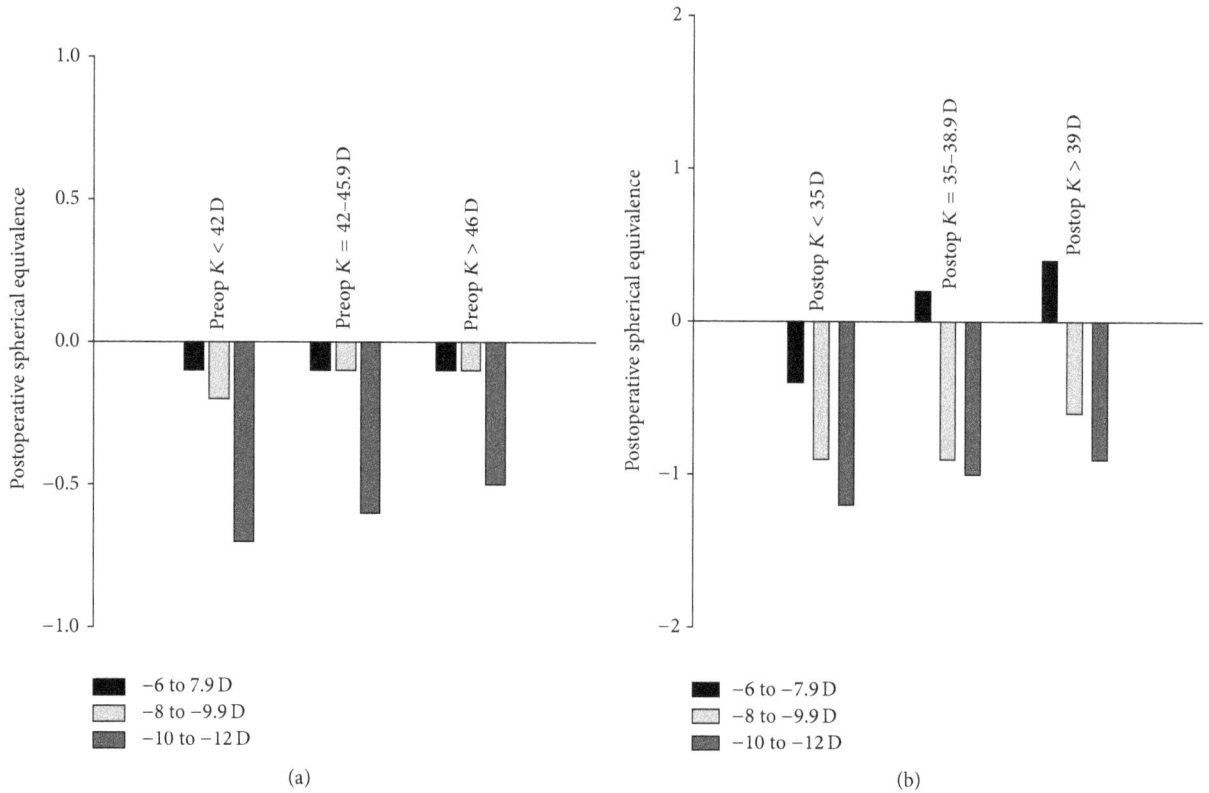

FIGURE 1: Postoperative spherical equivalence stratified by pre- and postoperative keratometry, respectively.

with similar preoperative myopia, greater undercorrection was noted in eyes with postoperative keratometry <35 D than in eyes with steeper corneas (keratometry > 39 D) (Figure 1(b)).

4.3. Change in Keratometry (ΔK).

The impact of change in corneal power was also addressed. The results showed that the larger the change in the keratometry between pre- and postoperative keratometric readings is, the more the postoperative spherical equivalence was affected. The postoperative SE was more when ΔK was higher in all groups of myopia as shown in Table 4.

4.4. Corneal Asphericity.

The results of Spearman correlation coefficient between the degree of pre- and postoperative keratometry and the Q-factor (pre- and postoperative) revealed

TABLE 4: Postoperative spherical equivalence stratified by change in keratometry.

Myopia group (D)	Postoperative SE (D) Mean ± SD			P value
	ΔK < 5 D	ΔK = 5–7.9 D	ΔK > 8 D	
−6 to −7.9 D	−0.4 ± 0.5	+0.2 ± 0.6	Nil	0.05*
−8 to −9.9 D	Nil	−0.9 ± 1.2	−0.6 ± 1.1	0.033*
−10 to −12 D	Nil	−1.0 ± 1.2	−0.9 ± 1.2	0.02*

ΔK: change in keratometry; SE: spherical equivalent; ANOVA: analysis of variance.

a correlation coefficient of 0.90 and 0.96, respectively, indicating a high correlation between the 2 variables; that is, the change in corneal asphericity increased with the degree of corneal curvature (Figure 2).

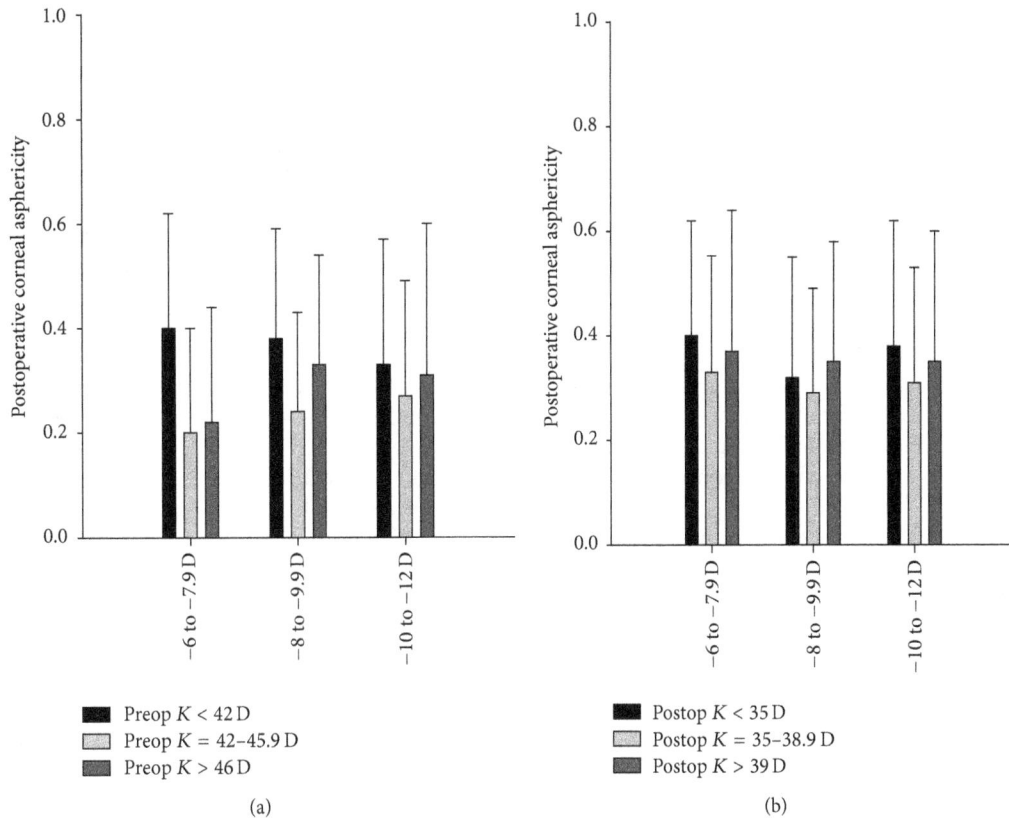

FIGURE 2: Postoperative corneal asphericity stratified by pre- and postoperative keratometry, respectively.

5. Discussion

The precision of refractive surgery for the correction of myopia has improved with the advent of LASIK, particularly for high myopia. However, marked variability in refractive outcomes still exists among individual patients [3, 5].

This study analyzed the relationship between preoperative and postoperative keratometry to postoperative spherical equivalence and corrected distance visual acuity in a cohort of 812 eyes having LASIK by a single surgeon, using a standardized treatment protocol for all patients. To the best of our knowledge, this is the first study to address the effect of both pre- and postoperative keratometry in cases of moderate and high myopia in a large group of patients. We also addressed the effect of preoperative and postoperative corneal power on corneal asphericity.

The relationship between preoperative keratometry (K) and visual outcomes in laser-assisted in situ keratomileusis (LASIK) has been studied in myopia as well as in hyperopia.

We noted a trend toward greater undercorrection in patients with keratometry <43.5 D than in those with keratometry >46 D in all myopia groups. The possibility of undercorrection resulting from treating flatter corneas with a standard protocol has been described in a neural network model [12]. Also, the loss of ablation efficiency at nonnormal incidence may explain many of the current findings: Considering the loss of efficiency in a pure myopia profile, the profile "shrinks," steepening the average slope and then slightly increasing the myopic power of the profile as well as inducing spherical aberrations [13–16].

Rao et al. [17] reported increased undercorrection in eyes with preoperative SE of −10.0 to −11.9 D and in eyes with flat corneas compared with steeper corneas. Perez-Santonja et al. [5] also reported a tendency toward undercorrection in eyes with flatter corneas that had received LASIK for the correction of high myopia of −8.00 to −20.00 D, while Christiansen et al. [18] studied moderately myopic eyes undergoing LASIK and their results suggested that flatter corneas have better visual outcomes than those with steeper corneas which disagreed with the previous studies as well as ours.

Other studies examining hyperopic LASIK agree with our results. Williams et al. [8] prospectively examined 6-month follow-up data and found an increased incidence of loss of BSCVA with eyes that had preoperative K > 44.0 D. Esquenazi and Mendoza [19] found that undercorrection occurred more frequently in eyes with preoperative K > 45.0 D.

Another study of the effect of keratometry on refractive outcome was carried out by de Benito-Llopis et al. [20] in LASEK cases on 1180 eyes and found that there is a weak positive correlation between preoperative keratometry and postoperative SE, mostly in the subgroup with steeper corneas and when the preoperative refractive error was higher. Yet they did not find a tendency toward undercorrection in flatter corneas, as some studies of LASIK have concluded. Studies by Hersh et al. [21], Blaker and Hersh [22], and Varssano et al. [23] yielded the same results in PRK patients as well. In contrast, Ditzen et al. [24] reported that preoperative K values affected outcomes of hyperopic LASIK. They found that flat, rather than steep, preoperative corneal keratometry led to greater regression and vision undercorrection.

The differences between the results of surface ablation and LASIK may be due to the fact that creating a stromal flap could be a confounding factor in LASIK. Flattening of the central cornea can result from cutting the peripheral stroma due to interlamellar forces [25, 26]. In non-femto-assisted LASIK, the microkeratome produces a meniscus shaped flap that is thinner in the center and thicker in the periphery [27, 28]. The preoperative corneal curvature seems to affect the profile of the stromal flap, while surface laser ablation alters only the corneal curvature, thus avoiding this potential confounding factor.

Another factor that might explain why the studies of PRK patients found no relationship between these 2 factors is the aggressive stromal healing response and epithelial remodeling in surface ablation. So, with less healing response in LASIK, any relationship between preoperative keratometry and final refraction may be more evident [29].

Rao et al. [17] suggest that because the change in corneal curvature is responsible for correcting myopia, more ablation might be required in a flatter cornea than a steeper cornea to produce a similar amount of effective change. Stark et al. [30] also suggest that the laser beam incises less perpendicularly the surface in the midperiphery of steep corneas than of flatter ones, which may cause a loss of ablative efficiency away from the corneal apex in steep corneas. This can result in deeper central ablation and shallower paracentral ablation leading to slightly greater myopic correction in steep corneas than in flat corneas.

As regards the effect of postoperative keratometry on refractive state, Jin et al. [31] found no association between postoperative K greater than 49.0 D and poor visual acuity in hyperopes. Cobo-Soriano et al. [32] also found that postoperative K did not affect outcomes and that postoperative K greater than 48.0 D had no effect on visual outcomes.

Tabbara et al. [33] supported the conclusion that rather than dependence on the preoperative or postoperative K values, the outcomes of hyperopic LASIK are dependent on intraoperative changes in K. Cobo-Soriano et al. as well found an association between K changes greater than 4.0 D and poor outcomes.

As regards corneal asphericity, Holladay et al. [34] found a high average rise in the Q-factor after refractive surgery, which declined over 6 months to a value that was still higher than the presurgery level.

Bottos et al. [35] investigated the asphericity change after wavefront-guided LASIK in 177 myopic eyes and found that there is a change in the direction of a more oblate profile which is in agreement with our results as well. Several studies revealed that corneal vertex centration resulted in less ocular aberrations and changes in asphericity. Because of the smaller angle between corneal vertex and pupil center associated with myopes compared with hyperopes, centration problems are less apparent [36, 37]. However, pupillary offset larger than

250 μm seems to be sufficiently large to be responsible for differences in ocular aberrations, yet not large enough to correlate this difference in ocular aberrations with functional vision [38–40].

We classified the myopic eyes into 3 groups to avoid masking the underlying relationship between keratometry and refractive outcome if it has been analyzed all in one group as the level of preoperative ametropia was proved to strongly affect the final outcome [3, 5, 17]. We understand that longer follow-up periods were warranted to shed light on the long term postoperative effects.

In conclusion, our data revealed the occurrence of greater undercorrection after LASIK in eyes with flatter preoperative keratometry and postoperative keratometry as well. Analysis of large group of patients allowed us to conclude that the effect of preoperative keratometry on the final refractive outcome appeared greater in eyes with higher myopia, and these differences were clinically significant in eyes with myopia greater than –10.0 D. Preoperative and postoperative keratometry appeared to influence the corneal asphericity as well. LASIK nomograms integrating corneal curvature would lead to better outcomes particularly in eyes with high myopia.

Disclosure

This research has been presented as a paper in the ASCRS 2014, Boston, USA.

Conflict of Interests

The author has no proprietary interests or conflict of interests related to this paper.

References

[1] K.-M. A. Tuan and D. Chernyak, "Corneal asphericity and visual function after wavefront-guided LASIK," *Optometry and Vision Science*, vol. 83, no. 8, pp. 605–610, 2006.

[2] G. Savini, K. J. Hoffer, M. Carbonelli, and P. Barboni, "Scheimpflug analysis of corneal power changes after myopic excimer laser surgery," *Journal of Cataract and Refractive Surgery*, vol. 39, no. 4, pp. 605–610, 2013.

[3] A. Maldonado-Bas and R. Onnis, "Results of laser in situ keratomileusis in different degrees of myopia," *Ophthalmology*, vol. 105, no. 4, pp. 606–611, 1998.

[4] R. J.-F. Tsai, "Laser in situ keratomileusis for myopia of -2 to -25 diopters," *Journal of Refractive Surgery*, vol. 13, no. 5, supplement, pp. S427–S429, 1997.

[5] J. J. Perez-Santonja, J. Bellot, P. Claramonte, M. M. Ismail, and J. L. Alio, "Laser in situ keratomileusis to correct high myopia," *Journal of Cataract and Refractive Surgery*, vol. 23, no. 3, pp. 372–385, 1997.

[6] K. Ditzen, A. Handzel, and S. Pieger, "Laser in situ keratomileusis nomogram development," *Journal of Refractive Surgery*, vol. 15, no. 2, supplement, pp. S197–S201, 1999.

[7] C. P. Lohmann and J. L. Güell, "Regression after LASIK for the treatment of myopia: the role of the corneal epithelium," *Seminars in Ophthalmology*, vol. 13, no. 2, pp. 79–82, 1998.

[8] L. B. Williams, S. B. Dave, and M. Moshirfar, "Correlation of visual outcome and patient satisfaction with preoperative keratometry after hyperopic laser in situ keratomileusis," *Journal of Cataract and Refractive Surgery*, vol. 34, no. 7, pp. 1083–1088, 2008.

[9] P. S. Binder, R. L. Lindstrom, R. D. Stulting et al., "Keratoconus and corneal ectasia after LASIK," *Journal of Cataract and Refractive Surgery*, vol. 31, no. 11, pp. 2035–2038, 2005.

[10] Y. S. Rabinowitz, "Videokeratographic indices to aid in screening for keratoconus," *Journal of Refractive Surgery*, vol. 11, no. 5, pp. 371–379, 1995.

[11] Y. S. Rabinowitz and P. J. McDonnell, "Computer-assisted corneal topography in keratoconus," *Refractive and Corneal Surgery*, vol. 5, no. 6, pp. 400–408, 1989.

[12] S. H. Yang, R. N. Van Gelder, and J. S. Pepose, "Neural network computer program to determine photorefractive keratectomy nomograms," *Journal of Cataract and Refractive Surgery*, vol. 24, no. 7, pp. 917–924, 1998.

[13] C. Dorronsoro, D. Cano, J. Merayo-Lloves, and S. Marcos, "Experiments on PMMA models to predict the impact of corneal refractive surgery on corneal shape," *Optics Express*, vol. 14, no. 13, pp. 6142–6156, 2006.

[14] M. Mrochen and T. Seiler, "Influence of corneal curvature on calculation of ablation patterns used in photorefractive laser surgery," *Journal of Refractive Surgery*, vol. 17, no. 5, pp. S584–S587, 2001.

[15] J. R. Jiménez, R. G. Anera, L. J. Del Barco, E. Hita, and F. Pérez-Ocón, "Correction factor for ablation algorithms used in corneal refractive surgery with gaussian-profile beams," *Optics Express*, vol. 13, no. 1, pp. 336–343, 2005.

[16] Y. Kwon and S. Bott, "Postsurgery corneal asphericity and spherical aberration due to ablation efficiency reduction and corneal remodelling in refractive surgeries," *Eye*, vol. 23, no. 9, pp. 1845–1850, 2009.

[17] S. K. Rao, A. C. K. Cheng, D. S. P. Fan, A. T. S. Leung, and D. S. C. Lam, "Effect of preoperative keratometry on refractive outcomes after laser in situ keratomileusis," *Journal of Cataract and Refractive Surgery*, vol. 27, no. 2, pp. 297–302, 2001.

[18] S. M. Christiansen, M. C. Neuffer, S. Sikder, R. T. Semnani, and M. Moshirfar, "The effect of preoperative keratometry on visual outcomes after moderate myopic LASIK," *Clinical Ophthalmology*, vol. 6, no. 1, pp. 459–464, 2012.

[19] S. Esquenazi and A. Mendoza, "Two-year follow-up of laser in situ keratomileusis for hyperopia," *Journal of Refractive Surgery*, vol. 15, no. 6, pp. 648–652, 1999.

[20] L. de Benito-Llopis, M. A. Teus, J. M. Sánchez-Pina, and R. Gil-Cazorla, "Influence of preoperative keratometry on refractive results after laser-assisted subepithelial keratectomy to correct myopia," *Journal of Cataract and Refractive Surgery*, vol. 34, no. 6, pp. 968–973, 2008.

[21] P. S. Hersh, O. D. Schein, R. Steinert et al., "Characteristics influencing outcomes of excimer laser photorefractive keratectomy," *Ophthalmology*, vol. 103, no. 11, pp. 1962–1969, 1996.

[22] J. W. Blaker and P. S. Hersh, "Theoretical and clinical effect of preoperative corneal curvature on excimer laser photorefractive keratectomy for myopia," *Journal of Refractive and Corneal Surgery*, vol. 10, no. 5, pp. 571–574, 1994.

[23] D. Varssano, M. Waisbourd, L. Minkev, T. Sela, M. Neudorfer, and P. S. Binder, "Visual acuity outcomes in eyes with flat corneas after PRK," *Journal of Refractive Surgery*, vol. 29, no. 6, pp. 384–389, 2013.

[24] K. Ditzen, H. Huschka, and S. Pieger, "Laser in situ keratomileusis for hyperopia," *Journal of Cataract and Refractive Surgery*, vol. 24, no. 1, pp. 42–47, 1998.

[25] C. Roberts, "Biomechanics of the cornea and wavefront-guided laser refractive surgery," *Journal of Refractive Surgery*, vol. 18, no. 5, pp. S589–S592, 2002.

[26] W. J. Dupps Jr. and S. E. Wilson, "Biomechanics and wound healing in the cornea," *Experimental Eye Research*, vol. 83, no. 4, pp. 709–720, 2006.

[27] L. P. Lasik, "Complications," in *Cornea*, J. M. M. Krachmer and E. J. Holland, Eds., Elsevier, Edinburgh, UK, 2nd edition, 2005.

[28] D. Z. Reinstein, H. F. S. Sutton, S. Srivannaboon, R. H. Silverman, T. J. Archer, and D. J. Coleman, "Evaluating microkeratome efficacy by 3D corneal lamellar flap thickness accuracy and reproducibility using Artemis VHF digital ultrasound arc-scanning," *Journal of Refractive Surgery*, vol. 22, no. 5, pp. 431–440, 2006.

[29] O. Gris, J. L. Guell, and A. Muller, "Keratomileusis update," *Journal of Cataract and Refractive Surgery*, vol. 22, no. 5, pp. 620–623, 1996.

[30] W. J. Stark, W. Chamon, M. T. Kamp, C. L. Enger, E. V. Rencs, and J. D. Gottsh, "Clinical follow-up of 193-nm ArF excimer laser photokeratectomy," *Ophthalmology*, vol. 99, no. 5, pp. 805–812, 1992.

[31] G. J. C. Jin, W. A. Lyle, and K. H. Merkley, "Laser in situ keratomileusis for primary hyperopia," *Journal of Cataract and Refractive Surgery*, vol. 31, no. 4, pp. 776–784, 2005.

[32] R. Cobo-Soriano, F. Llovet, F. González-López, B. Domingo, F. Gómez-Sanz, and J. Baviera, "Factors that influence outcomes of hyperopic laser in situ keratomileusis," *Journal of Cataract and Refractive Surgery*, vol. 28, no. 9, pp. 1530–1538, 2002.

[33] K. F. Tabbara, H. F. El-Sheikh, and S. M. Monowarul Islam, "Laser in situ keratomileusis for the correction of hyperopia from +0.50 to +11.50 Diopters with the keracor 117C laser," *Journal of Refractive Surgery*, vol. 17, no. 2, pp. 123–128, 2001.

[34] J. T. Holladay, D. R. Dudeja, and J. Chang, "Functional vision and corneal changes after laser in situ keratomileusis determined by contrast sensitivity, glare testing, and corneal topography," *Journal of Cataract and Refractive Surgery*, vol. 25, no. 5, pp. 663–669, 1999.

[35] K. M. Bottos, M. T. Leite, M. Aventura-Isidro et al., "Corneal asphericity and spherical aberration after refractive surgery," *Journal of Cataract and Refractive Surgery*, vol. 37, no. 6, pp. 1109–1115, 2011.

[36] M. Pande and J. S. Hillman, "Optical zone centration in keratorefractive surgery. Entrance pupil center, visual axis, coaxially sighted corneal reflex, or geometric corneal center?" *Ophthalmology*, vol. 100, no. 8, pp. 1230–1237, 1993.

[37] B. S. Wachler, T. S. Korn, N. S. Chandra, and F. K. Michel, "Decentration of the optical zone: centering on the pupil versus the coaxially sighted corneal light reflex in LASIK for hyperopia," *Journal of Refractive Surgery*, vol. 19, no. 4, pp. 464–465, 2003.

[38] R. B. Mandell, "Apparent pupil displacement in videokeratography," *The CLAO Journal*, vol. 20, no. 2, pp. 123–127, 1994.

[39] Y. Yang, K. Thompson, and S. A. Burns, "Pupil location under mesopic, photopic, and pharmacologically dilated conditions," *Investigative Ophthalmology and Visual Science*, vol. 43, no. 7, pp. 2508–2512, 2002.

[40] M. Bueeler, M. Mrochen, and T. Seiler, "Maximum permissible lateral decentration in aberration-sensing and wavefront-guided corneal ablation," *Journal of Cataract and Refractive Surgery*, vol. 29, no. 2, pp. 257–263, 2003.

23

Biodegradable PTLGA Terpolymers versus Collagen Implants Used as an Adjuvant in Trabeculectomy in Rabbit Eye

Weiran Niu,[1] Guanglin Shen,[1] Yuanzhi Yuan,[1] Xiaoping Ma,[1] Suming Li,[2] Jingzhao Wang,[2] Zhongyong Fan,[3] and Lan Liao[3]

[1]*Department of Ophthalmology, Zhongshan Hospital of Fudan University, Shanghai 200032, China*
[2]*Institute de High Performance Polymers, Qingdao University of Science and Technology, Qingdao 266042, China*
[3]*Department of Materials Science, Fudan University, Shanghai 200433, China*

Correspondence should be addressed to Xiaoping Ma; xiaopingma@126.com

Academic Editor: Antonio Ferreras

Purpose. To evaluate the effectiveness and safety of three biodegradable terpolymers prepared from L-lactide, trimethylene carbonate, and glycolide (PTLGA) as an aid for trabeculectomy compared with the Ologen (OLO). *Methods.* Trabeculectomy was carried out on rabbits with implantation made from OLO or three PTLGA terpolymers. Intraocular pressure (IOP) was recorded 1, 2, 3, and 6 months postoperatively and bleb evaluations were performed using ultrasound biomicroscopy (UBM) 3 months after surgery, optical coherence tomography (OCT) every month, and transmission electron microscopy (TEM) six months after surgery followed by histological examination 1, 2, 3, and 6 months postoperatively. *Result.* IOP was significantly reduced in all groups after surgery. There were no significant differences in the IOL between groups at any time after implantation. There was no significant difference between the groups examined by OCT, UBM, and TEM. Exposure of the implant was observed in one eye from the OLO group and one eye in the P1. Subconjunctiva hyperblastosis was observed in one eye from group P3 and two eyes from the OLO group. *Conclusions.* Subconjunctival implantation of filtering devices made from PTLGA may present a safe and effective additional surgical tool for the treatment of filtering surgery. Fewer complications were observed in the group with P2 implants compared to other groups.

1. Introduction

Since trabeculectomy was introduced in 1968, it has been the most common surgery to treat glaucoma [1]. Because scarring is still the major threat to the long-term success of glaucoma trabeculectomy surgery, mitomycin C (MMC) has been widely used as an antifibrotic agent to inhibit fibroblast proliferation and to maintain an ideal postoperative intraocular pressure (IOP) for more than two decades [2]. It has been proved that MMC raised the success rate of many types of glaucoma filtration surgery [3–5], and the use of MMC as a therapeutic agent has been well established as an effective clinical practice at achieving low final intraocular pressures (IOPs). However, severe complications such as leakage, infection, hypotony, and endophthalmitis with complete loss of vision may occur in surgeries with MMC, and surgery still fails in some individuals unfortunately [6, 7]. Less toxic antifibrotic agents or better therapeutic methods are needed.

Because of that, many promising new agents and implants to inhibit scar formation with fewer adverse effects have been evaluated in recent researches. Biodegradable implants such as Ologen (OLO), a porous collagen-glycosaminoglycan matrix, could potentially take the place of MMC to prevent the adhesion of the conjunctiva and sclera [8, 9] and the collapse of the subconjunctival space after trabeculectomy which leads to collagen deposition and microcyst formation after penetrating antiglaucomatous surgery. Use of OLO decreased early postoperative scarring and could be used to repair postoperative bleb leaks [10, 11]. Adverse effects of OLO included translocation or exposure of the implant or erosion of the conjunctiva.

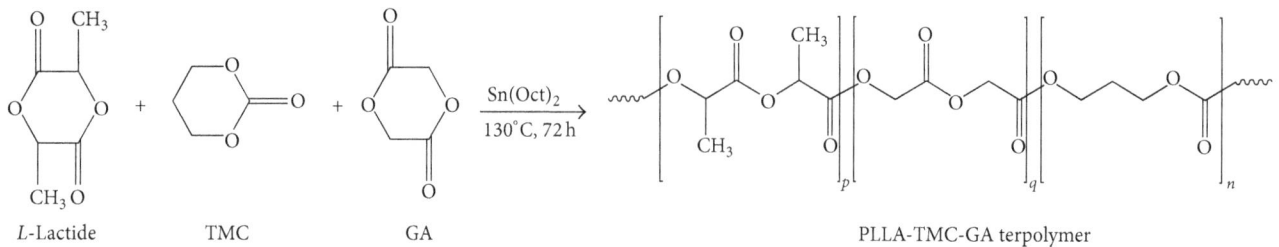

FIGURE 1: Synthesis route of PTLGA terpolymers. By permission from Shen et al. [12].

Biodegradable polymers such as poly(L-lactide) (PLLA), polyglycolide (PGA), poly(1,3-trimethylene carbonate) (PTMC), and their copolymers have attracted great attention for biomedical applications such as surgical implants, drug carrier, and tissue engineering scaffold because of their outstanding biocompatibility and biodegradability. In previous studies, terpolymers prepared from L-lactide, glycolide, and 1,3-trimethylene carbonate (PTLGA) have been successfully used as intravascular stent [12].

The goal of this study was to evaluate the efficacy and safety of PTLGA terpolymer in keeping the postoperative space between the conjunctiva and sclera functional and thus to maintain the filtering bleb active after trabeculectomy in rabbit eyes.

2. Materials and Methods

All experiments were carried out on the OD eye under a surgical microscope and general anesthesia. Rabbits weighing between 2.5 and 3.0 kg were anesthetized by intramuscular injection of ketamine hydrochloride (10 mg/kg) and xylazine (20 mg/kg). Topical anesthesia (0.5% proparacaine hydrochloride, Alcaine, Alcon-Couvreur, Belgium) was applied to the eyes. All rabbits were treated in accordance with the ARVO Statement on the Use of Animals in Ophthalmic and Vision Research, and the experimental protocol was approved by the Animal Care and Use Committee of Zhongshan Hospital, Fudan University.

2.1. Trabeculectomy in Rabbit Eyes.
Four groups of eight female rabbits underwent trabeculectomy (32 animals in total). A fornix-based conjunctival incision was made and a 3×3 mm scleral flap was created. Trabeculectomy was performed at the scleral spur, followed by iridectomy. A 5×6 mm implant sheet was placed on the scleral flap, the implant inserted over the flap. The scleral flap and conjunctival wound were sutured with 10-0 nylon. The implants included OLO and 3 different kinds of PTLGA terpolymers, P1, P2, and P3, in the study groups (see Section 2.2 below). No antifibrotic agent such as MMC was applied. Filtering bleb formation and inflammation of the anterior chamber were observed with slit-lamp microscopy by masked observers.

2.2. Materials.
PTLGA terpolymers [13] (Figure 1) were generously prepared [12] and provided by Dr. Suming Li and Dr. Zhongyong Fan. The implant has a shape of film and a thickness of 1 mm:

P1, PLLA : GA : TMC (95.8 : 5.4 : 4.2, mole : mole). Number average molecular weight is 232 KDa.

P2, PLLA : GA : TMC (60 : 13.2 : 22.8, mole : mole). Number average molecular weight is 45 KDa.

P3, PLLA : GA : TMC (2 : 1.19 : 0.8, mole : mole). Number average molecular weight is 28 KDa.

OLO (Ologen; Aeon Astron Group B.V. Leiden, the Netherlands). The implant size was 10 mm (W) × 10 mm (L) × 2 mm (H) (number 870051).

All implants were cut into 5 mm (W) × 6 mm (L) in the study.

2.3. Examining Methods

2.3.1. Intraocular Pressure (IOP) Measurements.
After topical anesthesia of 0.5% proparacaine hydrochloride Alcaine (Alcon-Couvreur, Belgium), IOP was measured using a Goldman applanation tonometry at baseline and twice a month for 1, 2, 3, and 6 months after surgery in all groups. IOP measurements were made by a blinded investigator. An average of three tonometer readings, with a maximum 5% standard deviation (SD), was recorded per eye. The IOP of all the experimental rabbits was measured at approximately 3 p.m.

2.3.2. Hematoxylin-Eosin Staining.
Rabbits were killed by excess ketamine (35 mg/kg) and xylazine (5 mg/kg) on months 1, 2, 3, and 6 after implantation. Eyes were quickly removed and fixed in 4% formaldehyde. The conjunctiva and implant with the underlying scleral bed were dissected, dehydrated, and embedded in paraffin. Sections were cut by a microtome at 7 micrometers and stained with hematoxylin and eosin (H&E) for general histologic observation.

2.3.3. Optical Coherence Tomography (OCT).
The subconjunctival fluid space was classified as none, single small, multiple small, or large and scored as 0, 1, 2, and 3, respectively, using a Zeiss Visante OCT (Model 1000, Carl Zeiss Meditec Inc., Dublin, CA). The upper lid was gently lifted by the operator to maximize bleb exposure as best as possible without pressing on the globe. Several radial and transverse sections were assessed.

TABLE 1: Comparison of IOP measurements between the Ologen group and PTLGA terpolymer groups.

Time points	n	OLO (mean ± SD)	P1 (mean ± SD)	P2 (mean ± SD)	P3 (mean ± SD)
Preoperative	8	15.5 ± 1.2	15.3 ± 1.3	15.4 ± 1.3	15.4 ± 1.1[×][*]
1 month after surgery	8	9.6 ± 1.1	9.3 ± 1.6	9.6 ± 1.5	9.7 ± 1.1[×][*]
2 months after surgery	6	13.5 ± 1.2	13.3 ± 2.0	13.6 ± 0.9	13.7 ± 1.0[*]
3 months after surgery	4	15.1 ± 1.1	14.5 ± 1.9	15.1 ± 1.3	15.2 ± 1.2
6 months after surgery	2	16.3 ± 0.6	13.9 ± 0.5	16.2 ± 0.1	15.9 ± 1.5

[×]$P = 0.000$, paired-sample t-test.
[*]$P < 0.05$, paired-sample t-test.
Data are presented as mean ± standard deviation.

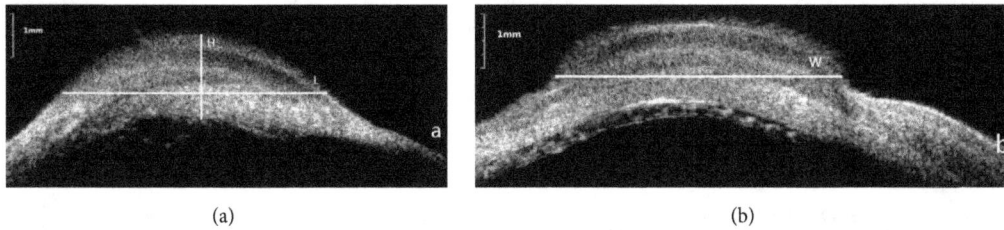

(a)   (b)

FIGURE 2: Imaging of UBM examination. (a) Horizontal section of the filtering bleb. (b) Vertical section of the filtering bleb.

2.3.4. Ultrasound Biomicroscopy (UBM). UBM (SW-3200, SUOER, Tianjin, China) was used to evaluate the height of the postoperative filtering blebs, and the maximum height of the filtering bleb including the eyeball wall in each scan was manually measured and automatically calculated with the device's software. The vertical line was drawn through the maximum height point of the filtering bleb at the corneal limbus, whereas a horizontal line through the same point was used as a base (Figure 2); the bleb area and height within this section of the bleb were used to estimate the volume of the bleb area and analyzed.

2.3.5. Transmission Electron Microscope Examination. Rabbits were euthanized six months after surgery. Eyes were quickly removed and fixed in 4% formaldehyde. Sections of conjunctiva and implant with the underlying scleral bed were cut to a thickness of 1 μm stained with uranyl acetate, followed by lead citrate. Slices were observed using an electron microscope (JEOL 1200, JEOL Co., Japan).

2.4. Statistical Analysis. Statistical analyses were performed using SPSS statistical software (Windows version 20.0; SPSS Inc., Chicago, IL, USA). One-way analyses of variance (One-way ANOVA) and Fisher's exact test were used to compare between the groups. In comparison of pre/postoperative results, paired Student's t-test was used. Complete resorption time was compared using the log rank test and survival curves (Kaplan-Meier curves). The results are expressed as mean ± standard deviation, and $P < 0.05$ was deemed to be statistically significant.

3. Results

3.1. IOP Measurements. No animals were excluded from this study since there were no intraoperative complications. One

month after surgery, postoperative mean intraocular pressure (IOP) was significantly lower ($P < 0.0001$) in all groups. At one, three, and six months after surgery, the mean IOP was not statistically ($P > 0.05$) different between groups (Table 1).

3.2. Morphology Observation. Only mild conjunctival hyperemia and edema were observed three to six days postoperatively and disappeared about two weeks later. No occurrence of keratitis, uveitis, or endophthalmitis was observed. During the postoperative follow-up observations, we did not detect allergy or translocation of the implants. Exposure of the implant was observed in one eye in the control group in the second week and group 1 in forth week. The implants were repositioned by conjunctival suture (Figure 3). Table 2 provided an overview of the recorded side effects between the OLO group and PTLGA terpolymer groups. Using the Kruskal-Wallis test, the frequency of postoperative complication did not significantly differ between the groups.

One month after surgery, the filtering bleb was obviously visible in all eyes. Three months later, the filtering blebs were observed flatter in eyes of the OLO group and groups P2 and P3 (Figure 4). Six months after surgery, except for group P1, it was quite difficult to observe the filtering blebs.

3.3. Histologic Evaluation. With hematoxylin-eosin staining we observed that all the biomaterials were found in the samples isolated at three months, except for P1 which had been observed at 3 months after surgery and undergone complete degradation six months after implantation. A weak fibrous capsule formation was observed around all of the biomaterials especially after one month after implantation (Figure 5). Three months after surgery, the fibrous capsule was difficult to observe in all eyes of group P3 and 3 eyes of the OLO group. Subconjunctiva hyperblastosis composed of fibroblasts, small vessels, and inflammatory cells was observed in one eye of

TABLE 2: Comparison of complications between the Ologen group and PTLGA terpolymer groups.

Complications	OLO number (%)	P1 number (%)	P2 number (%)	P3 number (%)	P
Mild conjunctival hyperemia	7 (87.5%)	8 (100%)	7 (87.5%)	7 (87.5%)	0.057
Mild conjunctival edema	2 (25%)	5 (62.5%)	3 (37.5%)	1 (12.5%)	1.000
Mild hyphema	0	0	0	0	—
Hypotony	0	0	0	0	—
Shallow anterior chamber	0	0	0	1 (12.5%)	0.057
Avascular cystic bleb	0	0	0	0	—
Cataract formation	0	0	0	0	—
Keratitis	0	0	0	0	—
Uveitis	0	0	0	0	—
Endophthalmitis	0	0	0	0	—
Choroidal detachment	0	0	0	0	—
Bleb leakage	1 (12.5%)	1 (12.5%)	0	1 (12.5%)	0.057
Implant exposure	1 (12.5%)	1 (12.5%)	0	0	0.086

Fisher's exact test.

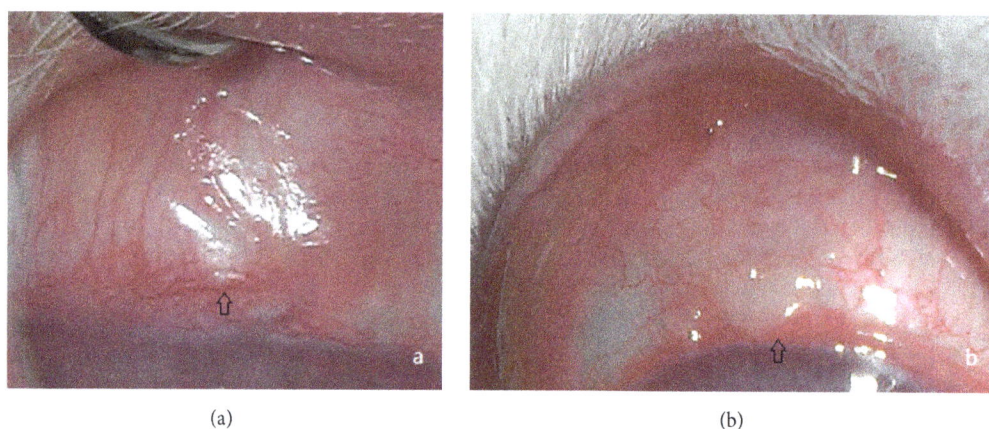

(a) (b)

FIGURE 3: Exposure of implant happened in 2 eyes; both of them were repositioned by conjunctival suture and recovered well. (a) Exposure of Ologen in control group. (b) Exposure of P1 in Group 1.

group P3 and 2 eyes of the OLO group even after the biomaterials were biodegraded (Figure 6).

3.4. Morphology Examination

3.4.1. Optical Coherence Tomography (OCT). Gradual resorption of the implant and subconjunctival fluid spaces was observed. The complete resorption time was 2 months in 10 eyes and 3 months in 14 eyes. The complete degradation time of group P1 was longer than others but not significantly different, 4 months in 2 eyes, 5 months in 1 eye, and 6 months in 1 eye; there were still implants left in 2 eyes when rabbits were executed. There were no significant differences of the Kaplan-Meier chart curves between the Ologen group and PTLGA terpolymer groups (log rank test, $P = 0.051$) (Figure 7). Three months after surgery, the OCT scores were not significantly ($F = 0.77$, $P = 0.53$) different between groups: 2 ± 1, 2.5 ± 0.6, 1.8 ± 0.5, and 2.0 ± 0.8 for the groups OLO, P1, P2, and P3, respectively. Because of its low depth of penetration, OCT could not be used to assess the route under

the scleral flap in some cases, but it is easy to examine if there are implantations left (Figure 8).

3.4.2. Ultrasound Biomicroscopy (UBM). There were no significant ($F = 2$, $P = 0.18$) differences in mean bleb volume at three months: $26 \pm 7 \, mm^3$, $21 \pm 7 \, mm^3$, $33 \pm 3 \, mm^3$, and $30 \pm 11 \, mm^3$, for groups OLO, P1, P2, and P3, respectively.

3.5. Transmission Electron Microscope. A weak fibrous capsule formation was observed around all of the four biomaterials, and small amounts of macrophages were observed nearby (Figure 9).

4. Discussion

As stated in the introduction, trabeculectomy is the most common antiglaucoma surgical procedure. Although both of MMC and OLO had a good record of higher achievement ratio in the surgery [14, 15], because of some adverse effects of them, investigators have developed new materials to take

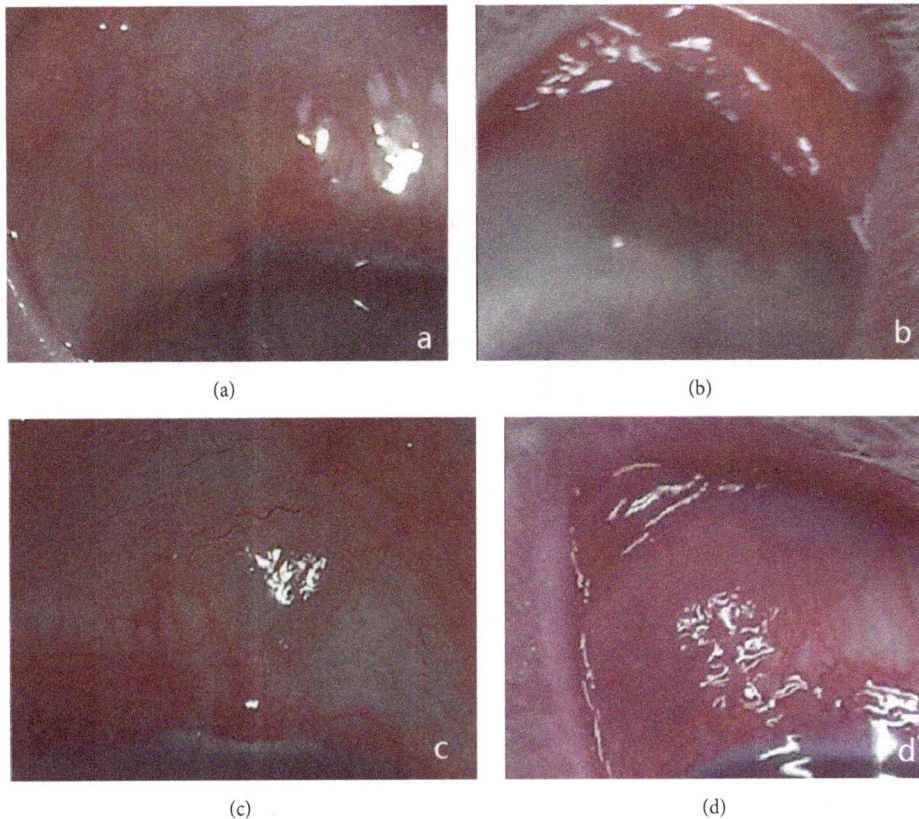

(a)   (b)

(c)   (d)

FIGURE 4: Morphology observation of the filtering bleb 3 months after surgery. (a) Control group. (b) Group 1. Implant under the conjunctiva still can be seen. (c) Group 2. (d) Group 3.

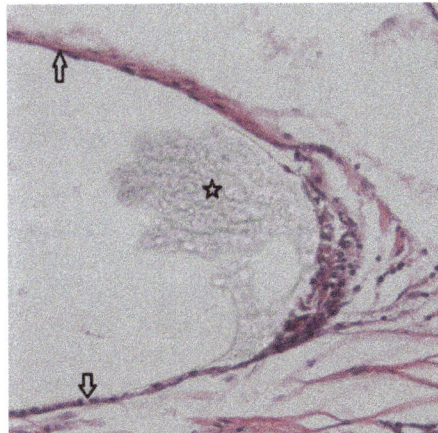

FIGURE 5: Weak fibrous capsule around the biomaterials marked by arrows.

their place. One intravascular stent material, PTLGA terpolymer, which has a good record of safety and histocompatibility [12], was tested as a biodegradable implant compared to OLO.

Published studies of our department had proved that there are reasons why trabeculectomy with Ologen has been a safe and effective procedure in patients with glaucoma even during a five-year follow-up. First, the structure of Ologen contained thousands of microscopic pores and can induce fibroblast growth, leading to a well organized and healthy healing process. Second, with a thickness of 2 mm and placed directly over the scleral flap and under the subconjunctival space, Ologen could provide space with a dynamic and physiological aqueous reservoir system. Subsequently, Ologen is biodegraded by the body within 90~180 days from its implantation which offered enough time to create a mature bleb structure [16]. In this study, we tested the PTLGA terpolymers, which have a similar structure and a similar degradation time to Ologen and have a thinner thickness

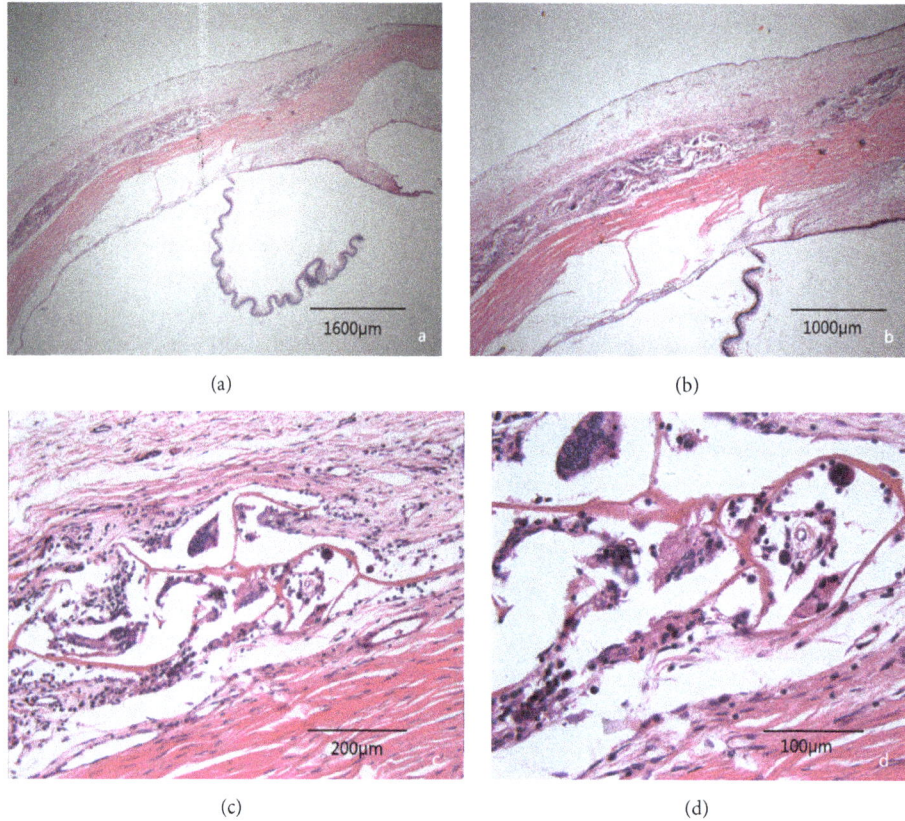

(a)   (b)

(c)   (d)

FIGURE 6: Subconjunctiva hyperblastosis composed of fibroblasts, small vessels, and inflammatory cells had been observed in the control group; the biomaterials (Ologen) had already degraded. Hematoxylin-Eosin staining, (a) ×25. (b) ×40. (c) ×200. (d) ×400.

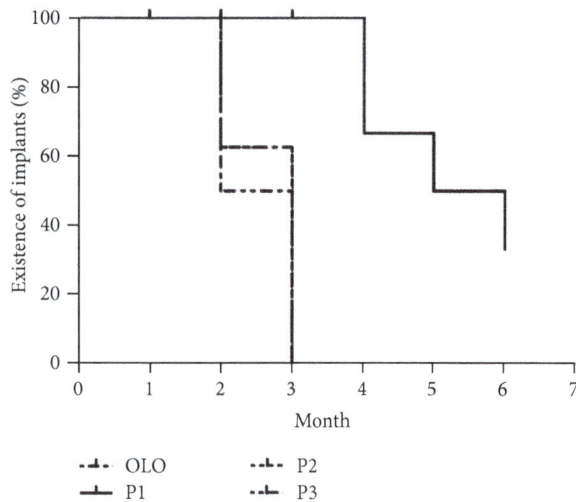

FIGURE 7: The Kaplan-Meier chart of complete resorption time between the Ologen group and PTLGA terpolymer groups. There were no significant differences of the curves between those groups (log rank test, $P = 0.051$).

of 1 mm, so, theoretically, these implants can get the similar outcome as Ologen in improving the surgical success of trabeculectomy without the adjunctive use of antifibrotic agents.

In this study, biodegradable implants made of PTLGA terpolymers were as safe as those made of OLO. Implants of PTLGA terpolymers were as effective as those made of OLO in achieving a low target IOP level. It was encouraging to confirm that P1 and P2 maintained the size of filtering blebs, even though there might be no strong correlation between IOP and bleb height [17]. The differences of the physical and chemical properties between the PTLGA terpolymers were due to the different percentages of components in the PTLGA terpolymer. The results of examinations and complications in the study included that the efficacy and safety of P2 made it the most suitable implant among the three kinds of PTLGA terpolymers.

Exposure of the implant was one of the complications we found. Exposure in the OLO group may have been due to the thickness of implant. Exposure of implant made from P1 may be due to the hardness of P1 with sharp edges, cusp angles, and a long biodegradation procedure. There were no significant differences of complete resorption time between the groups (we did not take the two rabbits killed before complete resorption of implants into account as perfect biodegraded); we presume that differences would be found and the longest complete resorption time would be seen in the P1 group, if our study has a bigger sample and a longer follow-up time. And we also presume that if the P1 implants were roundish shaped and with a blunt edge, the exposure of P1 would be avoidable.

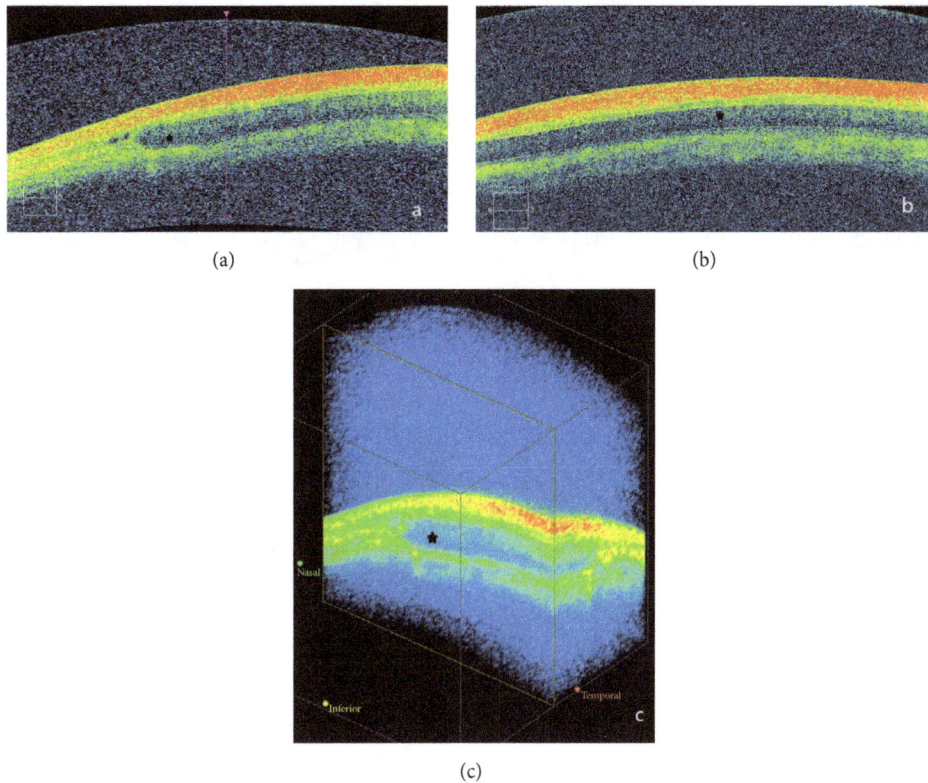

(a)

(b)

(c)

FIGURE 8: Imaging of OCT examination. (a) Horizontal section of the subconjunctival fluid space. (b) Three-dimensional reconstruction of the subconjunctival fluid space. (c) Vertical section of the subconjunctival fluid space.

Subconjunctiva hyperblastosis was a unique complication observed in our study which may be due to the response of the conjunctiva to the long-term stimulus from the more acid decomposition product of P3, because P3 has the highest percentage of GA. Subconjunctiva hyperblastosis has been observed in both P3 and OLO groups; however, it is arduous to find such reports in published studies; there may be some reasons behind this: in the first place, OLO has a fair histocompatibility itself; the low occurrence of subconjunctiva hyperblastosis could make it difficult to be observed; then, the subconjunctiva hyperblastosis did not raise the IOP so obviously or so frequently after the operation; third, there might be an absorption of it; the hyperblastosis could only be observed in a short time; the last, it might be hard to be observed by other testing methods. Although the subconjunctiva hyperblastosis in our research did not cause the significant difference of success rate between the groups, we cannot help but conceive the idea that when the subconjunctiva hyperblastosis grows large enough to block the aqueous humor outflow channel, the surgery might end in failure. Longer time follow-up observation was needed to confirm whether there will be a regression or a growth of the subconjunctiva hyperblastosis later, to find what stimulated the development of subconjunctiva hyperblastosis and what strategy is needed for avoiding it or controlling it.

There was a good control of IOP after surgery and no significantly different frequency of complications in all the 4 groups. In particular, complications such as exposure were not observed for implants made of P2, as supposed, due to the thin and soft characteristic of it, and there was no subconjunctiva hyperblastosis observed in the P2 group either, which has a chance to block the aqueous humor outflow of the artificial channel built in the trabeculectomy and cause the IOP to rise rapidly. All these results suggested that P2 may be an ideal material as a new choice of antifibrotic agents. Due to the low incidence of complications and small sample size of our study, more studies are needed to confirm this idea.

OCT measurements were more reproducible and easier to perform than those of UBM. Because of its low depth of penetration, although OCT could not be used to assess the route under the scleral flap in some cases, it is competent enough to observe the residue of implants under the conjunctiva. Detailed anatomic assessment of bleb morphology was made using UBM and OCT. Several investigators have established that UBM and OCT can be used to identify morphologic changes in blebs related to wound healing and to identify parameters for the functional prognosis of the filter blebs [18–22]. The complementary use of OCT and UBM made them irreplaceable.

It is widely accepted that OLO keeps an outstanding postoperative IOP; according to the results of our study, all the three kinds of PTLGA terpolymers played a similar role in the control of IOP after antiglaucoma surgical procedure. Results also implied that there were fewer adverse events in PTLGA terpolymer groups happening than that in the OLO group. Since P2 manifested the fewest complications among

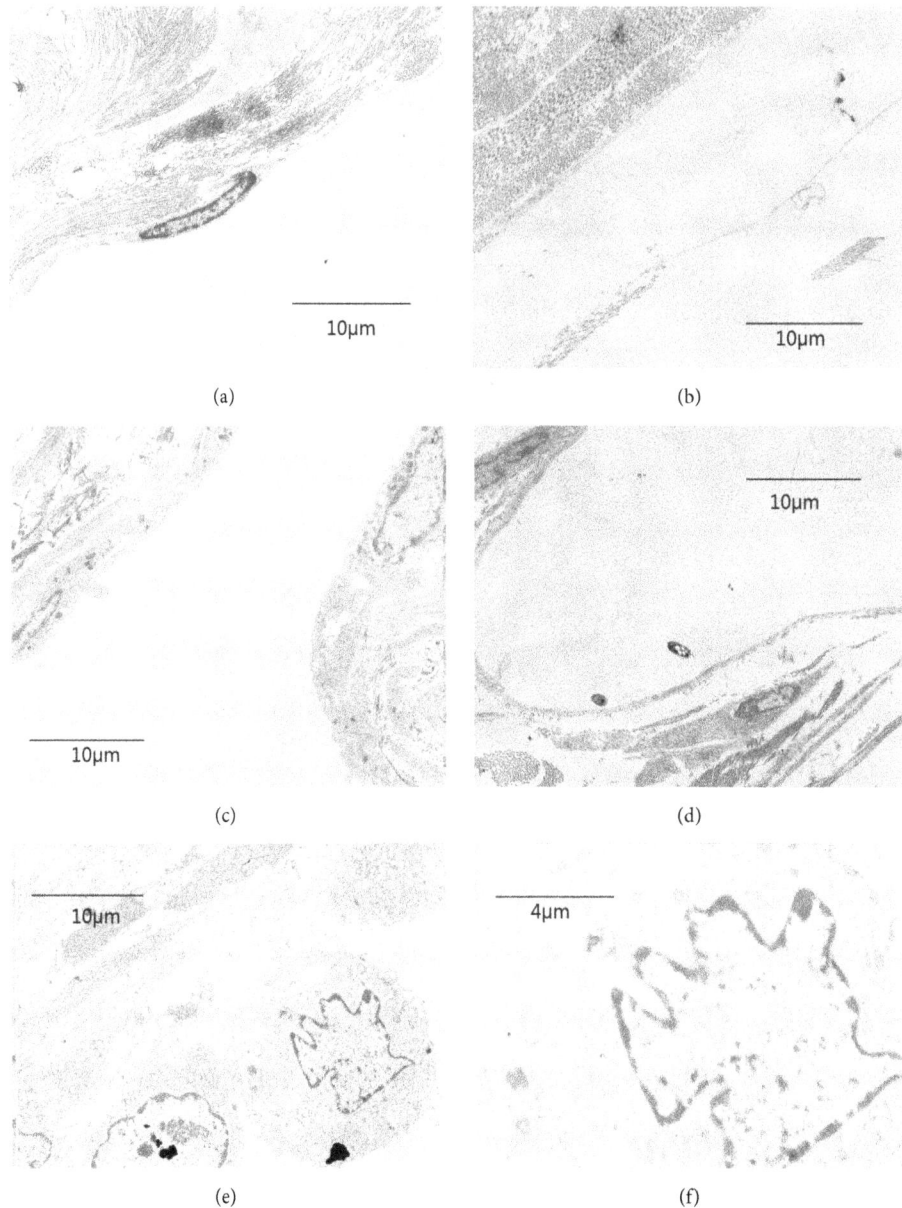

(a)

(b)

(c)

(d)

(e)

(f)

FIGURE 9: Transmission electron microscope. A weak fibrous capsule formation marked by arrows was observed around all of the 4 biomaterials: (a) control group, ×2500; (b) group 1, ×2500; (c) group 2, ×2500; (d) group 3, ×2500. And small amounts of macrophages marked by arrows had been observed nearby ((e) ×2500, (f) ×5000).

all the agents, consequently it has been considered as the most promising adjuvant in trabeculectomy.

Our study had several limitations. Our sample size was relatively small, and the study reported short-term outcomes.

5. Conclusions

In conclusion, OCT and UBM were useful tools to measure filtering blebs. Subconjunctival implants made from PTLGA may present a safe and effective additional surgical tool for the maintenance of filtering blebs in antiglaucoma surgery. Fewer complications were observed in the group with P2 implants.

Longer-term observations of bigger sample size studies are needed to fully evaluate this new PTLGA terpolymer.

Conflict of Interests

The authors have no proprietary or commercial interest in any materials discussed in this paper.

References

[1] J. E. Cairns, "Trabeculectomy. Preliminary report of a new method," *American Journal of Ophthalmology*, vol. 66, no. 4, pp. 673–679, 1968.

[2] G. L. Skuta and R. K. Parrish II, "Wound healing in glaucoma filtering surgery," *Survey of Ophthalmology*, vol. 32, no. 3, pp. 149–170, 1987.

[3] J. Matlach, E. Panidou, F. Grehn, and T. Klink, "Large-area versus small-area application of mitomycin C during trabeculectomy," *European Journal of Ophthalmology*, vol. 23, no. 5, pp. 670–677, 2013.

[4] L. M. Meyer, N. E. Graf, S. Philipp et al., "Two-year outcome of repeat trabeculectomy with mitomycin C in primary open-angle and PEX glaucoma," *European Journal of Ophthalmology*, vol. 25, no. 3, pp. 185–191, 2015.

[5] S. Suominen, M. Harju, L. Kurvinen, and E. Vesti, "Deep sclerectomy in normal-tension glaucoma with and without mitomycin-c," *Acta Ophthalmologica*, vol. 92, no. 7, pp. 701–706, 2014.

[6] D. Z. Chen, V. Koh, C. Sng, M. C. Aquino, P. Chew, and S. Bhattacharya, "Complications and outcomes of primary phacotrabeculectomy with mitomycin C in a multi-ethnic asian population," *PLoS ONE*, vol. 10, no. 3, Article ID e0118852, 2015.

[7] N. Anand, S. Arora, and M. Clowes, "Mitomycin C augmented glaucoma surgery: evolution of filtering bleb avascularity, transconjunctival oozing, and leaks," *British Journal of Ophthalmology*, vol. 90, no. 2, pp. 175–180, 2006.

[8] A. Rosentreter, A. M. Schild, J. F. Jordan, G. K. Krieglstein, and T. S. Dietlein, "A prospective randomised trial of trabeculectomy using mitomycin C vs an ologen implant in open angle glaucoma," *Eye*, vol. 24, no. 9, pp. 1449–1457, 2010.

[9] D. Tanuj, S. Amit, M. Saptorshi, and G. Meenakshi, "Combined subconjunctival and subscleral ologen implant insertion in trabeculectomy," *Eye*, vol. 27, no. 7, p. 889, 2013.

[10] H. S.-L. Chen, R. Ritch, T. Krupin, and W.-C. Hsu, "Control of filtering bleb structure through tissue bioengineering: an animal model," *Investigative Ophthalmology and Visual Science*, vol. 47, no. 12, pp. 5310–5314, 2006.

[11] W.-C. Hsu, R. Ritch, T. Krupin, and H. S.-L. Chen, "Tissue bioengineering for surgical bleb defects: an animal study," *Graefe's Archive for Clinical and Experimental Ophthalmology*, vol. 246, no. 5, pp. 709–717, 2008.

[12] X. Shen, F. Su, J. Dong, Z. Fan, Y. Duan, and S. Li, "*In vitro* biocompatibility evaluation of bioresorbable copolymers prepared from L-lactide, 1, 3-trimethylene carbonate, and glycolide for cardiovascular applications," *Journal of Biomaterials Science, Polymer Edition*, vol. 26, no. 8, pp. 497–514, 2015.

[13] Y. Yuan, X. Jin, Z. Fan, S. Li, and Z. Lu, "In vivo degradation of copolymers prepared from l-lactide, 1,3-trimethylene carbonate and glycolide as coronary stent materials," *Journal of Materials Science: Materials in Medicine*, vol. 26, no. 3, p. 139, 2015.

[14] M. S. Johnson and S. R. Sarkisian Jr., "Using a collagen matrix implant (Ologen) versus mitomycin-C as a wound healing modulator in trabeculectomy with the Ex-PRESS mini glaucoma device: a 12-month retrospective review," *Journal of Glaucoma*, vol. 23, no. 9, pp. 649–652, 2014.

[15] T. Dada, R. Kusumesh, S. J. Bali et al., "Trabeculectomy with combined use of subconjunctival collagen implant and low-dose mitomycin C," *Journal of Glaucoma*, vol. 22, no. 8, pp. 659–662, 2013.

[16] F. Yuan, L. Li, X. Chen, X. Yan, and L. Wang, "Biodegradable 3D-porous collagen matrix (ologen) compared with mitomycin c for treatment of primary open-angle glaucoma: results at 5 years," *Journal of Ophthalmology*, vol. 2015, Article ID 637537, 7 pages, 2015.

[17] R. Fernández-Buenaga, G. Rebolleda, P. Casas-Llera, F. J. Muñoz-Negrete, and M. Pérez-López, "A comparison of intrascleral bleb height by anterior segment OCT using three different implants in deep sclerectomy," *Eye*, vol. 26, no. 4, pp. 552–556, 2012.

[18] D. Kazakova, S. Roters, C. C. Schnyder et al., "Ultrasound biomicroscopy images: long-term results after deep sclerectomy with collagen implant," *Graefe's Archive for Clinical and Experimental Ophthalmology*, vol. 240, no. 11, pp. 918–923, 2002.

[19] A. Labbé, P. Hamard, V. Iordanidou, S. Dupont-Monod, and C. Baudouin, "Utility of the Visante OCT in the follow-up of glaucoma surgery," *Journal Francais d'Ophtalmologie*, vol. 30, no. 3, pp. 225–231, 2007.

[20] G. Savini, M. Zanini, and P. Barboni, "Filtering blebs imaging by optical coherence tomography," *Clinical and Experimental Ophthalmology*, vol. 33, no. 5, pp. 483–489, 2005.

[21] M. Singh, T. Aung, D. S. Friedman et al., "Anterior segment optical coherence tomography imaging of trabeculectomy blebs before and after laser suture lysis," *American Journal of Ophthalmology*, vol. 143, no. 5, pp. 873–875, 2007.

[22] F. Aptel, S. Dumas, and P. Denis, "Ultrasound biomicroscopy and optical coherence tomography imaging of filtering blebs after deep sclerectomy with new collagen implant," *European Journal of Ophthalmology*, vol. 19, no. 2, pp. 223–230, 2009.

24

Microperimetric Biofeedback Training Improved Visual Acuity after Successful Macular Hole Surgery

Tomoko Ueda-Consolvo, Mitsuya Otsuka, Yumiko Hayashi, Masaaki Ishida, and Atsushi Hayashi

Department of Ophthalmology, Graduate School of Medicine and Pharmaceutical Sciences, University of Toyama, 2630 Sugitani, Toyama 930-0194, Japan

Correspondence should be addressed to Atsushi Hayashi; ahayashi@med.u-toyama.ac.jp

Academic Editor: Enzo M. Vingolo

Purpose. To evaluate the efficacy of setting a preferred retinal locus relocation target (PRT) and performing Macular Integrity Assessment (MAIA) biofeedback training in patients showing insufficient recovery of best corrected visual acuity (BCVA) despite successful closure of an idiopathic macular hole (MH). *Methods.* Retrospective interventional case series. Nine eyes of 9 consecutive patients with the decimal BCVA of less than 0.6 at more than 3 months after successful MH surgery were included. A PRT was chosen based on MAIA microperimetry and the patients underwent MAIA biofeedback training. BCVA, reading speed, fixation stability, and 63% bivariate contour ellipse area (BCEA) were evaluated before and after the training. Statistical analysis was carried out using paired Student's t-test. *Results.* PRT was chosen on the nasal side of the closed MH fovea in 8 patients. After the MAIA training, BCVA improved in all patients. The mean logMAR value of BCVA significantly improved from 0.33 to 0.12 ($p = 0.007$). Reading speed improved in all patients ($p = 0.29$), fixation stability improved in 5 patients ($p = 0.70$), and 63% BCEA improved in 7 patients ($p = 0.21$), although these improvements were not statistically significant. *Conclusion.* MAIA biofeedback training improved visual acuity in patients with insufficient recovery of BCVA after successful MH surgery.

1. Introduction

Vision impairment and metamorphopsia are major symptoms of patients with an idiopathic macular hole (MH). MH surgery has been improved since Kelly and Wendel first reported successful closure of MHs by use of pars plana vitrectomy with gas-fluid exchange [1]. A technique of internal limiting membrane (ILM) peeling improved visual outcomes and the closure rate in MH surgeries [2, 3]. Microincision vitrectomy surgery has shortened the operating time and improved patient comfort and visual recovery time [4]. Numerous studies have reported preoperative predictive factors for visual outcomes following MH surgery, including stage and size of MH [5], duration of symptoms [6], preoperative visual acuity [7], retinal sensitivity, fixation status [8], and optical coherence tomography (OCT) parameters such as minimum diameter of MH, base hole diameter, the hole form factor, MH index, and inner segment/outer segment junction

defect length [9]. These factors are not enough, however, to predict visual outcomes precisely. Visual outcomes are often worse than expected despite successful MH surgery.

Recently, foveal displacement following MH surgery has been reported [10–13]. After ILM peeling and gas tamponade, the retina is displaced toward the optic disc [10–13]. Ishida et al. showed that the ratio of retinal displacement in the temporal field was significantly correlated with the basal diameter of the MH [11]. We hypothesized that the foveal displacement might be one of the reasons for poor visual recovery after successful MH surgery. Helping patients to fix at the point of the best visual acuity after the closure of MH might improve their visual performances.

Biofeedback training by means of a microperimeter has been reported as an efficient method to improve the visual performance of patients with macular diseases such as age-related macular degeneration, Stargardt's disease, cone dystrophy, vitelliform dystrophy, and posttraumatic macular

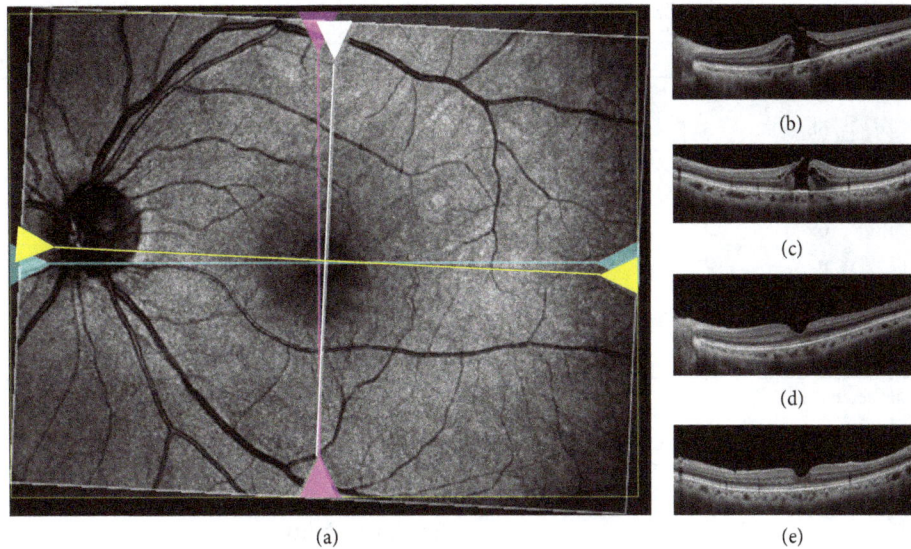

FIGURE 1: (a) Composite infrared image made by overlapping preoperative and postoperative images (case 6). Yellow line and white line indicate preoperative location of the horizontal and vertical scan (b, c). Blue line and pink line indicate postoperative location of the horizontal and vertical scan (d, e). Center of MH and fovea were identified by moving the location of scans (yellow, white, blue, and pink lines). The fovea has shifted toward the optic disc after MH surgery.

scar [14–16]. The training helped the patients stably fix their gaze at the preferred retinal locus relocation target (PRT) near the fovea.

In this study, we performed biofeedback training using a Macular Integrity Assessment (MAIA) microperimeter to provide an efficient PRT and to improve visual performance in patients who had insufficient visual recovery after successful closure of a MH.

2. Methods

2.1. Inclusion and Exclusion Criteria. We recruited 9 eyes of 9 consecutive patients (4 men and 5 women), who had undergone MH surgery at Toyama University Hospital between May 2013 and June 2014. Inclusion criteria were (1) patients with idiopathic MH, (2) patients in whom closure of MH was confirmed with optical coherence tomography (OCT) by the first MH surgery, (3) patients with visual acuity of 0.6 or less after 3 months of the MH surgery, (4) patients who could undergo OCT examinations with a single spectral domain OCT machine (RS-3000 Advance, NIDEK Co., Ltd., Aichi, Japan) before and after the MH surgery, and (5) patients who agreed with the MAIA training and were followed up for more than 3 months. Exclusion criteria were the presence of ocular complications that could affect visual performance, such as macular degeneration, rhegmatogenous retinal detachment, diabetic retinopathy, glaucoma, and corneal diseases.

2.2. Ophthalmic Examinations. All patients underwent comprehensive ophthalmologic examinations, including measurement of the decimal best corrected visual acuity (BCVA),

reading speed test, intraocular pressure, slit-lamp biomicroscopy with a contact lens, OCT, and fixation stability test. Axial length was measured in all eyes preoperatively (OA-1000, Tomey, Aichi, Japan). The single spectral domain OCT machine (RS-3000 Advance) was used to evaluate tomographic features through the macula. The macula was scanned with the macula map mode of 9 mm × 9 mm scan (512 × 128) or 9 mm × 12 mm scan (256 × 128) by RS-3000 Advance. The basal diameter of each MH was measured with a caliper built in the software of the OCT machine.

All eyes underwent a standard pars plana vitrectomy with three 25-gauge ports. All patients underwent ILM peeling around the MH in the same manner. Sulfur hexafluoride gas (20%) was used as a tamponade gas at the end of the surgery and the patients were asked to adopt face-down position for at least one hour after the surgery.

The distance of foveal displacement in each eye was measured after the closure of MH according to the methods of Kawano et al. [10]. Briefly, infrared fundus images were taken together with OCT images. The center of the MH was marked in the preoperative infrared fundus image by referencing OCT images (Figures 1(a), 1(b), and 1(c)), and the length on the image was corrected with the axial length. Postoperatively, the center of foveal depression was similarly marked in the infrared fundus image by reference with OCT images within 3 months after the MH surgery (Figures 1(a), 1(d), and 1(e)). The two marked infrared fundus images were overlapped manually (Figure 1(a)) and the distance of foveal displacement between the marks was measured using ImageJ software (National Institutes of Health, Bethesda, MD, available at http://imagej.nih.gov/ij/).

Reading speed was measured by reading Japanese words written in black on white background at a distance of 30 cm with appropriate refractive correction (MNRead-J, Handaya,

TABLE 1: Preoperative clinical characteristics.

Patient number	Sex	Age (years)	Stage	Duration of symptoms (months)	Basal diameter (μm)	Preoperative decimal BCVA
1	F	64	3	1	571	0.2
2	M	66	3	Unknown	615	0.4
3	F	75	4	2	483	0.8
4	M	70	3	1.5	949	0.15
5	M	69	3	1	457	0.1
6	F	65	3	1	837	0.2
7	F	67	3	2	459	0.15
8	M	64	3	2	588	0.15
9	F	64	3	1	369	0.15

BCVA: best corrected visual acuity.

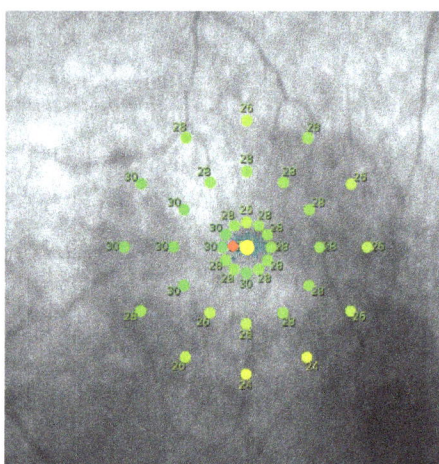

FIGURE 2: Each colored dot indicates retinal threshold sensitivity (case 8). We chose a region within the 2-degree ring that had the highest potential retinal sensitivity and set the new PRT (red dot) within that area.

Tokyo, Japan). Patients were asked to read the letters aloud as fast as possible without skipping any letters. The sentences contained high-frequency, nontechnical words. A fixation stability test was performed with an MAIA microperimeter (Topcon, Tokyo, Japan). The percentage of fixation points located within the 2-degree circle of the PRT was measured.

Sixty-three percent of bivariate contour ellipse area (BCEA) was also measured to evaluate fixation stability. The 63% BCEA is the elliptical area which encompasses 63% of fixation points during one fixation trial. A smaller BCEA correlates to more stable fixation. Square degree (Sqd) was used as the unit for the 63% BCEA.

2.3. Defining Preferred Retinal Locus Relocation Target (PRT).
Before starting biofeedback training, macular threshold sensitivity and fixation stability were assessed with a MAIA microperimeter using an automated program. Retinal threshold sensitivity was displayed within a 10-degree range of the gravitational center of all fixation points. We chose a region within the 2-degree ring that had the highest potential retinal sensitivity and set the new PRT within that area (Figure 2). If the retinal threshold sensitivity did not exhibit

any difference within 2-degree ring, 6 points were screened as candidate PRTs and one point was selected according to fixation stability.

2.4. MAIA Biofeedback Training.
MAIA biofeedback training was performed using a PRL training module for 10 minutes each session and repeated at least three times within three months. Before beginning the MAIA biofeedback training, the patients were asked to fix their gaze at the PRT by themselves according to an audio feedback program equipped with MAIA. This audio feedback program advised the patients whether or not they were getting closer to the PRT. All the procedures were checked by the examiner.

2.5. Statistical Analysis.
All statistical analyses were carried out using JMP statistical discovery software (Version 9; SAS Institute, Cary, NC). Paired Student's t-test was used to compare the differences between values before and after the training. Spearman correlation coefficient was used to investigate correlations between 63% BCEA and BCVA. Statistical significance was defined as $p < 0.05$. The BCVA was measured with a Landolt C chart in decimal units and converted to a logarithm of the minimum angle of resolution (logMAR) for statistical analysis.

3. Results

3.1. Characteristics of the Patients.
Nine eyes of 9 patients were examined. The preoperative characteristics of the patients are listed in Table 1. The patients' ages ranged from 64 years old to 75 years old (67.2 ± 3.4 years old, mean $\pm$ standard deviation (SD)). The decimal BCVA before idiopathic MH surgery ranged from 0.1 to 0.8. There were 8 eyes with stage 3 macular holes and 1 eye with stage 4 macular hole. In the preoperative OCT images, the basal diameter of the macular hole ranged from 369 μm to 949 μm ($592 \pm 178 \mu$m; mean $\pm$ SD). Anatomical closure of the MH was confirmed by OCT examination and no recurrence of MH occurred in any patients in this study. The mean distance of foveal displacement was $155.4 \pm 102.6 \mu$m (range: 35.7 μm to 387.6 μm). Eight of the 9 eyes revealed displacement of the foveal center in the nasal direction and in the one eye the foveal center displaced in the temporal direction.

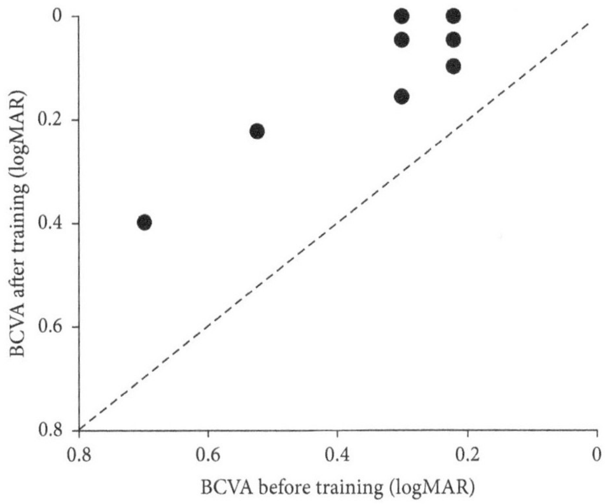

FIGURE 3: Scatter plot of best corrected visual acuity (BCVA) before and after MAIA biofeedback training.

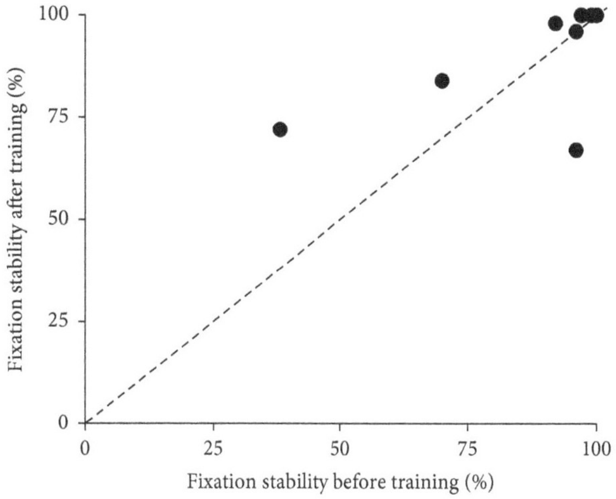

FIGURE 4: Scatter plot of fixation stability before and after MAIA biofeedback training.

The PRT in each patient was selected according to the sensitivity of the results of microperimetry and the patient's responses. The PRT was selected on the nasal side of the foveal center of the closed MH within 2 degrees in 8 of the 9 patients and in the other patient the PRT was chosen superior to the foveal center of the closed MH within 2 degrees. The patients started MAIA biofeedback training at 3 to 9 months (4.6 ± 1.9 months) after the MH surgery (Table 2). When the patients wished to continue the MAIA biofeedback training after completing 3 sessions, we allowed them to continue it. Five patients ended MAIA training after 3 sessions, while 2 patients performed 4 sessions and 2 patients completed 5 sessions (3.7 ± 0.8 times; mean ± SD). The training period ranged from 1.5 to 4 months (2.3 ± 0.7 months; mean ± SD) (Table 2).

3.2. Visual Acuity. BCVA improved in all patients after the MAIA biofeedback training (Figure 3). The mean logMAR value of BCVA was 0.33 at the baseline, but it significantly improved to 0.12 after 3 MAIA training sessions ($p = 0.007$) (Table 2). Five patients showed rapid improvement of BCVA after the initial MAIA training.

3.3. Reading Speed. The MAIA biofeedback training accelerated the reading speed in all patients. The reading speed before the training was 339 ± 72 words/min and slightly improved to 378 ± 71 words/min at the end of the training, a difference that was not statistically significant ($p = 0.29$) (Table 2).

3.4. Fixation Stability. Fixation stability was improved in five patients (patients 1, 2, 4, 5, and 6 in Table 2). In three patients (7–9 in Table 2), fixation stability was unchanged following the training. Two of those patients (patients 8 and 9 in Table 2) showed 100% fixation sensitivity before the start of MAIA training. In one patient (patient 3 in Table 2), fixation stability worsened. The mean fixation stability slightly

improved from 88 ± 20% before the training to 91 ± 12% after the training, a difference that was not statistically significant ($p = 0.70$) (Table 2 and Figure 4).

The 63% BCEA was improved in 7 of 9 patients. In one patient the 63% BCEA was unchanged. The 63% BCEA was worsened in one patient. The mean 63% BCEA improved from 0.96 ± 0.91 Sqd before the training to 0.42 ± 0.49 Sqd after the training, although it was not statistically significant ($p = 0.21$) (Table 2). There was no correlation between 63% BCEA and BCVA before the training (Spearman correlation coefficients, $r = 0.36$; $p = 0.34$) or after the training ($r = 0.27$; $p = 0.49$).

4. Discussion

The current study demonstrated that biofeedback training using MAIA microperimetry effectively improved the visual acuity of patients when the visual acuity had not fully recovered after successful closure of the MH.

Microperimetric biofeedback training has been performed to improve visual performance of patients with several diseases such as age-related macular degeneration, Stargardt's disease, cone dystrophy, macular myopic degeneration, vitelliform dystrophy, and posttraumatic macular scars [14–16]. Patients with these diseases lost the fixation at the central fovea and were trained to fix at an extrafoveal area (PRT) to improve their visual acuity. In this study, we examined the possibility of biofeedback training to improve the BCVA and visual performances in patients with insufficient recovery of visual acuity after the successful closure of a MH.

One of the advantages using MAIA biofeedback training was that the patients could easily understand and repeat the training with the aid of the audio feedback informing them whether or not they were getting closer to the PRT. Sound perception increases the conscious attention of patients [17], and the increased attention helps the brain fix the PRT [14, 18]. Vingolo et al. reported that audio feedback

TABLE 2: Visual performance before and after the training.

Patient number	Period after operation (months)	Training (number of sessions)	Distance of foveal displacement (μm)	Decimal BCVA		Reading speed (words/min)		Fixation stability (%)		63% BCEA (square degree)	
				Pre	Post	Pre	Post	Pre	Post	Pre	Post
1	5	3	89.4	0.2	0.4	243	461	38	72	1.2	0.5
2	3	3	249.0	0.5	0.6	260	292	92	98	0.8	0.2
3	3	3	387.6	0.6	1.0	319	338	96	67	0.3	1.6
4	3	5	35.7	0.3	0.6	279	280	70	84	0.4	0.2
5	6	5	82.7	0.5	1.0	477	486	99	100	0.9	0.1
6	3	4	152.0	0.6	1.0	326	328	97	100	3.3	0.1
7	9	4	192.8	0.5	1.0	387	429	96	96	1.2	0.9
8	4	3	132.7	0.6	0.8	344	360	100	100	0.1	0.1
9	5	3	77.2	0.6	0.8	418	430	100	100	0.4	0.1

BCVA: best corrected visual acuity;
Pre: baseline values;
Post: values at the end of training;
BCEA: bivariate contour ellipse area.

facilitated stimuli transmission between intraterinal neurons as well as between the retina and the brain and supports a "remapping phenomenon" [15]. The second advantage was that the examiner could select an appropriate PRT in the macula according to the results of the microperimetry and the patients could repeat the training at the same PRT every time.

Kawano et al. reported that the center of the macula area moved toward the optic disc an average distance of 0.1 disc diameter after vitrectomy with ILM peeling [10]. Ishida et al. showed that the ratio of the displacement of the temporal vessel was significantly correlated with the maximum size of the preoperative MH [11]. Nakagomi et al. showed that the postoperative fovea-to-disc distance (3.82 ± 0.34 mm) was significantly shorter than the preoperative one (4.00 ± 0.33 mm, $p < 0.0001$) [13]. These results suggest that the center of the fovea shifted after successful MH surgery with ILM peeling in most patients. Foveal displacement following MH surgery might be one of the reasons for insufficient visual recovery after the closure of MH, and introducing a PRT near the anatomical center of the fovea might result in better visual performance such as visual acuity, reading speed, and fixation stability for those patients. In our study, careful selection of a new PRT, followed by MAIA biofeedback training, improved visual acuity in all patients.

The mean distance of foveal displacement in this study did not differ from those in previous studies [10, 11, 13]. Therefore, patients who showed insufficient recovery of visual acuity were not categorized into a specific group of patients. In addition, the correlation between the location of the PRT and the distance of foveal displacement was unclear. This might be due to the fact that the preferred retinal locus was located on any margin of the preoperative macular hole [19]. In this study, however, the PRT was located slightly to the nasal side of the foveal center in 8 patients (89%). It appears that the fovea with the highest visual acuity might shift to the nasal side of the retina after successful closure of MH.

Visual recovery after macular hole surgery sometimes requires more than 3 months. We cannot exclude the possibility that the visual acuity in our cases improved as part of the natural course during MAIA biofeedback training. In our investigation, however, BCVA immediately improved after the initial MAIA training in 5 of 9 patients and improved further after the completion of 3 MAIA training sessions.

The patients did not show a significant improvement of reading speed, fixation stability, nor 63% BCEA after MAIA biofeedback training. Cappello et al. reported that the maximum reading speed was significantly improved after MH surgery [20]. Another group showed that the mean maximum reading speeds were comparable for eyes with closed MHs and their healthy fellow eyes [21]. Because we examined reading speed, fixation stability, and 63% BCEA of the patients with successful closure of the MH, a significant improvement was not detected even though all patients showed a tendency to improve their visual performance after MAIA biofeedback training. Tarita-Nistor et al. reported that change in fixation stability was a strong predictor of visual outcome after successful closure of the macular hole in 10

patients [22]. As shown in Table 2, patients 1 and 4 improved their fixation stability more than 14% by MAIA biofeedback training.

In patient 3, fixation stability and 63% BCEA worsened after the training. It was possible that the point of PRT became inapt while retinal sensitivity was improved nonuniformly during the training. This case suggested that we should recalibrate PRT even during the training when fixation stability or 63% BCEA worsen.

Limitations of this study are the small sample size and the nonrandomized comparison. The effective number of training session and intervals between each training session are also unknown. However, most of the patients experienced an immediate improvement in visual performance after the first MAIA biofeedback training in this study. MAIA biofeedback training was easy for most patients and could be an option for patients whose recovery of visual acuity after successful MH surgery is insufficient.

Further studies with larger numbers of patients are needed to identify the most effective locations of the PRT and compare different methods of PRT location.

Conflict of Interests

None of the authors have any proprietary interests in this study.

Acknowledgment

The authors would like to express their gratitude for Toshihiko Oiwake's invaluable assistance with data analysis.

References

[1] N. E. Kelly and R. T. Wendel, "Vitreous surgery for idiopathic macular holes. Results of a pilot study," *Archives of Ophthalmology*, vol. 109, no. 5, pp. 654–659, 1991.

[2] D. W. Park, J. O. Sipperley, S. R. Sneed, P. U. Dugel, and J. Jacobsen, "Macular hole surgery with internal-limiting membrane peeling and intravitreous air," *Ophthalmology*, vol. 106, no. 7, pp. 1392–1398, 1999.

[3] H. L. Brooks Jr., "Macular hole surgery with and without internal limiting membrane peeling," *Ophthalmology*, vol. 107, no. 10, pp. 1939–1949, 2000.

[4] I. D. Fabian and J. Moisseiev, "Sutureless vitrectomy: evolution and current practices," *British Journal of Ophthalmology*, vol. 95, no. 3, pp. 318–324, 2011.

[5] S. Ullrich, C. Haritoglou, C. Gass, M. Schaumberger, M. W. Ulbig, and A. Kampik, "Macular hole size as a prognostic factor in macular hole surgery," *British Journal of Ophthalmology*, vol. 86, no. 4, pp. 390–393, 2002.

[6] L. A. Stec, R. D. Ross, G. A. Williams, M. T. Trese, R. R. Margherio, and M. S. Cox Jr., "Vitrectomy for chronic macular holes," *Retina*, vol. 24, no. 3, pp. 341–347, 2004.

[7] S. Kusuhara and A. Negi, "Predicting visual outcome following surgery for idiopathic macular holes," *Ophthalmologica*, vol. 231, no. 3, pp. 125–132, 2014.

[8] Z. Sun, D. Gan, C. Jiang et al., "Effect of preoperative retinal sensitivity and fixation on long-term prognosis for idiopathic

macular holes," *Graefe's Archive for Clinical and Experimental Ophthalmology*, vol. 250, no. 11, pp. 1587–1596, 2012.

[9] J. M. Ruiz-Moreno, C. Staicu, D. P. Piñero, J. Montero, F. Lugo, and P. Amat, "Optical coherence tomography predictive factors for macular hole surgery outcome," *British Journal of Ophthalmology*, vol. 92, no. 5, pp. 640–644, 2008.

[10] K. Kawano, Y. Ito, M. Kondo et al., "Displacement of foveal area toward optic disc after macular hole surgery with internal limiting membrane peeling," *Eye*, vol. 27, no. 7, pp. 871–877, 2013.

[11] M. Ishida, Y. Ichikawa, R. Higashida, Y. Tsutsumi, A. Ishikawa, and Y. Imamura, "Retinal displacement toward optic disc after internal limiting membrane peeling for idiopathic macular hole," *American Journal of Ophthalmology*, vol. 157, no. 5, pp. 971–977, 2014.

[12] Y. Itoh, M. Inoue, T. Rii, Y. Ando, and A. Hirakata, "Asymmetrical recovery of cone outer segment tips line and foveal displacement after successful macular hole surgery," *Investigative Ophthalmology & Visual Science*, vol. 55, no. 5, pp. 3003–3011, 2014.

[13] T. Nakagomi, T. Goto, Y. Tateno, T. Oshiro, and H. Iijima, "Macular slippage after macular hole surgery with internal limiting membrane peeling," *Current Eye Research*, vol. 38, no. 12, pp. 1255–1260, 2013.

[14] E. M. Vingolo, S. Cavarretta, D. Domanico, F. Parisi, and R. Malagola, "Microperimetric biofeedback in AMD patients," *Applied Psychophysiology Biofeedback*, vol. 32, no. 3-4, pp. 185–189, 2007.

[15] E. M. Vingolo, S. Salvatore, and S. Cavarretta, "Low-vision rehabilitation by means of MP-1 biofeedback examination in patients with different macular diseases: a pilot study," *Applied Psychophysiology Biofeedback*, vol. 34, no. 2, pp. 127–133, 2009.

[16] M. D. Crossland, L. E. Culham, S. A. Kabanarou, and G. S. Rubin, "Preferred retinal locus development in patients with macular disease," *Ophthalmology*, vol. 112, no. 9, pp. 1579–1585, 2005.

[17] C. Buia and P. Tiesinga, "Attentional modulation of firing rate and synchrony in a model cortical network," *Journal of Computational Neuroscience*, vol. 20, no. 3, pp. 247–264, 2006.

[18] E. Altpeter, M. Mackeben, and S. Trauzettel-Klosinski, "The importance of sustained attention for patients with maculopathies," *Vision Research*, vol. 40, no. 10-12, pp. 1539–1547, 2000.

[19] H. Ozdemir, M. Karacorlu, F. Senturk, S. A. Karacorlu, and O. Uysal, "Retinal sensitivity and fixation changes 1 year after triamcinolone acetonide assisted internal limiting membrane peeling for macular hole surgery—a MP-1 microperimetric study," *Acta Ophthalmologica*, vol. 88, no. 6, pp. e222–e227, 2010.

[20] E. Cappello, G. Virgili, L. Tollot, M. D. Borrello, U. Menchini, and M. Zemella, "Reading ability and retinal sensitivity after surgery for macular hole and macular pucker," *Retina*, vol. 29, no. 8, pp. 1111–1118, 2009.

[21] S. Richter-Mueksch, S. Sacu, E. Osarovsky-Sasin, E. Stifter, C. Kiss, and M. Velikay-Parel, "Visual performance 3 years after successful macular hole surgery," *British Journal of Ophthalmology*, vol. 93, no. 5, pp. 660–663, 2009.

[22] L. Tarita-Nistor, E. G. González, M. S. Mandelcorn, L. Lillakas, and M. J. Steinbach, "Fixation stability, fixation location, and visual acuity after successful macular hole surgery," *Investigative Ophthalmology & Visual Science*, vol. 50, no. 1, pp. 84–89, 2009.

25

Evaluation of Retinal Nerve Fiber Layer and Ganglion Cell Complex in Patients with Optic Neuritis or Neuromyelitis Optica Spectrum Disorders Using Optical Coherence Tomography in a Chinese Cohort

Guohong Tian,[1] Zhenxin Li,[2] Guixian Zhao,[2] Chaoyi Feng,[1] Mengwei Li,[1] Yongheng Huang,[1] and Xinghuai Sun[1]

[1]*Department of Ophthalmology, Eye, Ear, Nose, and Throat Hospital, Fudan University, Shanghai 200031, China*
[2]*Department of Neurology, Huashan Hospital, Fudan University, Shanghai 200040, China*

Correspondence should be addressed to Guohong Tian; valentian99@hotmail.com

Academic Editor: Jun Zhang

We evaluate a cohort of optic neuritis and neuromyelitis optica (NMO) spectrum disorders patients in a territory hospital in China. The peripapillary retinal nerve fiber layer (RNFL) and macular ganglion cell complex (GCC) were measured using spectral-domain OCT after 6 months of acute onset. The results showed that both the peripapillary RNFL and macular GCC were significantly thinner in all optic neuritis subtypes compared to controls. In addition, the recurrent optic neuritis and NMO groups showed more severe damage on the RNFL and GCC pattern.

1. Introduction

Acute optic neuritis may be the first manifestation of both multiple sclerosis (MS) and neuromyelitis optica (NMO), or some unknown etiology of disorders [1, 2]. In Chinese, the demographic and clinical features of optic neuritis spectrum disorder are less well-defined than that in Caucasus [3–5].

During the past few years, numerous studies showed that peripapillary RNFL and macular thickness analysis may be used to detect axonal loss in optic neuritis, neuromyelitis optica, and other forms of chronic relapsing optic neuritis [6–9]. In addition, it has been suggested that OCT abnormalities can help differentiate MS from NMO on the severity of axonal loss [10–14].

Due to the ethnic differences, optic neuritis in China shows more atypical features than those in western countries and the prognosis is not clearly described. The propose of this study was to evaluate the thickness of the RNFL and macular GCC using SD-OCT in different forms of optic neuritis in a cohort of Chinese patients and compare the pattern of damage in MS-ON, NMO-ON, and R-ON group.

2. Materials and Methods

2.1. Patients. The current study was a cross-sectional study. Patients who presented with acute optic neuritis in Neuroophthalmology Division in Eye Ear Nose and Throat hospital, Fudan University, Shanghai, between May 2013 and January 2014, were recruited. Paper consent forms were obtained for participation through a study protocol that was approved by the hospital institutional review board. All patients had their diagnosis confirmed by referred neurologists and neuroophthalmologists. After thorough ancillary tests and at least one-year of follow-up, patients were divided into 3 groups for evaluating the involved eye: MS-ON, R-ON, and NMO-ON.

MS-ON group patients included typical acute demyelinating optic neuritis with brain lesions fulfilling the revised McDonald criteria or clinical isolate syndrome (CIS) [15, 16]. Recurrent isolated optic neuritis (R-ON) was defined as unilateral or bilateral recurrence affecting optic nerves in patients whose clinical evidence showed no other brain lesion and seronegative AQP4-Ab. A diagnosis of NMO-ON was

TABLE 1: Demographics and clinical characteristics for MS-ON, R-ON, and NMO-ON group and control.

Group	Patients (n)	Age (year) (mean ± SD)	Course (month) (mean ± SD)	Bilateral%	Female%
MS-ON	62	30.47 ± 16.71	6.2 ± 3.0	33.3%	58.1%
R-ON	19	31.26 ± 11.20	20.0 ± 22.6	100%	68.4%
NMO-ON	37	40.54 ± 13.64	25.0 ± 33.4	34.7%	83.8%
Control	68	31.96 ± 13.78	NA	NA	64.7%
P value		$P = 0.007^a$	$P = 0.02^b$	$P = 0.01^c$	$P = 0.07^d$

NA: not applicable; a: the statistical difference between NMO-ON and other groups; b: the statistical difference between MS-ON and other ON subtypes; NMO-ON and other groups; c: the statistical difference between R-ON group and other ON subtypes; d: the statistical difference between ON subtypes and control.

given to patients who met established diagnostic criteria for NMO or NMO spectrum disorders (NMO-SD) published by Wingerchuk et al. [17]. The new onset eyes in three groups were included for OCT evaluating. As for acute bilateral involved patients, only one affected eye was randomly chosen for OCT evaluation. As for R-ON patients, the new attack eye was evaluated. All enrolled patients underwent the routine blood test including the infectious panel, the rheumatology panels. All patients underwent serum AQP4 antibody test in neurobiology laboratory using the ELISA methods (kit from ElisaRSR AQP4-Ab, RSR limited, UK). Neuroimaging was required to confirm the acute attack of the optic neuritis, evaluate brain demyelinating, and exclude the compressive optic neuropathy and anterior ischemic optic neuropathy.

Exclusion criteria included patients with pathologic myopia with spherical equivalent of the refractive error >6.0 diopters, a previous history of ocular disease (including macular degeneration, diabetic retinopathy, uveitis, and glaucoma), and neurodegenerative conditions that could impact OCT testing results (Parkinson's disease, Alzheimer's disease), and subjects with poor vision having difficulty maintaining fixation were excluded from analyses.

The group of control was recruited from volunteers of hospital staffs and patient's companions at the time duration of the follow-up. Inclusion criteria included best-corrected visual acuity of at least 20/20, spherical equivalent of the refractive error <6.0 diopters (highly myopic), without presence of any ophthalmic or neurological diseases known to affect RNFL thickness. One eye was randomly chosen for evaluation.

2.2. Optical Coherence Tomography. Spectral-domain optical coherence tomography (SD-OCT) was performed using 3D Disc, ONH, GCC protocols provided by the RTVue-100 4.0.7.5 version (Optovue Inc, Fremont, CA). An internal fixation target was used to improve reproducibility. Scan was accepted only if the images with a signal strength index were greater than 35. The peripapillary RNFL thickness was measured automatically using a RNFL 3.45 scan mode, where 4 circular scans (1024 A-scans/scan) acquired 3.45 mm from the center of the optic disc. The RNFL was divided into temporal (316°–45°), superior (46°–135°), nasal (136°–225°), and inferior (226°–315°) quadrants. A RNFL progression analysis is also available for follow-up.

The GCC scan technique provides inner retinal thickness values which consist of ganglion cell layer (GCL) and inner

plexiform layer (IPL). Scan mode for GCC analysis, which acquires 14 928A scans over a 7 mm square area in 0.58 seconds with 15 vertical scans collected at 0.5-mm intervals. The center of the scan was shifted 1.0 mm temporally to improve sampling of the temporal periphery. The GCC within the central 6 mm diameter area of the macular was calculated. All the data were measured and collected in acute optic neuritis patients 6 month after attack.

2.3. Statistical Analysis. Demographic variants were described and compared by ANOVA test (numeration variables) if the variance was homogeneity or chi-square test (categorical variables). The peripapillary RNFL data measured according to 4 quadrants was analyzed using repeat measurement analysis of variance due to the correlation intereye within patient. The difference between each group was statistic and compared with controls. GCC values were analyzed by independent-samples t test between groups. A P value of less than 0.05 was considered statistically significant. All analyses were conducted using IBM SPSS statistics for windows, Version 19.0 (IBM Corp, Chicago, USA).

3. Results

3.1. Demographics. A total of 118 patients, including MS-ON ($n = 62$), R-ON ($n = 19$), NMO-ON ($n = 37$), and 68 healthy controls were evaluated. The demographic and clinical characteristics are summarized in Table 1. Among the MS-ON group, 6 patients were diagnosed with clinical definite MS with optic neuritis; 4 patients had presented with CIS with brain or brainstem demyelinated lesion and subsequently got optic neuritis; the other 52 patients presented with isolated acute optic neuritis fulfilling the idiopathic demyelinating etiology after thorough ancillary work-up. Among the 19 R-ON patients, the recurrent times differ from 8 to 3. Among the 37 NMO-ON patients, 5 had previous myelitis and all patients showed a seropositive for AQP4-Ab.

The mean age in NMO-ON group was significantly older than other groups ($P = 0.01$), whereas there was no difference in age between MS-ON, R-ON, and control. The mean disease duration was significantly longer in R-ON and NMO-ON groups compared to MS-ON ($P = 0.02$). R-ON group showed high prevalence of bilateral involvement than MS-ON and NMO-ON group ($P = 0.01$). There was no statistic difference in female prevalence in all groups.

TABLE 2: Peripapillary RNFL thicknesses (μm) for eyes of patients in each group.

RNFL	MS-ON	R-ON	NMO-ON	Control
Average	79.12 ± 15.64	56.06 ± 9.83	63.94 ± 11.86	112.01 ± 10.93
Temporal	57.94 ± 14.57	48.37 ± 11.25	46.59 ± 12.10	139.93 ± 19.27
Superior	100.43 ± 22.51	80.74 ± 9.50	79.45 ± 16.47	120.43 ± 30.71
Nasal	59.84 ± 17.59	48.37 ± 8.90	48.91 ± 14.08	81.28 ± 13.05
Inferior	98.29 ± 21.57	82.76 ± 17.87	80.82 ± 17.40	141.76 ± 20.19

3.2. RNFL Measurement. Because age is known to influence retinal thickness parameters, first of all, covariance was analyzed using a linear regression model and the results showed there was no significant relation between age and RNFL thickness in our groups of subjects. Peripapillary RNFL thickness measured in 3 optic neuropathy groups was significantly thinning compared to healthy controls (Table 2). After repeat measurement of variance of 4 quadrants in each group, the mean difference showed an average of RNFL loss in MS-ON, R-ON, and NMO-ON groups of 32.8 μm, 46.9 μm, and 43.8 μm, respectively, compared to healthy control (Table 3). Furthermore, the R-ON and NMO-ON patients showed significant decreased RNFL in eyes in all quadrants compared with MS-ON, whereas there was no significant difference between R-ON and NMO-ON group.

3.3. Macular GCC Measurement. For the macular GCC, the tendency was the same as the peripapillary RNFL pattern, which showed significantly reduced in 3 optic neuritis groups compared to control (Figure 1). An average GCC thinning in MS-ON, R-ON, and NMO-ON groups was of 24.2 μm, 28.5 μm, and 28.5 μm, respectively, compared to healthy control. There were no statistic differences for the GCC between R-ON and NMO-ON.

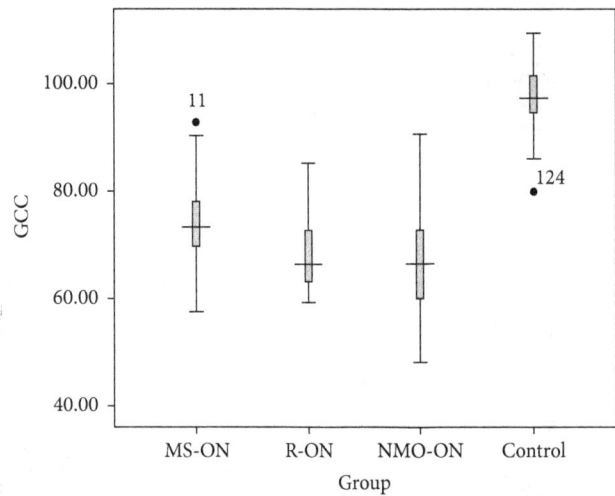

FIGURE 1: The boxplot analysis representing the macular GCC thickness in MS-ON, R-ON, NMO-ON, and control group. Mean values and 5% and 95% percentiles are shown. The difference between the 4 groups was statistically significant (P < 0.001), whereas there was no significant difference between R-ON and NMO-ON group (P = 0.725).

4. Discussion

Optic neuritis is one of the common optic neuropathies, which lead to visual loss in young Chinese and the underline etiologies have not been full clarified [1]. Our cohort study composed of a group of typical MS related optic neuritis patients, as well as atypical forms like R-ON and NMO-ON. Most of these patients presented as first attack which can be a manifestation of MS, NMO, or other unknown inflammatory disorders. Although the clinical characteristics and laboratory tests can help differentiating some of the etiology, the board spectrum of optic neuritis made it difficult to a definite diagnosis in a short term after one optic neuritis episode.

SD-OCT is a very useful and objective method to provide data on RNFL and macular GCC thickness and volumes. Also the eye tracking systems permit perfect repositioning in longitudinal studies for investigators to capture subtle changes on the order of a few micrometers.

The up to date cross-sectional studies and longitudinal investigations on OCT showed a significant alteration pattern in NMOSD patients with optic neuritis compared to MS-ON and healthy controls [18, 19]. A meta-analysis showed a loss of approximately 20 m in the affected eye in relapsing-remitting MS compared to healthy controls [20]. Bichuetti et al. [12]

research also showed that, in patients with NMO and chronic relapsing inflammatory optic neuritis, the RNFL tend to have significantly lower thickness than patients with MS-ON. Our findings also demonstrate the same OCT pattern that the peripapillary RNFL and macular GCC thickness decreased significantly 6 months after once attack of optic neuritis compared to healthy controls. Furthermore, the R-ON and NMO-ON groups showed more severe damage compared to patients with MS (Figure 2). Approximately 40 μm thinning of RNFL was found in NMO-ON and R-ON eyes compared to controls (approximately 30 μm thinning in MS-ON). The temporal quadrant damage tendency in MS-ON was not shown in our cohort according to Naismith et al. study [11].

The GCC measured in our study by RTVue-100 protocol provided a value of combined macular ganglion cell layer and inner plexiform layer, which can help estimate the retrograde of optic nerve after damage. Six months after attack, the GCC showed an nearly 30 μm thinning in NMO-ON and R-ON groups, as well as approximately 20 μm in MS-ON compared to controls. The profound loss of GCC, which is closely associated with visual disability in MS [21], can also help in differentiating NMO or R-ON from MS-ON in early stage, where the true peripapillary RNFL will not be available due to the swell of optic disc.

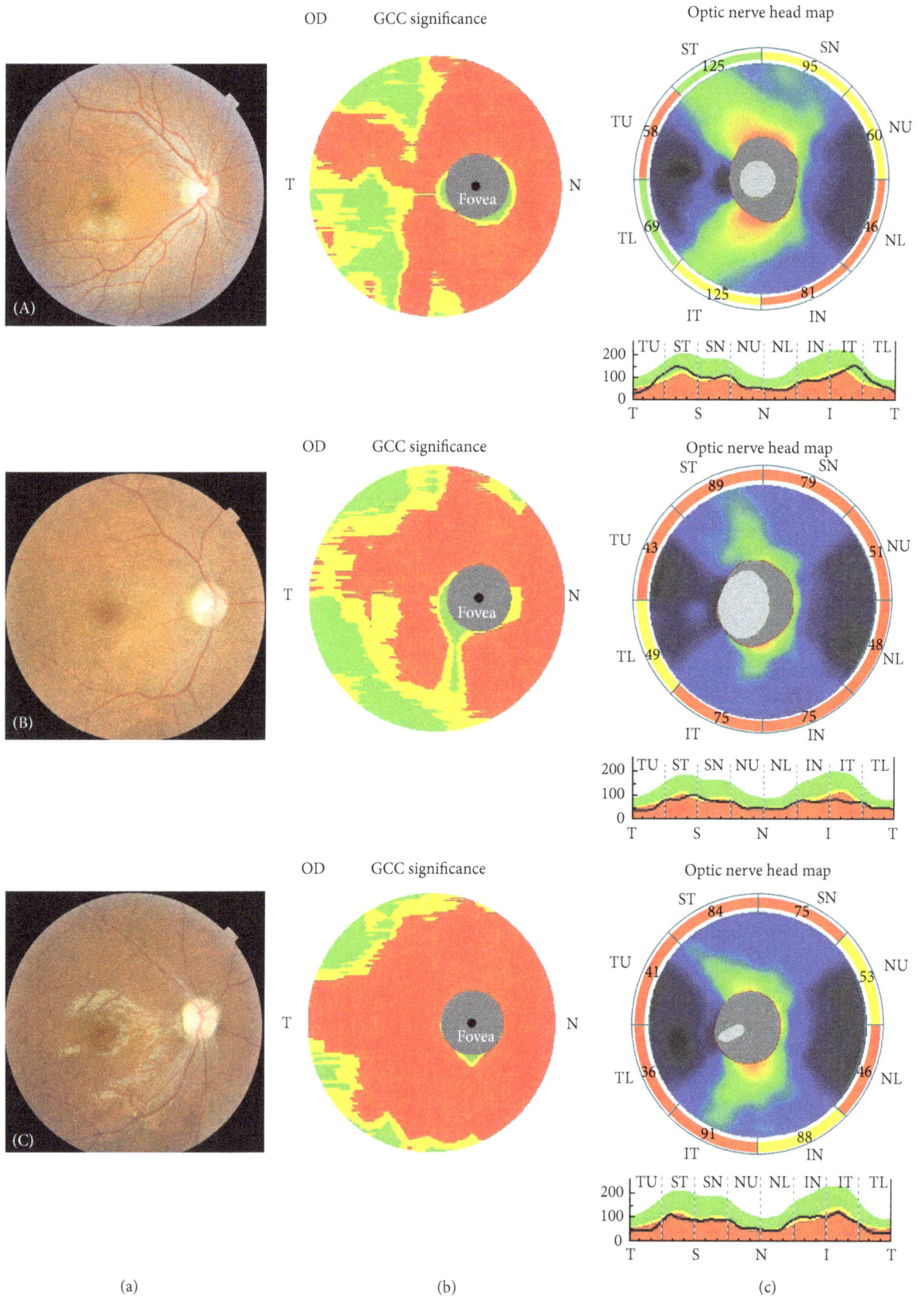

FIGURE 2: The fundus photograph (a) together with the corresponding macular GCC (b) and RNFL (c) measurements in MS-ON (A), R-ON (B), and NMO-ON (C) groups are showed, respectively.

TABLE 3: Repeated measures ANOVA of multiple comparisons of each group.

| (I) group | (J) group | Mean difference (I − J) | Std. error | Sig. | 95% confidence interval | |
					Lower bound	Upper bound
MS-ON	R-ON	14.087*	3.558	.000	7.066	21.108
	NMO-ON	10.998*	3.336	.001	4.415	17.581
	Control	−32.795*	2.312	.000	−37.358	−28.232
R-ON	NMO-ON	−3.089	4.278	.471	−11.531	5.353
	Control	−46.882*	3.547	.000	−53.881	−39.882
NMO-ON	Control	−43.793*	3.309	.000	−50.322	−37.263

*The mean difference is significant at the 0.05 level.

The profound loss of peripapillary RNFL and macular GCC in R-ON group, whose pattern is similar to NMO-ON, to some extent, indicate that they share the some underline etiology. In addition, the OCT technique makes it possible to measure the single layer of ganglion cell around macular, which will give accurate thickness of the neurons. Further prospective longitudinal investigations will be needed to illustrate the change in OCT pattern as a structure marker for axonal degeneration and neuronal loss.

Conflict of Interests

The authors have no proprietary or commercial interest in any of the materials discussed in this paper.

Acknowledgment

The authors thank Ms. Heng Fan (Department of Biostatistics, School of Public Health, Fudan University) for statistical analysis consultation.

References

[1] A. T. Toosy, D. F. Mason, and D. H. Miller, "Optic neuritis," *The Lancet Neurology*, vol. 13, no. 1, pp. 83–99, 2014.

[2] F. A. Warren, "Atypical optic neuritis," *Journal of Neuro-Ophthalmology*, vol. 34, no. 4, pp. e12–e13, 2014.

[3] J. T. Peng, H. R. Cong, R. Yan et al., "Neurological outcome and predictive factors of idiopathic optic neuritis in China," *Journal of the Neurological Sciences*, vol. 349, no. 1-2, pp. 94–98, 2015.

[4] C. Lai, G. Tian, W. Liu, W. Wei, T. Takahashi, and X. Zhang, "Clinical characteristics, therapeutic outcomes of isolated atypical optic neuritis in China," *Journal of the Neurological Sciences*, vol. 305, no. 1-2, pp. 38–40, 2011.

[5] A. C. O. Cheng, N. C. Y. Chan, and C. K. M. Chan, "Acute and subacute inflammation of the optic nerve and its sheath: clinical features in Chinese patients," *Hong Kong Medical Journal*, vol. 18, no. 2, pp. 115–122, 2012.

[6] S. B. Syc, S. Saidha, S. D. Newsome et al., "Optical coherence tomography segmentation reveals ganglion cell layer pathology after optic neuritis," *Brain*, vol. 135, no. 2, pp. 521–533, 2012.

[7] D. B. Fernandes, A. S. Raza, R. G. Nogueira et al., "Evaluation of inner retinal layers in patients with multiple sclerosis or neuromyelitis optica using optical coherence tomography," *Ophthalmology*, vol. 120, no. 2, pp. 387–394, 2013.

[8] M. L. R. Monteiro, D. B. Fernandes, S. L. Apóstolos-Pereira, and D. Callegaro, "Quantification of retinal neural loss in patients with neuromyelitis optica and multiple sclerosis with or without optic neuritis using fourier-domain optical coherence tomography," *Investigative Ophthalmology and Visual Science*, vol. 53, no. 7, pp. 3959–3966, 2012.

[9] H. Merle, S. Olindo, A. Donnio, R. Richer, D. Smadja, and P. Cabre, "Retinal peripapillary nerve fiber layer thickness in neuromyelitis optica," *Investigative Ophthalmology and Visual Science*, vol. 49, no. 10, pp. 4412–4417, 2008.

[10] J. N. Ratchford, M. E. Quigg, A. Conger et al., "Optical coherence tomography helps differentiate neuromyelitis optica and MS optic neuropathies," *Neurology*, vol. 73, no. 4, pp. 302–308, 2009.

[11] R. T. Naismith, N. T. Tutlam, J. Xu et al., "Optical coherence tomography differs in neuromyelitis optica compared with multiple sclerosis," *Neurology*, vol. 72, no. 12, pp. 1077–1082, 2009.

[12] D. B. Bichuetti, A. S. de Camargo, A. B. Falcão, F. F. Gonçalves, I. M. Tavares, and E. M. L. de Oliveira, "The retinal nerve fiber layer of patients with neuromyelitis optica and chronic relapsing optic neuritis is more severely damaged than patients with multiple sclerosis," *Journal of Neuro-Ophthalmology*, vol. 33, no. 3, pp. 220–224, 2013.

[13] E. Schneider, H. Zimmermann, T. Oberwahrenbrock et al., "Optical coherence tomography reveals distinct patterns of retinal damage in neuromyelitis optica and multiple sclerosis," *PLoS ONE*, vol. 8, no. 6, Article ID e66151, 2013.

[14] K.-A. Park, J. Kim, and S. Y. Oh, "Analysis of spectral domain optical coherence tomography measurements in optic neuritis: Differences in neuromyelitis optica, multiple sclerosis, isolated optic neuritis and normal healthy controls," *Acta Ophthalmologica*, vol. 92, no. 1, pp. e57–e65, 2014.

[15] C. H. Polman, S. C. Reingold, B. Banwell et al., "Diagnostic criteria for multiple sclerosis: 2010 revisions to the McDonald criteria," *Annals of Neurology*, vol. 69, no. 2, pp. 292–302, 2011.

[16] D. H. Miller, D. T. Chard, and O. Ciccarelli, "Clinically isolated syndromes," *The Lancet Neurology*, vol. 11, no. 2, pp. 157–169, 2012.

[17] D. M. Wingerchuk, V. A. Lennon, C. F. Lucchinetti, S. J. Pittock, and B. G. Weinshenker, "The spectrum of neuromyelitis optica," *The Lancet Neurology*, vol. 6, no. 9, pp. 805–815, 2007.

[18] L. J. Balk and A. Petzold, "Current and future potential of retinal optical coherence tomography in multiple sclerosis with and without optic neuritis," *Neurodegenerative Disease Management*, vol. 4, no. 2, pp. 165–176, 2014.

[19] J. Bennett, J. de Seze, M. Lana-Peixoto et al., "Neuromyelitis optica and multiple sclerosis: seeing differences through optical

coherence tomography," *Multiple Sclerosis Journal*, vol. 21, no. 6, pp. 678–688, 2015.

[20] A. Petzold, J. F. de Boer, S. Schippling et al., "Optical coherence tomography in multiple sclerosis: a systematic review and meta-analysis," *The Lancet Neurology*, vol. 9, no. 9, pp. 921–932, 2010.

[21] S. D. Walter, H. Ishikawa, K. M. Galetta et al., "Ganglion cell loss in relation to visual disability in multiple sclerosis," *Ophthalmology*, vol. 119, no. 6, pp. 1250–1257, 2012.

26

Prophylactic Circumferential Retinal Cryopexy to Prevent Pseudophakic Retinal Detachment after Posterior Capsule Rupture during Phacoemulsification

T. Bertelmann, C. Heun, C. Paul, E. Bari-Kacik, W. Sekundo, and S. Schulze

Department of Ophthalmology, Philipps-University Marburg, Baldingerstraße, 35043 Marburg, Germany

Correspondence should be addressed to T. Bertelmann; thomas.bertelmann@staff.uni-marburg.de

Academic Editor: Mauricio Maia

Purpose. To evaluate whether prophylactic circumferential retinal cryopexy (CRC) can prevent pseudophakic retinal detachment (PRD) development after posterior capsule rupture (PCR) during phacoemulsification. *Methods.* Retrospective patient chart analysis of eyes experiencing a PCR during phacoemulsification. Comparison of PRD development between eyes receiving CRC (cryo+ group) or not (cryo− group). *Results.* Overall 106 patients were analyzed, thereof 61 (58%) in the cryo+ and 45 (42%) in the cryo− group. In both clusters a total of 10 PRDs (9.4%) occurred, thereof 3 (30%) in the cryo+ as well as 7 (70%) in the cryo− group ($p = 0.087$), 79.8 ± 81.58 weeks after PCR. Relative/absolute risk reduction in CRC-treated eyes was calculated to be 68%/11%. Prophylactic CRC reduced PRD development 0.3-fold. Number needed to treat was estimated to be 9.4. *Conclusion.* Prophylactic CRC might be a useful treatment option in eyes with PCR to hamper PRD development in the further course. Further research is indicated to evaluate this beneficial effect between eyes with and without a rupture of the anterior vitreous cortex and accompanying vitreous loss in an expanding number of eyes.

1. Introduction

Cataract is the most common cause of reversible vision loss in the world. Many advances have been made within the last decades to improve the surgical lens removal procedure, such as phacoemulsification technique, small incision surgery, the use of viscoelastics, and the development of intraocular lenses [1]. This ensures a less traumatic approach to the eye, reduces complication rates, and backs up rapid visual recovery in most cases [1, 2]. Therefor cataract surgery has ascended to be the most frequently performed surgical intervention in developed countries nowadays [3]. Despite these major improvements various complications, including endophthalmitis, acute corneal decompensation, raised intraocular pressure (IOP), or postsurgical cystoid macular edema, may occur [4]. Posterior capsule rupture (PCR) during the surgical maneuver is another major complication raising the risk for pseudophakic retinal detachment (PRD) in the further postsurgical course [5]. Former research described a protective effect of prophylactic circumferential

retinal cryopexy (CRC) in aphakic eyes [6] or in eyes with peripheral retinal breaks [7] in respect to retinal detachment (RD) development. Thus, the purpose of this investigation was to evaluate whether prophylactic CRC after PCR during a complicated phacoemulsification procedure can prevent PRD development.

2. Material and Methods

A retrospective patient chart analysis was performed including all phacoemulsification cases performed at Department of Ophthalmology, Philipps-University Marburg, Germany, in which a PCR occurred during the operation between July 1996 and December 2012. To be included into this investigation, patients needed to be 40 years of age or older scheduled for a routine age-related cataract removal procedure using phacoemulsification technique. The postsurgical observation period needed to extend 2 years at a minimum. Exclusion criteria were eyes with an axial length (AL) of more than 25 mm, congenital or traumatic cataract formation,

TABLE 1: Baseline characteristics of patients receiving prophylactic circumferential retinal cryopexy (cryo+) or not (cryo−) after posterior capsule rupture during phacoemulsification.

	Cryo+ group ($n = 61/58\%$)	Cryo− group ($n = 45/42\%$)	p value
Gender (male/female)	31 (51%)/30 (49%)	37 (55%)/30 (45%)	0.771
Age (phacoemulsification)	75.1 ± 8.3 years	75 ± 8.6 years	0.931
Eye affected (right/left)	32 (52%)/29 (48%)	27 (60%)/18 (40%)	0.285
Axial length (mm)	23.16 ± 0.78	23.14 ± 0.96	0.977

previously vitrectomized eyes, and any combination of the phacoemulsification procedure with other ocular surgical procedures, such as keratoplasty, glaucoma operations, or posterior segment surgery.

2.1. Statistical Analysis. Tables were prepared using Microsoft Word 2007 (Microsoft©). Statistical analysis was performed with Office Excel 2007 (Microsoft©) and SPSS Statistics 20 (IBM©). To test baseline value differences between groups, binomial distribution test and Mann-Whitney U test were performed. To test the effect of retinal cryocoagulation in respect to PRD rates, logistic regression was executed including cryo+/−, axial length (AL), time till cryocoagulation, and patients' age and gender as covariates. Significant results were assumed if p values were less than 5% ($p < 0.05$).

3. Results

Overall 106 patients were included into this analysis, thereof 55 male (51.9%) and 51 female (48.1%) subjects with an overall age of 75.1 ± 8.4 years (mean value ± standard deviation). Patients were split into a cryocoagulation (cryo+) and a noncryocoagulation (cryo−) group depending on whether prophylactic CRC was performed after PCR or not. Patients' baseline characteristics of each group are displayed in Table 1.

In the cryo+ group prophylactic CRC was performed 11.6 ± 27.2 weeks after PCR. A total of 10 (9.4%) PRD occurred in both groups, thereof 3 (30%) in the cryo+ as well as 7 (70%) in the cryo− group ($p = 0.087$). Relative/absolute risk reduction in CRC-treated eyes was calculated to be 68%/11%. Prophylactic CRC reduced PRD development 0.3-fold. Number needed to treat (NNT) was estimated to be 9.4. Axial length ($p = 0.484$), time till cryocoagulation ($p = 0.657$), and patients' age ($p = 0.394$) and gender ($p = 0.498$) did not have a significant impact on PRD development.

Overall PRD occurred 79.8 ± 81.58 weeks after the eventful phacoemulsification. In all cases pars plana vitrectomy (ppV) was performed for successful RD repair.

4. Discussion

Major improvements in extracapsular cataract extraction (ECCE) procedures have been made within the last decades, especially the replacement of manual nuclear extraction by phacoemulsification [8]. Additionally, a stepwise improvement of the latter resulted in a further significant decrease of complication rates. Hereby, the number of posterior capsule ruptures (PCR) and anterior vitrectomies (AV) halved despite

substantially increasing procedure counts [8]. PCRs were reported to occur in between 0.45% and 16% of all phacoemulsification procedures mostly dependent on surgical experience [4, 9–11] and other various risk factors [12]. Thus, PCRs remain one of the most common complications in cataract surgery with a major risk of compromised final visual outcome [4, 9]. PCRs oftentimes occur during the phacoemulsification (roughly 60%) or irrigation/aspiration (about 25%) process [4]. Accompanying vitreous loss (VL) is associated with an even poorer visual acuity (VA) outcome and typically occurs, in about 1.0% to 75% of PCR cases, during nuclear disassembly and removal [4, 11, 13].

Former reports indicated a fivefold increase of retinal detachments in pseudophakic eyes in which a PCR and VL occurred during the phacoemulsification procedure in comparison to uncomplicated cataract surgeries [4, 5]. Contrariwise, prophylactic circumferential retinal cryopexy (CRC) was successfully used in eyes prior to cataract surgery in patients prone to retinal detachments [14] and in several patients undergoing pars plana vitrectomy [15, 16]. Prophylactic CRC is also administered for various peripheral lesions like retinal breaks, tears, and others such as lattice degeneration to prevent RD development [17], if not addressable with laser photocoagulation. Thus, the question arises, whether prophylactic CRC after an eventful phacoemulsification procedure can reduce PRD development in the further course. As demonstrated herein there was a meaningful reduction in PRD development in the cryo+ group (relative/absolute risk reduction in prophylactic CRC-treated eyes of 68%/11%) although statistical significance failed. This in turn is essentially attributed to the marginal number of overall PRD developments of 9.4% (cryo+: 3 PRDs in 61 PCR cases; cryo−: 7 PRDs in 45 PCR events) in this series. According to this data, calculation of number of cases to show statistically significant differences revealed group sizes of 139/179 PCR cases in each group to reach a statistical power of 80%/90%. In particular the NNT of 9.4 cases emphasizes the benefits of prophylactic CRC in routine patient care when comparing with NNT of 25 for prophylactic warfarin intake to prevent stroke in atrial fibrillation [18] for instance. This in turn awards a positive risk-benefit profile of prophylactic CRC in PCR cases. Nevertheless there are potential risks such as macular pucker formation, proliferative vitreoretinopathy (PVR), or surgically induced scleritis [17, 19], and therefore, individual risks and benefits for each patient have to be weighted. In this regard the technique of CRC is also important and a mild CRC (just visible whitening of the retina) should be preferred over distinctive freezing [20, 21]. Alternatively 360° laser retinopexy might be another option to prevent PRD development as laser treatment is routinely used to seal peripheral retinal breaks or degenerative areas prone to RD accruement, at least if they are symptomatic [22]. So far there is no report in the literature about the efficacy of prophylactic 360° laser retinopexy in eyes with PCR during phacoemulsification. Specific complications in the anterior [23] as well as posterior segment [24] can occur and have been reported as well. Contrariwise laser retinopexy is less traumatic to the eye and therefore a prospective study using laser instead of cold for prophylactic retinal treatment is indicated.

In theory, CRC can be used to induce permanent chorioretinal scar development and thus "glue" the retina to the underlying choroid. This could be of importance after a PCR due to the anterior movement of the vitreous towards the anterior segment of the eye. This anterior shift is additionally increased after anterior vitreous cortex (AVC) rupture with vitreous loss and a consequently performed anterior vitrectomy [25]. As the vitreous cortex is attached to the peripheral retina, the anteriorly directed drive of the vitreous body causes vitreoretinal traction and can induce retinal break or tear formation and thus induce PRD development [25, 26]. Thus a prophylactic CRC seems reasonable and the data herein support its routine use.

The strength of this evaluation is, to the best of our knowledge, to be the first investigation to evaluate whether prophylactic CRC after PCR during a complicated phacoemulsification procedure can prevent PRD development. A reasonable number of patients were included and observed over a long postoperative time. The limitation is the retrospective study design. Furthermore, the effect of prophylactic CRC may differ between eyes with and without AVC rupture and accompanying vitreous loss. Performing anterior vitrectomy in these scenarios can additionally prevent PRD significantly [27]. The position of the lens implanted (sulcus ciliaris, in the bag, optic capture) and whether the eye stays (temporarily) aphakic or not [11] might also be of key interest in this regard. Due to the small number of PCR and accompanying PRD cases eligible for this evaluation within a 16.5 years' observation period, a separated and additional evaluation of these unanswered questions was not possible and would need some decades to gain enough patients. Nevertheless, these essential questions need further evaluation on a larger number of eyes affected in the future.

Conflict of Interests

Thomas Bertelmann is Medical Advisor at Novartis Pharma GmbH, Nuremberg, and scientific staff of Philipps-University Marburg, Germany.

References

[1] P. A. Asbell, I. Dualan, J. Mindel, D. Brocks, M. Ahmad, and S. Epstein, "Age-related cataract," *The Lancet*, vol. 365, no. 9459, pp. 599–609, 2005.

[2] J. Alió, J. L. Rodriguez-Prats, and A. Galal, "Advances in microincision cataract surgery intraocular lenses," *Current Opinion in Ophthalmology*, vol. 17, no. 1, pp. 80–93, 2006.

[3] J. C. Erie, "Rising cataract surgery rates: demand and supply," *Ophthalmology*, vol. 121, no. 1, pp. 2–4, 2014.

[4] S.-E. Ti, Y.-N. Yang, S. S. Lang, and S. P. Chee, "A 5-year audit of cataract surgery outcomes after posterior capsule rupture and risk factors affecting visual acuity," *American Journal of Ophthalmology*, vol. 157, no. 1, pp. 180–185.e1, 2014.

[5] N. Lois and D. Wong, "Pseudophakic retinal detachment," *Survey of Ophthalmology*, vol. 48, no. 5, pp. 467–487, 2003.

[6] G. M. Gombos and M. M. Gomobs, "Prevention of aphakic retinal detachment by retinocryocoagulation," *Annals of Ophthalmology*, vol. 16, no. 12, pp. 1124–1126, 1984.

[7] S. G. Kramer and W. E. Benson, "Prophylactic therapy of retinal breaks," *Survey of Ophthalmology*, vol. 22, no. 1, pp. 41–47, 1977.

[8] P. Jaycock, R. L. Johnston, H. Taylor et al., "The Cataract National Dataset electronic multi-centre audit of 55,567 operations: updating benchmark standards of care in the United Kingdom and internationally," *Eye*, vol. 23, no. 1, pp. 38–49, 2009.

[9] P. B. Greenberg, V. L. Tseng, W.-C. Wu et al., "Prevalence and predictors of ocular complications associated with cataract surgery in United States veterans," *Ophthalmology*, vol. 118, no. 3, pp. 507–514, 2011.

[10] R. L. Johnston, H. Taylor, R. Smith, and J. M. Sparrow, "The Cataract National Dataset electronic multi-centre audit of 55,567 operations: variation in posterior capsule rupture rates between surgeons," *Eye*, vol. 24, no. 5, pp. 888–893, 2010.

[11] H. V. Gimbel, R. Sun, M. Ferensowicz, E. Anderson Penno, and A. Kamal, "Intraoperative management of posterior capsule tears in phacoemulsification and intraocular lens implantation," *Ophthalmology*, vol. 108, no. 12, pp. 2186–2189, 2001.

[12] N. Narendran, P. Jaycock, R. L. Johnston et al., "The Cataract National Dataset electronic multicentre audit of 55,567 operations: risk stratification for posterior capsule rupture and vitreous loss," *Eye*, vol. 23, no. 1, pp. 31–37, 2009.

[13] R. B. Vajpayee, N. Sharma, T. Dada, V. Gupta, A. Kumar, and V. K. Dada, "Management of posterior capsule tears," *Survey of Ophthalmology*, vol. 45, no. 6, pp. 473–488, 2001.

[14] C. J. Campbell and M. C. Rittler, "Cataract extraction in the retinal detachment-prone patient," *American Journal of Ophthalmology*, vol. 73, no. 1, pp. 17–24, 1972.

[15] S. Schulze, N. Zaki, and P. Kroll, "Advantages and disadvantages of the circumferential retinal cryocoagulation before vitrectomy in proliferative diabetic vitreoretinopathy," *Klinische Monatsblätter für Augenheilkunde*, vol. 224, no. 8, pp. 647–652, 2007.

[16] A. Hager, S. Ehrich, and W. Wiegand, "Vitreoretinal secondary procedures following elective macular surgery," *Ophthalmologe*, vol. 101, no. 1, pp. 39–44, 2004.

[17] K. Watanabe, H. Ideta, J. Nakatake, K. Shinagawa, S. Demizu, and C. Takenaka, "Anterior chamber inflammation after transconjunctival cryosurgery," *Graefe's Archive for Clinical and Experimental Ophthalmology*, vol. 233, no. 2, pp. 71–73, 1995.

[18] M. I. Aguilar and R. Hart, "Oral anticoagulants for preventing stroke in patients with non-valvular atrial fibrillation and no previous history of stroke or transient ischemic attacks," *Cochrane Database of Systematic Reviews*, vol. 3, Article ID CD001927, 2005.

[19] A. H. Chignell, I. H. Revie, and R. S. Clemett, "Complications of retinal cryotherapy," *Transactions of the Ophthalmological Societies of the United Kingdom*, vol. 91, pp. 635–651, 1971.

[20] J. A. A. Govan, "Prophylactic circumferential cryopexy: a retrospective study of 106 eyes," *British Journal of Ophthalmology*, vol. 65, no. 5, pp. 364–370, 1981.

[21] M. Brihaye and J. A. Oosterhuis, "Experimental transscleral cryocoagulation of the retina," *Klinische Monatsblatter fur Augenheilkunde*, vol. 158, no. 2, pp. 171–184, 1971.

[22] S. Blindbæk and J. Grauslund, "Prophylactic treatment of retinal breaks—a systematic review," *Acta Ophthalmologica*, vol. 93, no. 1, pp. 3–8, 2015.

[23] N. Bouheraoua, L. Hrarat, C. F. Parsa et al., "Decreased corneal sensation and subbasal nerve density, and thinned corneal epithelium as a result of 360-degree laser retinopexy," *Ophthalmology*, vol. 122, no. 10, pp. 2095–2102, 2015.

[24] U. Mester, B. Volker, P. Kroll, and P. Berg, "Complications of prophylactic argon laser treatment of retinal breaks and degenerations in 2,000 eyes," *Ophthalmic Surgery*, vol. 19, no. 7, pp. 482–484, 1988.

[25] T. Bertelmann, M. Witteborn, and S. Mennel, "Pseudophakic cystoid macular oedema," *Klinische Monatsblätter für Augenheilkunde*, vol. 229, no. 8, pp. 798–811, 2012.

[26] F. Kuhn and B. Aylward, "Rhegmatogenous retinal detachment: a reappraisal of its pathophysiology and treatment," *Ophthalmic Research*, vol. 51, no. 1, pp. 15–31, 2013.

[27] M. Russell, B. Gaskin, D. Russell, and P. J. Polkinghorne, "Pseudophakic retinal detachment after phacoemulsification cataract surgery: ten-year retrospective review," *Journal of Cataract and Refractive Surgery*, vol. 32, no. 3, pp. 442–445, 2006.

27

Suppression of *In Vivo* Neovascularization by the Loss of TRPV1 in Mouse Cornea

**Katsuo Tomoyose,[1] Yuka Okada,[1] Takayoshi Sumioka,[1]
Masayasu Miyajima,[2] Kathleen C. Flanders,[3] Kumi Shirai,[1] Tomoya Morii,[1]
Peter S. Reinach,[4] Osamu Yamanaka,[1] and Shizuya Saika[1]**

[1]*Department of Ophthalmology, Wakayama Medical University, 811-1 Kimiidera, Wakayama 641-0012, Japan*
[2]*Laboratory Animal Center, Wakayama Medical University, 811-1 Kimiidera, Wakayama 641-0012, Japan*
[3]*Laboratory of Cell Regulation and Carcinogenesis, National Cancer Institute, National Institutes of Health, Bethesda, MD, USA*
[4]*Wenzhou Medical University School of Ophthalmology and Optometry, Wenzhou, China*

Correspondence should be addressed to Yuka Okada; yokada@wakayama-med.ac.jp

Academic Editor: Caio V. Regatieri

To investigate the effects of loss of transient receptor potential vanilloid receptor 1 (TRPV1) on the development of neovascularization in corneal stroma in mice. Blocking TRPV1 receptor did not affect VEGF-dependent neovascularization in cell culture. Lacking TRPV1 inhibited neovascularization in corneal stroma following cauterization. Immunohistochemistry showed that immunoreactivity for active form of TGFβ1 and VEGF was detected in subepithelial stroma at the site of cauterization in both genotypes of mice, but the immunoreactivity seemed less marked in mice lacking TRPV1. mRNA expression of VEGF and TGFβ1 in a mouse cornea was suppressed by the loss of TRPV1. TRPV1 gene ablation did not affect invasion of neutrophils and macrophage in a cauterized mouse cornea. Blocking TRPV1 signal does not affect angiogenic effects by HUVECs *in vitro*. TRPV1 signal is, however, involved in expression of angiogenic growth factors in a cauterized mouse cornea and is required for neovascularization in the corneal stroma *in vivo*.

1. Introduction

The cornea is a unique ocular tissue of avascularity and transparency for proper vision. It is susceptible to neovascularization-inducing intervention, that is, microbial infection or ocular surface damage. Such unfavorable neovascularization potentially impairs vision. The process of the new vessel formation in an injured cornea is orchestrated by a complex system of various growth factor signaling [1–5]. Resident corneal cells and inflammatory cells invaded to an injured tissue express growth factors and cytokines involved in injury-induced neovascularization. Such factors include vascular endothelial growth factor (VEGF), transforming growth factor β (TGFβ), and fibroblast growth factor (FGF) [6–10].

Members of the transient receptor potential (TRP) channel superfamily are polymodal receptors that are activated by a host of stimuli to mediate sensory transduction. The family is divided into 7 different subfamilies and composed of 28 different genes [11–14]. TRP vanilloid subtype 1 (TRPV1), the capsaicin receptor, is a nociceptor and one of the prototypes of TRPV subfamily. It elicits responses to a variety of noxious stimuli including chemical irritants besides capsaicin, inflammatory mediators, tissue injury, an alteration in pH, and moderate heat (≥43°C). TRPV1 activation leads to nociception and evokes pain or pain-related behaviors and reportedly induces release of tachykinin neuropeptides from sensory nerves, inducing neurogenic inflammation in the surrounding area [15–17]. Various nonneuronal cell linages, that is, epidermal keratinocyte or corneal epithelium and keratocytes, also express TRPV1, which presumably exerts a variety of biological responses to external stimuli [18–24]. We previously reported that lacking TRPV1 counteracted inflammatory and fibrogenic reactions in corneal stroma following an alkali burn [24]. The phenotype of less-inflammation/fibrosis was found to depend on the loss of keratocytes in the affected stroma, but not on inflammatory cells as revealed by reciprocal bone marrow transplantation experiments. Stromal neovascularization is also a component of the biological reaction observed in an injured cornea. In our previous study on an alkali-burned cornea, however, we failed to extract the effects of the loss of TRPV1 on injury-induced neovascularization in an alkali-burned cornea due to complex tissue reaction in the stroma. It was reported that capsiate and piperine, both TRPV1 agonists, suppress angiogenic behaviors of vascular endothelial cells cultured in the absence of inflammatory components *in vitro* [25, 26]. *In vivo* role of TRPV1 signal in modulation of neovascularization is to be assessed in *in vivo* condition. In the present study we examined the roles of TRPV1 signal in the activity of neovascularization development by using TRPV1-null (KO) mice and *in vitro* human umbilical vein endothelial cell (HUVEC) culture model of neovascularization.

2. Materials and Methods

In vivo experiments were approved by the DNA Recombination Experiment Committee and the Animal Care and Use Committee of Wakayama Medical University and performed in accordance with the Association for Research in Vision and Ophthalmology Statement for the Use of Animals in Ophthalmic and Vision Research.

2.1. Coculture Experiment of Tube-Like Structure Formation by HUVECs. We first employed *in vitro* assay of angiogenic activity of HUVECs. The degree of tube-like structure formation by HUVECs on a fibroblast feeder layer was employed to assess the effects of each agent on neovascularization activity of the cells. The detailed procedure was reported in our previous publications [8, 27]. HUVECs were seeded on the fibroblast feeder layer as the manufacture suggested (NV kit, Kurabo, Tokyo, Japan). Then the culture was maintained in the routine culture condition in the presence of vascular endothelial cell growth factor- (VEGF-) A (10.0 ng/ml, Kurabo, Tokyo, Japan) as an angiogenesis inducer in the presence or absence of a TRPV1 antagonist, SB366791 (10 μM, Sigma-Aldrich). HUVECs did not develop tube-like structure in the absence of VEGF (data not shown). Eight wells were prepared for each culture condition. After 11 days of culture the cells were processed for immunohistochemistry for CD31 (a marker for vascular endothelium) according to the manufacture's protocol. Color development was performed by 3,3'-diaminobentidine (DAB) reaction [8, 27]. Average length and the average number of bifurcations (the number of branching points) were counted in three central fields in each well in a blinded fashion by an investigator. The mean value of the data from these three fields represented the data of each well. Statistical analysis of the data from eight wells was conducted by employing Tukey-Kramer test and $p < 0.05$ was taken as significant.

2.2. Induction of Stromal Neovascularization by Cauterization of the Central Cornea in Mice. We then performed an *in vivo*

neovascularization assessment experiment by using a wild-type (WT) of C57Bl/6 ($n = 52$) or KO mouse of C57Bl/6 background ($n = 65$) as previously reported [8]. KO mice were healthy without any obvious general abnormalities and were fertile. There was no difference in the histological findings in an uninjured cornea between a WT and KO mice as previously reported [24]. Corneal stromal neovascularization from the limbal vessels was induced by cauterization of the central cornea of an eye of both WT and KO mice by disposable cauterization tool as previously reported [8].

We first observed the morphology of neovascularization at day 3 after cauterization in whole-mounted specimens by using CD34 immunostaining. Four WT and 4 KO mice were used. Mice were sacrificed at day 3 after cauterization in the central cornea by CO_2 asphyxia. The eye was enucleated, processed for whole-mounted immunostaining. The eyes were fixed in 4% paraformaldehyde for 48 hrs. After washing in phosphate-buffered saline (PBS), the specimens were treated in 0.5% Triton X for 1 hr to facilitate the antibody penetration into the tissue. After rinsing in PBS, the samples were allowed to react with a monoclonal anti-CD31 antibody (1 : 100 in PBS, Santa Cruz Biotechnology Inc., Santa Cruz, CA, USA) for 24 hrs at 4°C. After washing the antibody the tissues were then treated with a FITC-labeled secondary antibody (Southern Biotechnology, Birmingham, Alabama, USA) for 12 hrs at 4°C, mounted in Fluoromount-G after another wash in PBS, and observed under Carl Zeiss Apotome. 2 AxioVision 4.8 fluorescence microscopy.

We then examined the length of neovascularization from limbus toward the center of the cornea following cauterization in histological section. For this purpose, 15, 16, or 8 WT mice and 21, 21, or 10 KO mice were used for assessment at day 3, 7, or 14, respectively. Mice were sacrificed at days 3, 7, and 14 after cauterization in the central cornea by CO_2 asphyxia. The eye was enucleated, processed for cryosections, and used for immunohistochemistry for CD31 (monoclonal, 1 : 100 in PBS, Santa Cruz Biotechnology Inc.) as previously reported [28]. The length of corneal stromal neovascularization was measured as follows: length between limbus and the tip of neovascularization was measured in both sides of the limbus in three cryosections produced from one eye. The average value of the six data represented the neovascularization in one cornea. Statistical analysis was conducted with the use of Mann-Whitney U test, and $p < 0.05$ was taken as significant.

2.3. Immunohistochemistry. Cornea of three eyes of each genotype of mice was also cauterized and then processed for paraffin section immunohistochemistry for active form of TGFβ1, VEGF, substance P, and F4/80 macrophage antigen as previously reported. As described below we semiquantified mRNA expression of TGFβ1 in treated corneas and TGFβ1 exerts its action after processing to the active form. We therefore used an antibody that reacts the active, but not inactive, form of TGFβ1 in the current study [24, 29].

2.4. Gene Expression Analysis. We examined the expression of mRNAs of neovascularization-related growth factors and the degree of inflammation in *in vivo* mouse cornea. We considered mRNA level quantification was essential because our

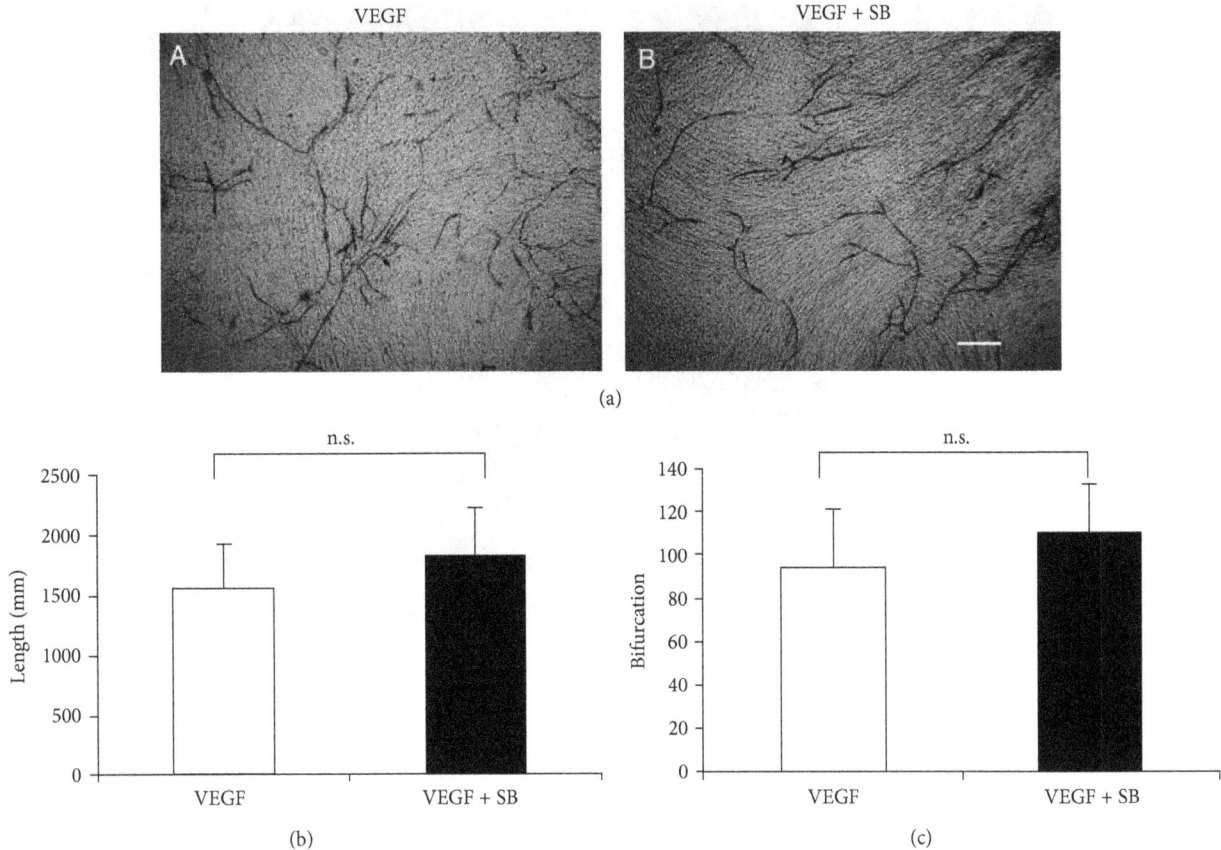

FIGURE 1: Tube-like structure formation by human umbilical vein endothelial cells (HUVECs). (a) The HUVEC culture on fibroblast feeder was processed for CD31 immunocytochemistry at day 11. In control vascular endothelial growth factor- (VEGF-) plus, culture HUVEC forms CD31-labeled tube-like tissue (A). VEGF action of tube-like structure formation is not affected by supplementation of a TRPV1 antagonist, SB366791 (10 μM) (B). Measurement of total length (b) and the number of branching points (c) of CD31-labeled structure coincide with the findings shown in frame (a). $^*p < 0.05$, bar, 1 mm.

preliminary immunohistochemistry for VEGF and TGFβ1 showed very faint staining with minimal difference of the staining in central corneal stroma between a WT and a KO mouse. Centrally cauterized cornea ($n = 6$ in each of WT or KO group) was excised at day 3. Total RNA was extracted from these tissues and processed for TaqMan real-time reverse transcription-polymerase chain reaction (RT-PCR) for VEGF, TGFβ1, myeloperoxidase (MPO) and F4/80 macrophage antigen and as previously reported [24]. Delta/delta CT method by Applied Biosystem Inc. was employed with the internal control of glyceraldehyde 3-phosphate dehydrogenase (GAPDH) expression. Primers (Applied Biosystem Inc.) used were described in the following list. Data were statistically analyzed by employing Mann-Whitney U test.

Primers Used (Applied Biosystem Inc.). Consider

vascular endothelial growth factor: Mm01281447_ml;

transforming growth factor β1: Mm03024053_ml;

substance P: Mm01166996_ml;

interleukin-6: Mm01210732_gl;

myeloperoxidase: Mm01298422_gl;

F4/80: Mm00802524_ml.

3. Results

3.1. In Vitro Experiment of Tube-Like Structure Formation by HUVECs. Dense CD31 immunoreactivity was detected in tissue where HUVECs formed a vessel-like tube structure. Without exogenous VEGF, HUVECs grown on the fibroblast feeder layer did not form a vessel-like tube tissue. The HUVEC culture was processed for CD31 immunocytochemistry at day 11 (Figure 1(a)). The angiogenic behaviors of HUVECs were evaluated by measurement of the mean total length of the structure (Figure 1(b)) and of the men number of bifurcations (Figure 1(c)) in randomly selected fields of the culture as described above. In the culture with VEGF-A (10 μg/ml) CD31-labeled tube-like structure was observed. Supplementation of a TRPV1 antagonist, SB366791 (10 μM), did not affect VEGF-A action on tube-like structure formation by HUVECs (Figure 1).

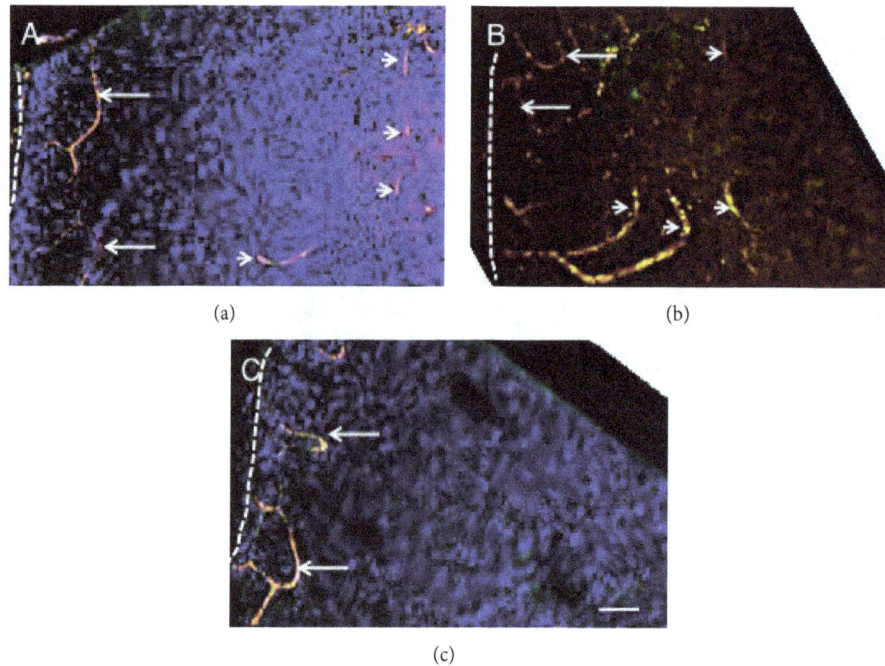

(a)

(b)

(c)

FIGURE 2: Neovascularization in corneal stroma as observed in whole-mounted specimens. We first observed the morphology of neovascularization in whole-mounted specimens by employing CD34 immunostaining. WT ((a), (b)) and KO (c) corneas at day 3 show loop-like distribution of blood limbal vasculature (arrows in (a), (b), and (c)). In WT corneas neovascularization was observed in the stroma apart from the limbus (arrowheads in (a) and (b)), although the staining procedure did not figure the continuous elongation of the vessels. Dotted lines, limbal corneoscleral border; bar, 100 μm.

3.2. Neovascularization in Corneal Stroma. We first observed the morphology of neovascularization in whole-mounted specimens by employing CD31 immunostaining. Figure 2 shows the morphology of limbal vasculature of WT and KO corneas at day 3. In both WT (Figures 2(a) and 2(b)) and KO (Figure 2(c)) corneas loop-like distributions of blood vessels were observed. In WT corneas neovascularization was observed in the stroma apart from the limbus, although the staining procedure did not figure the continuous elongation of the vessels (Figures 2(a) and 2(b)).

We then measured the length of neovascularization in the stroma in histology section. CD31 immunostaining was performed in cryosections of the mouse cornea (Figure 3(a)). In WT mouse corneas, development of the CD31-labeled neovascularization from the limbus in the corneal stroma was detected in the peripheral cornea as early as at day 3 (Figure 3(a)). The length of the neovascularization between the limbus (arrowheads) and the tip (arrows) of new vessels in the corneal stroma was measured at each timepoint.

The length of neovascularization was shorter in KO mice as compared with WT mice at day 3 and day 7, but not at day 14 (Figure 3(b)).

3.3. Expression of Inflammatory and Angiogenic Components in Centrally Cauterized Cornea. Immunohistochemistry showed that active forms of TGFβ1, VEGF, and substance P were not detected in untreated cornea of both genotypes of mice (not shown). Active form of TGFβ1 was detected in stroma just beneath the epithelium in the area of

cauterization at days 3 and 7 in WT mice (Figures 4(a) and 4(c)). Its immunoreactivity was quite less marked in cornea of KO mice (Figures 4(b) and 4(d)). VEGF was also not detected in uninjured corneas of both genotypes of mice. At day 1 after cauterization very faint VEGF immunoreactivity was observed in basal cells of corneal epithelia in cauterization area of both WT and KO mice (Figures 4(e) and 4(f)). At day 3 the basal epithelial cells with VEGF immunoreactivity were more frequently observed in a WT cornea as compared with a KO mouse (Figures 4(g) and 4(h)). Immunoreactivity for substance P was detected in basal layer of corneal epithelium with no obvious difference in intensity between WT and KO mice at days 1 and 3 (Figures 4(i), 4(j), 4(k), and 4(l)).

We then examined mRNA expression of VEGF and TGFβ1, the major two growth factors reportedly involved in corneal neovascularization in day 3 specimens by using real-time RT-PCR. Expression of mRNAs of both VEGF (Figure 5(a)) and TGFβ1 was significantly less in a KO cornea as compared with a WT cornea at day 3 (Figure 5(b)). TRPV1 signal is reportedly involved in expression of substance P and interleukin-6 (IL-6), both involved in local tissue inflammation. However, in the present study the loss of TRPV1 did not affect mRNA expression level of substance P (Figure 5(c)) and IL-6 (Figure 5(d)) in the centrally cauterized cornea at this timepoint.

3.4. Expression of Inflammatory Cell Markers in Centrally Cauterized Cornea. We previously reported that cauterization in the central cornea induced inflammation in the affected area

(a)

(b)

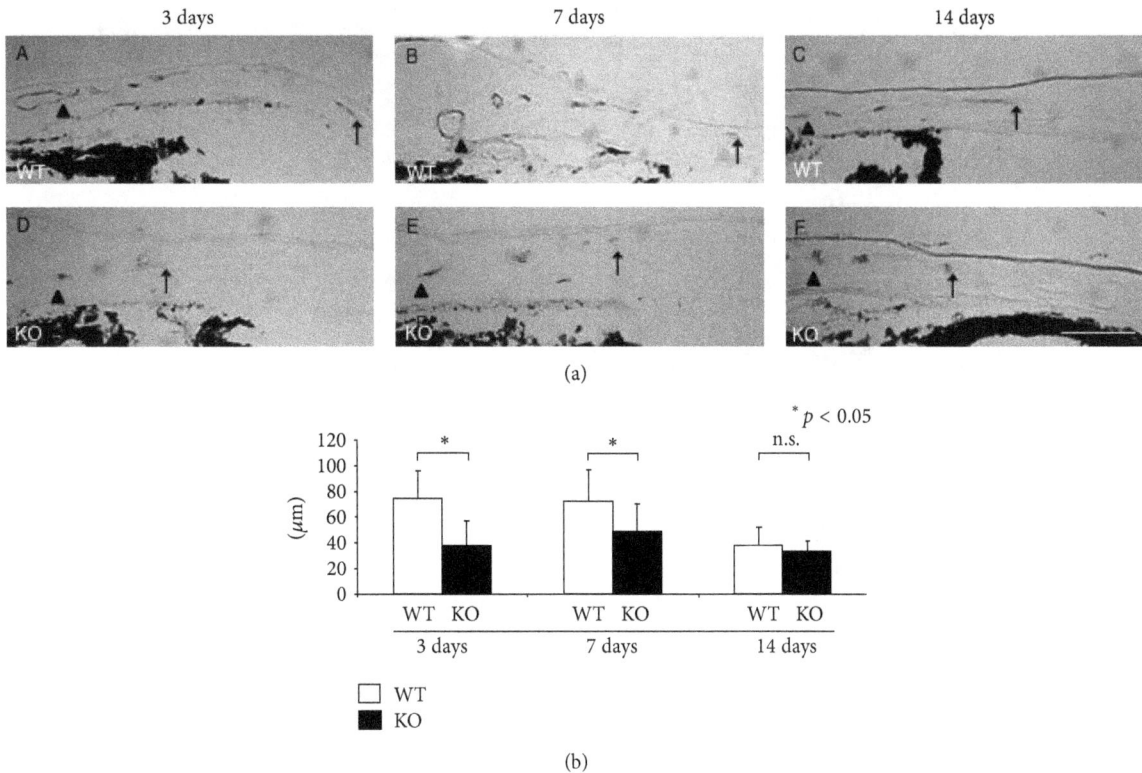

FIGURE 3: Neovascularization in corneal stroma in histology and evaluation of its length. (a) CD31 immunostaining was performed in cryosections of the mouse cornea. In WT mouse corneas, formation of CD31-labeled neovascularization (arrows) from the limbal vessels (arrowheads) in the corneal stroma was detected in the peripheral cornea at days 3 and 7. The length of the neovascularization was less in KO mice as compared with WT mice at day 3 and day 7 (b). $^*p < 0.05$; n.s.: not significant. Bar, 100 μm.

of tissues. We therefore first examined distribution of F4/80-labeled macrophages by using immunohistochemistry and saw difference of distribution of F4/80-labeled macrophages (Figure 6(a)). We then semiquantified the invasion of neutrophils and macrophages in tissues by conducting real-time RT-PCRs for mRNAs of MPO, a neutrophil marker, and F4/80. The loss of TRPV1 exhibited no remarkable effect on mRNA expression of these cell markers (Figures 6(b) and 6(c)).

4. Discussion

The present experiments first showed that lacking TRPV1 cation channel receptor suppressed stromal neovascularization in an *in vivo* mouse cornea following receiving a cauterization injury at the central cornea. Neovascularization was found to sprout from the loop-shaped vessels of the limbus toward the center of the corneal stroma in whole-mounted samples of WT tissues, while such neovascularization was much less in a KO cornea at day 3. The distance between limbus and the tip of the neovascularization in the stroma was significantly shorter in a KO cornea and compared with a WT mouse. Cell culture experiment showed that blockage of TRPV1 receptor did not affect VEGF angiogenic action on HUVECs. HUVECs do not reportedly express TRPV1 [26], and thus the present *in vivo* finding of less

angiogenesis observed in a KO cornea was not attributed to the direct effects of the loss of TRPV1 on vascular endothelial cells. Although various growth factors that potentially affect neovascularization activity are expressed in an injured cornea during tissue repair [29–32], expression of such components is reportedly modulated by ion channel receptor signaling, that is, signaling derived from TRP family members.

To analyze the mechanism of antiangiogenic effect of lacking TRPV1 in *in vivo* corneal stroma we conducted further experiments. Because TRPV1 signal is involved in inflammation in response to external stimuli, which potentially affect formation of neovascularization, we ran real-time RT-PCR for inflammatory/angiogenic growth factors and inflammation/wound healing-related components. The results showed that mRNA expression of VEGF and TGFβ1 in cauterized cornea was suppressed by lacking TRPV1, but expression of mRNA of IL-6 was not affected by the loss of TRPV1. Immunohistochemistry also showed that deposition of active form of TGFβ1 in the stroma beneath the regenerated epithelium and VEGF expression in the basal epithelial cells in the central cornea both seemed less in amount in a KO tissue as compared with a WT mouse. We reported that TGFβ1 is expressed in corneal epithelium and is deposited in stroma beneath the regenerated epithelium as an active form [33]. Thus, reduced accumulation of active form of TGFβ1 in the KO cornea might be attributable to the suppression

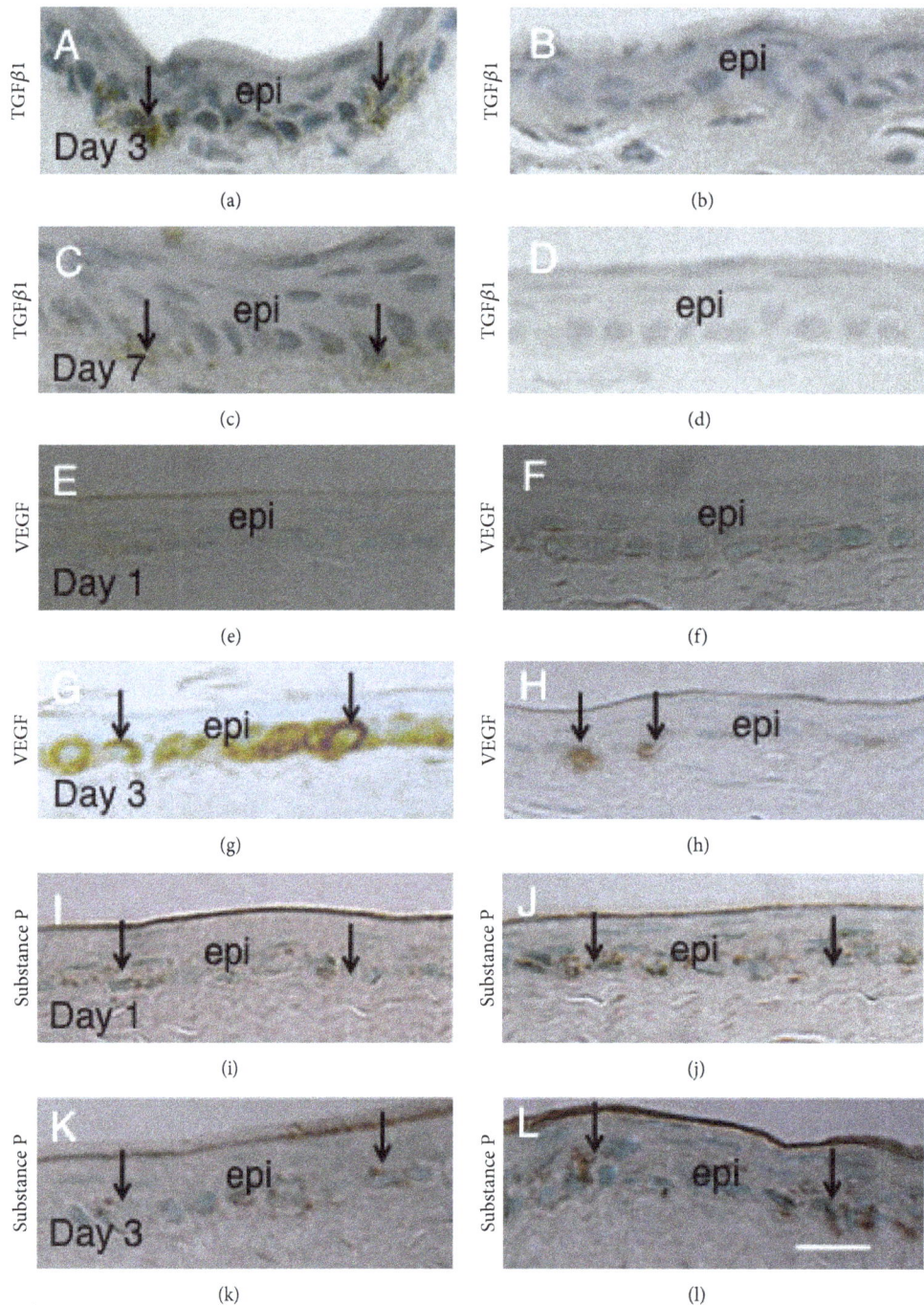

FIGURE 4: Immunohistochemical detection of angiogenic or inflammatory components in centrally cauterized cornea. Active form of TGFβ1 was detected in stroma just beneath the epithelium in the area of cauterization at days 3 and 7 in WT mice (arrows in (a) and (c)). Its immunoreactivity was quite less marked in cornea of KO mice ((b) and (d)). At day 1 after cauterization very faint VEGF immunoreactivity was observed in basal cells of corneal epithelia in cauterization area of both WT (e) and KO (f) mice. At day 3 the basal epithelial cell with VEGF immunoreactivity was more frequently observed in a WT cornea (e) as compared with a KO mouse (f). Immunoreactivity for substance P was detected in basal layer of corneal epithelium with no obvious difference in intensity between WT and KO mice at days 1 and 3 ((g)–(l)). Bar, 20 μm.

of TGFβ1 expression in epithelium after cauterization by the loss of TRPV1. Similarly, postcauterization VEGF expression in corneal epithelium was suppressed by lacking TRPV1. IL-6 was not detected by immunohistochemistry presumably because the protein might be secreted out from the cells.

We also examined the level of inflammation in cornea. Immunohistochemistry did not show difference of F4/80-labeled macrophage infiltration. We then ran semiquantification by real-time RT-PCR. The present assessment of inflammatory cell markers, that is, MPO and F4/40, indicated

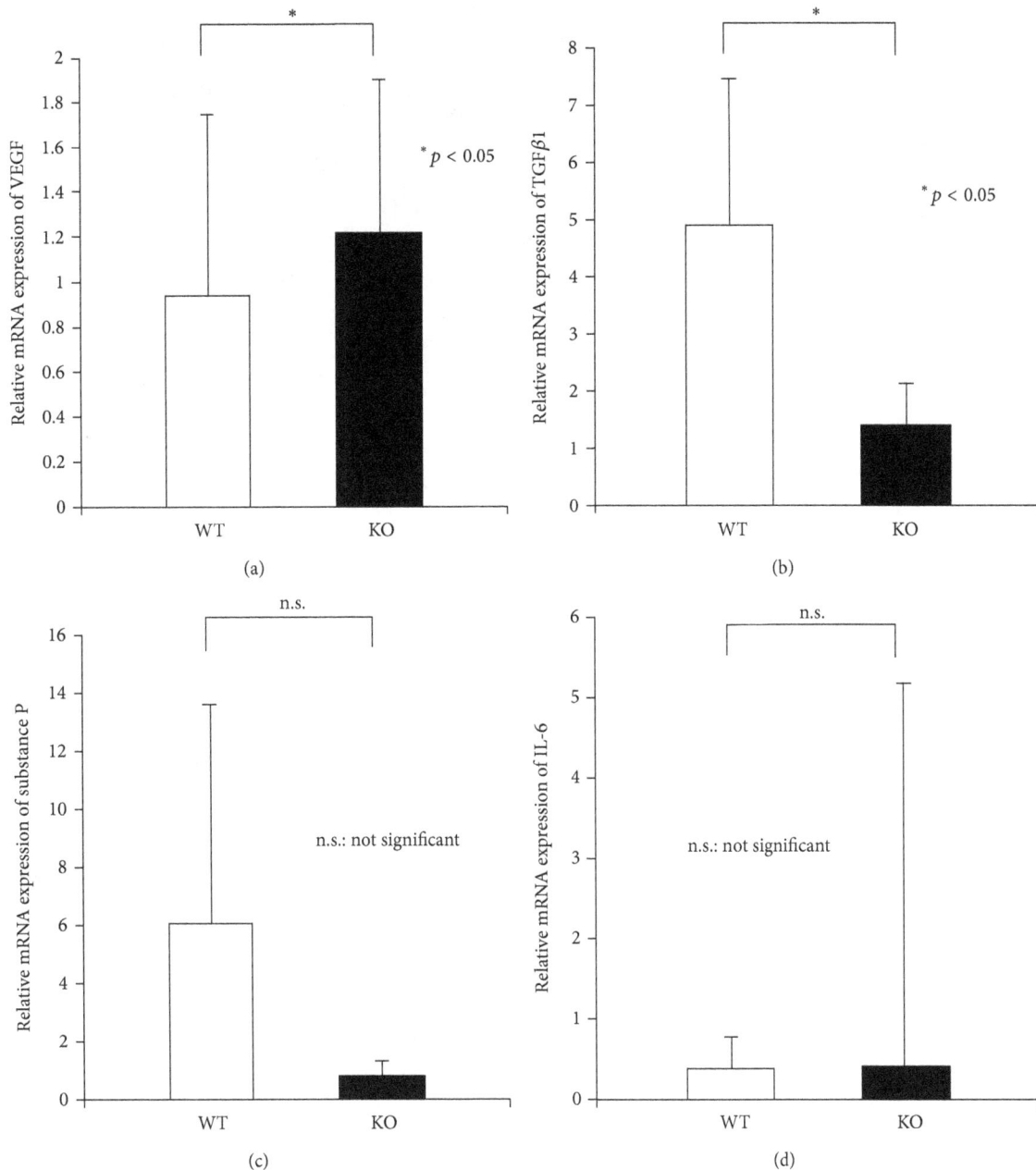

FIGURE 5: Expression of mRNAs of angiogenic or inflammatory components in centrally cauterized cornea at day 3. mRNA expression of vascular endothelial growth factor (VEGF, (a)) and transforming growth factor β1 (TGFβ1, (b)) mRNAs in the affected cornea of wild-type (WT) was more marked as compared with that in TRPV1-null (KO) mice at day 3 after cauterization. The loss of TRPV1 did not affect mRNA expression level of substance P (c) and IL-6 (d) in the centrally cauterized cornea at this timepoint. $^{*}p < 0.05$; n.s.: not significant.

that following cauterization in the central cornea the loss of TRPV1 did not affect infiltration of neutrophil leukocytes and macrophages. Data from these real-time RT-PCR results suggest that less expression of angiogenic growth factors, that is, VEGF and TGFβ1, is unattributed to the alteration of the level of inflammatory cell infiltration following cauterization in a KO tissue and presumably is dependent on the effects of lacking TRPV1 on the gene expression in resident corneal cells, that is, corneal epithelial cells. Involvement of keratocytes in the suppression of neovascularization in the KO mouse is to be further investigated. TRPV1 in sensory nerve

fibers reportedly mediates expression of neuroinflammatory mediators, for example, substance P [34, 35]. In the present study protein and mRNA expressions of substance P were similar in WT and KO corneas after cauterization.

In conclusion, blocking TRPV1 signal might be beneficial in suppression of neovascularization in cornea.

Disclosure

The abstract of the current study was presented by Dr. Tomoyose in the Annual Meeting of the Association for

(a)

(b)

(c)

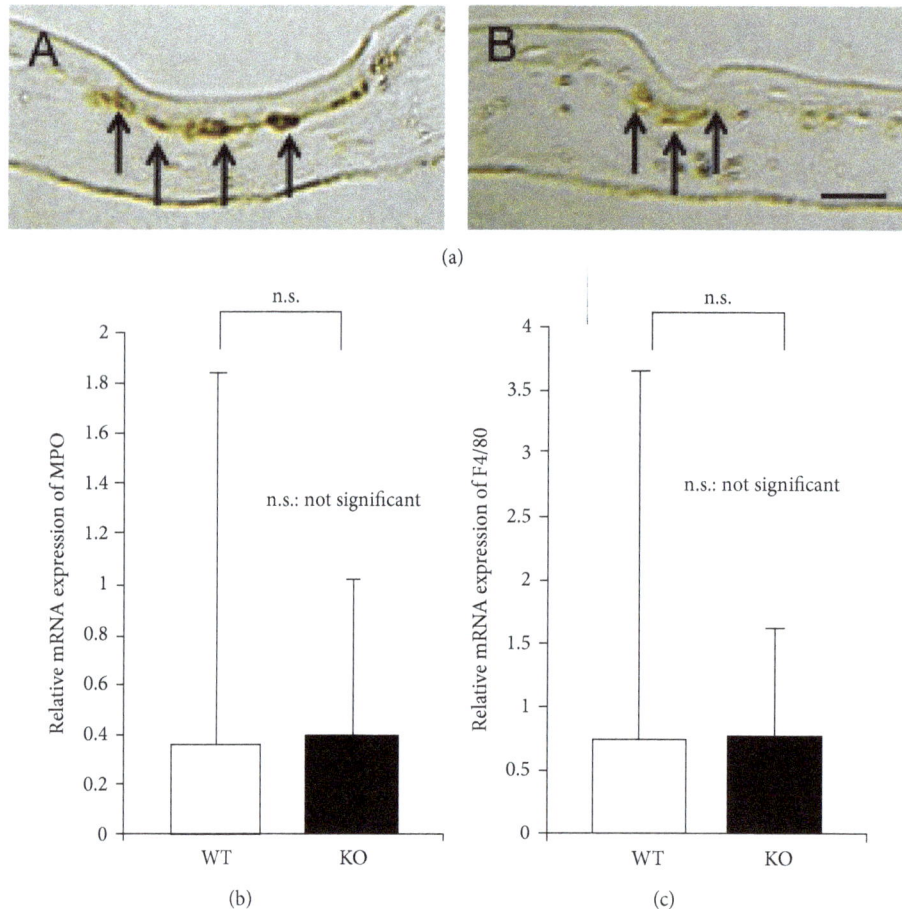

FIGURE 6: Inflammatory cells in centrally cauterized cornea of WT and KO mice. (a) Immunohistochemistry detected F4/80 labeled macrophages (arrows) beneath the epithelium in the central cornea of both WT (A) and KO (B) corneas at day 7. There is no difference in mRNA expression of myeloperoxidase (MPO), a neutrophil marker (b), and F4/80 macrophage antigen (c) between wild-type (WT) and TRPV1-null (KO) corneas at day 3 after cauterization. n.s.: not significant, bar, 50 μm.

Research in Vision and Ophthalmology (ARVO 2013, Seattle).

Conflict of Interests

The authors have declared that there is no conflict of interests regarding the paper.

Acknowledgment

This study was supported by grant from the Ministry of Education, Science, Sports and Culture of Japan (C40433362 to Takayoshi Sumioka, C21592241 to Yuka Okada, and C19592036 to Shizuya Saika).

References

[1] F. Bock, K. Maruyama, B. Regenfuss et al., "Novel anti(lymph) angiogenic treatment strategies for corneal and ocular surface diseases," Progress in Retinal and Eye Research, vol. 34, no. 1, pp. 89–124, 2013.

[2] J. L. Clements and R. Dana, "Inflammatory corneal neovascularization: etiopathogenesis," Seminars in Ophthalmology, vol. 26, no. 4-5, pp. 235–245, 2011.

[3] D. Meller, R. T. F. Pires, R. J. S. Mack et al., "Amniotic membrane transplantation for acute chemical or thermal burns," Ophthalmology, vol. 107, no. 5, pp. 980–989, 2000.

[4] S. Saika, O. Yamanaka, T. Sumioka et al., "Fibrotic disorders in the eye: targets of gene therapy," Progress in Retinal and Eye Research, vol. 27, no. 2, pp. 177–196, 2008.

[5] D. T. Azar, "Corneal angiogenic privilege: angiogenic and antiangiogenic factors in corneal avascularity, vasculogenesis, and wound healing (an American Ophthalmological Society Thesis)," Transactions of the American Ophthalmological Society, vol. 104, pp. 264–302, 2006.

[6] M. Papathanassiou, P. G. Theodossiadis, V. S. Liarakos, A. Rouvas, E. J. Giamarellos-Bourboulis, and I. A. Vergados, "Inhibition of corneal neovascularization by subconjunctival bevacizumab in an animal model," American Journal of Ophthalmology, vol. 145, no. 3, pp. 424.e1–431.e1, 2008.

[7] S. Saika, "TGFβ pathobiology in the eye," Laboratory Investigation, vol. 86, no. 2, pp. 106–115, 2006.

[8] S. Fujita, S. Saika, W. W.-Y. Kao et al., "Endogenous TNFα suppression of neovascularization in corneal stroma in mice,"

Investigative Ophthalmology and Visual Science, vol. 48, no. 7, pp. 3051–3055, 2007.

[9] W. Stevenson, S.-F. Cheng, M. H. Dastjerdi, G. Ferrari, and R. Dana, "Corneal neovascularization and the utility of topical VEGF inhibition: ranibizumab (Lucentis) Vs bevacizumab (Avastin)," *Ocular Surface*, vol. 10, no. 2, pp. 67–83, 2012.

[10] M. E. Francis, S. Uriel, and E. M. Brey, "Endothelial cell-matrix interactions in neovascularization," *Tissue Engineering Part B: Reviews*, vol. 14, no. 1, pp. 19–32, 2008.

[11] S. F. Pedersen, G. Owsianik, and B. Nilius, "TRP channels: an overview," *Cell Calcium*, vol. 38, no. 3-4, pp. 233–252, 2005.

[12] I. S. Ramsey, M. Delling, and D. E. Clapham, "An introduction to TRP channels," *Annual Review of Physiology*, vol. 68, pp. 619–647, 2006.

[13] G. Owsianik, K. Talavera, T. Voets, and B. Nilius, "Permeation and selectivity of TRP channels," *Annual Review of Physiology*, vol. 68, pp. 685–717, 2006.

[14] C. Montell, L. Birnbaumer, and V. Flockerzi, "The TRP channels, a remarkably functional family," *Cell*, vol. 108, no. 5, pp. 595–598, 2002.

[15] M. J. Caterina, M. A. Schumacher, M. Tominaga, T. A. Rosen, J. D. Levine, and D. Julius, "The capsaicin receptor: a heat-activated ion channel in the pain pathway," *Nature*, vol. 389, no. 6653, pp. 816–824, 1997.

[16] M. J. Caterina, A. Leffler, A. B. Malmberg et al., "Impaired nociception and pain sensation in mice lacking the capsaicin receptor," *Science*, vol. 288, no. 5464, pp. 306–313, 2000.

[17] J. B. Davis, J. Gray, M. J. Gunthorpe et al., "Vanilloid receptor-1 is essential for inflammatory thermal hyperalgesia," *Nature*, vol. 405, no. 6783, pp. 183–187, 2000.

[18] F. Zhang, H. Yang, Z. Wang et al., "Transient receptor potential vanilloid 1 activation induces inflammatory cytokine release in corneal epithelium through MAPK signaling," *Journal of Cellular Physiology*, vol. 213, no. 3, pp. 730–739, 2007.

[19] H. Yang, Z. Wang, J. E. Capó-Aponte, F. Zhang, Z. Pan, and P. S. Reinach, "Epidermal growth factor receptor transactivation by the cannabinoid receptor (CB1) and transient receptor potential vanilloid 1 (TRPV1) induces differential responses in corneal epithelial cells," *Experimental Eye Research*, vol. 91, no. 3, pp. 462–471, 2010.

[20] Z. Pan, Z. Wang, H. Yang, F. Zhang, and P. S. Reinach, "TRPV1 activation is required for hypertonicity-stimulated inflammatory cytokine release in human corneal epithelial cells," *Investigative Ophthalmology & Visual Science*, vol. 52, no. 1, pp. 485–493, 2011.

[21] Z. Wang, Y. Yang, H. Yang et al., "NF-κB feedback control of JNK1 activation modulates TRPV1-induced increases in IL-6 and IL-8 release by human corneal epithelial cells," *Molecular Vision*, vol. 17, pp. 3137–3146, 2011.

[22] Y. Yang, H. Yang, Z. Wang et al., "Cannabinoid receptor 1 suppresses transient receptor potential vanilloid 1-induced inflammatory responses to corneal injury," *Cellular Signalling*, vol. 25, no. 2, pp. 501–511, 2013.

[23] Y. M. Lee, S. M. Kang, and J. H. Chung, "The role of TRPV1 channel in aged human skin," *Journal of Dermatological Science*, vol. 65, no. 2, pp. 81–85, 2012.

[24] Y. Okada, P. S. Reinach, K. Shirai et al., "TRPV1 involvement in inflammatory tissue fibrosis in mice," *The American Journal of Pathology*, vol. 178, no. 6, pp. 2654–2664, 2011.

[25] B.-J. Pyun, S. Choi, Y. Lee et al., "Capsiate, a nonpungent capsaicin-like compound, inhibits angiogenesis and vascular permeability via a direct inhibition of Src kinase activity," *Cancer Research*, vol. 68, no. 1, pp. 227–235, 2008.

[26] C. D. Doucette, A. L. Hilchie, R. Liwski, and D. W. Hoskin, "Piperine, a dietary phytochemical, inhibits angiogenesis," *Journal of Nutritional Biochemistry*, vol. 24, no. 1, pp. 231–239, 2013.

[27] K. Fujita, T. Miyamoto, and S. Saika, "Sonic hedgehog: its expression in a healing cornea and its role in neovascularization," *Molecular Vision*, vol. 15, pp. 1036–1044, 2009.

[28] T. Sumioka, N. Fujita, A. Kitano, Y. Okada, and S. Saika, "Impaired angiogenic response in the cornea of mice lacking tenascin C," *Investigative Ophthalmology and Visual Science*, vol. 52, no. 5, pp. 2462–2467, 2011.

[29] S. Saika, T. Miyamoto, O. Yamanaka et al., "Therapeutic effect of topical administration of SN50, an inhibitor of nuclear factor-κB, in treatment of corneal alkali burns in mice," *The American Journal of Pathology*, vol. 166, no. 5, pp. 1393–1403, 2005.

[30] S. Saika, K. Ikeda, O. Yamanaka et al., "Therapeutic effects of adenoviral gene transfer of bone morphogenic protein-7 on a corneal alkali injury model in mice," *Laboratory Investigation*, vol. 85, no. 4, pp. 474–486, 2005.

[31] S. Saika, K. Ikeda, O. Yamanaka et al., "Expression of Smad7 in mouse eyes accelerates healing of corneal tissue after exposure to alkali," *The American Journal of Pathology*, vol. 166, no. 5, pp. 1405–1418, 2005.

[32] S. Saika, K. Ikeda, O. Yamanaka et al., "Loss of tumor necrosis factor α potentiates transforming growth factor β-mediated pathogenic tissue response during wound healing," *American Journal of Pathology*, vol. 168, no. 6, pp. 1848–1860, 2006.

[33] S. Saika, "TGF-β signal transduction in corneal wound healing as a therapeutic target," *Cornea*, vol. 23, no. 8, supplement, pp. S25–S30, 2004.

[34] M. A. Engel, M. Khalil, S. M. Mueller-Tribbensee et al., "The proximodistal aggravation of colitis depends on substance P released from TRPV1-expressing sensory neurons," *Journal of Gastroenterology*, vol. 47, no. 3, pp. 256–265, 2012.

[35] R. J. Steagall, A. L. Sipe, C. A. Williams, W. L. Joyner, and K. Singh, "Substance P release in response to cardiac ischemia from rat thoracic spinal dorsal horn is mediated by TRPV1," *Neuroscience*, vol. 214, pp. 106–119, 2012.

28

Blood Pressure and Heart Rate Variability to Detect Vascular Dysregulation in Glaucoma

Eva Charlotte Koch,[1] Johanna Staab,[1] Matthias Fuest,[1] Katharina Witt,[2] Andreas Voss,[2] and Niklas Plange[1]

[1]Department of Ophthalmology, RWTH Aachen University, Pauwelsstraße 30, 52072 Aachen, Germany
[2]Department of Medical Engineering and Biotechnology, Ernst-Abbe-Hochschule Jena, 07745 Jena, Germany

Correspondence should be addressed to Eva Charlotte Koch; eva.koch@rwth-aachen.de

Academic Editor: Gianluca Manni

Purpose. To investigate blood pressure and heart rate variability in patients with primary open-angle glaucoma (POAG) to detect disturbed blood pressure regulation. *Methods.* Thirty-one patients with POAG (mean age 68 ± 10 years) and 48 control subjects (mean age 66 ± 10 years) were included in a prospective study. Continuous blood pressure and heart rate were simultaneously and noninvasively recorded over 30 min (Glaucoscreen, aviant GmbH, Jena, Germany). Data were analyzed calculating univariate linear (time domain and frequency domain), nonlinear (Symbolic Dynamics, SD) and bivariate (Joint Symbolic Dynamics, JSD) indices. *Results.* Using nonlinear methods, glaucoma patients were separated with more parameters compared to linear methods. In POAG, nonlinear univariate indices (pW113 and pW120_Sys) were increased while the indices pTH10_Sys and pTH11_Sys reflect a reduction of dominant patterns. Bivariate indices (JSDdia29, JSDdia50, and JSDdia52; coupling between heart rate and diastolic blood pressure) were increased in POAG. The optimum set consisting of six parameters (JSDdia29, JSDdia58, pTH9_Sys, pW231, pW110_Sys and pW120_Sys) revealed a sensitivity of 83.3% and specificity of 80.6%. *Conclusions.* Nonlinear uni- and bivariate indices of continuous recordings of blood pressure and heart rate are altered in glaucoma. Abnormal blood pressure variability suggests disturbed autonomic regulation in patients with glaucoma.

1. Introduction

Glaucoma is a multifactorial chronic progressive disease, characterized by the loss of ganglion cells which leads to typical damage of the optic nerve and to visual field loss. The pathogenic concepts of glaucoma may be divided into a mechanical, pressure-related, and a vascular approach. It is well established that the main risk factor for glaucoma is individually elevated intraocular pressure. In addition, systemic vascular factors like arterial hypertension and hypotension, cardiovascular diseases, vasospasms, and others have been identified to play a significant role in the disease as well as impaired ocular blood flow [1–3].

In this context, disturbed vascular regulation may increase the susceptibility of the optic nerve and the ganglion cells to fluctuations in ocular perfusion pressure. Systemic blood pressure regulation and local mechanisms

(autoregulation) need to maintain ocular blood flow at a constant level despite changes in perfusion pressure [4, 5]. It has been shown that low ocular perfusion pressure is a risk factor for the prevalence of glaucoma. Abnormal perfusion and the following ischemia of the optic nerve are supposed to lead to glaucomatous damage [6, 7]. Disturbed autoregulation was observed in several studies in glaucoma [4, 8, 9]. The mechanisms may be related to primary vascular dysregulation, endothelial dysfunction, astrocyte activation, or increased intraocular pressure [7, 10]. In a previous study on 24 h blood pressure monitoring in glaucoma, an increased night-time blood pressure variability was found suggesting disturbed systemic blood pressure regulation [11].

The present prospective pilot study investigates the autonomic blood pressure regulation in patients with primary open-angle glaucoma (POAG) and controls. Systolic and diastolic blood pressure and heart rate variability was noninvasively and continuously assessed to characterize systemic vascular dysregulations using linear and nonlinear methods. The hypothesis is that POAG patients exhibit a different pattern of blood pressure and heart rate variability compared to controls as defined by using nonlinear analyzing methods.

2. Methods

Thirty-one patients with POAG and 48 age-matched controls were included in a prospective pilot study. All patients with POAG had a detailed ophthalmological examination; intraocular pressure was measured using Goldmann applanation tonometry. Patient's history was explored with special interest on cardiovascular risk factors (diagnosis of treated hypertension, arterial hypotension, history of cardiovascular events, nicotine abuse, and obesity). The systemic medications were recorded, but only the status of treated arterial hypertension was included in the analysis. Participants were recruited from the Department of Ophthalmology at the University of Aachen. Informed consent was obtained from all subjects. Adherence to the Declaration of Helsinki for research involving human subjects is confirmed. Ethics approval was granted by the committee of ethics at the University of Aachen.

To measure cardiovascular biosignals, blood pressure, and electrocardiogram, the diagnostic system "Glaucoscreen" (aviant GmbH, Jena, Germany) was used.

Synchronous ECG and blood pressure time series were continuously recorded over a period of 30 minutes in a lying position at rest using Glaucoscreen (aviant GmbH, Jena, Germany); see Figures 1 and 2. The method focusses on the detection of abnormal fluctuations of the cardiovascular system and the mechanisms of systemic autonomic regulation in patients without any physical activity. This system allows simultaneous and continuous multichannel registration of diastolic and systolic blood pressure and heart rate. Participants avoided activities that could alter the blood pressure or heart rate 30 min before examination. Nicotine or caffeine intake was not allowed on the day of the examination. For preparing the recording, at first electrodes were fixed on subject's body to record the electrocardiogram. For calibration, blood pressure was measured once before starting the recording using the upper arm. During the period of 30 minutes, blood pressure was measured continuously at two fingers, applying the noninvasive CNAP OEM Module (CNSystems Medizintechnik AG, Austria). The recording was started automatically controlled by the computer software. All recordings were performed under resting conditions (supine position, quiet environment, and the same location) and patients were instructed to lie calmly and to avoid speaking.

Systemic blood pressure variability (BPV) and heart rate variability (HRV) were analyzed offline (Ernst-Abbe-Hochschule Jena, Department of Medical Engineering and Biotechnology, Jena, Germany). For data preprocessing, the time series of successive beat-to-beat intervals (BBIs) and of systolic as well as diastolic pressure values were extracted.

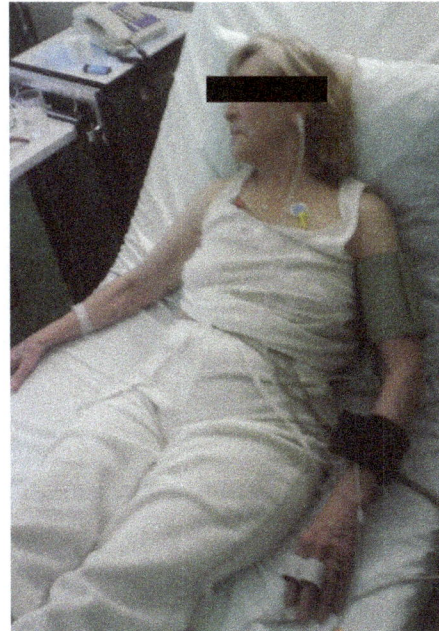

FIGURE 1: Simultaneous and continuous multichannel registration of diastolic and systolic blood pressure and heart rate in a lying position at rest.

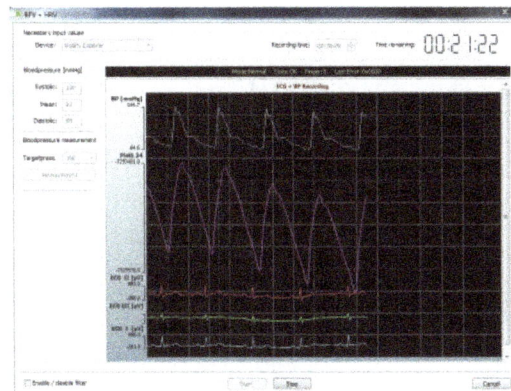

FIGURE 2: Synchronous ECG and blood pressure time series were continuously recorded and computer controlled.

HRV is the BBI length variability also called RR variability (where R represents the peak of the QRS complex of the ECG complex and RR is a time interval between two successive R peaks) whereas BPV represents the variability of successive systolic or diastolic blood pressure values corresponding to the related heart beats. In a further step, artefacts and/or ectopic beats and other disturbances (either R peaks recognized incorrectly or R peaks generated not in sinus rhythm) were detected within the RR time series and replaced (applying an adaptive filter) by interpolated "normal" beats to generate normal-to-normal (NN) beat time series representing normal sinus rhythm of the heart.

HRV and systolic and diastolic BPV standard parameters were calculated from time (Table 1) and frequency domain (Table 2) according to the Task Force of the European Society of Cardiology and the North American Society of Pacing and Voss et al. [12, 13].

TABLE 1: Description of parameters calculated by time domain analysis. Parameters were calculated for heart rate and systolic and diastolic blood pressure.

Method	Parameter	Description
Time domain	MEANNN	Mean value of all NN intervals
	SDNN	Standard deviation of all NN intervals
	CVNN	Coefficient of variation of all NN intervals
	SDANN1	Standard deviation of the averages of NN intervals in all 1-minute segments of the entire recording
	SDANN5	Standard deviation of the averages of NN intervals in all 5-minute segments of the entire recording
	SDANN10	Standard deviation of the averages of NN intervals in all 10-minute segments of the entire recording
	RMSSD	Square root of the mean squared differences of successive NN intervals
	PNN50	Proportion derived by dividing the number of interval differences of successive NN intervals greater than 50 ms by the total number of NN intervals
	PNN100	Proportion derived by dividing the number of interval differences of successive NN intervals greater than 100 ms by the total number of NN intervals
	PNN200	Proportion derived by dividing the number of interval differences of successive NN intervals greater than 200 ms by the total number of NN intervals
	PNNL10	Portion of NN interval differences <10 ms in all NN intervals
	PNNL20	Portion of NN interval differences <20 ms in all NN intervals
	PNNL30	Portion of NN interval differences <30 ms in all NN intervals
	PNNL50	Portion of NN interval differences <50 ms in all NN intervals
	RENYI2	Renyi entropy of the histogram with (order) alpha = 2
	RENYI4	Renyi entropy of the histogram with alpha = 4
	RENYI025	Renyi entropy of the histogram with alpha = 0.25
	SHANNON	Shannon entropy of the histogram

TABLE 2: Description of parameters calculated by frequency domain analysis. Parameters were calculated for heart rate and systolic and diastolic blood pressure.

Method	Parameter	Description
Frequency domain	ULF	Power (=variability) in "ultra low frequency" range (0–0.0033 Hz)
	VLF	Power (=variability) in "very low frequency" range (0.0033–0.04 Hz)
	LF	Power (=variability) in "low frequency" range (0.04–0.15 Hz)
	HF	Power (=variability) in "high frequency" range (0.15–0.4 Hz)
	XHF	Extended high frequency band from 0.15 to 0.6 Hz
	XF	Frequency band from 0.12 to 0.18 Hz
	P	Total power density spectra (variance of all NN intervals ≤0.4 Hz)
	LF/HF	Ratio of LF and HF
	LF/P	Ratio of LF and P
	HF/P	Ratio of HF and P
	XHF/PX	Ratio of XHF and the extended total power (variance of all NN intervals ≤0.6 Hz)
	VLF/P	Ratio of VLF and P
	ULF/P	Ratio of ULF and P
	(ULF + VLF + LF)/P	Ratio of (ULF + VLF + LF) and P
	(ULF + VLF)/P	Ratio of (ULF + VLF) and P
	UVLF	Sum of ULF, VLF, and LF (≤0.15 Hz)
	LFN	Normalized low frequency
	HFN	Normalized high frequency

In addition to these linear analysis methods, Symbolic Dynamics (SyD) and Joint Symbolic Dynamics (JSD), two nonlinear methods were applied in this study. Results of SyD analysis have been shown to be sufficient for the investigation of complex systems and describe dynamic aspects within time series. SyD is a nonlinear method which describes the global short- and long-term dynamics of beat-to-beat variability on the basis of symbolization and was introduced by Kurths and Voss et al. [14, 15]. The SyD method converts the NN interval time series into an alphabet of four predefined symbols (0, 1, 2, and 3) according to the transformation rules based on consecutive comparison of successive NN intervals.

The symbols "0" and "2" reflect slight deviations (<10% increase, resp., 10% decrease) from the mean NN interval, and the symbols "1" and "3" reflect stronger deviations (>10% increase, resp., 10% decrease) from the mean NN interval.

Then, the symbol strings are transformed into word series where each word consists of three successive symbols. This leads to a range of 64 different word types (xxx = 000, 001,..., 333). Then, estimates from the word distribution using the probability of occurrence (pWxxx) of each word type within NN interval time series are calculated (the summarized probability of all word types is normalized to 1).

On the basis of these word types, the number of all word types with a probability of occurrence of more than yyy percent (pTHyyy for HRV and _ pTHyyy _Sys/Dia for BPV) was separately counted (e.g., pTH13_Sys means the number of word types with a probability of occurrence greater than 13% in systolic blood pressure time series).

The SyD indices were all calculated for the heart rate and systolic and diastolic blood pressure time series.

The JSD (Figure 3) [16] is a bivariate method investigating interactions between BBI time series and systolic or diastolic time series. JSD was applied to quantify the short-term bivariate nonlinear behavior of the cardiovascular system. Similar to the SyD, JSD transforms BBIs, diastolic, and systolic blood pressure time series into symbol sequences of different words W according to the transformation rules using an alphabet $A = \{0, 1\}$. Thereby, symbol "1" represents increasing values (the actual value is greater than the previous one) and symbol "0" decreasing and unchanged values (the actual value is less than or equal to the previous one) applying a threshold level equal to zero.

Afterwards, short patterns (words of length consisting of 3 symbols) were formed ($k = 64$) in detail; see Figure 3.

The analysis method of JSD included the evaluation of 64 parameters for characterization of systolic blood pressure interaction with heart rate and 64 parameters for the interaction of diastolic blood pressure and heart rate.

2.1. Statistical Analysis. The analysis was performed on the basis of the HRV/BPV indices (time and frequency domain, methods from nonlinear dynamics). The nonparametric Mann-Whitney U test (SPSS 21) was applied for statistical analysis to figure out significant ($p < 0.05$) and highly significant ($p < 0.001$) parameters differentiating between patients with glaucoma and controls. For highly significant parameters, the multivariate stepwise discriminant function

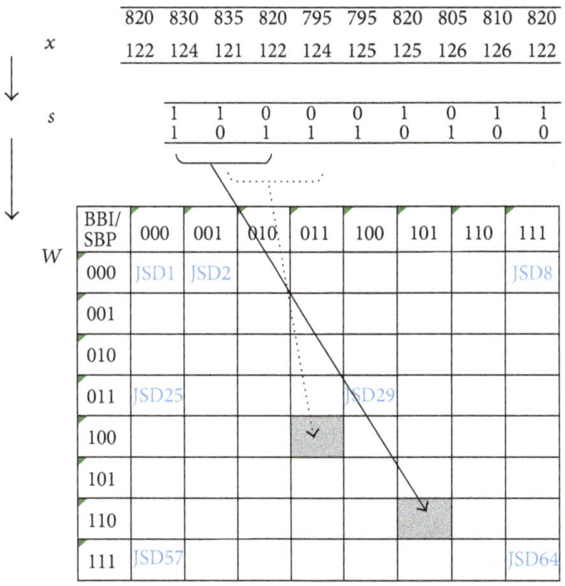

FIGURE 3: The method of Joint Symbolic Dynamics (JSD) quantifies the short-term bivariate nonlinear behavior (coupling) of blood pressure and heart rate. JSD transforms BBIs (beat-to-beat intervals) and diastolic or systolic blood pressure time series into symbol sequences of different words (3 successive symbols are one word) according to the pattern of change (increase or decrease) [14]. Top: x as time series of BBI (in ms) and systolic blood pressure values (in mmHg). Middle: s as symbol vector. Bottom: W as word type matrix with BBI (columns); SP, systolic blood pressure (rows). With JSD1...JSD64 as coupling indices.

analysis was performed to calculate the specific sensitivity and specificity and the area under the receiver operating characteristics (ROC) curve (AUC) applying the best set of six parameters.

3. Patients

Thirty-one patients with POAG and 48 age-matched volunteers were included in this prospective pilot study. Patients with POAG had a glaucomatous excavation of the optic disc and glaucomatous visual field defects as defined by the European Glaucoma Society [17]. The diagnostic criteria for glaucomatous visual field loss are as follows. Field loss was considered significant when (a) glaucoma hemifield test was abnormal, (b) 3 points were confirmed with $p < 0.05$ probability of being normal (one of which should have $p < 0.01$), not contiguous with the blind spot, or (c) corrected pattern standard deviation (CPSD) was abnormal with $p < 0.05$. All parameters were confirmed on two consecutive visual fields performed with Humphrey Field Analyzer. All patients with POAG had IOP values above 21 mmHg without treatment in their medical history. Visual field examinations were performed with the Humphrey Field Analyzer (Model 750, Humphrey-Zeiss, San Leandro, California, SITA program 24-2).

The control subjects did not have any ophthalmologic disease, showed IOP values below 22 mmHg, and did not

TABLE 3: Clinical data of patients with POAG and control subjects.

	POAG	Controls
Age (years)	68 ± 10	66 ± 10
Treated arterial hypertension	18/31	17/48
Diabetes mellitus	4/31	3/48
Cardiovascular or Cerebrovascular events	5/31	0/48
Adiposity (body mass index >30 kg/m^2)	1/31	9/48
Hypotonia/Raynaud's Phenomenon	5/31	0/48
Nicotine abuse	4/31	11/48

TABLE 4: Analysis methods and amount of significant parameter ($p < 0.05$) for controls versus POAG for each time series.

Time series and used analysis method	Amount of significant parameter controls versus POAG
Heart rate variability	
Time domain	0 out of 18
Frequency domain	1 out of 18
Symbolic Dynamics	5 out of 99
Systolic blood pressure	
Time domain	1 out of 18
Frequency domain	0 out of 18
Symbolic Dynamics	11 out of 99
Diastolic blood pressure	
Time domain	0 out of 18
Frequency domain	0 out of 18
Symbolic Dynamics	1 out of 99
Systolic JSD	1 out of 64
Diastolic JSD	7 out of 64

receive any topical treatment. Visual field examinations did not reveal any significant visual field loss. Visual field parameters (mean deviation (MD) and pattern SD (PSD), Humphrey Visual Field Analyzer) were within normal range and the glaucoma hemifield test was within normal limits. Healthy controls presented in funduscopy a normal optic nerve head appearance (no thinning or notching of neuroretinal rim, no bared circumlinear vessels, and no disc hemorrhages).

Volunteers and patients with POAG with an acute cardiovascular or cerebrovascular event within the last 6 months or with known heart rhythm disorders were excluded from this study.

Patients with glaucoma and controls were matched for age, sex, and treated arterial hypertension. All patients with glaucoma were on topical IOP lowering therapy that might influence the results.

4. Results

Thirty-one patients with POAG (mean age 66 ± 10 years; 17 men, 14 women) and 48 control subjects (mean age 68 ± 10 years; 24 men, 24 women) were included in this study.

Patients with POAG had on the right eye a mean IOD of 15 ± 3 mmHg (minimum 8 mmHg, maximum 36 mmHg) and on the left eye a mean IOD of 17 ± 5 mmHg (minimum 10 mmHg, maximum 33 mmHg). IOD of the healthy controls was never above 21 mmHg; mean IOD for the right eye was 15 ± 3 mmHg and for the left eye 14 ± 3 mmHg. All patients suffering from POAG were on topical IOP lowering medications. Seventeen patients used carbonic anhydrase inhibitors, 24 patients ß-blockers, 6 patients brimonidine, and 19 patients prostaglandins. Twenty-nine patients with POAG and 23 controls confirmed in their medical history treated arterial hypertension. The clinical data (systemic vascular risk factors by medical history) of both groups are shown in Table 3.

In the group of POAG, patients had a mean diastolic blood pressure of 89 ± 9 mmHg and a mean systolic blood pressure of 145 ± 17 mmHg. The controls showed a mean diastolic blood pressure of 86 ± 12 mmHg and a mean systolic blood pressure of 147 ± 17 mmHg. Mean heart rate in the group of POAG was 68 ± 10/min; healthy controls showed a mean heart rate of 67 ± 10/min. The mean as well as

standard deviation of the heart rate and diastolic and systolic blood pressure did not significantly differ between the two investigated groups.

Looking at the time series of heart rate and systolic blood pressure, more parameters belonging to the nonlinear analysis methods (SyD) were able to significantly separate control subjects and patients with POAG compared to the time series of diastolic blood pressure, where only one SyD parameter could separate the two groups significantly (Table 4).

Applying the method of JSD, more significant parameters were detected when analyzing the interaction of the time series diastolic blood pressure and heart rate compared to the interaction of time series systolic blood pressure and heart rate. The univariate indices pW113 and pW120_Sys (probability of occurrence of the specific word types: 113 for beat-to-beat intervals and 120 for systolic blood pressure) were increased in POAG. That means an increase of patterns with a valley-like behavior of heart rate patterns and an increase of systolic BPV patterns with a start of a plateau phase.

The univariate indices pTH10_Sys and pTH11_Sys (number of systolic BPV word types with a probability of occurrence higher than 10, resp., 11 percent) reflect a reduction of dominant patterns at the expense of an increased probability of occurrence of other word types (an increase of pTH3). That means that POAG exhibit a higher systolic BPV than controls.

Finally, the indices JSDdia29, JSDdia50, and JSDdia52 were increased in POAG. These indices characterize the coupling between heart rate and diastolic blood pressure. Interestingly all these indices may be found directly or in neighborhood to the word types representing diametric behavior (e.g., 011,100 or 110,001). These word types

TABLE 5: Significant parameters (p value, mean value, and standard deviation) separating controls versus patients with POAG according to time series and analysis methods.

Time series and analysis method	Significant parameters	Controls versus POAG	Controls		POAG	
			Mean	Std.	Mean	Std.
Heart rate						
Frequency domain	LFP	**4.81E − 02**	0.2025	0.0986	0.2534	0.1222
Heart rate						
	pW031	4.71E − 02	0.0001	0.0002	0.0001	0.0003
	pW113	**3.93E − 03**	0.0000	0.0001	0.0004	0.0016
Symbolic Dynamics	pW231	1.01E − 02	0.0001	0.0003	0.0003	0.0004
	pW310	3.45E − 02	0.0001	0.0002	0.0003	0.0006
Blood pressure systolic						
Time domain	renyi4_Sys	4.26E − 02	1.9573	0.4239	1.7789	0.4075
Blood pressure systolic						
	pW003_Sys	3.98E − 02	0.0006	0.0013	0.0012	0.0021
	pW011_Sys	2.00E − 02	0.0184	0.0082	0.0150	0.0073
	pW110_Sys	2.42E − 02	0.0181	0.0079	0.0150	0.0076
	pW120_Sys	**5.07E − 04**	0.0005	0.0010	0.0011	0.0015
	pTH3_Sys	4.20E − 02	7.3333	1.6417	8.0323	1.6829
Symbolic Dynamics	pTH8_Sys	1.13E − 02	3.1458	1.0717	2.5484	0.7229
	pTH9_Sys	1.59E − 02	2.8125	1.0033	2.2903	0.5287
	pTH10_Sys	**1.50E − 03**	2.5000	0.9453	2.0323	0.1796
	pTH11_Sys	**5.00E − 03**	2.3333	0.9070	1.8710	0.4995
	pTH12_Sys	1.51E − 02	2.1875	0.6410	1.8710	0.4995
	pTH13_Sys	4.71E − 02	2.1042	0.6601	1.8387	0.5829
Blood pressure diastolic						
Symbolic Dynamics	pW202_Dia	1.55E − 02	0.0212	0.0121	0.0280	0.0146
Joint Symbolic Dynamics systolic blood pressure, heart rate	JSD30	3.23E − 02	0.0116	0.0067	0.0141	0.0059
	JSDdia29	**9.74E − 03**	0.0283	0.0145	0.0417	0.0239
	JSDdia33	2.17E − 02	0.0183	0.0097	0.0130	0.0069
Joint Symbolic Dynamics diastolic blood pressure, heart rate	JSDdia37	3.58E − 02	0.0107	0.0112	0.0072	0.0044
	JSDdia50	**8.11E − 03**	0.0276	0.0145	0.0392	0.0217
	JSDdia52	**9.23E − 03**	0.0118	0.0085	0.0169	0.0111
	JSDdia53	2.49E − 02	0.0197	0.0136	0.0137	0.0087
	JSDdia58	2.62E − 02	0.0055	0.0040	0.0083	0.0055

demonstrate a behavior oppositional to the typical baroreflex response (e.g., 001,001 or 110,110).

Overall, only single linear indices from time and frequency domain analysis showed significant differences between groups. All significant parameters are shown in Tables 4 and 5.

The optimum set consisting of six parameters (JSDdia29, JSDdia58, pTH9_Sys, pW231, pW110_Sys, and pW120_Sys) revealed a sensitivity of 83.3%, a specificity of 80.6%, and an AUC of 82.3%.

5. Discussion

Ocular blood flow is an important factor in glaucomatous optic neuropathy and, together with ocular perfusion pressure, is directly affected by systemic blood pressure [3, 18]. The influence of systemic blood pressure on glaucomatous optic neuropathy has been investigated in several studies before [1, 11, 19, 20]. Systemic blood pressure has different fluctuation rhythms under physiological conditions. Systemic blood pressure has different fluctuation rhythms under physiological conditions, that is, seasonal variability with lower blood pressure values in winter times, short-time fluctuation patterns during day and night and the physiological night-time blood pressure depression [11]. There is evidence that excessive dipping could be associated with development or progression of glaucoma [21]. Sung et al. examined the relationship between 24 h mean ocular perfusion pressure and visual field progression in patients with normal tension glaucoma. In that retrospective study, 101 patients had at least a 4-year follow-up, and blood pressure and IOP were evaluated over 24 hours in each patient. Sung et al. showed that elevated 24 h mean arterial pressure and increased 24 h mean ocular perfusion pressure fluctuations were a significant risk factor for glaucoma progression [19].

Local blood flow of the optic nerve head is organized by autoregulation [22]. Autoregulation is the physiological phenomenon in which the resistance changes dynamically to keep blood flow at a constant level which is required by the local and metabolic activity despite changes in perfusion pressure. In healthy subjects, retinal blood flow is autoregulated to provide a constant blood flow regardless of changes in ocular perfusion pressure [4, 5]. Earlier studies have suggested that glaucoma patients show abnormal autoregulation especially in response to acute changes in ocular perfusion pressure [21, 22]. In glaucoma, autoregulatory dysfunction may be related to fluctuations in ocular perfusion pressure, via changes in either systemic blood pressure or intraocular pressure, leading to changes in retinal and optic nerve head perfusion [21, 23, 24]. The concept of altered ocular blood flow has been postulated to be a major component of glaucoma pathogenesis in normal tension glaucoma. However, disturbed blood flow has been found to be relevant in primary open-angle glaucoma also [3, 25–27].

In addition to the concept of autoregulation, systemic blood pressure and heart rate are influenced by systemic mechanisms of regulation. The concept of systemic vascular dysregulation in glaucoma affecting recurrent ischemic episodes of the optic nerve caused by an impaired capacity to compensate low perfusion pressures has been described before [10, 21]. The concept of disturbed blood flow regulation in glaucoma has been investigated in various studies using different approaches provoking the capability of systemic and local mechanisms of blood flow regulation. Stimuli such as carbon dioxide, oxygen, cold stress, isometric exercise, brachial arterial occlusion, or light flicker were used to examine blood flow regulation in patients with normal tension and primary open-angle glaucoma [9, 22, 28]. However, until today, no standard method to measure vascular dysregulation has been established. In contrast to provocation methods that focus on autoregulation of ocular blood flow, the concept of the present study is to quantify the extent of defective or abnormal systemic vascular regulation of blood pressure and heart rate without any stimulus given. Using this approach, the autonomic system may be characterized without any influence ab externo.

In our study, blood pressure and heart rate variability was noninvasively assessed to characterize systemic vascular dysregulation in glaucoma patients and controls. Nonlinear analyzing parameters of blood pressure and heart rate data were significantly different. The nonlinear model was designed to account for complex interactions of the continuously gained values characterizing systemic blood pressure and heart rate variability and dysregulation. In contrast, only singular linear indices from time and frequency domain showed significances. However, these indices could not contribute to the discrimination between glaucoma and controls in the same level as the nonlinear methods SyD and JSD. The optimum set consisting of 6 indices revealed a sensitivity of 83.3% and a specificity of 80.6%. Interestingly, in this set only, indices from nonlinear dynamics (Symbolic Dynamics) were included. In this context, we should emphasize that we do not believe that the identification of abnormal blood pressure or heart rate patterns would probably be a tool to identify glaucoma patients. But the measurement of systemic autonomic dysregulation might be an important method to identify patients with an increased risk for progression due to an impaired capacity of optic nerve head perfusion.

Methods of heart rate variability (HRV) and BPV based on nonlinear system theory and beat-to-beat dynamics have gained recent interest as they may reveal dedicated changes of autonomic regulations. These methods have been already used in other studies, investigating risk estimation for sudden cardiac death in patients with cardiomyopathy [15] or examining heart rate variability in normal pregnancy [16].

There are various types of different fractal scaling measures, complexity measures, power law analysis, measures of Symbolic Dynamics, turbulence, and acceleration/deceleration of heart rate and blood pressure and they have been studied in various patient populations [29, 30].

In this study, especially indices from SyD (univariate) and JSD (bivariate, coupling) exhibit significant impairments in the cardiovascular regulation in glaucoma patients. These results support the idea that glaucoma is not just a process involving the eye but may be a manifestation of a more generalized autonomic dysfunction that is in agreement with the findings of Brown et al. and others [31, 32]. Andrikopoulos et al. [33] summarized that PEX syndrome may be linked to impaired heart and blood vessels function, systemic and ocular blood flow changes, altered parasympathetic vascular control and baroreflex sensitivity, increased vascular resistance and decreased blood flow velocity, arterial endothelial dysfunction, high levels of plasma homocysteine, and arterial hypertension. These partly complex linked impairments might be a reason for the found coupling impairments in POAG in this study. In general, an increased blood pressure variability is associated with cardiovascular disorders [34]. An increased variability of systolic blood pressure represents also a strong predictor of early carotid atherosclerosis progression in general population [35]. In a 3-year follow-up study, progression of intima-media wall thickness was significantly greater in the patients with increased systolic BPV even after adjustment for other risk factors. Moreover, especially an increased daytime systemic BPV was associated with a greater risk of cardiovascular events [35]. We could confirm such an increased systemic BPV in this study. The reduced values of pTH10 and pTH11 (a lower number of dominating word types leading to a more broadly distributed variability) and the increased values of pWsys120 (representing an increased number of alternating patterns of the systolic blood pressure) are typical signs of an increased BPV. These patterns are related to an increased number of downregulations of the heart rate and to more temporal limitations of blood pressure increases. Both together might reflect an increased number of baroreflex activities to short-term down- regulated systolic blood pressure.

Even the sensitivity of baroreflex control of heart rate is depressed in glaucoma patients [31]; the number of tachycardic baroreflexes seems to be increased. Higher values of JSDdia29, JSDdia50, and JSDdia58 indicate enhanced occurrences of baroreflex regulations (couplings between diastolic blood pressure and heart rate) and, therefore, impaired short-term blood pressure regulation in glaucoma patients. Diastolic blood pressure variability and baroreflex characterize the short-term behavior of the cardiovascular system and are mainly determined by respiratory influences on the blood pressure and heart rate. Therefore, coupling analyses might uncover impairments of the autonomic blood pressure regulation [36].

However, it might be too early for this method for a more specific interpretation of the data. Further studies have to show if our pilot results can be reproduced in a larger scaled investigation. A major limiting factor of this prospective study is the possible influence of other systemic vascular diseases and topical and systemic medications possibly affecting ocular blood flow. A large controlled prospective study would be appropriate to investigate such confounding factors and to validate the results of this study. Secondly, this approach has to be investigated in patients with normal tension glaucoma as well, to learn if the same or other parameters will be found to be altered in these patients.

6. Conclusions

In conclusion, these alterations in blood pressure variability and coupling with heart rate suggest modified autonomic regulation due to a vascular dysfunction in patients suffering from glaucoma. The importance of the vascular influence for the pathogenesis of glaucoma is again emphasized by this study. Further studies need to show if the method is valuable to identify systemic autonomic dysfunction in glaucoma. Patients with systemic autonomic dysfunction might be at higher risk for progression of the disease due to a higher susceptibility of the optic nerve to fluctuations in intraocular pressure or ocular perfusion pressure.

Conflict of Interests

The authors declare that there is no conflict of interests regarding the publication of this paper.

References

[1] S. S. Hayreh, "Role of nocturnal arterial hypotension in the development of ocular manifestations of systemic arterial hypertension," *Current Opinion in Ophthalmology*, vol. 10, no. 6, pp. 474–482, 1999.

[2] O. Arend, N. Plange, W. E. Sponsel, and A. Remky, "Pathogenetic aspects of the glaucomatous optic neuropathy: fluorescein angiographic findings in patients with primary open angle glaucoma," *Brain Research Bulletin*, vol. 62, no. 6, pp. 517–524, 2004.

[3] N. Plange, M. Kaup, K. Huber, A. Remky, and O. Arend, "Fluorescein filling defects of the optic nerve head in normal tension glaucoma, primary open-angle glaucoma, ocular hypertension

and healthy controls," *Ophthalmic and Physiological Optics*, vol. 26, no. 1, pp. 26–32, 2006.

[4] C. E. Riva, S. H. Sinclair, and J. E. Grunwald, "Autoregulation of retinal circulation in response to decrease of perfusion pressure," *Investigative Ophthalmology and Visual Science*, vol. 21, no. 1, pp. 34–38, 1981.

[5] N. Plange, M. Kaup, A. Remky, and K. O. Arend, "Prolonged retinal arteriovenous passage time is correlated to ocular perfusion pressure in normal tension glaucoma," *Graefe's Archive for Clinical and Experimental Ophthalmology*, vol. 246, no. 8, pp. 1147–1152, 2008.

[6] U. J. M. Tielsch, J. Katz, A. Sommer, H. A. Quigley, and J. C. Javitt, "Hypertension, perfusion pressure, and primary open-angle glaucoma. A population-based assessment," *Archives of Ophthalmology*, vol. 113, no. 2, pp. 216–221, 1995.

[7] A. P. Cherecheanu, G. Garhofer, D. Schmidl, R. Werkmeister, and L. Schmetterer, "Ocular perfusion pressure and ocular blood flow in glaucoma," *Current Opinion in Pharmacology*, vol. 13, no. 1, pp. 36–42, 2013.

[8] J. E. Grunwald, C. A. Riva, R. A. Stone, E. U. Keates, and B. L. Petrig, "Retinal autoregulation in open-angle glaucoma," *Ophthalmology*, vol. 91, no. 12, pp. 1690–1694, 1984.

[9] N. Plange, M. Bienert, A. Harris, A. Remky, and K. O. Arend, "Color Doppler sonography of retrobulbar vessels and hypercapnia in normal tension glaucoma," *Ophthalmologe*, vol. 109, no. 3, pp. 250–256, 2012.

[10] D. Schmidl, G. Garhofer, and L. Schmetterer, "The complex interaction between ocular perfusion pressure and ocular blood flow—relevance for glaucoma," *Experimental Eye Research*, vol. 93, no. 2, pp. 141–155, 2011.

[11] N. Plange, M. Kaup, L. Daneljan, H. G. Predel, A. Remky, and O. Arend, "24-h blood pressure monitoring in normal tension glaucoma: night-time blood pressure variability," *Journal of Human Hypertension*, vol. 20, no. 2, pp. 137–142, 2006.

[12] American TFoTESoCaTN and Electrophysiology SoPa, "Heart rate variability; Standards of measurement, physiological interpretation, and clinical use," *European Heart Journal*, vol. 17, pp. 354–381, 1996.

[13] B. A. Voss, S. Schulz, R. Schroeder, M. Baumert, and P. Caminal, "Methods derived from nonlinear dynamics for analysing heart rate variability," *Philosophical Transactions of the Royal Society A: Mathematical, Physical and Engineering Sciences*, vol. 367, no. 1887, pp. 277–296, 2009.

[14] J. Kurths, A. Voss, P. Saparin, A. Witt, H. J. Kleiner, and N. Wessel, "Quantitative analysis of heart rate variability," *Chaos*, vol. 5, no. 1, pp. 88–94, 1995.

[15] A. Voss, J. Kurths, H. J. Kleiner et al., "The application of methods of non-linear dynamics for the improved and predictive recognition of patients threatened by sudden cardiac death," *Cardiovascular Research*, vol. 31, no. 3, pp. 419–433, 1996.

[16] M. Baumert, T. Walther, J. Hopfe, H. Stepan, R. Faber, and A. Voss, "Joint symbolic dynamic analysis of beat-to-beat interactions of heart rate and systolic blood pressure in normal pregnancy," *Medical & Biological Engineering & Computing*, vol. 40, no. 2, pp. 241–245, 2002.

[17] European Glaucoma Society, *Terminology and Guidelines for Glaucoma*, Editrice DOGMA, Savona, Italy, 2008.

[18] J. Flammer and S. Orgül, "Optic nerve blood-flow abnormalities in glaucoma," *Progress in Retinal and Eye Research*, vol. 17, no. 2, pp. 267–289, 1998.

[19] K. R. Sung, S. Lee, S. B. Park et al., "Twenty-four hour ocular perfusion pressure fluctuation and risk of normal-tension glaucoma progression," *Investigative Ophthalmology & Visual Science*, vol. 50, no. 11, pp. 5266–5274, 2009.

[20] G. Garhöfer, G. Fuchsjäger-Mayrl, C. Vass, B. Pemp, A. Hommer, and L. Schmetterer, "Retrobulbar blood flow velocities in open angle glaucoma and their association with mean arterial blood pressure," *Investigative Ophthalmology and Visual Science*, vol. 51, no. 12, pp. 6652–6657, 2010.

[21] V. P. Costa, A. Harris, D. Anderson et al., "Ocular perfusion pressure in glaucoma," *Acta Ophthalmologica*, vol. 92, no. 4, pp. e252–e266, 2014.

[22] S. T. Venkataraman, J. G. Flanagan, and C. Hudson, "Vascular reactivity of optic nerve head and retinal blood vessels in glaucoma—a review," *Microcirculation*, vol. 17, pp. 568–581, 2010.

[23] A. Harris, C. Jonescu-Cuypers, B. Martin, L. Kagemann, M. Zalish, and H. J. Garzozi, "Simultaneous management of blood flow and IOP in glaucoma," *Acta Ophthalmologica Scandinavica*, vol. 79, pp. 336–341, 2001.

[24] J. Flammer, K. Konieczka, and A. J. Flammer, "The primary vascular dysregulation syndrome: implications for eye diseases," *The EPMA Journal*, vol. 4, no. 1, article 14, 2013.

[25] L. A. Tobe, A. Harris, R. M. Hussain et al., "The role of retrobulbar and retinal circulation on optic nerve head and retinal nerve fibre layer structure in patients with open-angle glaucoma over an 18-month period," *British Journal of Ophthalmology*, vol. 99, no. 5, pp. 609–612, 2015.

[26] N. Plange, M. Bienert, A. Remky, and K. O. Arend, "Optic disc fluorescein leakage and intraocular pressure in primary open-angle glaucoma," *Current Eye Research*, vol. 37, no. 6, pp. 508–512, 2012.

[27] N. Plange, M. Kaup, O. Arend, and A. Remky, "Asymmetric visual field loss and retrobulbar haemodynamics in primary open-angle glaucoma," *Graefe's Archive for Clinical and Experimental Ophthalmology*, vol. 244, no. 8, pp. 978–983, 2006.

[28] J. Wierzbowska, S. Wojtkiewicz, A. Zbieć, R. Wierzbowski, A. Liebert, and R. Maniewski, "Prolonged postocclusive hyperemia response in patients with normal-tension glaucoma," *Medical Science Monitor*, vol. 20, pp. 2607–2616, 2014.

[29] A. Voss, H. Malberg, A. Schumann et al., "Baroreflex sensitivity, heart rate, and blood pressure variability in normal pregnancy," *The American Journal of Hypertension*, vol. 13, no. 11, pp. 1218–1225, 2000.

[30] A. Voss, R. Schroeder, S. Truebner, M. Goernig, H. R. Figulla, and A. Schirdewan, "Comparison of nonlinear methods symbolic dynamics, detrended fluctuation, and Poincaré plot analysis in risk stratification in patients with dilated cardiomyopathy," *Chaos*, vol. 17, no. 1, Article ID 015120, 2007.

[31] C. M. Brown, M. Dütsch, G. Michelson, B. Neundörfer, and M. J. Hilz, "Impaired cardiovascular responses to baroreflex stimulation in open-angle and normal-pressure glaucoma," *Clinical Science*, vol. 102, no. 6, pp. 623–630, 2002.

[32] Z. Visontai, B. Merisch, M. Kollai, and G. Holló, "Increase of carotid artery stiffness and decrease of baroreflex sensitivity in exfoliation syndrome and glaucoma," *British Journal of Ophthalmology*, vol. 90, no. 5, pp. 563–567, 2006.

[33] G. K. Andrikopoulos, D. K. Alexopoulos, and S. P. Gartaganis, "Pseudoexfoliation syndrome and cardiovascular diseases," *World Journal of Cardiology*, vol. 6, pp. 847–854, 2014.

[34] M. Jíra, E. Závodná, Z. Nováková, B. Fišer, and N. Honzíková, "Reproducibility of blood pressure and inter-beat interval variability in man," *Physiological Research*, vol. 59, supplement 1, pp. S113–S121, 2010.

[35] D. Sander, C. Kukla, J. Klingelhöfer, K. Winbeck, and B. Conrad, "Relationship between circadian blood pressure patterns and progression of early carotid atherosclerosis: a 3-year follow-up study," *Circulation*, vol. 102, no. 13, pp. 1536–1541, 2000.

[36] H. Malberg, R. Bauernschmitt, A. Voss et al., "Analysis of cardiovascular oscillations: a new approach to the early prediction of pre-eclampsia," *Chaos*, vol. 17, no. 1, Article ID 015113, 2007.

29

Accuracy of Intraocular Lens Power Formulas Involving 148 Eyes with Long Axial Lengths: A Retrospective Chart-Review Study

Chong Chen, Xian Xu, Yuyu Miao, Gaoxin Zheng, Yong Sun, and Xun Xu

Department of Ophthalmology, Shanghai Key Laboratory of Fundus Disease, Shanghai General Hospital Affiliated to Shanghai Jiao Tong University, Shanghai 200080, China

Correspondence should be addressed to Yong Sun; drsunyong@aliyun.com

Academic Editor: Kaevalin Lekhanont

Purpose. This study aims to compare the accuracy of intraocular lens power calculation formulas in eyes with long axial lengths from Chinese patients subjected to cataract surgery. *Methods.* A total of 148 eyes with an axial length of >26 mm from 148 patients who underwent phacoemulsification with intraocular lens implantation were included. The Haigis, Hoffer Q, Holladay 1, and SRK/T formulas were used to calculate the refractive power of the intraocular lenses and the postoperative estimated power. *Results.* Overall, the Haigis formula achieved the lowest level of median absolute error 1.025 D ($P < 0.01$ for Haigis versus each of the other formulas), followed by SRK/T formula (1.040 D). All formulas were least accurate when eyes were with axial length of >33 mm, and median absolute errors were significantly higher for those eyes than eyes with axial length = 26.01–30.00 mm. Absolute error was correlated with axial length for the SRK/T ($r = 0.212$, $P = 0.010$) and Hoffer Q ($r = 0.223$, $P = 0.007$) formulas. For axial lengths > 33 mm, eyes exhibited a postoperative hyperopic refractive error. *Conclusions.* The Haigis and SRK/T formulas may be more suitable for calculating intraocular lens power for eyes with axial lengths ranging from 26 to 33 mm. And for axial length over 33 mm, the Haigis formula could be more accurate.

1. Introduction

Myopia is a worldwide health concern, especially in East Asia [1, 2]. In urban areas of Asia, such as Singapore, China, Japan, and Korea, 80–90% of children who complete high school are myopic, and 10–20% have high myopia [3]. Similar trends are seen throughout the world, although they are generally less dramatic. In the United States, the prevalence of myopia, high myopia (−5.01 to −10.00 diopters [D]), and extremely high myopia (more than −10.00 D) are 46.4%, 3.2%, and 0.2%, respectively. Extremely high myopia is also very rare in Europe (1.2%) and Australia (0.3%) [4, 5].

Myopia is commonly defined as spherical equivalent (SE) more than −0.5 D, whereas the definition of high myopia is variable, with a cutoff range of −5.0 to −10.0 D [1]. Some authors [6] define extremely high myopia as an axial length (AL) of >27 mm and a refractive power of more than −10.0 D. However, other authors [7, 8] define extremely high myopia

as requiring the implantation of negative-power intraocular lenses (IOLs).

With advances in medical techniques, cataract surgeries are now refractive surgeries rather than rehabilitation surgeries. Thus, accurate IOL power calculations have become extremely important. It is generally accepted that most modern theoretical IOL formulas perform well for eyes of average axial myopia (22.0–24.5 mm) [9]. In cases of high or extremely high axial myopia, the postoperative refractive error may be greater because of difficulties in measuring the AL (the posterior staphyloma makes biometry more difficult) and problems associated with current IOL formulas [5].

In this study, we examined the postoperative refractive status of Chinese patients with an AL of >26 mm after phacoemulsification and IOL implantation, paying particular attention to patients with an AL of >33 mm. We compared the accuracy of several commonly used IOL formulas for predicting postoperative refractive error for individuals with high or extremely high axial myopia. Furthermore, we assessed correlations between AL and postoperative absolute error, which is the absolute value of the postoperative SE minus the predicted postoperative SE.

2. Methods

2.1. Study Design. This was a retrospective chart-review study. Data were obtained from patient charts and the IOLMaster-500 (Carl Zeiss Meditec, Jena, Germany) at the Shanghai General Hospital Affiliated to Shanghai Jiao Tong University (the National Key Discipline, Shanghai Medical Center for Vision Rehabilitation, Shanghai Eye Institute, Shanghai Key Laboratory of Ocular Fundus Diseases). The IOLMaster uses partial coherence interferometry technology for AL measurements; besides, the automated keratometry (K) and anterior chamber depth (ACD, corneal epithelium to lens) measurements allow rapid, noncontact, and accurate measurements of all the required parameters for IOL power calculation [10, 11].

Patient information was anonymized and deidentified prior to analysis. The study was approved by the Ethics Committee of the Shanghai General Hospital Affiliated to Shanghai Jiao Tong University and was conducted in accordance with the Declaration of Helsinki of the World Medical Association.

2.2. Participants. Medical records of patients who had undergone phacoemulsification and IOL implantation were reviewed. Patients with an AL of >26 mm (measured using the IOLMaster) were included in the study. In order to avoid duplication/compounding of data with bilateral eyes, only one eye from each study subject was included [12].

Patients were excluded if they had a previous ocular surgery, an eventful cataract surgery, keratoconus, endothelial dystrophy, uveitis, or glaucoma, were with grade IV or above cataract (Lens Opacities Classification System III, LOCS III), or were unable to measure the AL by IOLMaster.

2.3. Surgical Procedures. All surgeries were performed by one surgeon (Dr. YS) in the Ophthalmology Department of the General Hospital Affiliated to Shanghai Jiao Tong University. All surgical procedures were conducted under local infiltration anesthesia. A 3 mm wide incision was created in the superior corneal limbus. Phacoemulsification and IOL implantation were performed with continuous curvilinear capsulorhexis. The IOLs were Alcon Acrysofs (MA60MA/SA60AT, Alcon Laboratories, Ft. Worth, TX, USA) or AMO Sensars (AR40E/AR40e/AR40m, Abbott Medical Optics, Irvine, CA USA) with their corresponding optimization constants derived from the manufacturer. The lenses were implanted into the capsular bag.

2.4. Main Outcome Measures. An IOLMaster was used to measure the corneal curvature, ACD and AL. Four formulas were used to calculate the refractive power of the IOLs, as well as the estimated postoperative refraction of the eyes by

IOLMaster, namely the Haigis [13], Hoffer Q [14], Holladay 1 [15], and SRK/T [16] formulas.

The main assessed parameters were AL, K, refractive error (a negative difference implied that the postoperative refractive status was myopic, whereas a positive difference indicated hyperopia), median absolute error (MedAE), and the percentage of eyes with absolute errors within 0.5, 1.0, 2.0, or 3.0 D. Eyes were divided into four groups based on AL, which are across a range of 2.0 mm or 3.0 mm: Group A: AL = 26.01–28.00 mm, Group B: AL = 28.01–30.00 mm, Group C: AL = 30.01–33.00 mm, and Group D: AL = 33.01–36.00 mm.

2.5. Statistical Analyses. All statistical analyses were performed using SPSS software, version 22.0 (SPSS, Chicago, USA). Values were recorded as mean ± standard deviation (SD) or median (when data are not a Gaussian distribution) and a 95% confidence interval. A repeated-measures analysis of variance (ANOVA) was performed to assess the overall difference in absolute error among the four formulas and the effect of AL on absolute error in subgroup analyses. The Chi-square test was performed to assess differences between the percentages of eyes with absolute errors of different diopters. Post hoc tests adjusting for multiple comparisons were performed for pairwise comparisons between two formulas. The one-way ANOVA was performed to assess between-group differences in age and corneal power. Correlation between AL and absolute error was evaluated using linear regression analysis. P values < 0.05 were considered statistically significant.

3. Results

3.1. Study Population. A total of 148 eyes from 148 patients who were examined consecutively andmet the inclusion criteria were analyzed. All had undergone phacoemulsification and IOL implantation surgeries. Of the 148 patients, 78 (52.7%) were female. Patient ages ranged from 40 to 88 years (mean = 66.16 ± 10.37 years). The cataract grade ranged from I to III (LOCS III). In general, the study population had a broad range of anatomical variability, with ALs from 26.01 to 35.93 mm (mean = 29.03 ± 2.05 mm) and preoperative corneal curvatures from 39.94 to 47.88 D (mean = 44.15 ± 1.70 D).

For subgroup analyses, eyes were divided into four groups based on AL. There were 57 eyes in Group A, 48 eyes in Group B, 37 eyes in Group C, and 6 eyes in Group D. There were significant differences in age among the four groups (P = 0.017; one-way ANOVA). Patients in Group D were significantly younger than patients in Groups A and B (P = 0.015 and 0.029, resp.). Besides, there were no significant differences in corneal curvatures among groups (P = 0.195; one-way ANOVA). All eyes in Group D had significant posterior scleral staphyloma. Baseline characteristics of the study are summarized in Table 1.

3.2. Comparison of Formula Accuracy. For the main outcome of MedAE, the Haigis formula achieved the lowest error of 1.025 D (95% confidence interval = 1.297–1.816 D; P < 0.01 for Haigis versus each of the other formulas, Table 2 and

TABLE 1: Baseline characteristics of eyes included in the study.

AL (mm)	Eyes (number)	Patient age (yr)	Mean AL (mm)	Mean K (D)
Group A				
26.01–27.00	24	68.92 ± 10.15	26.39 ± 0.33	44.28 ± 1.92
27.01–28.00	33	67.67 ± 9.24	27.46 ± 0.32	44.06 ± 1.97
Subtotal	**57**	**68.19 ± 9.56**	**27.01 ± 0.63**	**44.15 ± 1.94**
P value[†]		**0.015***	**/**	**0.137**
Group B				
28.01–29.00	17	68.29 ± 11.85	28.54 ± 0.29	44.61 ± 1.84
29.01–30.00	31	66.58 ± 10.45	29.49 ± 0.24	44.39 ± 1.32
Subtotal	**48**	**67.19 ± 10.87**	**29.16 ± 0.53**	**44.47 ± 1.51**
P value[†]		**0.029***	**/**	**0.057**
Group C				
30.01–31.00	18	63.50 ± 10.55	30.45 ± 0.34	43.67 ± 1.70
31.01–32.00	13	64.92 ± 10.89	31.45 ± 0.30	44.17 ± 1.73
32.01–33.00	6	58.00 ± 9.83	32.61 ± 0.26	44.22 ± 0.86
Subtotal	**37**	**63.11 ± 10.47**	**31.15 ± 0.86**	**43.93 ± 1.59**
P value[†]		**0.210**	**/**	**0.244**
Group D				
33.01–36.00	6	57.50 ± 4.68	34.02 ± 1.09	43.07 ± 0.58
Subtotal	**6**	**57.50 ± 4.68**	**34.02 ± 1.09**	**43.07 ± 0.58**
Total	**148**	66.16 ± 10.37	29.03 ± 2.05	44.15 ± 1.70
P value[‡]		**0.017***	**/**	**0.195**

AL, axial length; K, keratometric reading; D, diopters.
[†]Compared with Group D (one-way ANOVA).
[‡]Compared among the four groups (one-way ANOVA).
* indicates $P < 0.05$.

TABLE 2: Absolute error (D) for each formula.

Formula	Median absolute error[†]	95% CI	Range	P value[‡]
Haigis	1.025	1.297–1.816	0.01–5.92	/
Hoffer Q	1.635	1.925–2.042	0.04–7.37	<0.001***
Holladay 1	1.435	1.610–2.149	0.04–6.87	<0.001***
SRK/T	1.040	1.479–2.042	0.04–6.61	0.002**

[†]Absolute error = actual postoperative spherical equivalent − predicted spherical equivalent.
[‡]Compared with results achieved using the Haigis formula (repeated-measures ANOVA).
D, diopters; CI, confidence interval.
** indicates $P < 0.01$; *** indicates $P < 0.001$.

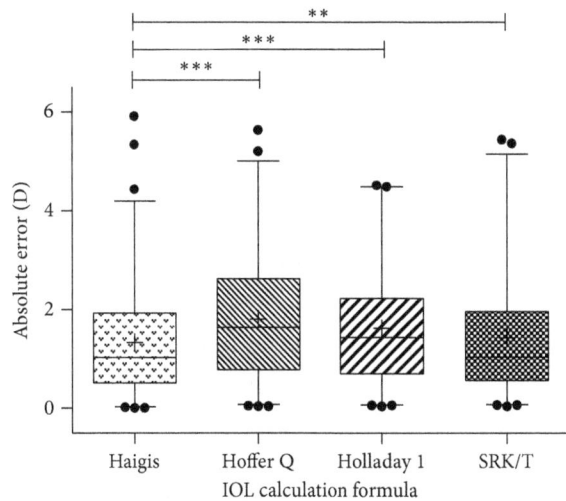

FIGURE 1: Comparisons of absolute errors in all eyes ($n = 148$). Absolute errors for the four intraocular lens (IOL) calculation formulas. The horizontal lines below and above the main box (whiskers) for each formula represent 2.5 and 97.5 percentile. The symbol + indicates mean absolute error, ** indicates $P < 0.01$, and *** indicates $P < 0.001$, as determined by a repeated-measures ANOVA test. D, diopters.

Figure 1). In addition, for eyes with absolute errors within 0.5 D of the target, all formulas performed similarly (around 20%), whereas 49.32% and 47.97% of eyes were within 1.0 D of the target using the Haigis and SRK/T formula—42% ∼ 52% more than the Hoffer Q formula (33.78%) and Holladay 1 formula (32.43%) ($P = 0.007$ and 0.003 for Haigis versus Hoffer Q and Holladay 1, resp.). These results were essentially consistent across all endpoints for 2.0-D and 3.0-D postoperative refractive thresholds (Table 3).

All four formulas were least accurate for eyes within Group D (Figure 2 and Table 4). The MedAE was significantly higher for Group D than for Groups A, B, and C ($P = 0.002$, 0.002, and 0.010, resp.; Table 4). Additionally, for Groups A, B, and C, Haigis and SRK/T formulas were more accurate in calculating the IOL power than the other two formulas ($P < 0.05$, repeated-measures ANOVA; Table 4), while there

TABLE 3: Percentages of eyes with different absolute errors at different refractive thresholds.

Formula	Percentages of eyes with indicated absolute error (P value[†])			
	<0.5 D	<1.0 D	<2.0 D	<3.0 D
Haigis	23.65%	49.32%	77.03%	91.89%
Hoffer Q	16.89% (0.148)	33.78% (0.007)	63.51% (0.011)	81.76% (0.010)
Holladay 1	18.24% (0.253)	32.43% (0.003)	68.24% (0.090)	87.16% (0.184)
SRK/T	19.60% (0.397)	47.97% (0.816)	76.35% (0.891)	89.86% (0.545)

[†]Compared with results achieved using the Haigis formula (Chi-square test). D, diopters.

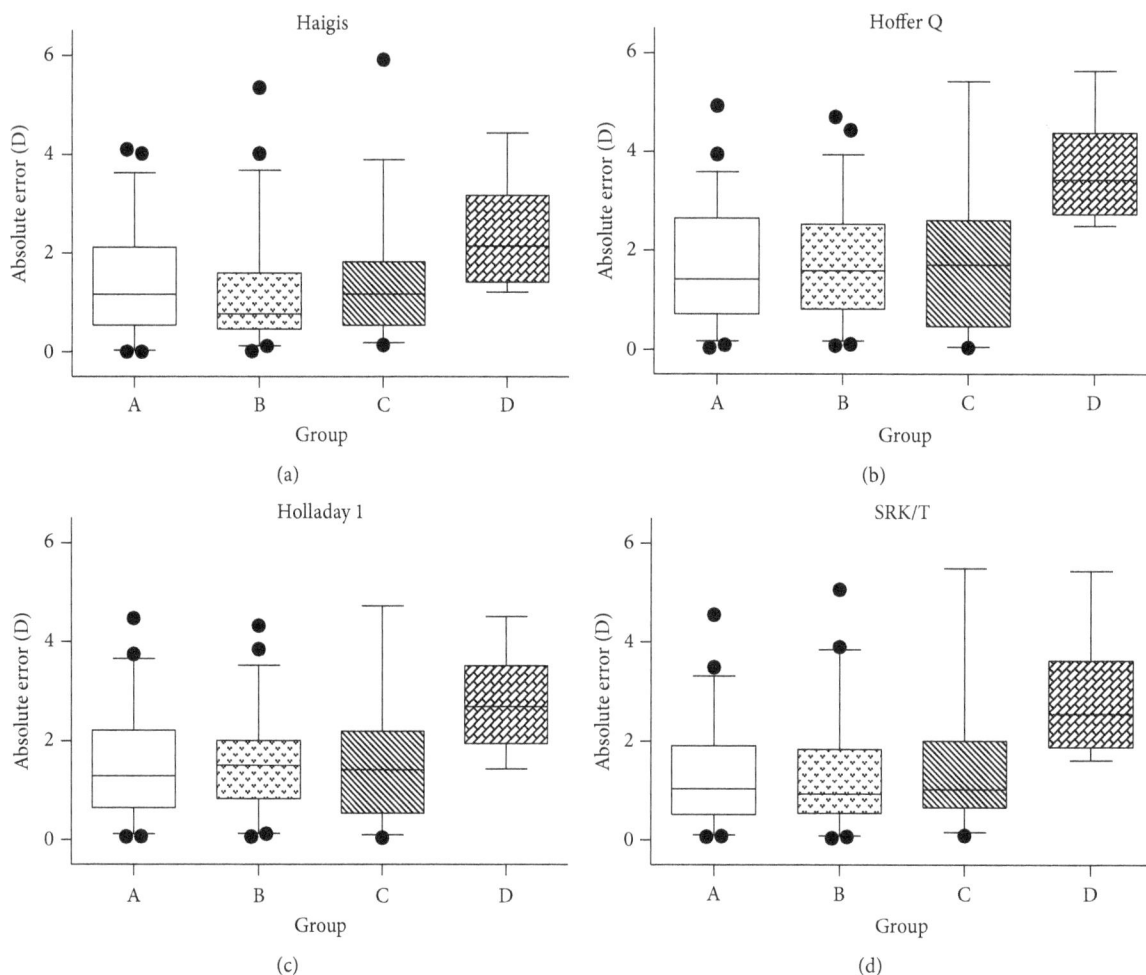

FIGURE 2: Subgroup analysis: absolute errors for Groups A–D calculated using the four IOL formulas. All four formulas were least accurate for eyes within Group D. The overall median absolute error was significantly higher for Group D than for Groups A, B, and C ($P = 0.002$, 0.002 and 0.010, resp., as determined by a repeated-measures ANOVA test). The whiskers indicate 5 and 95 percentile of absolute errors in each group. D, diopters.

were no significant differences between Haigis and SRK/T formulas ($P > 0.05$). However, for Group D, Haigis was more accurate than each of the other formula ($P < 0.01$). Three months after the operation, all the six eyes in Group D were hyperopic, for which the IOL power was calculated using the four formulas.

3.3. Correlation between AL and Absolute Error. To determine whether AL correlates with postoperative refractive outcome, the correlation between AL and absolute error was evaluated using linear regression analysis. Absolute error was associated with AL when the Hoffer Q or SRK/T formulas were used (SRK/T: Pearson correlation $r = 0.212$, $P = 0.010$; Hoffer Q: $r = 0.223$, $P = 0.007$; Figures 3(a) and 3(b)). None of the other formulas revealed significant associations between AL and absolute error (Holladay 1: $r = 0.150$ and $P = 0.070$; Haigis: $r = 0.106$ and $P = 0.198$). When we focused on data from Group D, much stronger associations between

TABLE 4: Median absolute errors (D) calculated by each formula for Groups A–D.

Formula	Group A (n = 57)	Group B (n = 48)	Group C (n = 37)	Group D (n = 6)
Haigis	1.080	0.805	1.160	2.145
Hoffer Q	1.420	1.635	1.710	3.430
Holladay	1.290	1.530	1.410	2.695
SRK/T	1.040	0.975	0.990	2.555
P-value[†]	0.002	0.002	0.010	/

[†]Compared with the results achieved with Group D (repeated-measures ANOVA).
Group A: AL = 26.01–28.00 mm, Group B: AL = 28.01–30.00 mm, Group C: AL = 30.01–33.00 mm, and Group D: AL = 33.01–36.00 mm.
D, diopters.

AL and absolute error were found (SRK/T: r = 0.926 and P = 0.008; Hoffer Q: r = 0.928 and P = 0.008; Figures 3(c) and 3(d)).

4. Discussion

Refractive status is a complex variable determined by the optical power of the cornea and the lens and the AL of the eye (with its component parts ACD, lens thickness, and vitreous chamber depth) [3]. Although there is no clear definition of extremely high axial myopia, it is well established that the higher the refractive power and the longer the AL are, the more significant the deviation in AL measurement and the refractive power of the IOL calculation will be [17, 18].

The widespread application of phacoemulsification and IOL implantation cataract surgery has led to improved surgical techniques and fewer surgical complications. Thus, the postoperative refractive status is less affected by surgical factors than it has been in the past. Accuracy of the IOL power calculation is now the most important factor affecting the postoperative refractive status. Moreover, the choice of IOL formula is closely related to the accuracy of IOL power calculation.

In 1990, Sanders et al. [19] reported that the SRK/T formula is marginally better for eyes with high axial myopia. That study, however, included very few eyes with an AL of ≥28.4 mm, because among these patients from Europe and America the proportion of eyes with an AL of >27 mm or >28.4 mm was only 1.0% or 0.1%, respectively. However, China has a very high percentage of people with a long AL and extremely high axial myopia [3].

During the past decade, relationships between eyes with a long AL and postoperative refractive error have been examined in a range of ethnicities [18, 20–25]. These analyses did not, however, produce a consensus concerning the most accurate formula in predicting postoperative refractive error in long eyes. Importantly, the eyes evaluated rarely had an AL of >30 mm.

Our study found that, overall, the Haigis formula resulted in the lowest MedAE (1.025 D) in high and extremely high myopic Chinese eyes with an AL of >26 mm (mean AL = 29.02 mm). The SRK/T formula generated the second most accurate results (1.040 D), whereas the Hoffer Q was the least

accurate in all subgroups. The Haigis formula is a fourth-generation formula and may have performed better in highly myopic eyes because it uses three constants, a_0, a_1, and a_2, to predict the effective lens position (ELP), where ELP = a_0 + ($a_1 \times$ ACD$_{preoperative}$) + ($a_2 \times$ AL). Third-generation formulas, such as Hoffer Q, Holladay 1, and SRK/T, rely on AL and central corneal power to calculate the ELP without actually measuring the ACD. This approach may be less accurate for short or long eyes [13, 18].

We further illustrated that longer ocular ALs are associated with less-accurate predictions of postoperative refractive status, especially for eyes with an AL of >33 mm. We draw this conclusion from the regression equations shown in Figure 3. For the SRK/T and Hoffer Q formulas, a 1 mm increase in AL resulted in an absolute error increase of ~0.1 D (for AL > 26 mm). For eyes with an AL of >33 mm, however, a 1 mm increase in AL resulted in an absolute error increase of 1.15 D for SRK/T and 0.94 D for Hoffer Q.

In addition, our results confirmed earlier findings that the implantation of low-power IOLs (including negatively powered IOLs) into highly myopic eyes resulted in hyperopic refractive errors [17, 18, 20, 26–29]. We found that most eyes with an AL of >33 mm presented with postoperative hyperopia of +2.0 D to +3.0 D. Haigis [5, 17] indicated that plus-IOLs and minus-IOLs should be characterized by different sets of IOL constants. It has recently been demonstrated that AL-dependent hyperopic refractive errors are primarily caused by the use of positive-power IOL constants for both positive-power and negative-power IOLs [17].

We recommend that, for eyes with extremely long ALs, preservation of postoperative myopia of −2.0 to −3.0 D (or more) should be a preoperative consideration when calculating the refractive power of the implanted IOLs. This is consistent with the near-sighted lifestyle of patients and can reduce the possibility of postoperative hyperopia resulting from errors associated with AL measurement and current IOL formulas. Furthermore, extremely long ALs are often associated with fundus lesions, which reduce distance vision. As distance vision for these patients is probably critically reduced, trying to improve postoperative near vision may represent a good option.

5. Conclusions

Our findings suggest that the Haigis and SRK/T formulas perform better for calculating the IOL power for Chinese patients whose eyes have an AL ranging within 26~33 mm (MedAEs ~ 1.0 D; Table 4). Therefore, to achieve a target refraction of −3.00 D in Chinese eyes with an AL of 26.01–33.00 mm, we suggest setting a postoperative target around −4.00 D, using Haigis or SRK/T formulas. In addition, the Haigis may be the best formula for eyes with an AL of >33 mm; however, the postoperative absolute error increased to ~2.0 D even when using the Haigis formula (Table 4). Hence, for eyes with an AL of 33.00–36.00 mm, we recommend setting a postoperative target around −5.00 D using Haigis formula. Selecting higher IOL powers is often preferred, leaving the patient slightly myopic rather than hyperopic.

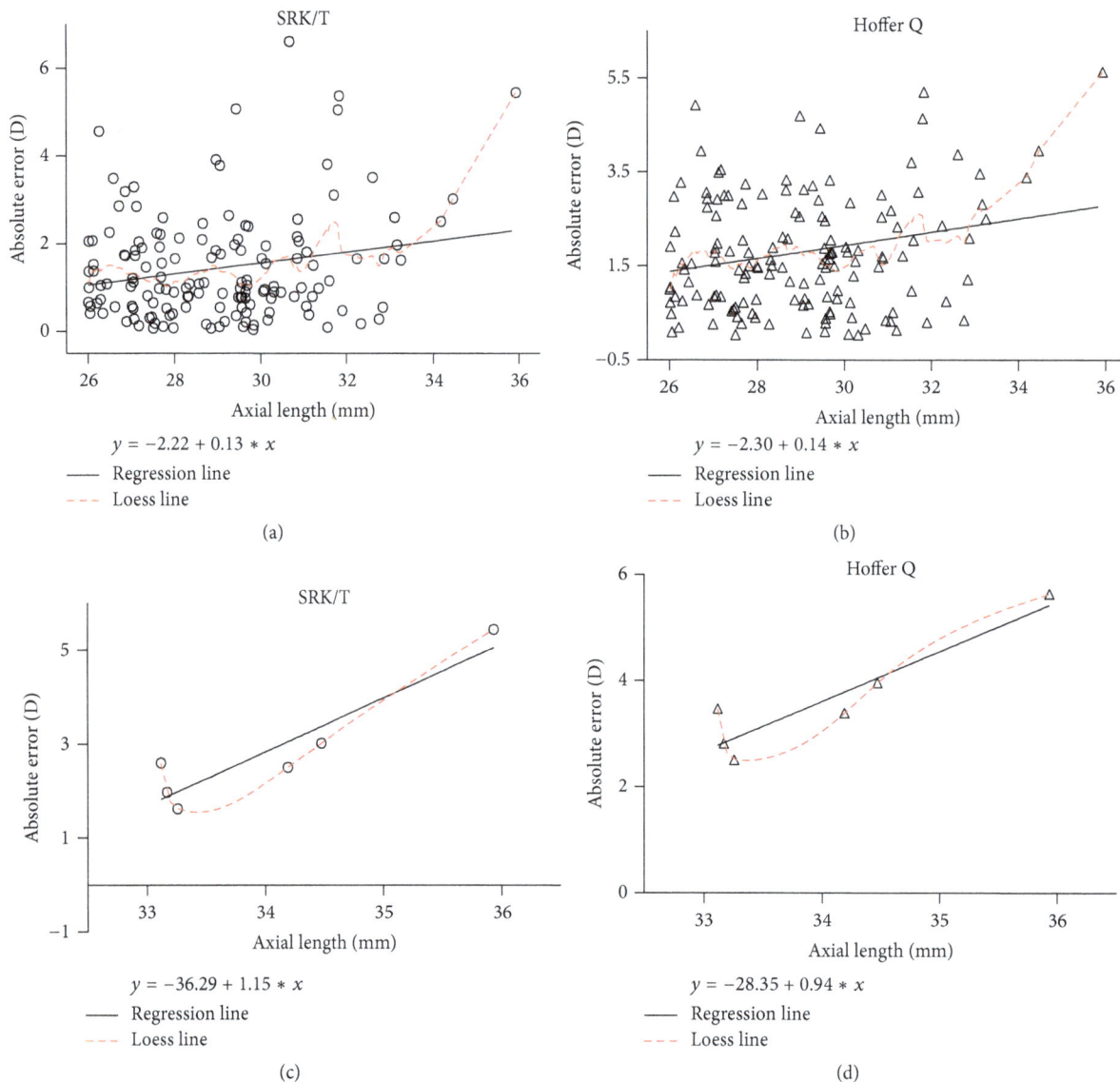

FIGURE 3: Correlations between axial length and absolute error. The associations between axial length and absolute error were analyzed using absolute errors derived from (a) the SRK/T formula ($r = 0.212$; $P = 0.010$; regression equation: $y = -2.22 + 0.13x$) and (b) the Hoffer Q formula ($r = 0.223$; $P = 0.007$; regression equation: $y = -2.30 + 0.14x$). Similar analyses were carried out with Group D data only using (c) the SRK/T formula ($r = 0.926$; $P = 0.008$; regression equation: $y = -36.29 + 1.15x$) and (d) the Hoffer Q formula ($r = 0.928$; $P = 0.008$; regression equation: $y = -28.35 + 0.94x$).

Further studies using other IOL calculating formulas should be conducted to compare the accuracy for extremely high axial myopia [10], and predictive models should be improved to increase the accuracy of IOL calculations.

Conflict of Interests

The authors declare that they have no competing interests.

Authors' Contribution

Xun Xu conceived and designed the experiments and supervised the project. Yong Sun designed the research, carried out the surgical procedures, and helped to draft the paper. Chong Chen performed the experiments and the statistical analysis and drafted the paper. Xian Xu participated in the data analysis. Yuyu Miao participated in the design of the study and performed the experiments. Gaoxin Zheng provided technical support and conceptual advice. All authors read and approved the final paper.

Acknowledgments

This work was supported by grants from the National Science and Technology Pillar Program of the Twelfth Five-Year Plan (2011ZX09302-007-02) and the Research Fund for the

National Natural Science Foundation of China (nos. 81273424 and 81170862).

References

[1] S.-M. Saw, Y.-H. Chan, W.-L. Wong et al., "Prevalence and risk factors for refractive errors in the singapore malay eye survey," *Ophthalmology*, vol. 115, no. 10, pp. 1713–1719, 2008.

[2] L. Hyman, "Myopic and hyperopic refractive error in adults: an overview," *Ophthalmic Epidemiology*, vol. 14, no. 4, pp. 192–197, 2007.

[3] I. G. Morgan, K. Ohno-Matsui, and S.-M. Saw, "Myopia," *The Lancet*, vol. 379, no. 9827, pp. 1739–1748, 2012.

[4] C. A. McCarty, P. M. Livingston, and H. R. Taylor, "Prevalence of myopia in adults: implications for refractive surgeons," *Journal of Refractive Surgery*, vol. 13, no. 3, pp. 229–234, 1997.

[5] W. Haigis, "Biometry and intraocular lens calculation in extreme myopia," *Acta Clinica Croatica*, vol. 51, supplement 1, pp. 65–69, 2012.

[6] J. S. Lee, B. S. Oum, B. J. Lee, and S. H. Lee, "Photorefractive keratectomy for astigmatism greater than −2.00 diopters in eyes with low, high, or extreme myopia," *Journal of Cataract and Refractive Surgery*, vol. 24, no. 11, pp. 1456–1463, 1998.

[7] Y.-H. Ji, Y. Lu, G.-S. Lu, Y. Luo, and M. Wang, "Phacoemulsification and the negative power intraocular lenses in extremely myopic eyes," *Zhonghua Yan Ke Za Zhi*, vol. 41, no. 3, pp. 196–199, 2005.

[8] I. Jimenez-Alfaro, S. Miguelez, J. L. Bueno, and P. Puy, "Clear lens extraction and implantation of negative-power posterior chamber intraocular lenses to correct extreme myopia," *Journal of Cataract and Refractive Surgery*, vol. 24, no. 10, pp. 1310–1316, 1998.

[9] W. E. Hill and S. F. Byrne, "Complex axial length measurements and unusual IOL power calculation," in *Clinical Modules for Ophthalmologists*, F. Points, Ed., pp. 22–29, American Academy of Ophthalmology, San Francisco, Calif, USA, 2004.

[10] O. Reitblat, E. I. Assia, G. Kleinmann, A. Levy, G. D. Barrett, and A. Abulafia, "Accuracy of predicted refraction with multifocal intraocular lenses using two biometry measurement devices and multiple intraocular lens power calculation formulas," *Clinical and Experimental Ophthalmology*, vol. 43, no. 4, pp. 328–334, 2015.

[11] P. J. Buckhurst, J. S. Wolffsohn, S. Shah, S. A. Naroo, L. N. Davies, and E. J. Berrow, "A new optical low coherence reflectometry device for ocular biometry in cataract patients," *British Journal of Ophthalmology*, vol. 93, no. 7, pp. 949–953, 2009.

[12] K. J. Hoffer, J. Aramberri, W. Haigis et al., "Protocols for studies of intraocular lens formula accuracy," *American Journal of Ophthalmology*, vol. 160, no. 3, pp. 403.e1–405.e1, 2015.

[13] W. Haigis, "The Haigis formula," in *Intraocular Lens Power Calculations*, H. J. Shammas, Ed., pp. 41–57, Slack Inc, Thorofare, NJ, USA, 2003.

[14] K. J. Hoffer, "The Hoffer Q formula: a comparison of theoretic and regression formulas," *Journal of Cataract and Refractive Surgery*, vol. 19, no. 6, pp. 700–712, 1993, Erratam in: *Journal of Cataract and Refractive Surgery*, vol. 20, pp. 677, 1994, and vol. 33, pp. 2-3, 2007.

[15] J. T. Holladay, T. C. Prager, T. Y. Chandler, K. H. Musgrove, J. W. Lewis, and R. S. Ruiz, "A three-part system for refining intraocular lens power calculations," *Journal of Cataract and Refractive Surgery*, vol. 14, no. 1, pp. 17–24, 1988.

[16] J. A. Retzlaff, D. R. Sanders, and M. C. Kraff, "Development of the SRK/T intraocular lens implant power calculation formula," *Journal of Cataract & Refractive Surgery*, vol. 16, no. 3, pp. 333–340, 1990, Erratum in: *Journal of Cataract & Refractive Surgery*, vol. 16, p. 528, 1990.

[17] W. Haigis, "Intraocular lens calculation in extreme myopia," *Journal of Cataract and Refractive Surgery*, vol. 35, no. 5, pp. 906–911, 2009.

[18] S. Bang, E. Edell, Q. Yu, K. Pratzer, and W. Stark, "Accuracy of intraocular lens calculations using the IOLMaster in eyes with long axial length and a comparison of various formulas," *Ophthalmology*, vol. 118, no. 3, pp. 503–506, 2011.

[19] D. R. Sanders, J. A. Retzlaff, M. C. Kraff, and H. V. M. G. Gimbel Raanan, "Comparison of the SRK/T formula and other theoretical and regression formulas," *Journal of Cataract and Refractive Surgery*, vol. 16, no. 3, pp. 341–346, 1990.

[20] C. S. L. Tsang, G. S. L. Chong, E. P. F. Yiu, and C. K. Ho, "Intraocular lens power calculation formulas in Chinese eyes with high axial myopia," *Journal of Cataract and Refractive Surgery*, vol. 29, no. 7, pp. 1358–1364, 2003.

[21] R. Donoso, J. J. Mura, M. López, and A. Papic, "Emmetropization at cataract surgery. Looking for the best IOL power calculation formula according to the eye length," *Archivos de la Sociedad Española de Oftalmología*, vol. 78, pp. 477–480, 2003.

[22] J.-K. Wang, C.-Y. Hu, and S.-W. Chang, "Intraocular lens power calculation using the IOLMaster and various formulas in eyes with long axial length," *Journal of Cataract and Refractive Surgery*, vol. 34, no. 2, pp. 262–267, 2008.

[23] M. A. Kapamajian and K. M. Miller, "Efficacy and safety of cataract extraction with negative power intraocular lens implantation," *The Open Ophthalmology Journal*, vol. 2, no. 1, pp. 15–19, 2008.

[24] P. Aristodemou, N. E. K. Cartwright, J. M. Sparrow, and R. L. Johnston, "Formula choice: Hoffer Q, Holladay 1, or SRK/T and refractive outcomes in 8108 eyes after cataract surgery with biometry by partial coherence interferometry," *Journal of Cataract & Refractive Surgery*, vol. 37, no. 1, pp. 63–71, 2011.

[25] L. Wang, M. Shirayama, X. J. Ma, T. Kohnen, and D. D. Koch, "Optimizing intraocular lens power calculations in eyes with axial lengths above 25.0 mm," *Journal of Cataract and Refractive Surgery*, vol. 37, no. 11, pp. 2018–2027, 2011.

[26] R. Zaldivar, M. C. Shultz, J. M. Davidorf, and J. T. Holladay, "Intraocular lens power calculations in patients with extreme myopia," *Journal of Cataract and Refractive Surgery*, vol. 26, no. 5, pp. 668–674, 2000.

[27] B. Zuberbuhler, M. Seyedian, and S. Tuft, "Phacoemulsification in eyes with extreme axial myopia," *Journal of Cataract and Refractive Surgery*, vol. 35, no. 2, pp. 335–340, 2009.

[28] A. Ghanem and H. El-Sayed, "Accuracy of intraocular lens power calculation in high myopia," *Oman Journal of Ophthalmology*, vol. 3, no. 3, pp. 126–130, 2010.

[29] T. Yokoi, M. Moriyama, K. Hayashi, N. Shimada, and K. Ohno-Matsui, "Evaluation of refractive error after cataract surgery in highly myopic eyes," *International Ophthalmology*, vol. 33, no. 4, pp. 343–348, 2013.

30

Antiproliferative, Apoptotic, and Autophagic Activity of Ranibizumab, Bevacizumab, Pegaptanib, and Aflibercept on Fibroblasts: Implication for Choroidal Neovascularization

Lyubomyr Lytvynchuk,[1,2,3] Andrii Sergienko,[1] Galina Lavrenchuk,[4] and Goran Petrovski[2,3]

[1]Professor Sergienko Eye Clinic, 47 A Pirogova Street, 21008 Vinnycia, Ukraine
[2]Department of Ophthalmology, Faculty of Medicine, Albert Szent-Györgyi Clinical Center, University of Szeged, Korányi fasor Ulica 10-11, 6720 Szeged, Hungary
[3]Stem Cells and Eye Research Laboratory, Department of Biochemistry and Molecular Biology, Faculty of Medicine, University of Debrecen, Egyetem Téren 1, 4032 Debrecen, Hungary
[4]State Institution "Research Center for Radiation Medicine of Academy of Medical Sciences of Ukraine", Laboratory of Cell Radiobiology, 53 Melnykova Street, 04050 Kyiv, Ukraine

Correspondence should be addressed to Goran Petrovski; gokipepo@gmail.com

Academic Editor: Juliana L. Dreyfuss

Purpose. Choroidal neovascularization (CNV) is one of the most common complications of retinal diseases accompanied by elevated secretion of vascular endothelial growth factor (VEGF). Intravitreal anti-VEGFs (ranibizumab, bevacizumab, pegaptanib, and aflibercept) can suppress neovascularization, decrease vascular permeability and CNV size, and, thereby, improve visual function. The antiproliferative, apoptotic, and autophagic effect of anti-VEGF drugs on fibroblasts found in CNVs has not been yet explored. *Methods.* Concentration-dependent cellular effects of the four anti-VEGFs were examined in L929 fibroblasts over a 5-day period. The cell survival, mitotic and polykaryocytic indices, the level of apoptosis and autophagy, and the cellular growth kinetics were all assessed. *Results.* The anti-VEGFs could inhibit the survival, mitotic activity, and proliferation as well as increase the cellular heterogeneity, apoptosis, and autophagy of the fibroblasts in a dose-dependent manner. Cellular growth kinetics showed ranibizumab to be less aggressive, but three other anti-VEGFs showed higher antiproliferative and apoptotic activity and expressed negative cellular growth kinetics. *Conclusions.* The antiproliferative, apoptotic, and autophagic activity of anti-VEGFs upon fibroblasts may explain the cellular response and the etiology of CNV involution *in vivo* and serve as a good study model for CNV *in vitro*.

1. Introduction

The development of choroidal neovascularization (CNV) is one of the most sight threatening complications of different retinal diseases such as age-related macular degeneration, pathologic myopia, angioid streaks, and choroidal rupture. Foveal or extrafoveal location of CNV limits the use of lasers due to its potential side effects on the surrounding healthy tissue. The effectiveness of intravitreal administration of different antivascular endothelial growth factors (anti-VEGFs) is well known in the treatment of CNV of different origin [1–4]. The mechanism how intravitreal injections (IVIs) of such

drugs work is complex and involves blocking of various types of VEGFs, decreased permeability of newly formed blood vessel walls, and reduced swelling of the retinal layers. Our optical coherence tomography (OCT) and fluorescein angiography (FA) performed before and after IVI of anti-VEGF drugs have revealed significant involution and decrease of CNV size (Figure 1).

The exact mechanism which leads to decrease of the CNV dimensions is not well understood. During recent years, a number of studies have published the impact of anti-VEGF drugs upon different cellular cultures *in vitro* [5–10]. Fibroblasts and myofibroblasts being among the most common

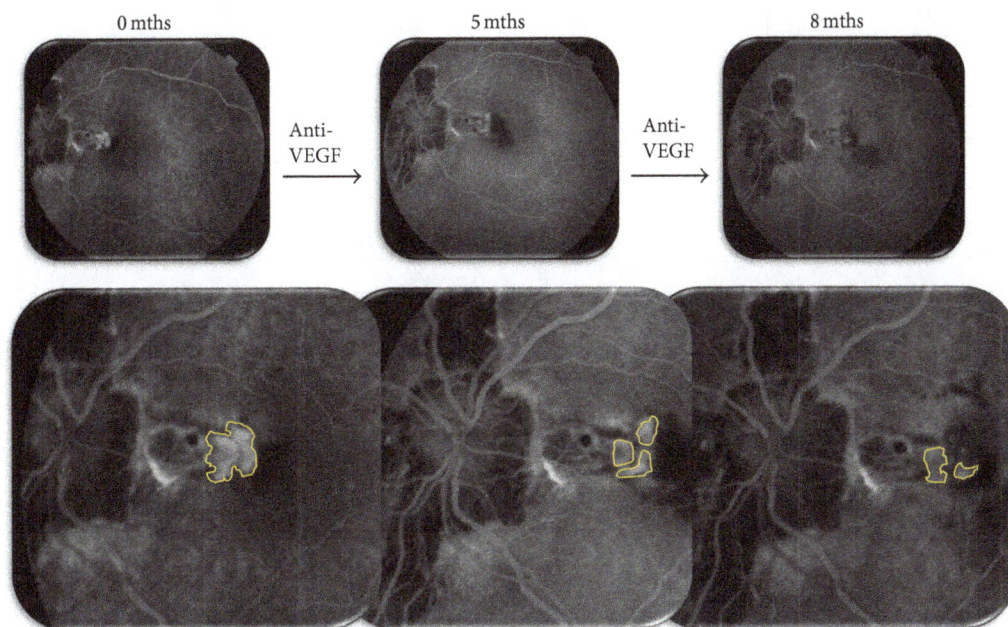

FIGURE 1: Choroidal neovascularization (CNV) dynamics after repeated anti-VEGF therapy (CNV size is circumscribed with yellow color; images shown are at the 40th second of fluorescein angiography).

cells found within the cellular matrix of CNVs and known to have high mitotic activity [7] have not been examined for their cellular effects upon anti-VEGF drug treatment. Our goal was to investigate the antiproliferative, apoptotic, and autophagic effects of anti-VEGF drugs on a fibroblast-like cell strain which can serve as *in vitro* model for CNV cellular matrix formation and to analyze the dose dependence regarding antiproliferative activity.

2. Materials and Methods

2.1. Cell Culture and Treatment Regimes. In vitro studies were performed using a fibroblast-like mouse cell strain L929 obtained from ATCC and cultivated according to conventional methods [11, 12] and nutrient medium composed of RPMI-1640 supplemented with fetal calf serum (10%) and gentamicin (10 mg/mL). Cultivation of the cell strain with different concentration of anti-VEGF drugs was performed as described below.

Ranibizumab (Lucentis, Novartis, Switzerland), a fragment of a human monoclonal antibody against VEGF-A, which is secreted by recombinant strain of *Escherichia coli* and its isoforms selectively bind to VEGF-A (VEGF$_{110}$, VEGF$_{121}$, and VEGF$_{165}$), was added to the culture 24 hours after fresh cell plating in concentrations of 12.5, 50, 125, and 250 μg/mL.

Bevacizumab (Avastin, Genetech/Roche, USA), a monoclonal antibody against VEGF, which is used off-label to treat various eye diseases in which increased concentration of VEGF is found and neovascularization is present, was added to the culture 24 hours after fresh cell plating at concentrations of 0.65, 3.13, 6.5, and 12.5 μg/mL.

Pegaptanib (Macugen, Pfizer, USA), a pegylated modified oligonucleotide that binds selectively and with high affinity to an extracellular VEGF$_{165}$, was added to the culture 24 hours after fresh cell plating at concentrations of 0.075, 0.15, 0.3, 0.75, and 1.5 μg/mL.

Aflibercept (Eylea, Bayer HealthCare, Germany), a fusion protein approved in the United States and Europe for the treatment of wet form of age-related macular degeneration, working by binding to circulating VEGF (subtypes VEGF-A and VEGF-B), as well as to placental growth factor (PGF), thus inhibiting growth of new blood vessels in the choriocapillaris [2], was added to the culture 24 hours after cell plating at concentrations of 0.04, 0.08, 0.2, 0.4, and 0.5 μg/mL.

Minimal drug concentrations were established according to the appearance of a multiplex of cellular effects (cellular proliferation, mitotic activity, polykaryocytic index, and apoptosis) and applied into the study, while maximal concentrations were determined with relevance and close approximation to the ones used in clinical practice (e.g., 0.5 mg/4 mL vitreous volume for ranibizumab; 1.25 mg/4 mL vitreous volume for bevacizumab; 0.3 mg/4 mL vitreous volume for pegaptanib; 2.0 mg/4 mL vitreous volume for aflibercept; all of the anti-VEGFs are used clinically at 1–3-month interval).

2.2. Cellular Vital Parameters. Different cellular responses were evaluated on a daily basis up to 5 days. The following cellular vital activity indices were evaluated: cellular growth/ expansion and mitotic and polykaryocytic indices (PKI). For cultivation, 5×10^4 cells were added to the cell culture dishes covered by culture glass slides (size 16 × 8 mm) and filled up to 1 mL of medium and then left to form monolayers within 5 days. Anti-VEGFs were added to the cultures 24 hours after cell plating in different concentrations specified accordingly.

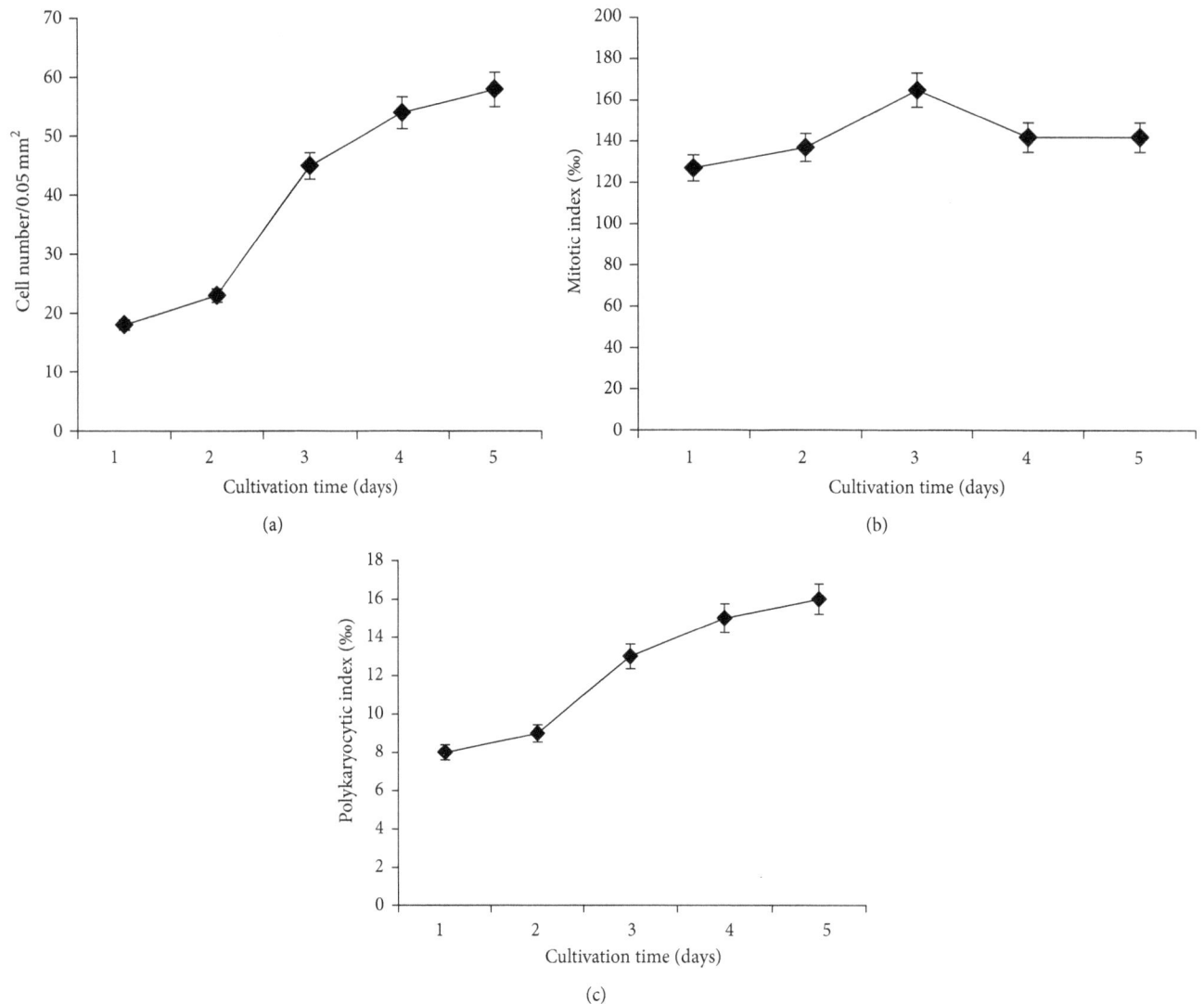

FIGURE 2: Kinetics of the cellular survival (a) and mitotic (b) and polykaryocytic indices (c) in untreated, control L929 cells.

The samples were fixed for analysis in 96% ethanol and then stained by hematoxylin and eosin (H&E). The total number of cells and the count of mitoses and polykaryocytes (2 or more nuclei) were determined under optical microscope (Axioscope, Germany) at 1000x magnification within a grid area of 0.05 mm². Mitotic index and PKI were adjusted to 1000 cells (‰). Parallely, cellular vital indices were evaluated within the intact cellular culture.

2.3. Detection of Apoptosis and Autophagy. The level of apoptosis was determined on the same cultures in which the cellular vital indices were analyzed. The cells were first washed in phosphate buffered saline (PBS) and then detached for 10 minutes in trypsin and suspended again in PBS. Consequently, centrifugation (1400 rpm, 5 min) and resuspension of the cells in propidium iodide (1 μg/mL) were performed. The level of apoptosis was determined according to the number of apoptotic cells in pre-G1 phase using ductal cytofluorimeter FACStar Plus (Becton Dickinson, USA).

Anti-LC3 polyclonal antibody was purchased from Novus Biologicals, USA (NB100-2220-0.1) for analysis of autophagy. Cell lysates were prepared from each condition after which equal amounts of protein were loaded onto the gel. Proteins were separated on a NuPAGE 15% Bis-Tris polyacrylamide gel and then transferred onto Immobilon-P Transfer Membrane (Millipore, IPVH00010). Membranes were blocked in Tris buffered saline containing 0.05% Tween-20 (TBS-T) and 5% nonfat dry milk (BioRad, 170-6435, 170-6531, and 100-04504-MSDS) for 1 hour. After blocking, membranes were probed overnight at 4°C with the anti-LC3 antibody in dilution buffer (TBS-T containing 1% nonfat dry milk), followed by 1-hour incubation with a peroxidase-conjugated rat anti-rabbit secondary antibody (Sigma, A6154) for 1 hour at room temperature. Peroxidase activity was detected with SuperSignal West Femto Maximum Sensitivity Chemiluminescent Substrate (Pierce, 34095) using a Lumi-Imager (Roche Diagnostics, Mannheim, Germany).

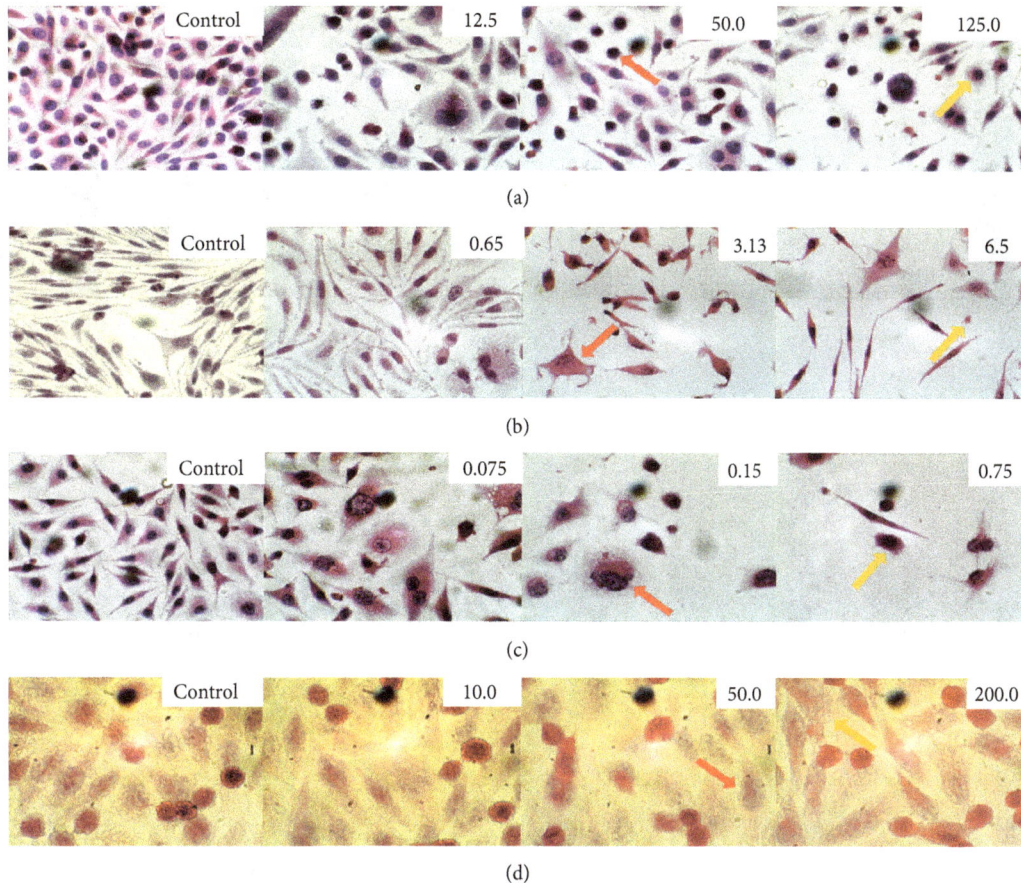

FIGURE 3: Cellular effects of ranibizumab (a), bevacizumab (b), pegaptanib (c), and aflibercept (d) on L929 cells. Cells shown are at Day 5 of various treatment concentrations (H&E staining, magnification ×1000).

2.4. Cellular Growth Kinetics. Proliferative activity of cells was determined according to their growth kinetics parameters: specific growth velocity (μ), population doubling time (t_d), and reproduction velocity (n) at Day 5 of the observation [13]. The specific growth velocity of the culture in phase of logarithmic growth was calculated using the formula $\mu = (\ln X - \ln X_o)t^{-1}$, where X is the cell quantity after certain time interval t (Day 5 of cultivation), X_o is the cell quantity on Day 1 of cultivation, and t is the time of observation (5 days of cultivation). Using specific growth velocity, population doubling time was calculated as $t_d = \ln 2/\mu = 0693\mu$. Reproduction velocity (n) was determined using the formula $n = 3.32 \log(X/X_o)$.

2.5. Statistical Analysis. Results were statistically analyzed by Student's t-test using Microsoft Excel and Biostat (Primer of Biostatistics, Version 4.03, by Stanton A. Glantz). $P < 0.05$ was considered significant. If not otherwise noted, all the experiments were performed three times independently.

3. Results

3.1. Morphological and Functional Characteristics of L929 Cells Treated by Anti-VEGFs. Under normal conditions, L929 cells form a dense cellular monolayer with the majority of the cells

acquiring polygonal and spindle shape morphology. The cells have relatively large nuclei, light cytoplasmic vacuoles, and small granules with occasional di- and trinucleated cells found in the culture. On average, 2 to 5 cells at different stages of mitosis can be detected per visual field in the untreated culture, assuming round shape, small cytoplasm, and hyperchromatic nuclei due to condensation of the chromatin under mitosis. The intact cells have a characteristic proliferative activity that increases from Day 1 to Day 5 of cultivation (logarithmic growth phase), reaching growth plateau at Day 6 (stationary growth phase), when the density of the cellular monolayer becomes highest ($58.0 \pm 2.7/0.05$ mm^2) (Figure 2(a)). Maximum mitotic activity is observed at Day 3 of cultivation (166.0 ± 7.5‰), with a decrease in the mitotic index at Day 4 due to contact inhibition and confluency of the cellular culture. The PKI in the intact control cells varies between 8 and 12‰.

Incubation of the L929 cells with ranibizumab at a concentration of 12.5 μg/mL leads to decreased density of the culture monolayer by 3 times (Figures 3(a) and 4(a)), which is caused by the appearance of increased number of cells with apoptotic features—decreased cytoplasm and condensed chromatin in the nucleus (Figures 3(a) (red arrow) and 4(d)). The treated cells assume mainly spindle-shape morphology, while their PKI increases by 54‰ (Figure 4(c)), a sign of cell

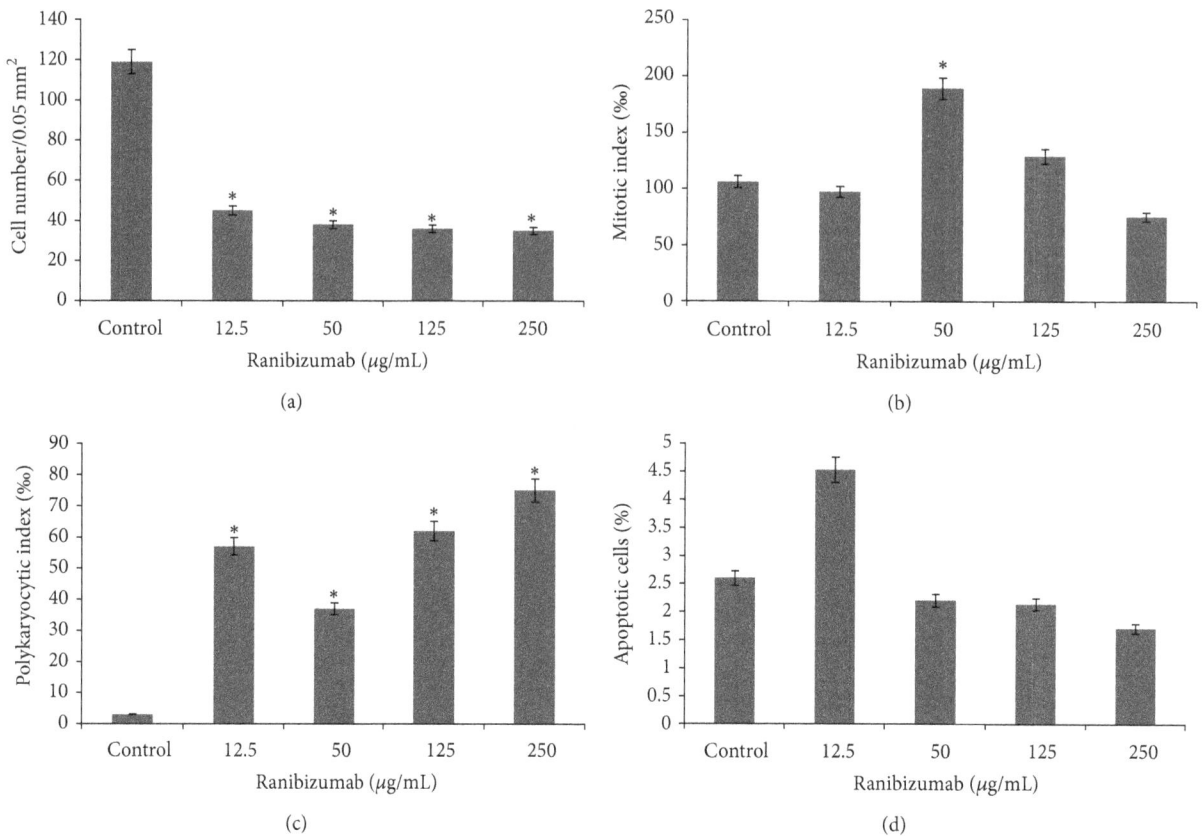

FIGURE 4: Kinetics of cellular proliferation (a), mitotic activity (b), polykaryocytic index (c), and apoptosis (d) in L929 cells treated by ranibizumab at different concentrations (data shown are at Day 5 of the treatment; $n = 3$, $^*P < 0.05$).

demise. At higher concentrations up to 125.0 μg/mL, the heterogeneity of the cell culture increases, with a predominant cellular morphology being round and polygonal (Figure 3(a) (yellow arrow)). The number of polykaryocytes markedly increases to 62‰, while the mitotic index remains relatively stable compared to the control (Figure 4(b)). Incubation of the L929 cells at a dose of 250 μg/mL results in severe degradation of the cellular structure and strong vacuolization of the cytoplasm.

Exposure to bevacizumab at concentration of 0.65 μg/mL induces no morphological changes in the L929 cells compared to the control (Figure 3(b)). Increasing the dose up to 3.13 μg/mL leads to an increase in the heterogeneity of cellular culture, with round and polygonal cellular morphology becoming more prominent (Figure 3(b) (red arrow)). A small number of mitotic cells with vacuolar cytoplasm can be observed compared to the control, while the number of polykaryocytes increases 6.3 times (Figure 5(c)), and the mitotic index and cell number decrease by 1.9 and 1.6 times, respectively, compared to the control (Figures 5(a) and 5(b)). At higher concentrations of bevacizumab (6.25 and 12.5 μg/mL), a severe degradation of cellular structure, with the cytoplasm becoming full of vacuoles, and a large number of apoptotic cells appear (38.0 ± 1.5 and 46.0 ± 2.2, resp.) (Figures 3(b) (yellow arrow) and 4(d)). A significant reduction

in the cell density and mitotic activity as well as increase in the PKI is noticed at concentrations higher than 0.625 μg/mL ($P < 0.05$) (Figure 5(c)).

Incubation of cells with pegaptanib shows pronounced antiproliferative effects of the drug from its lowest dose (0.075 μg/mL) (Figure 6(a)) and an almost doubling of the apoptotic cells in the culture. This is manifested by a significant decrease in the cell number and mitotic activity compared to the controls ($P < 0.05$) (Figures 6(a) and 6(b)). Increasing the dose up to 1.5 μg/mL increases the antiproliferative effect which is manifested through a reduction in the density of the cells and the appearance of vacuoles in the cytoplasm (Figure 3(c) (red arrow)). Cells with signs of apoptosis also appear at higher concentrations (Figure 3(c) (yellow arrow)), but their number, paradoxically, is similar to that of the control cells (Figure 6(d)), while the number of mitoses and presence of polykaryocytes decreases and increases, respectively (Figures 6(b) and 6(c)).

Exposure to aflibercept causes not much morphological difference in the L929 cells compared to the control; for example, the cells remain predominantly polygonal and spindle shaped with centrally situated well-colored round or oval nuclei (Figure 3(d) (red arrow)). The cytoplasm has mesh structure and becomes slightly vacuolized under aflibercept treatment (Figure 3(d) (yellow arrow)), with many cells

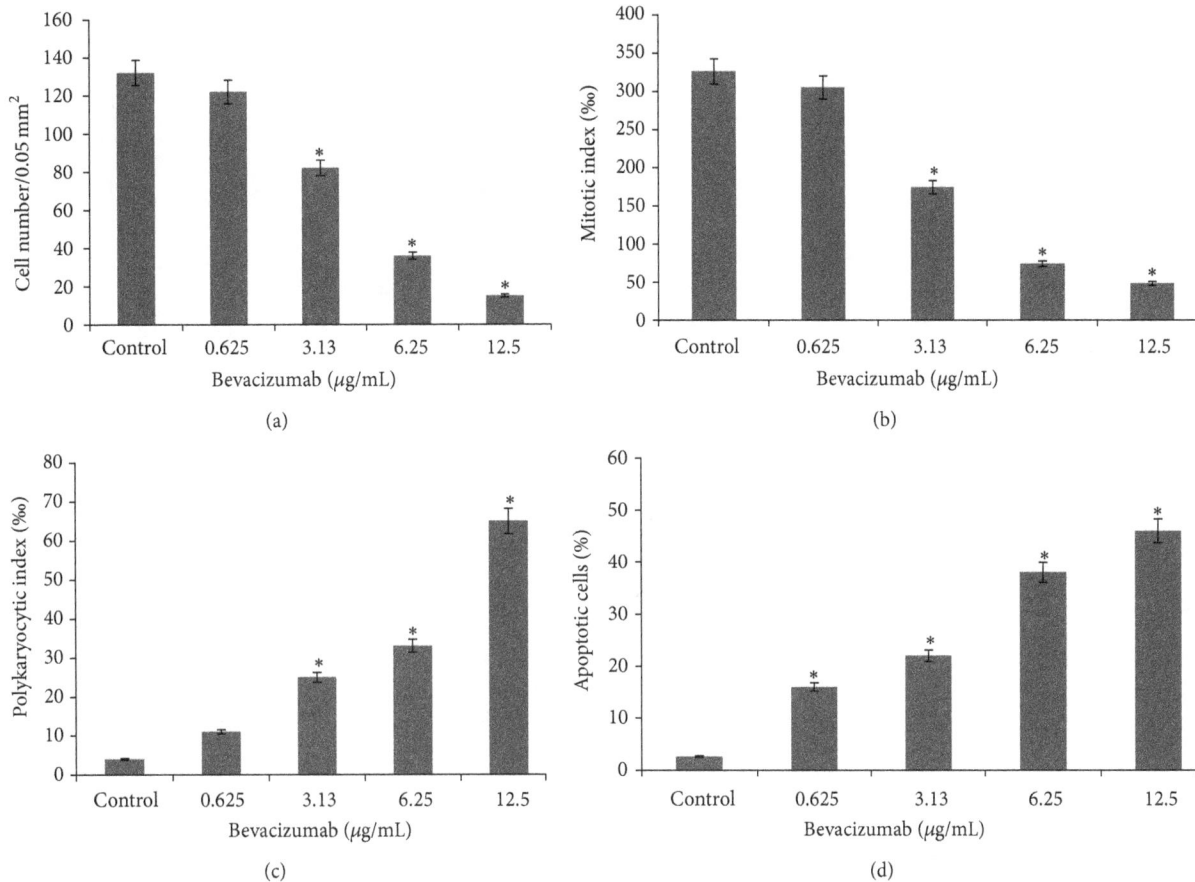

FIGURE 5: Kinetics of cellular proliferation (a), mitotic activity (b), polykaryocytic index (c), and apoptosis (d) in L929 cells treated by bevacizumab at different concentrations (data shown are at Day 5 of the treatment; $n = 3$, $^*P < 0.05$).

appearing at different stages of mitosis and, under certain concentrations, an entire absence of polykaryocytes' formation is seen compared to control (Figure 7(c)). The cell number is reduced by at least 1.6-fold with drug concentration of 10 μg/mL and by 2.2-fold when exposed to a maximum concentration of 200 μg/mL (Figure 7(a)). Interestingly, the mitotic index does not change compared to the control, which corresponds well to the morphological cellular stability observed (Figure 7(b)). Furthermore, complete lack of polykaryocytes is observed under certain concentrations (10 and 100 μg/mL) (Figure 7(c)). There is no statistical difference between PKI of control cells and under 50 or 200 μg/mL treatment with aflibercept ($P < 0.05$). The number of apoptotic cells (Figure 7(d)) increases and depends in a nonlinear manner on the drug concentration.

3.2. Cellular Growth Kinetics of L929 Cells under Different Treatments.
Comparison of the cellular growth effect of different concentrations of anti-VEGF drugs is shown in Figure 8. According to the cellular growth kinetic parameters (specific growth velocity (μ), population doubling time (t_d), and cell reproduction velocity (n)), ranibizumab seems to be less aggressive compared to the rest of the anti-VEGFs studied, the cellular death being compensated by cellular reproduction in its case (Figure 8(a)) [13]. Minimal concentrations

of bevacizumab cause faster cellular proliferation than death (Figure 8(b)); however, this turns around under higher concentrations, when generalized cell death through initiation of apoptosis occurs. The action of pegaptanib appears to be antiproliferative at lowest concentrations, while the balance between survival, reproductive activity, and death is shifted towards death at higher concentrations, meaning that the destruction in cellular culture runs faster than cellular mitosis (Figure 8(c)). Treatment by aflibercept (Figure 8(d)) causes statistically significant reduction in the cell number, in particular, concentrations of 50 to 200 μg/mL, while, at the same time, the population doubling time decreases (at 50 μg/mL), and the rate of cell proliferation increases. This indicates a shift of the balance of cellular growth and death in the culture towards death, and, according to the determination of number of apoptotic cells (Figure 8(d)), this death is mainly caused by apoptosis. Concentration of 200 μg/mL slows down the progression of cellular growth, which indicates linking of the reproductive death (pathologic mitosis) to apoptosis.

3.3. Induction of Autophagy by Ranibizumab and Bevacizumab in L929 Cells.
The appearance of vacuoles in the cytoplasm of L929 cells under different treatments by ranibizumab and bevacizumab was further examined for the presence of autophagy. Both treatment modalities induce

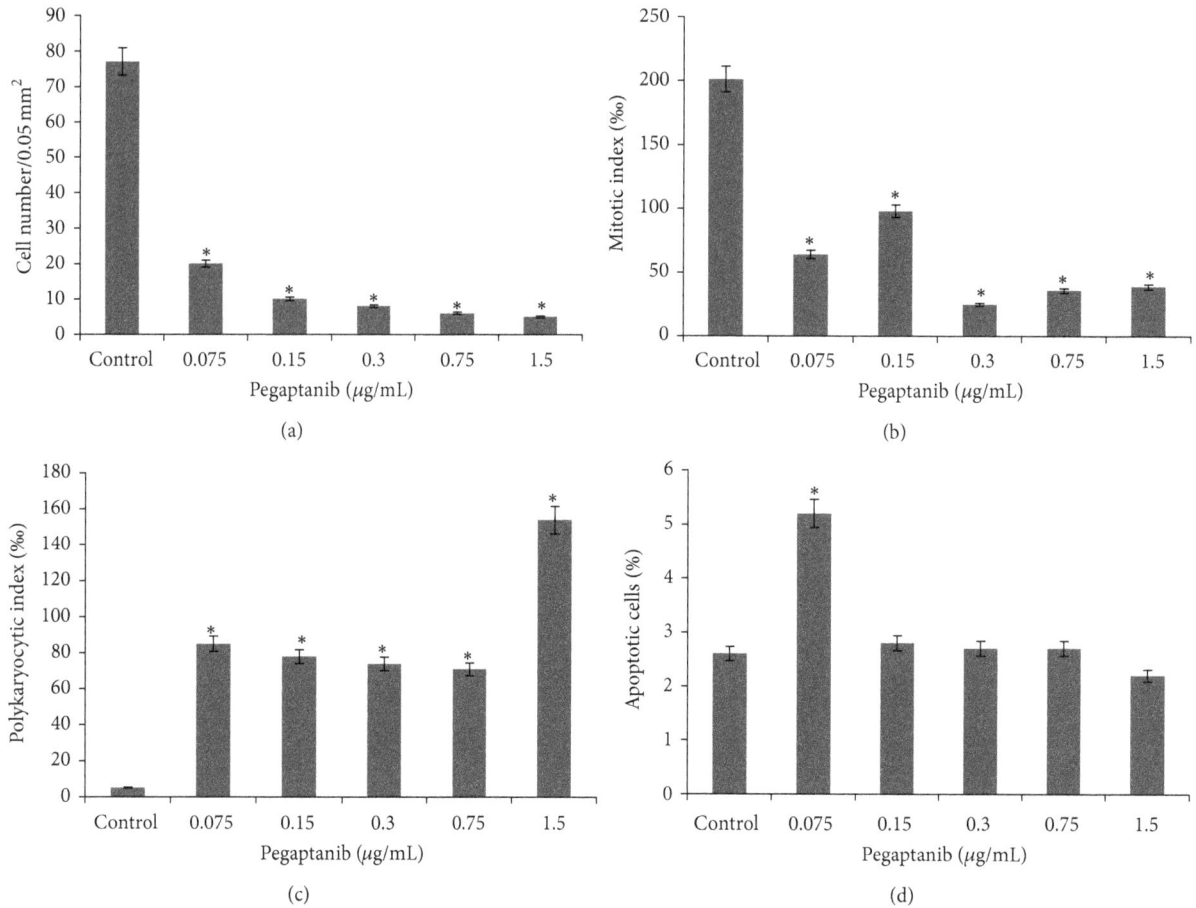

(a)

(b)

(c)

(d)

FIGURE 6: Kinetics of cellular proliferation (a), mitotic activity (b), polykaryocytic index (c), and apoptosis (d) in L929 cells treated by pegaptanib at different concentrations (data shown are at Day 5 of the treatment; $n = 3$, $^{*}P < 0.05$).

conversion of the cytoplasmic form of the myosin light chain kinase 3 (LC3) I into the autophagic vacuoles-bound LC3 II, with the highest concentrations of each drug inducing highest conversion of LC3 I to LC3 II (quantification data not shown) (Figure 9).

4. Discussion

Over the past decade, IVIs of anti-VEGF drugs take the leading place among the treatment modalities used for retinal diseases with increased production of VEGF [1–4]. However, only a few studies are dedicated to the side effects these drugs have on ocular tissues being exposed [5–10]. To our knowledge, this is the first study which compares antiproliferative action of ranibizumab, bevacizumab, pegaptanib, and aflibercept on fibroblast-like cells in vitro to elucidate the different dose-dependent properties and implications for CNV.

Our data show that all four anti-VEGFs demonstrate antiproliferative activity on the L929 cells over a 5-day study period. Starting from the lowest concentrations used, the heterogeneity of the cellular monolayer increases as a result of depression of mitosis and survival, while the number of apoptotic cells increases. Increasing the concentrations of each of

the four anti-VEGFs results in exacerbation of the above-mentioned effects.

The growth kinetic analysis reveals concentration-dependent antiproliferative and apoptotic effects of all anti-VEGFs, except for ranibizumab, where higher cellular reproduction occurs with concentration increase, and, therefore, the concentration-dependent cellular growth is partially compensated by reproduction. The ranibizumab proves, therefore, to be less aggressive than other anti-VEGFs in regard to its antiproliferative activity.

A recent study compared the antiproliferative and cytotoxic effects of bevacizumab, pegaptanib, and ranibizumab on different ocular cells, except fibroblasts [8]. Ranibizumab reduced the cell proliferation by 44.1%, while bevacizumab and pegaptanib reduced it by 38.2% and 35.1%, respectively, when applied to choroidal epithelial cells (CECs), although the difference was not found to be statistically significant. A slight antiproliferative effect of bevacizumab and pegaptanib was also revealed on adult retinal pigment epithelium (ARPE19 cell line). Ranibizumab neither had the same effect on cell proliferation of ARPE19 cells nor did it have cytotoxicity on retinal ganglion cells (RGC5), CECs, and ARPE19 cells. It could also efficiently block migration, but not proliferation

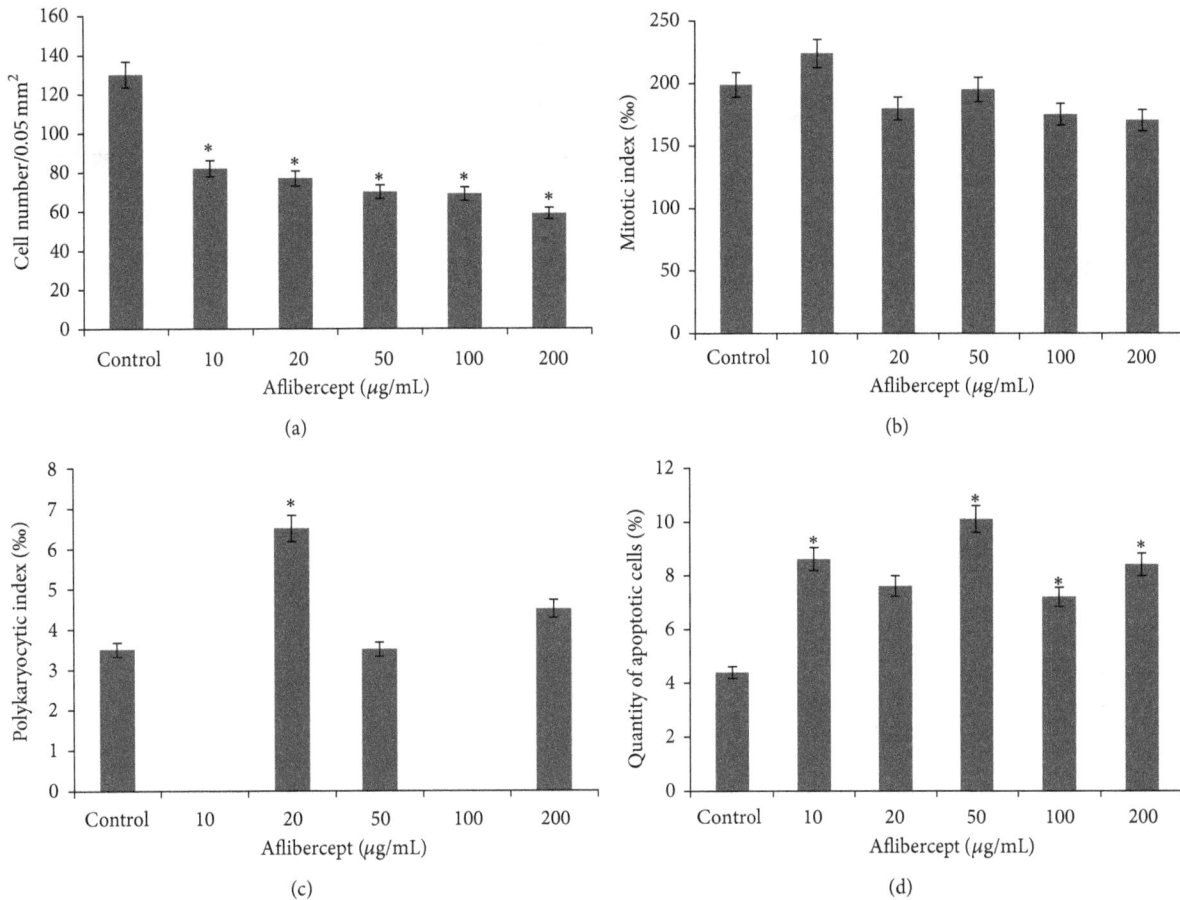

FIGURE 7: Kinetics of cellular proliferation (a), mitotic activity (b), polykaryocytic index (c), and apoptosis (d) in L929 cells treated by aflibercept at different concentrations (data shown are at Day 5 of the treatment; $n = 3$ $^*P < 0.05$).

induced by growth factor combinations, including VEGF in retinal endothelial cells.

Another study collated the effects of ranibizumab, pegaptanib, and bevacizumab on the different stages of angiogenesis using cultivation of drugs on human umbilical vein endothelial cells (HUVEC) [5]. According to the results, apoptosis of HUVEC was markedly increased by ranibizumab and bevacizumab. Clinically used doses of these drugs, but not pegaptanib, caused significantly reduced cellular proliferation without causing cytotoxic effects at all concentrations used. Finally, incubation of HUVEC with anti-VEGF drugs caused a decreased expression of the active form of the VEGF receptor-2, with bevacizumab causing 66% of control and ranibizumab and pegaptanib causing 86% decrease compared to the control.

A separate study compared the cytotoxicity and antiproliferative activity of aflibercept, bevacizumab, and ranibizumab on different ocular cells (ARPE19, RGC-5, and 661W) [7] and concluded that aflibercept does not affect cellular viability or induce apoptosis. Albeit aflibercept had slight upregulation and downregulation effects on certain VEGF-related factors, however, those were not significant when compared to bevacizumab and ranibizumab.

Our experimental study explored the cellular effects of four different anti-VEGFs on L929 cells as a model of the

fibroblast-based cellular matrix of CNV *in vitro*. The results revealed their effect on the proliferative activity (survival, proliferative and mitotic activity, and apoptosis) and their hormesis; that is, small doses of the drugs (ranibizumab 12.5 μg/mL, bevacizumab 3.13 μg/mL, pegaptanib 0.15 μg/mL, and aflibercept 0.04 μg/mL) exhibited a pronounced antiproliferative effect on the cellular culture, while bevacizumab in all concentrations increased apoptosis of the L929 cells. Inhibition of the proliferation and increased heterogeneity of these cells under anti-VEGF treatment are a sign of reproductive cellular death.

When cultured with bevacizumab, pegaptanib, and aflibercept, the L929 cells showed marked dose-dependent effects which were manifested by an increase in the antiproliferative action with increasing dose. Inversely, ranibizumab caused compensation of the antiproliferative and apoptotic action by cellular proliferation in spite of increasing drug concentration. This compensation can probably be partially due to autophagy, which is a self-digestive or self-recycling mechanism found in cells.

The reasons why L929 cell strain was chosen in this study were the absence of background VEGF secretion, as well as exploring the alternative cellular effects of anti-VEGF drugs as an *in vitro* model for CNV. Indeed, the most highly proliferating cell types amid the cellular types in CNV are

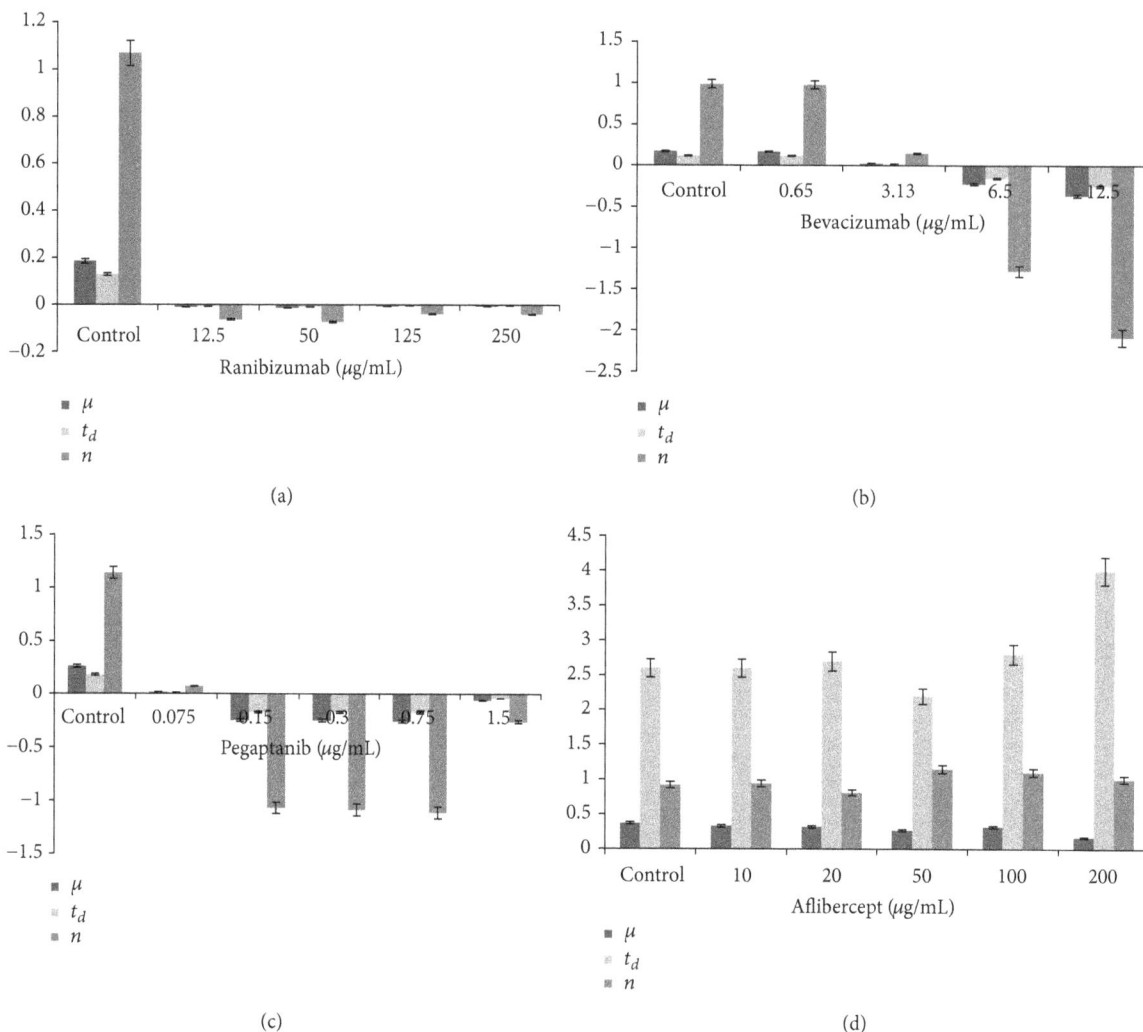

FIGURE 8: Comparison of the cellular growth kinetics in L929. Specific growth velocity (μ), population doubling time (t_d), and cell reproduction velocity (n) are shown under treatment with ranibizumab (a), bevacizumab (b), pegaptanib (c), and aflibercept (d) at different concentrations (data shown are at Day 5 of the treatment; $n = 3$).

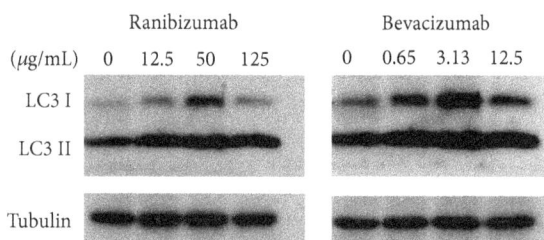

FIGURE 9: Induction of autophagy by ranibizumab and bevacizumab in L929 cells.

fibroblasts and myofibroblasts [14]. L929 cells have also been used as *in vitro* model for vital cell, allowing to judge cellular effects of different drugs upon vital, highly proliferating cells.

Although the data regarding presence of absence of VEGF receptors on the cellular membrane of fibroblast-like cells in CNV is missing, other studies have shown VEGF receptor presence on joint fibroblasts extracted from humans as well as

expression of VEGF by inflammatory stimulation of fibroblast-like cells that infiltrate the joint in a collagen-induced arthritis [15]. An obvious limitation of this study is the resemblance of the *in vitro* findings to clinical conditions, for example, CNV.

Antiproliferative and apoptotic properties of anti-VEGF drugs on fibroblast-like cells can explain an alternative, beneficial mechanism of their action on such cells and myofibroblasts found in CNV [14]. Inhibition of the cellular survival and mitosis by ranibizumab, bevacizumab, pegaptanib, and aflibercept in different concentrations has to be taken into consideration while using them in patients. Only ranibizumab, amid all anti-VEGFs studied, exhibits the slightest antiproliferative activity which allows for compensation of apoptosis by increased proliferation. The complete absence of polykaryocytes revealed after cultivation with aflibercept at concentrations of 10 and 100 μg/mL may indicate the influence of the drug on the signal transfer from the membrane to the nucleus.

The identified properties of these drugs require further investigation of their action *in vitro* and *in vivo*. Additionally, further research pertaining to hormesis of anti-VEGFs needs to be performed to eliminate possible side effects on healthy retinal tissues.

Conflict of Interests

The authors declare that they have no competing interests.

Acknowledgments

The work has been supported by the Hungarian Scientific Research Fund (OTKA PD 101316) and TÁMOP-4.2.2A-11/1/KONV-2012-0023 Grant, project implemented through the New Hungary Development Plan and cofinanced by the European Social Fund.

References

[1] P. Biswas, S. Sengupta, R. Choudhary, S. Home, A. Paul, and S. Sinha, "Comparative role of intravitreal ranibizumab versus bevacizumab in choroidal neovascular membrane in age-related macular degeneration," *Indian Journal of Ophthalmology*, vol. 59, no. 3, pp. 191–196, 2011.

[2] D. J. Browning, P. K. Kaiser, P. J. Rosenfeld, and M. W. Stewart, "Aflibercept for age-related macular degeneration: a game-changer or quiet addition?" *American Journal of Ophthalmology*, vol. 154, no. 2, pp. 222–226, 2012.

[3] S. Grisanti and F. Ziemssen, "Bevacizumab: off-label use in ophthalmology," *Indian Journal of Ophthalmology*, vol. 55, no. 6, pp. 417–420, 2007.

[4] N. Kumaran, D. A. Sim, and A. Tufail, "Long-term remission of myopic choroidal neovascular membrane after treatment with ranibizumab: a case report," *Journal of Medical Case Reports*, vol. 3, article 84, 2009.

[5] Â. Carneirob, M. Falcão, A. Pirraco, P. Milheiro-Oliveira, F. Falcão-Reis, and R. Soaresa, "Comparative effects of bevacizumab, ranibizumab and pegaptanib at intravitreal dose range on endothelial cells," *Experimental Eye Research*, vol. 88, no. 3, pp. 522–527, 2009.

[6] S. Kaempf, S. Johnen, A. K. Salz, A. Weinberger, P. Walter, and G. Thumann, "Effects of bevacizumab (avastin) on retinal cells in organotypic culture," *Investigative Ophthalmology & Visual Science*, vol. 49, no. 7, pp. 3164–3171, 2008.

[7] S. Schnichels, U. Hagemann, K. Januschowski et al., "Comparative toxicity and proliferation testing of aflibercept, bevacizumab and ranibizumab on different ocular cells," *British Journal of Ophthalmology*, vol. 97, no. 7, pp. 917–923, 2013.

[8] M. S. Spitzer, E. Yoeruek, A. Sierra et al., "Comparative antiproliferative and cytotoxic profile of bevacizumab (Avastin), pegaptanib (Macugen) and ranibizumab (Lucentis) on different ocular cells," *Graefe's Archive for Clinical and Experimental Ophthalmology*, vol. 245, no. 12, pp. 1837–1842, 2007.

[9] M. S. Spitzer, B. Wallenfels-Thilo, A. Sierra et al., "Antiproliferative and cytotoxic properties of bevacizumab on different ocular cells," *British Journal of Ophthalmology*, vol. 90, no. 10, pp. 1316–1321, 2006.

[10] Y. Wang, D. Fei, M. Vanderlaan, and A. Song, "Biological activity of bevacizumab, a humanized anti-VEGF antibody in vitro," *Angiogenesis*, vol. 7, no. 4, pp. 335–345, 2004.

[11] L. P. Dyakonov, Ed., *Animal Cells in Culture (Methods and Application of Biotechnology)*, Sputnik, Moscow, Russia, 2009.

[12] H. Hay and J. Cohen, "Studies on the specificity of the L929 cell bioassay for the measurement of tumor necrosis factor," *Journal of Clinical and Laboratory Immunology*, vol. 29, pp. 151–155, 1989.

[13] I. Freshney, *Animal Cell Culture, A Practical Approach*, IRL Press Oxford, Washington, DC, USA, 1986.

[14] A. Scupola, L. Ventura, A. C. Tiberti, D. D'Andrea, and E. Balestrazzi, "Histological findings of a surgically excised myopic choroidal neovascular membrane after photodynamic therapy. A case report," *Graefe's Archive for Clinical and Experimental Ophthalmology*, vol. 242, no. 7, pp. 605–610, 2004.

[15] J. Lu, T. Kasama, K. Kobayashi et al., "Vascular endothelial growth factor expression and regulation of murine collagen-induced arthritis," *Journal of Immunology*, vol. 164, no. 11, pp. 5922–5927, 2000.

31

Effects of Laser Peripheral Iridotomy in Subgroups of Primary Angle Closure Based on Iris Insertion

Sung-Cheol Yun,[1] Ji Wook Hong,[2] Kyung Rim Sung,[2] and Jin Young Lee[2]

[1]*Department of Clinical Epidemiology and Biostatistics, Asan Medical Center, College of Medicine, University of Ulsan, Seoul 138736, Republic of Korea*
[2]*Department of Ophthalmology, Asan Medical Center, College of Medicine, University of Ulsan, Seoul 138736, Republic of Korea*

Correspondence should be addressed to Kyung Rim Sung; sungeye@gmail.com

Academic Editor: Dexter Leung

Purpose. To investigate the effect of laser peripheral iridotomy (LPI) in subgroups of primary angle closure based on iris insertion configuration. *Methods.* Anterior segment optical coherence tomography (AS-OCT) images were obtained before and two weeks after LPI. Qualitative classification of angle closure eyes according to iris insertion (basal insertion group (BG) and nonbasal insertion group (NBG)) was performed. Anterior chamber depth (ACD), lens vault (LV), iris curvature, iris area, iris thickness (IT_{750}), and angle opening distance (AOD_{750}) 750 microns from scleral spur were calculated. Uni- and multivariate regression analysis was carried out to evaluate factors associated with AOD_{750} before and after LPI. *Results.* Ninety-two eyes of 92 subjects were categorized as NBG (39 eyes) or BG (53 eyes). The mean change after LPI was not significantly different between two groups in all parameters. In both groups, AOD_{750} was affected by ACD ($p < 0.001$, $p = 0.044$) before LPI. AOD_{750} was affected by LV ($p = 0.012$) in NBG, but by ACD ($p < 0.001$) and IT_{750} ($p = 0.039$) in BG after LPI. *Conclusions.* The outcomes of LPI are not significantly different between angle closure subgroups with different iris insertions. However, factors affecting AOD_{750} show differences between two subgroups after LPI.

1. Introduction

Primary angle closure glaucoma (PACG) is one of the leading causes of visual loss in Asians [1–3]. Previous studies have reported the several anatomical features of the eyes with PACG including short axial length and shallow anterior chamber [4–7].

In the past, angle closure was entirely diagnosed by gonioscopic examination. Gonioscopic examination is still the reference standard for primary angle closure (PAC) diagnosis, but recent advances in imaging devices have allowed various anterior segment (AS) parameters to be measured. AS optical coherence tomography (AS-OCT) quantitatively measures AS parameters using a noncontact method with the subject in a sitting position [8, 9]. Among the several AS parameters, iris-related parameters have become a focus of recent studies. Wang et al. reported that iris curvature (IC), iris area (IA), and iris thickness (IT) are independently associated with the existence of a narrow angle [10, 11]. Furthermore, in several

recent papers the peripheral iris thickness was reported as an important predictor of the successful outcome of laser peripheral iridotomy (LPI) [12, 13].

Another point of interest is the location of the iris insertion into ciliary body. The area of the peripheral iris insertion into the ciliary body is very close to the trabecular meshwork, and, thus, characteristics of iris insertion may affect the configuration of the anterior chamber angle and the amount of pupillary block. LPI is performed to open the closed anterior chamber angle by resolving the pupillary block in PAC eyes. Hence, we intended to evaluate whether the effect of LPI is different in subgroups of PAC based on iris insertion configuration using AS-OCT images.

2. Methods

2.1. Subjects. PAC suspect (PACS) or PAC patients who visited the glaucoma clinic of Asan Medical Center, Seoul,

Korea, were seen by a single glaucoma specialist (Kyung Rim Sung) and met the inclusion criteria below which were consecutively included in this study based on a medical record review. The study was approved by the Institutional Review Board of Asan Medical Center and followed the tenets of the Declaration of Helsinki. All participants underwent a complete ophthalmic examination, including a review of their medical history, measurement of best-corrected visual acuity (BCVA), slit-lamp biomicroscopy, Goldmann applanation tonometry, gonioscopy, fundoscopic examination using a 90- or 78-diopter lens, stereoscopic optic disc photography, retinal nerve fiber layer photography, a visual field (VF) test (Humphrey field analyzer, Swedish Interactive Threshold Algorithm (SITA) 24-2; Carl Zeiss Meditec, Dublin, CA), Cirrus HD-OCT (Carl Zeiss Meditec), and AS-OCT (Visante OCT, Carl Zeiss Meditec).

PACS and PAC were diagnosed by gonioscopic examination. Eyes with appositional contact between the peripheral iris and the posterior trabecular meshwork of greater than 270° were included in the PACS group [14]. Eyes with an occludable angle and exhibiting features indicating trabecular obstruction by the peripheral iris were considered to have PAC [14]. PAC was considered present when an eye had an occludable angle (appositional contact between the peripheral iris and the posterior trabecular meshwork of >270°) and exhibited features indicative of trabecular obstruction by the peripheral iris, such as elevated intraocular pressure (IOP), iris whorling (distortion of radially orientated iris fibers), "glaukomflecken" lens opacity, or excessive pigment deposition on the trabecular surface, but without the development of a glaucomatous optic disc or any VF change [14]. We combined both PACS and PAC eyes and defined them as having "angle closure" for our current analysis in particular. Only reliable VF test results (false-positive errors <15%, false-negative errors <15%, and fixation loss <20%) were included in the analysis. Eyes with peripheral anterior synechiae (PAS) in anterior chamber (AC) angle were excluded. We excluded patients with a history or current use of topical or systemic medications (antihistamines, antiepileptics, antiparkinsonian agents, antispasmolytic drugs, mydriatic agents, and sympathetic agents) that could affect the angle or the pupillary reflex [15]; those with a history of previous intraocular surgery (including cataract surgery, laser trabeculoplasty, laser iridoplasty, and laser iridotomy); and those unable to fixate prior to the AS-OCT examination. Among the abovementioned criteria for PAC, patients with a history of acute PAC, defined by the presence of ocular or periocular pain, nausea, or vomiting, and a history of intermittent blurring of vision with haloes; an intraocular pressure (IOP) >30 mmHg; and the presence of at least three of the following: conjunctival injection, corneal epithelial edema, middilated unreactive pupil, and shallow AC, were also excluded [16]. Eyes diagnosed with secondary angle closure, such as those with neovascular or uveitic glaucoma, were also excluded. All eyes were newly diagnosed cases, and AS-OCT imaging was performed before starting any glaucoma medication, laser treatment, or intraocular surgery.

2.2. Gonioscopy. Prior to AS-OCT imaging, all patients underwent a slit-lamp examination and gonioscopy, conducted by an independent observer (Kyung Rim Sung) who has extensive experience in the performance of such examinations. All eyes were examined using a Sussman lens in a darkened room ($0.5 \, \text{cd/m}^2$). Both static gonioscopy and dynamic gonioscopy were performed using a Sussman lens with the eye in the primary gaze position. Indentation gonioscopy was performed to determine whether angle closure was attributable to apposition or to PAS. Care was taken to ensure that light did not fall on the pupil during the examinations.

2.3. AS-OCT Imaging. All participants were imaged in terms of the nasal and temporal angle (0–180°) using AS-OCT (Visante OCT, version 2.0; Carl Zeiss Meditec) operating in the enhanced AS single mode (scan length 16 mm; 256 A-scans). To confirm the consistency of the iris root insertion according to the pupillary reaction, four sessions using four different standardized lighting conditions (3.25, 100.8, 426, and $1420 \, \text{cd/m}^2$), grading from dark to light, was performed by a single well-trained operator. The room in which AS-OCT imaging was performed had four-graded lighting controlled by four-leveled switches. The lighting condition was changed by turning the switch at each session. Thus, the same four light level conditions were provided to all participants. Participants were asked to sit back after imaging and wait for 30 seconds, during which the lighting conditions were changed. After 30 seconds of adaptation to the new lighting conditions, imaging was resumed. Thus, four images, obtained under four different lighting conditions, were obtained from each participant. Among the four images obtained in each session, the images obtained at $3.25 \, \text{cd/m}^2$ were used for the analysis [17]. AS parameters in each image were evaluated by an independent examiner (Ji Wook Hong) who was blind to all other test results and the clinical information for the participants.

All parameters were determined using Image J software (ver. 1.44, National Institutes of Health, Bethesda, MD). The analyzed parameters are described in Figure 1. Anterior chamber depth (ACD) was defined as the distance from the corneal endothelium to the anterior surface of the lens. The scleral spur was defined as the point at which a change in curvature of the inner surface of the angle wall became apparent and often presented as an inward protrusion of the sclera [18]. After determination of the scleral spur location, iris thickness 750 μm from the scleral spur (IT_{750}) was measured [11]. Iris area (IA) was defined as the cross-sectional area of the iris. Anterior chamber area (AA) was defined as the cross-sectional area bordered at the corneal endothelium and anterior surface of the lens and iris. Iris curvature (IC) was defined as the maximum perpendicular distance between the iris pigment epithelium and a line connecting the most peripheral to the most central point of the epithelium [11]. The lens vault (LV) was defined as the perpendicular distance between the anterior pole of the crystalline lens and a horizontal line joining the two scleral spurs [19]. Angle opening distances (AOD_{750}) which were defined as the linear distance between the point of the inner corneoscleral wall

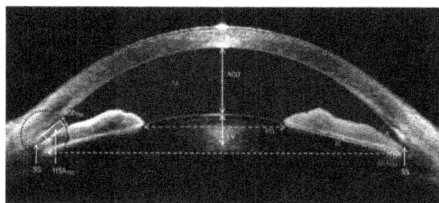

FIGURE 1: Anterior segment parameters determined by anterior segment optical coherence tomography. Abbreviation: ACD: anterior chamber depth, SS: scleral spur, IT750: iris thickness 750 μm from the scleral spur, IA: cross-sectional area of iris, AA: anterior chamber area, IC: iris curvature, LV: lens vault, AOD_{750}: angle opening distance 750 μm anterior to the scleral spur, ARA_{750},: angle recess area, triangular area formed by the AOD_{750}, $TISA_{750}$: trabecular-iris space area—trapezoidal area with the following boundaries; anteriorly, the AOD_{750} and posteriorly, a line drawn from the scleral spur perpendicular to the plane of the inner sclera wall to the opposing iris; superiorly, the inner corneoscleral wall; and inferiorly, the iris surface, PD: pupillary distance.

(750 μm anterior to the scleral spur) and the iris, were also assessed. The ARA_{750} was defined as the triangular area formed by the AOD_{750}. The corners of the triangle were the angle recess (the apex), the iris surface, and the inner corneoscleral wall. $TISA_{750}$ was defined as the trapezoidal area with the following boundaries: anteriorly, the AOD_{750}; posteriorly, a line drawn from the scleral spur perpendicular to the plane of the inner scleral wall to the opposing iris; superiorly, the inner corneoscleral wall; and, inferiorly, the iris surface. Measurement variability of the parameters was checked prior to the full analysis by calculating the intraclass correlation coefficients (ICCs). Intraexaminer ICC values for various AS parameters ranged between 0.933 and 0.951 [20].

The image acquisition procedure and analysis methods have been previously described in detail [20–22]. All parameters except for ACD, LV, AA, and pupillary distance (PD) were measured on both nasal and temporal sides and the average of the two values was used for analysis. Iris root insertion configuration was independently assessed by two glaucoma experts (Kyung Rim Sung and Jin Young Lee) who were blind to other AS-OCT parameters and all other test results including the clinical information of the participants. Four images at different lighting conditions were reviewed by two experts. Iris root insertion was categorized into two groups, a nonbasal group (NBG) and a basal insertion group (BG), according to the presence of a space between scleral spur and iris root (Figure 2). Each grader classified each eye as NBG or BG. If the opinions of the two observers differed, the eye in question was excluded.

2.4. *Laser Peripheral Iridotomy (LPI)*. LPI was performed in the superior region of the iris (from 10 to 2 o'clock) by sequential argon and neodymium-yttrium-aluminum-garnet laser after pretreatment with 2% pilocarpine instilled into the eye one hour before the LPI. The power settings used were 500–1000 mW with a spot size of 50 μm for a duration of 0.05 seconds with the argon laser and 2–5 mJ with

the yttrium-aluminum-garnet laser. Topical medications that could affect the angle measurement were not prescribed at the post-LPI.

2.5. *Statistical Analysis*. The Wilk-Shapiro test was used to explore the distribution of the numerical data. An unpaired Student's t-test was used for comparisons between NBG and BG of age, baseline IOP, spherical equivalent (SE), Cirrus HD OCT measured retinal nerve fiber layer (RNFL) thickness, and PD. Categorical variables were compared by Chi square test. We used a mixed-effects regression to calculate the pre-post AS-OCT parameter's mean difference and relative mean difference, the latter defined by (preparameter − postparameter)/preparameter × 100. For each outcome we also calculated pre-post outcome change adjusted for age, gender, SE, PD, and the pre-post PD difference. Residual diagnostic plots were used to detect features of concern in the model. Exploratory analyses of the residuals suggested that the chosen models were appropriate for all parameters. Univariate and multivariate regression analysis was performed to evaluate the factors associated with AC angle narrowing in each group. Univariate analyses were performed separately for each variable. Variables with a probability value ≤0.20 in univariate analyses were included in the multivariate analysis. AC angle narrowing was defined as AOD_{750}. All reported p-values were two-sided, and a value of $p <$ 0.05 was considered statistically significant. SAS software, version 9.2 (SAS Institute, Inc., Cary, NC) and SPSS version 15.0 (SPSS Inc., Chicago, IL), was used for the statistical analyses.

3. Results

Ninety-two PAC (60) or PACS subjects (32) were imaged and subcategorized as NBG (39 eyes) or BG (53 eyes). Three eyes were excluded due to different opinions between graders regarding the assessment AS-OCT image. All were East Asians (77 women: 15 men). There was a significant difference in age between the groups, with NBG subjects being older (62.7 ± 5.7 versus 59.8 ± 7.3 years, $p = 0.043$). NBG eyes were more hyperopic (1.29 ± 1.17 versus 0.813 ± 1.00 diopter, $p = 0.039$). The baseline IOP was marginally higher in BG eyes (16.6 ± 5.2 versus 14.8 ± 3.4 mmHg, $p = 0.063$). The average RNFL thickness and VF mean deviation were not different between the two groups. The demographic features and baseline status of the study subjects are listed in Table 1.

The mean differences of the AS-OCT parameters obtained at pre- and post-LPI were not significantly different between the BG and NBG eyes. In addition, there were no differences in the percentage changes in any parameter between the two groups after LPI (Table 2).

In both groups, AOD_{750} was affected by ACD (NBG; $p < 0.001$, BG; $p = 0.044$) before LPI (Tables 3 and 4). However, anatomical factors affecting the AOD_{750} did show a difference between the two groups after LPI. AOD_{750} was affected by LV ($p = 0.012$) in NBG (Table 5) but by ACD ($p < 0.001$) and IT_{750} ($p = 0.039$) in BG after LPI (Table 6).

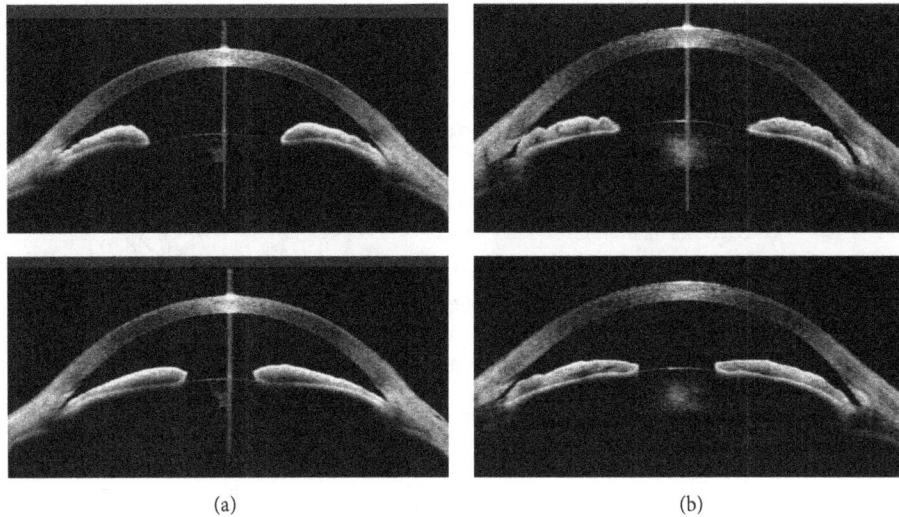

FIGURE 2: Categorization of primary angle closure eyes according to the location of iris root insertion. (a) Basal insertion (upper; dark, lower; light lighting conditions). (b) Nonbasal insertion (upper; dark, lower; light lighting conditions).

TABLE 1: Demographic features and baseline status of the study subjects.

	NBG ($n = 39$)	BG ($n = 53$)	p-value
Age (years)	62.7 ± 5.7	59.8 ± 7.3	0.043[†]
Sex (male/female)	5/34	10/43	0.217[‡]
Spherical equivalent (diopter)	1.29 ± 1.17	0.81 ± 1.00	0.039[†]
Baseline IOP (mmHg)	14.8 ± 3.4	16.6 ± 5.2	0.063[†]
VF MD (decibel)	−2.60 ± 2.99	−2.26 ± 4.03	0.662[†]
Average RNFL thickness (micron)	77.1 (±35.9)	82.7 (±29.3)	0.419

Abbreviations: BG; basal insertion group, NBG; nonbasal insertion group, IOP; intraocular pressure, VF MD; visual field mean deviation, RNFL; retinal nerve fiber layer; †: t-test, ‡: Chi-square test.

TABLE 2: Mean difference in the AS-OCT parameters in the two study groups at pre- and post-LPI.

	Pre-LPI		Post-LPI		p-value (difference)	p-value (difference, ratio)
	NBG	BG	NBG	BG		
ACD (mm)	2.100 ± 0.211	2.110 ± 0.301	2.092 ± 0.208	2.113 ± 0.307	0.3624	0.4208
LV (mm)	0.982 ± 0.200	0.889 ± 0.245	1.071 ± 0.234	0.967 ± 0.266	0.1444	0.1511
IC (mm)	0.354 ± 0.077	0.320 ± 0.076	0.131 ± 0.059	0.104 ± 0.045	0.9582	0.2412
IA (mm^2)	1.516 ± 0.268	1.588 ± 0.235	1.632 ± 0.297	1.674 ± 0.246	0.9107	0.8769
ARA$_{750}$ (mm^2)	0.154 ± 0.081	0.116 ± 0.079	0.193 ± 0.070	0.149 ± 0.088	0.8848	0.1536
TISA$_{750}$ (mm^2)	0.122 ± 0.063	0.099 ± 0.067	0.164 ± 0.058	0.132 ± 0.073	0.7420	0.0568
AOD$_{750}$ (mm)	0.229 ± 0.083	0.239 ± 0.098	0.314 ± 0.102	0.284 ± 0.136	0.0584	0.2082
IT$_{750}$ (mm)	0.359 ± 0.065	0.378 ± 0.082	0.369 ± 0.067	0.381 ± 0.066	0.5110	0.6178

[*] A mixed-effects model was used to compare the pre-post AS-OCT parameter's mean difference and relative difference between the two groups, adjusted for age, gender, SE, PD and the difference of pre-post-PD.
Abbreviations: AS-OCT: anterior segment optical coherence tomography; BG: basal insertion group; NBG: nonbasal insertion group; ACD: anterior chamber depth; IT$_{750}$: iris thickness from the scleral spur (at 750 m from the scleral spur); IA: cross-sectional area of the iris; IC: iris curvature; LV: lens vault; AOD$_{750}$: angle opening distances (corneoscleral wall 750 m anterior to the scleral spur); ARA$_{750}$: angle recess area formed by the AOD$_{750}$; TISA$_{750}$: trabecular-iris space area, trapezoidal area with the following boundaries: anteriorly, the AOD$_{750}$; posteriorly, a line drawn from the scleral spur perpendicular to the plane of the inner sclera wall to the opposing iris; superiorly, the inner corneoscleral wall; and inferiorly, the iris surface; PD: pupillary distance.

4. Discussion

The mechanism of angle closure involves the interplay between anatomic predisposition and physiological factors. Recent studies of anterior chamber parameters obtained by AS-OCT have led to the identification of several novel anatomic risk factors for angle closure, such as increased iris thickness and area, greater lens vault, and smaller anterior chamber width [10, 11, 19, 23]. Moreover, physical variations of the iris and ciliary body structures may play a role in

TABLE 3: Uni- and multivariate linear regression analysis of the association between various parameters and anterior chamber angle narrowing (AOD_{750}) assessed pre-LPI in the NBG subjects.

	Univariate			Multivariate		
	SE	B coefficient (95% CI)	p-value	SE	B coefficient (95% CI)	p-value
ACD, mm	0.052	0.218 (0.113, 0.323)	<0.001			
LV, mm	0.057	−0.084 (−0.216, 0.048)	0.207			
IC, mm	0.171	−0.132 (−0.478, 0.215)	0.293	0.052	0.218 (0.113, 0.323)	<0.001
IA, mm^2	0.048	−0.050 (−0.147, 0.047)	0.300			
IT$_{750}$, mm	0.200	0.219 (−0.187, 0.626)	0.281			
PD, mm	0.020	−0.010 (−0.051, 0.031)	0.614			

Abbreviations: NBG: nonbasal insertion group; ACD: anterior chamber depth; IT$_{750}$: iris thickness from the scleral spur (at 750 m from the scleral spur); IA: cross-sectional area of the iris; IC: iris curvature; LV: lens vault; AOD_{750}: angle opening distances (corneoscleral wall 750 m anterior to the scleral spur); PD: pupillary distance; SE: standard error; CI: confidence interval; LPI: laser peripheral iridotomy.

TABLE 4: Uni- and multivariate linear regression analysis of the association between various parameters and anterior chamber angle narrowing (AOD_{750}) assessed pre-LPI in the BG subjects.

	Univariate			Multivariate		
	SE	B coefficient (95% CI)	p-value	SE	B coefficient (95% CI)	p-value
ACD, mm	0.048	0.092 (−0.005, 0.190)	0.063			
LV, mm	0.061	−0.075 (−0.203, 0.051)	0.235	0.087	0.174 (0.007, 0.333)	0.044
IC, mm	0.177	−0.141 (−0.497, 0.215)	0.430			
IA, mm^2	0.053	−0.091 (−0.198, 0.017)	0.096			
IT$_{750}$, mm	0.162	0.050 (−0.277, 0.376)	0.761	0.045	−0.084 (−0.175, 0.007)	0.071
PD, mm	0.018	−0.020 (−0.056, 0.016)	0.268			

Abbreviations: BG: basal insertion group; ACD: anterior chamber depth; IT$_{750}$: iris thickness from the scleral spur (at 750 m from the scleral spur); IA: cross-sectional area of the iris; IC: iris curvature; LV: lens vault; AOD_{750}: angle opening distances (corneoscleral wall 750 m anterior to the scleral spur); PD: pupillary distance; SE: standard error; CI: confidence interval; LPI: laser peripheral iridotomy.

TABLE 5: Uni- and multivariate linear regression analysis of the association between various parameters and anterior chamber angle narrowing (AOD_{750}) assessed post-LPI in the NBG subjects.

	Univariate			Multivariate		
	SE	B coefficient (95.0% CI)	p-value	SE	B coefficient (95.0% CI)	p-value
ACD, mm	0.077	0.168 (0.011, 0.325)	0.036	0.086	0.076 (−0.098, 0.251)	0.381
LV, mm	−0.191	−0.191 (−0.322, −0.059)	0.006	0.065	−0.191 (−0.305, −0.040)	0.012
IC, mm	0.286	0.111 (−0.469, 0.691)	0.701			
IA, mm^2	0.053	−0.098 (−0.206, 0.010)	0.075			
IT$_{750}$, mm	0.250	−0.284 (−0.792, 0.223)	0.263	0.051	−0.071 (−0.174, 0.031)	0.168
PD, mm	0.019	−0.012 (−0.027, 0.051)	0.540			

Abbreviations: NBG: nonbasal insertion group; ACD: anterior chamber depth; IT$_{750}$: iris thickness from the scleral spur (at 750 m from the scleral spur); IA: cross-sectional area of the iris; IC: iris curvature; LV: lens vault; AOD_{750}: angle opening distances (corneoscleral wall 750 m anterior to the scleral spur); PD: pupillary distance; SE: standard error; CI: confidence interval; LPI: laser peripheral iridotomy.

TABLE 6: Uni- and multivariate linear regression analysis of the association between various parameters and anterior chamber angle narrowing (AOD_{750}) assessed post-LPI in the BG subjects.

	Univariate			Multivariate		
	SE	B coefficient (95.0% CI)	p-value	SE	B coefficient (95.0% CI)	p-value
ACD, mm	0.092	0.185 (0.000, 0.370)	0.050			
LV, mm	0.104	−0.059 (−0.270, −0.151)	0.572	0.050	0.217 (0.116, 0.318)	<0.001
IC, mm	0.459	−0.261 (−1.184, 0.662)	0.572			
IA, mm^2	0.099	−0.051 (−0.249, 0.148)	0.608			
IT$_{750}$, mm	0.280	−0.483 (−1.047, 0.080)	0.091	0.235	−0.500 (−0.973, −0.028)	0.039
PD, mm	0.028	−0.003 (−0.059, 0.053)	0.918			

Abbreviations: BG: basal insertion group; ACD: anterior chamber depth; IT$_{750}$: iris thickness from the scleral spur (at 750 m from the scleral spur); IA: cross-sectional area of the iris; IC: iris curvature; LV: lens vault; AOD_{750}: angle opening distances (corneoscleral wall 750 m anterior to the scleral spur); PD: pupillary distance; SE: standard error; CI: confidence interval; LPI: laser peripheral iridotomy.

the development of angle closure. It is conceivable that basal iris insertion contributes to angle crowding more than non-basal insertion and, thus, predisposes an eye with crowded anterior chamber characteristics (such as a short axial length [24, 25], smaller anterior chamber width [23], or greater lens vault [19]) to pupillary block and subsequent PAC. In our current study, we aimed to categorize PAC eyes according to the configuration of iris insertion into the ciliary body and to analyze whether the effect of the LPI is different in PAC subgroups based on iris insertion. Also, we investigated anatomic risk factors for angle closure in such subgroups based on iris insertion characteristics.

Iris insertion was categorized in our study into two groups, NBG and BG, according to the presence of a space between the scleral spur and the peripheral side of the basal iris. NBG and BG subjects had some different features; that is, NBG cases were older and hyperopic. The IOP was marginally higher in BG eyes. Interestingly, the mean change after an LPI was not significantly different between our two groups in any AS-OCT parameter, nor did the percentage changes differ between the two groups in any parameter. In other words, pupillary block is considered to exist in both groups, and thus the effect of pupillary block on angle closure might not be different between the two groups, since LPI was expected to resolve the pupillary block. Additionally, factors that affect the angle narrowing were rather similar in the two groups prior to the LPI, showing that ACD was the most important factor for angle narrowing. However, factors affecting angle narrowing were different between the two groups after the LPI. In the NBG cases, a greater LV was associated with angle narrowing while a thicker peripheral iris was associated with the BG. The mean age of the NBG was older than that of the BG. Aging is reported to significantly increase LV, and a higher LV may play an important role in the mechanism of angle closure [22]. This effect may result from the induction of the forward movement of the lens due to zonular laxity or increases in lens thickness, which can cause an elevated LV. Also, increased LV can directly induce narrowing of the peripheral angle or increase pupillary block by expanding iridolenticular contact.

A thicker peripheral iris was found to be associated with a narrow angle in the BG eyes after a resolution of the pupillary block, indicating that this would contribute to angle crowding in these cases. A thicker peripheral iris is likely to contribute to angle closure, because the peripheral iris would be in closer proximity to the angle [10]. This finding supports the concept that increased thickness and bulk of the iris root anterior to the plane of the scleral spur push the peripheral iris against the trabecular meshwork, thereby worsening angle crowding in an already predisposed eye.

Multiple pathogenic mechanisms are expected to contribute to PAC. The outcomes of LPI differed between angle closure subgroups with different anatomical characteristics, suggesting that the pathogenic mechanism of angle closure may differ among subgroups [26]. In previous studies, a considerable portion of the PAC eyes analyzed showed a closed angle despite a successful LPI, and those eyes that underwent LPI showed progressive narrowing afterwards [22, 25, 27]. These earlier studies suggested that the nonpupillary block mechanism may substantially contribute to PAC. Hence, predicting which factor is more important in the development of angle closure in specific eyes would be beneficial. Our current results may provide some clue that the contributing factors may be different according to the iris insertion configurations.

The limitations of our study must be acknowledged. First, although two experienced clinicians qualitatively graded iris insertion and peripheral iris configuration, subjective identification of anatomic landmarks could lead to inaccurate determination of reference points and may result in misclassification. However, we tried to minimize the variability by using standard photographs for comparison and to create a consensus between the two graders. In a dilated state, the iris root insertion was not differentiated in some eyes, so we acquired 4 serial images with different lighting conditions and reviewed all 4 images to determine the location of the iris root insertion. By performing image acquisitions at 4 light levels, we believe that we reduced the possibility of misclassification.

Second, AS-OCT images have a limited resolution and some features such as the position of the ciliary processes and iris angulation are thus difficult to identify with this modality. In this context, ultrasound biomicroscopy (UBM) offers better imagery, and several previous publications have nicely categorized PAC using UBM [27–29]. Those studies categorized iris insertion configurations into three categories (apical, mid, and basal configuration). Since AS-OCT does not show the whole feature of the ciliary body, discerning an apical versus mid insertion was difficult. We instead used two classifications: basal and nonbasal insertions. Finally, the relatively small sample size we used may have affected our ability to detect subtle differences in the AS-OCT parameters.

5. Conclusions

Our current findings indicate that the outcome of the LPI shows no significant difference between angle closure subgroups classified according to the iris root insertion into the ciliary body. However, anatomical factors affecting the AOD_{750} do show a difference between these two subgroups after LPI. This suggests that identification of the iris insertion may provide some clues to further understanding the anatomical factors that contribute to angle closure after LPI.

Conflict of Interests

The authors have no proprietary interests in or financial support for the development or marketing of instruments or equipment mentioned in this paper or any competing instruments or equipment.

References

[1] P. J. Foster, J. Baasanhu, P. H. Alsbirk, D. Munkhbayar, D. Uranchimeg, and G. J. Johnson, "Glaucoma in Mongolia: a population-based survey in Hovsgol province, northern Mongolia," Archives of Ophthalmology, vol. 114, no. 10, pp. 1235–1241, 1996.

[2] P. J. Foster and G. J. Johnson, "Glaucoma in china: how big is the problem?" *The British Journal of Ophthalmology*, vol. 85, no. 11, pp. 1277–1282, 2001.

[3] N. Congdon, F. Wang, and J. M. Tielsch, "Issues in the epidemiology and population-based screening of primary angle-closure glaucoma," *Survey of Ophthalmology*, vol. 36, no. 6, pp. 411–423, 1992.

[4] R. F. Lowe, "Aetiology of the anatomical basis for primary angle-closure glaucoma. Biometrical comparisons between normal eyes and eyes with primary angle-closure glaucoma," *British Journal of Ophthalmology*, vol. 54, no. 3, pp. 161–169, 1970.

[5] R. Sihota, N. C. Lakshmaiah, H. C. Agarwal, R. M. Pandey, and J. S. Titiyal, "Ocular parameters in the subgroups of angle closure glaucoma," *Clinical & Experimental Ophthalmology*, vol. 28, no. 4, pp. 253–258, 2000.

[6] R. George, P. G. Paul, M. Baskaran et al., "Ocular biometry in occludable angles and angle closure glaucoma: a population based survey," *The British Journal of Ophthalmology*, vol. 87, no. 4, pp. 399–402, 2003.

[7] T. Aung, W. P. Nolan, D. Machin et al., "Anterior chamber depth and the risk of primary angle closure in 2 East Asian populations," *Archives of Ophthalmology*, vol. 123, no. 4, pp. 527–532, 2005.

[8] M. H. Cheon, K. R. Sung, E. H. Choi et al., "Effect of age on anterior chamber angle configuration in Asians determined by anterior segment optical coherence tomography; clinic-based study," *Acta Ophthalmologica*, vol. 88, no. 6, pp. e205–e210, 2010.

[9] D. Y. Kim, K. R. Sung, S. Y. Kang et al., "Characteristics and reproducibility of anterior chamber angle assessment by anterior-segment optical coherence tomography," *Acta Ophthalmologica*, vol. 89, no. 5, pp. 435–441, 2011.

[10] B.-S. Wang, A. Narayanaswamy, N. Amerasinghe et al., "Increased iris thickness and association with primary angle closure glaucoma," *The British Journal of Ophthalmology*, vol. 95, no. 1, pp. 46–50, 2011.

[11] B. Wang, L. M. Sakata, D. S. Friedman et al., "Quantitative iris parameters and association with narrow angles," *Ophthalmology*, vol. 117, no. 1, pp. 11–17, 2010.

[12] K. R. Sung, K. S. Lee, and J. W. Hong, "Baseline anterior segment parameters associated with the long-term outcome of laser peripheral iridotomy," *Current Eye Research*, 2014.

[13] R. Y. Lee, T. Kasuga, Q. N. Cui et al., "Association between baseline iris thickness and prophylactic laser peripheral iridotomy outcomes in primary angle-closure suspects," *Ophthalmology*, vol. 121, no. 6, pp. 1194–1202, 2014.

[14] P. J. Foster, R. Buhrmann, H. A. Quigley, and G. J. Johnson, "The definition and classification of glaucoma in prevalence surveys," *The British Journal of Ophthalmology*, vol. 86, no. 2, pp. 238–242, 2002.

[15] J. S. M. Lai and R. A. Gangwani, "Medication-induced acute angle closure attack," *Hong Kong Medical Journal*, vol. 18, no. 2, pp. 139–145, 2012.

[16] K. Y. C. Lee, F. Rensch, T. Aung et al., "Peripapillary atrophy after acute primary angle closure," *The British Journal of Ophthalmology*, vol. 91, no. 8, pp. 1059–1061, 2007.

[17] Y. Lee, K. R. Sung, J. H. Na, and J. H. Sun, "Dynamic changes in anterior segment (AS) parameters in eyes with primary angle closure (PAC) and PAC glaucoma and open-angle eyes assessed using as optical coherence tomography," *Investigative Ophthalmology & Visual Science*, vol. 53, no. 2, pp. 693–697, 2012.

[18] L. M. Sakata, R. Lavanya, D. S. Friedman et al., "Assessment of the scleral spur in anterior segment optical coherence tomography images," *Archives of Ophthalmology*, vol. 126, no. 2, pp. 181–185, 2008.

[19] M. E. Nongpiur, M. He, N. Amerasinghe et al., "Lens vault, thickness, and position in chinese subjects with angle closure," *Ophthalmology*, vol. 118, no. 3, pp. 474–479, 2011.

[20] S. Baek, K. R. Sung, J. H. Sun et al., "A hierarchical cluster analysis of primary angle closure classification using anterior segment optical coherence tomography parameters," *Investigative Ophthalmology & Visual Science*, vol. 54, no. 1, pp. 848–853, 2013.

[21] K. S. Lee, K. R. Sung, K. Shon, J. H. Sun, and J. R. Lee, "Longitudinal changes in anterior segment parameters after laser peripheral iridotomy assessed by anterior segment optical coherence tomography," *Investigative Ophthalmology & Visual Science*, vol. 54, no. 5, pp. 3166–3170, 2013.

[22] J. H. Sun, K. R. Sung, S.-C. Yun et al., "Factors associated with anterior chamber narrowing with age: an optical coherence tomography study," *Investigative Ophthalmology and Visual Science*, vol. 53, no. 6, pp. 2607–2610, 2012.

[23] M. E. Nongpiur, L. M. Sakata, D. S. Friedman et al., "Novel association of smaller anterior chamber width with angle closure in Singaporeans," *Ophthalmology*, vol. 117, no. 10, pp. 1967–1973, 2010.

[24] R. Wojciechowski, N. Congdon, W. Anninger, and A. T. Broman, "Age, gender, biometry, refractive error, and the anterior chamber angle among Alaskan Eskimos," *Ophthalmology*, vol. 110, no. 2, pp. 365–375, 2003.

[25] R. Lavanya, T.-Y. Wong, D. S. Friedman et al., "Determinants of angle closure in older Singaporeans," *Archives of Ophthalmology*, vol. 126, no. 5, pp. 686–691, 2008.

[26] S. Han, K. R. Sung, K. S. Lee, and J. W. Hong, "Outcomes of laser peripheral iridotomy in angle closure subgroups according to anterior segment optical coherence tomography parameters," *Investigative Ophthalmology & Visual Science*, vol. 55, no. 10, pp. 6795–6801, 2014.

[27] Y. E. Wang, Y. Li, D. Wang, M. He, L. Wu, and S. C. Lin, "Comparison of iris insertion classification among American caucasian and ethnic Chinese using ultrasound biomicroscopy," *Investigative Ophthalmology & Visual Science*, vol. 54, no. 6, pp. 3837–3843, 2013.

[28] J. Y. Ku, M. E. Nongpiur, J. Park et al., "Qualitative evaluation of the iris and ciliary body by ultrasound biomicroscopy in subjects with angle closure," *Journal of Glaucoma*, vol. 23, no. 9, pp. 583–388, 2013.

[29] Y. Jiang, M. He, W. Huang, Q. Huang, J. Zhang, and P. J. Foster, "Qualitative assessment of ultrasound biomicroscopic images using standard photographs: the Liwan eye study," *Investigative Ophthalmology and Visual Science*, vol. 51, no. 4, pp. 2035–2042, 2010.

32

Aqueous Levels of Pigment Epithelium-Derived Factor and Macular Choroidal Thickness in High Myopia

Wei Chen,[1] **Yubo Guan,**[1] **Guanghui He,**[1] **Zhiwei Li,**[2] **Hui Song,**[1] **Shiyong Xie,**[1] **and Quanhong Han**[1]

[1] *Clinical College of Ophthalmology, Tianjin Medical University, No. 4, Gansu Road, Tianjin 300020, China*
[2] *Department of Ophthalmology, Shandong Provincial Hospital Affiliated to Shandong University, Jinan 250000, China*

Correspondence should be addressed to Quanhong Han; hanquanhong1968@163.com

Academic Editor: Ricardo Giordano

Purpose. To investigate the correlation between aqueous and serum levels of pigment epithelium-derived factor (PEDF) and macular choroidal thickness in high myopia patients, both with and without choroidal neovascularization (CNV). *Methods.* Serum and aqueous levels of PEDF were measured by enzyme-linked immunosorbent assay in 36 high myopia patients (36 eyes) with no CNV (non-CNV group), 14 high myopia patients (14 eyes) with CNV (CNV group), and 42 nonmyopia patients (42 eyes) (control group). Macular choroidal thickness was measured by enhanced-depth imaging optical coherence tomography. *Results.* Aqueous levels of PEDF were significantly higher in CNV group compared with non-CNV ($P < 0.001$) and control ($P < 0.001$) groups. Macular choroidal thicknesses were significantly decreased in the non-CNV and CNV groups compared with the control ($P < 0.001$) group. A statistically significant difference ($P = 0.012$) was found between the CNV and non-CNV groups. There was a positive correlation between aqueous PEDF and macular choroidal thickness in the non-CNV group ($P = 0.005$), but no correlation with the CNV group. No correlation between serum PEDF and macular choroidal thickness was detected in the three groups. *Conclusion.* Variations in aqueous PEDF levels coincide with changes in macular choroidal thickness in high myopia patients with no CNV, while no such relationship exists in high myopia patients with CNV.

1. Introduction

High myopia, which accounts for 27–33% of all myopia, is a major cause of legal blindness in numerous developed countries worldwide [1], with a prevalence of ~2% in the general population. Pathologically, myopia is characterized by excessive and progressive elongation of the globe (axial length, >26.5 mm) [2] and is associated with degenerative changes of the retina, choroid, and sclera at the posterior segment [3]. Myopic chorioretinal atrophy and choroidal neovascularization (CNV) are common causes of visual loss in high myopes. Since prevention of myopia is presently unachievable, it is of great importance to investigate the underlying mechanisms of and morphological changes associated with chorioretinal atrophy and CNV in highly myopic eyes.

Pigment epithelium-derived factor (PEDF), a secreted 50 kDa glycoprotein belonging to the superfamily of serine protease inhibitors, was first identified in conditioned media of cultured fetal human retinal pigment epithelial (RPE) cells [4]. PEDF not only is a more potent inhibitor of angiogenesis in the eye than are other endogenous antiangiogenic molecules [5], but also has neurotrophic/neuroprotective functions, playing roles in retinal differentiation, survival, and maintenance. Measurable variations in levels of aqueous PEDF in high myopia—with and without CNV—may indirectly reflect the nature and pathogenesis of these two phases of high myopia.

A new technique was recently implemented for improving depth imaging by optical coherence tomography (OCT). This technique—enhanced-depth imaging- (EDI-) OCT—has been shown to produce reliable images of full-thickness choroid [6]. EDI-OCT is, therefore, a most valuable tool for measuring choroidal thickness in highly myopic eyes. Wang et al. reported choroidal thickness to be a better indicator classifying myopic maculopathy than is either axial length or refractive error [7]. Using EDI-OCT, Ohsugi et al. revealed that choroidal thickness in all regions of highly myopic eyes was significantly reduced compared with normal refractive eyes [8].

Whether aqueous levels of PEDF are reflective of stages of chorioretinal atrophy and CNV in high myopia remains to be elucidated. The aim of our study was to determine how changes in choroidal thickness in high myopia contribute to the formation of myopic lesions in CNV. We investigated variations in aqueous and serum levels of PEDF in high myopia patients (with and without CNV) and correlated these variations with macular choroidal thickness. Results are expected to clarify the role of PEDF in the pathophysiology and morphology of high myopia.

2. Materials and Methods

2.1. Subjects. This observational, comparative, prospective study was carried out at the Tianjin Eye Hospital, Tianjin, China, between August and November 2013. The study conformed to the Declaration of Helsinki tenets for research involving human subjects and was approved by the Institutional Review Board of Tianjin Eye Hospital. Informed consent was obtained from all participants. Patients who had had surgery on both eyes were only enrolled at the time of the first surgery.

Patients were divided into groups based on myopia with and without CNV. The *non-CNV group* comprised 36 high myopia patients (n = 36 eyes) (with no CNV) who were in need of cataract surgery. Inclusion criteria included patients with eyes of axial lengths of ≥26.5 mm (Miller and Singerman, 2001) [9], refractive errors of >6 diopters (D), and no apparent macular abnormalities (e.g., choroidal neovascularization, macular holes) and who were 50–70 years of age. Exclusion criteria included poor image quality on OCT as a result of unstable fixation, severe cataract, previous ocular surgery, use of immunosuppressive drugs, eye diseases (e.g., glaucoma, age-related macular degeneration, and retinal detachment), and systemic diseases like serious heart, lung, liver, or kidney dysfunction. Patients with eyes in which the chorioscleral interface could not be clearly visualized were also excluded. The *CNV group* comprised 14 high myopia patients (n = 14 eyes) who were in need of intravitreal injections of ranibizumab (Lucentis, Novartis, Switzerland). Inclusion criteria comprised patients with eyes of axial lengths of ≥26.5 mm, refractive errors of >6 D, and choroidal neovascularization by fundus fluorescein angiography (FFA) and who were 50–70 years of age. Exclusion criteria were the same as those for the non-CNV group. Patients with secondary choroidal neovascular diseases, for example, angioid streaks and ocular trauma, were also excluded. All cases of CNV were confirmed by FFA. The *control group* comprised 42 normal patients (n = 42 eyes) who were in need of cataract surgery. Inclusion criteria comprised patients with healthy eyes with spherical equivalents of −3D–+3D. Exclusion criteria were the same as for the other groups.

2.2. Aqueous and Serum Samples. Samples of undiluted aqueous humor (100–200 μL) were collected by aspiration into a 1 mL syringe at the start of cataract surgery or before a single 0.05 mL intravitreal injection of ranibizumab. Serum specimens were collected prior to surgery. The levels of PEDF in aqueous humor and serum were measured using enzyme-linked immunosorbent assay (ELISA), according to the manufacturer's instructions (ChemiKine, Temecula, California, USA).

2.3. Ophthalmic Examination. All patients underwent a complete ophthalmic examination, including assessment of visual acuity (VA), refractive error, intraocular pressure (IOP), and axial length; OCT; dilated fundus examination by indirect ophthalmoscopy; and color fundus photographic assessment of myopic maculopathy. FFA was performed on all high myopia patients to confirm the presence or absence of CNV.

2.4. Measurements

2.4.1. Choroidal Thickness. The scan protocol of the Cirrus OCT (Carl Zeiss Meditec, Jena, Germany) generates a cube of data through a 9 mm line consisting of 4,096 A-scans around the macular region via a HD 5-line raster mode. EDI-OCT protocols have been described elsewhere [10]. Using the software-provided caliper system, choroidal thickness was measured from the outer surface of the hyperreflective line ascribed to the retinal pigment epithelium (RPE) to the hyperreflective line of the inner scleral border (Figure 1). Choroidal thicknesses were measured at the fovea, 3 mm superior and inferior to the fovea in vertical sections, and 3 mm temporal and nasal to the fovea in horizontal sections. The mean overall choroidal thickness, recorded as macular choroidal thickness, was obtained by calculating average choroidal thickness measurements from all measured areas. Two independent observers manually measured each choroidal thickness; both sets of measurements were averaged for analysis.

2.4.2. Axial Length, Refractive Error, and IOP. Axial length was measured using the Intraocular Lens Master (IOL-Master; Carl Zeiss Meditec, Dublin, CA). Refractive error was measured by autorefractometry (RK-3; Canon, Tokyo, Japan). IOP was measured by noncontact tonometry (TX-20 model; Canon, Tokyo, Japan).

2.5. Statistical Analysis. Statistical analyses were performed using version 17.0 SPSS software (SPSS, Inc., Chicago, IL, USA). All data were described as mean ± standard deviation (SD), with a 95% confidence interval (CI). An unpaired t-test was used to compare two independent groups with normal distribution; the Mann-Whitney U test was used to compare two independent groups without normal distribution; the Kruskal-Wallis H-test was used to compare variables among different groups; Fisher's exact t-test was used to compare noncontinuous variables; and Pearson's correlation test was used to analyze the correlation between aqueous PEDF concentrations, macular choroidal thickness, and serum PEDF

Table 1: Demographic and clinical characteristics.

Variables	Control group (n = 42)	High myopia without CNV group (n = 36)	High myopia with CNV group (n = 14)	P value
Mean age (years)	58.5 ± 5.3	59.6 ± 4.9	57.6 ± 5.4	0.573*
Axial length (mm)	24.3 ± 0.6	28.5 ± 1.1	29.6 ± 1.3	<0.001*
Refractive error (D)	−0.29 ± 1.42	−12.3 ± 4.7	−15.2 ± 3.1	<0.001*
Male gender (%)	42.9	44.4	42.9	0.916**
IOP (mmHg)	14.5 ± 2.8	15.8 ± 2.6	15.5 ± 3.2	0.357*

*Kruskal-Wallis H-test, compared among control, high myopia without CNV (non-CNV), and high myopia with CNV (CNV) groups.
**Fisher's exact t-test compared between control, non-CNV, and CNV groups.
CNV, choroidal neovascularization; D, diopters; IOP, intraocular pressure.

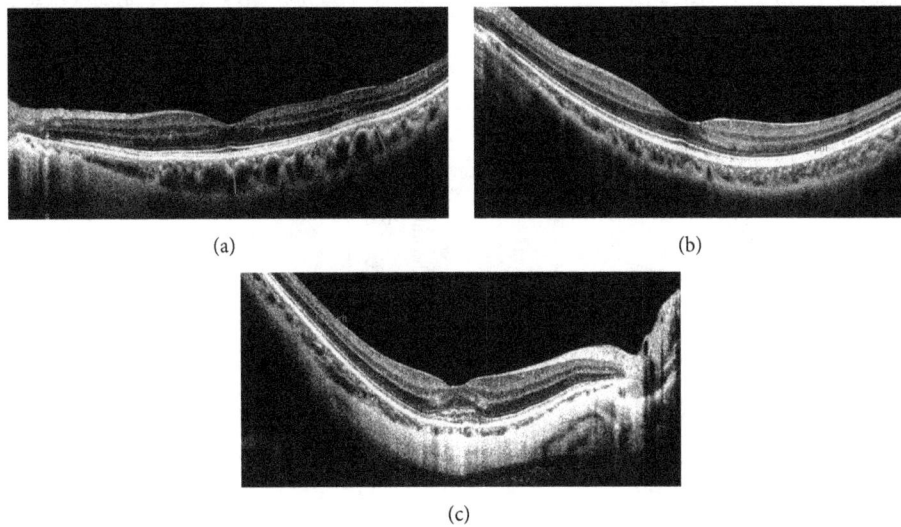

(a)

(b)

(c)

Figure 1: Optical coherence tomography (OCT) images using enhanced-depth imaging. The choroidal thickness (red line) is defined as the vertical from the outer surface of the hyperreflective line ascribed to the retinal pigment epithelium (RPE) to the hyperreflective line of the inner sclera border (a). Representative scan of a control individual (b). Representative scan of an individual with high myopia without choroidal neovascularization (CNV); note that the choroid is thinner than in the control but thicker than in high myopia with CNV (c). Representative scan of an individual with high myopia with CNV; note that the choroid is thinner than that of control or high myopia without CNV.

concentrations for the three groups. A $P < 0.05$ was considered statistically significant.

3. Results

Table 1 summarizes demographic and clinical characteristics. Average axial globe lengths were 24.3 ± 0.6, 28.5 ± 1.1, and 29.6 ± 1.3 mm for the control, non-CNV, and CNV groups, respectively. Average refractive errors (spherical equivalent refraction) were −0.29 ± 1.42, −12.3 ± 4.7, and −15.2 ± 3.1 D for the control, non-CNV, and CNV groups, respectively. Significant differences among the three groups were seen in axial length and refractive error ($P < 0.001$). Diffuse chorioretinal atrophy was present in 28 of 36 (77.8%) highly myopic eyes in the non-CNV group.

Aqueous levels of PEDF were significantly decreased in the non-CNV group (3.6 ± 1.3 ng/mL) compared with the control group (4.8 ± 1.8 ng/mL) ($P = 0.001$) and were significantly elevated in the CNV group (17.0 ± 5.8 ng/mL)

compared with the other two groups ($P < 0.001$) (Figure 2). Mean serum concentrations of PEDF were 5.8 ± 1.3, 5.4 ± 1.2, and 6.1 ± 1.5 µg/mL in the control, non-CNV, and CNV groups, respectively, with no statistically significant differences ($P = 0.632$). Aqueous levels of PEDF were significantly lower than serum levels of PEDF in all three groups ($P < 0.001$). Mean macular choroidal thicknesses were 230.6 ± 81.8, 111.1 ± 45.0, and 77.2 ± 26.9 µm in the control, non-CNV, and CNV groups, respectively. Differences were statistically significant for the non-CNV and CNV groups compared with the control group ($P < 0.001$), while a significant difference ($P = 0.012$) was also found between the non-CNV and CNV groups (Figure 2).

We studied the correlation between aqueous PEDF levels and macular choroidal thickness for the non-CNV group and found a significant, positive correlation ($R^2 = 0.211$, $P = 0.005$) (Figure 3), while no correlation was found for the CNV group ($R^2 = 0.108$, $P = 0.214$) (Figure 4). Conversely, no correlation between serum PEDF and macular choroidal

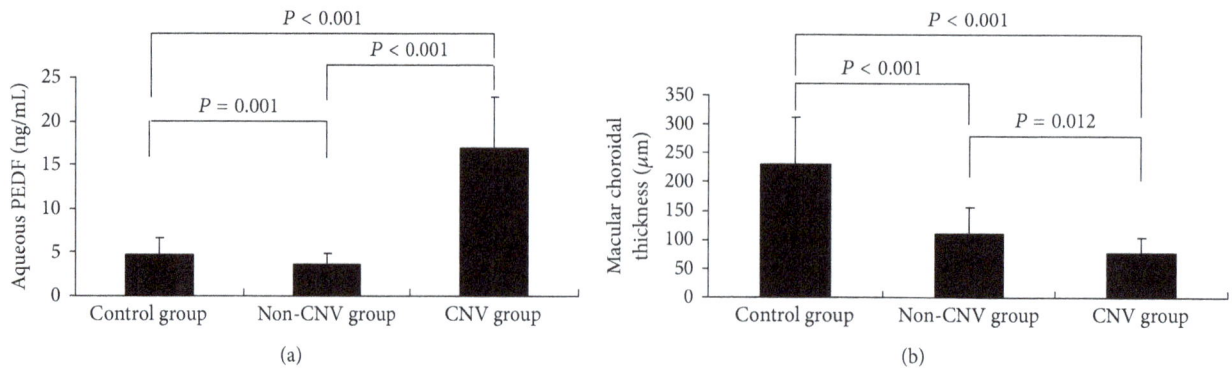

FIGURE 2: Aqueous pigment epithelium-derived factor (PEDF) levels in control and non-CNV groups (a) and in high myopia with CNV group. (b) Macular choroidal thickness in control, non-CNV, and CNV groups. Results are geometric mean (95% CI).

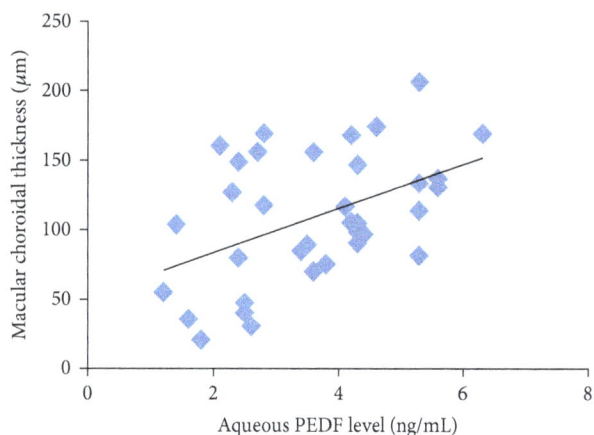

FIGURE 3: Scatterplots of aqueous PEDF levels and macular choroidal thickness in the non-CNV group show a significant positive correlation ($R^2 = 0.211$; $y = 15.852x + 51.986$; $P = 0.005$).

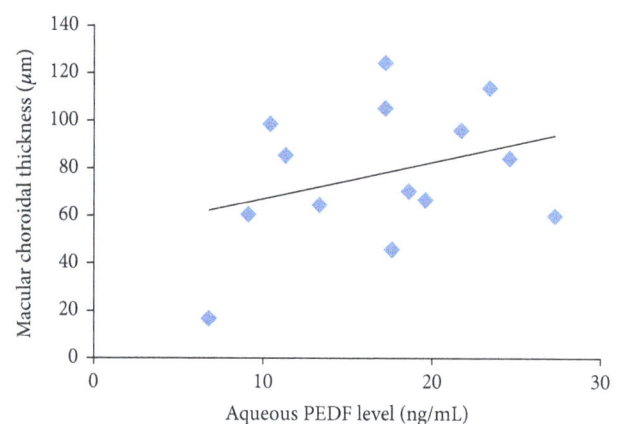

FIGURE 4: Scatterplots of aqueous PEDF levels and macular choroidal thickness in the CNV group show no correlation ($R^2 = 0.108$; $y = 1.5162x + 51.404$; $P = 0.214$).

thickness was detected for the non-CNV and CNV groups ($R^2 = 0.078$, $P = 0.674$; $R^2 = 0.0064$, $P = 0.720$, resp.). Also no correlation was found between aqueous and serum concentrations of PEDF for the non-CNV and CNV groups ($R^2 = 0.017$ and $R^2 = 0.0054$, resp.). There were also no correlations between aqueous PEDF, serum PEDF, and macular choroidal thickness for the control group.

4. Discussion

Pathologic myopia with progressive and excessive elongation of the eyeball results in a number of chorioretinal changes, including posterior staphyloma, chorioretinal atrophy, and pathologic CNV. Although the mechanisms underlying the development of chorioretinal atrophy and CNV remain unknown, dysfunctional RPE and RPE retraction—in the direction of radial traction line from its underlying glial tissue—are important contributors [11].

PEDF is synthesized and secreted by RPE and retinal ganglion cells and diffuses into the vitreous and aqueous humors [12]. In high myopia, the mechanical tissue strain caused by axial elongation could lead to the development

of choroidal ischemia, followed by RPE atrophy. There is a trend toward fewer photoreceptor cells and decreased RPE cell density in eyes with pathological myopia [13]. In addition, age-related functional deterioration of the RPE could result in altered PEDF expression, consequently decreasing inhibition of CNV growth [14].

In the present study, we found that levels of aqueous PEDF in non-CNV eyes were significantly lower (3.6 ± 1.3 ng/mL) than in the control group ($P = 0.001$). Ogata et al. also found the mean aqueous PEDF levels in high myopia to be significantly lower than in eyes with cataract alone [15]. However, Shin et al. reported that PEDF concentrations in highly myopic eyes did not differ significantly from those of control eyes [16]. We speculate that there are two reasons for the decrease found in the non-CNV group. First, because of the elongated axial length of highly myopic eyes, PEDF concentrations may be diluted as a result of the larger vitreous cavity, leading to decreased aqueous concentrations. Second, with chorioretinal atrophy-associated high myopia, decreased PEDF production may be a consequence of degenerated RPE and retinal ganglion cells, its two main sources in the eye.

Vascular endothelial growth factor (VEGF) and PEGF are two major cytokines in angiogenesis. VEGF not only is the major stimulator of neovascular growth and vascular permeability, but also maintains normal functions in many normal adult tissues. The aqueous level of VEGF has been analyzed in high myopia in another study of our group. We found aqueous levels of VEGF from non-CNV high myopia patients were significantly lower compared with those from control persons ($P < 0.001$); meanwhile aqueous levels of VEGF were significantly associated with both macular choroidal thickness ($P < 0.001$) and axial length ($P < 0.001$) [17]. Interestingly, in a similar study, Shin et al. reported that aqueous levels of VEGF in high myopia without CNV were significantly lower than levels in normal eyes [16].

Aqueous levels of PEDF were significantly increased in the CNV group compared with the non-CNV and control groups ($P < 0.001$). Ogata et al. demonstrated increased expression of both VEGF and PEDF in retinas with experimentally induced CNV [18]. However, Holekamp et al. demonstrated lower PEDF, but not VEGF, levels in the vitreous of patients with active CNV resulting from age-related macular degeneration (AMD) [19].

In the present study, we found no significant differences in serum PEDF levels among groups. Furthermore, there were no significant correlations between concentrations of aqueous and serum PEDF for the non-CNV and CNV groups. These findings suggest that, in high myopia, aqueous concentrations of PEDF are not determined by serum concentrations but, rather, by alterations in intraocular synthesis of PEDF.

In our study, macular choroidal thicknesses were 111.1 ± 45.0 and $77.2 \pm 26.9\,\mu m$ in the non-CNV and CNV groups, respectively, both significantly thinner than that of the control group ($P < 0.001$). In addition, Ikuno et al. reported that eyes with myopic CNV have a thinner choroid in comparison to the contralateral eye without CNV [20]. Chung et al. also speculated that a thinner choroid is a risk factor for CNV in eyes with high myopia [21]. We found that choroidal thickness differed significantly ($P = 0.012$) between highly myopic eyes with CNV and those with no CNV. Ikuno et al. also found choroidal thinning to be more prominent in eyes with myopic CNV compared with non-CNV eyes [20]. The association of choroidal thinning with development of myopic CNV is, as yet, unknown. One hypothesis is that choroidal thinning at the fovea leads to outer retinal hypoxic changes, resulting in release of VEGF—a critical mediator of angiogenesis in the eye [22].

To ensure consistency and to minimize any potential influence from diurnal fluctuation, we measured choroidal thickness between 9:00 a.m. and 12:00 p.m. Studies have shown the choroid to be thickest near midnight and thinnest near noon [23]. Using regression analysis, Margolis and Spaide reported an approximate decrease in choroidal thickness of $15\,\mu m$ every 10 years [24]. Thus, in order to reduce the influence of age, we chose patients who were 50–70 years old.

Although the primary regulatory role of the choroid in ocular physiology is well known, the in vivo clinical association of choroidal thickness with aqueous PEDF levels is unclear. We examined scatterplots of aqueous PEDF levels and macular choroidal thickness and found positive correlations for the non-CNV (Figure 3), but not the CNV (Figure 4), groups. There was no correlation for the CNV group, because PEDF could not be derived from the atrophic RPE cells in this stage.

Several limitations of our study should be mentioned. First, patients undergoing cataract surgery may differ from patients in general or high myopia patients and, accordingly, it is unclear whether the patients included in our study were representative of normal and high myopia patients. Second, choroidal thickness measurements were performed manually, as there exists no automated device for such measurements. In the present study, two masked readers performed measurements, with open negotiation if there was a difference of >15%. Third, RPE autofluorescence was not evaluated but may be an interesting variable to add to future studies.

In summary, variations in aqueous PEDF levels coincide with changes in macular choroidal thickness in high myopia patients with no CNV, while no such relationship exists in high myopia patients with CNV. Our findings suggest that in vivo macular choroidal thickness may be indicative of aqueous PEDF concentration in high myopia with no CNV, but no indication in high myopia with CNV. Nevertheless, based on previous studies showing that age, refractive error, and/or axial length could significantly influence choroidal thickness, the use of macular choroidal thickness as an indirect assessment of aqueous PEDF concentration might be of limited clinical application. Large-scale studies are recommended, particularly to examine the potential prognostic value of aqueous PEDF levels and choroidal changes.

Disclosure

Wei Chen and Yubo Guan are co-first authors.

Conflict of Interests

The authors declare that there is no conflict of interests regarding the publication of this paper.

References

[1] J. H. Kempen, "The prevalence of refractive errors among adults in the United States, Western Europe, and Australia," *Archives of Ophthalmology*, vol. 122, no. 4, pp. 495–505, 2004.

[2] Verteporfin in Photodynamic Therapy (VIP) Study Group, "Photodynamic therapy of subfoveal choroidal neovascularization in pathologic myopia with verteporfin: 1-year results of a randomized clinical trial VIP report no. 1," *Ophthalmology*, vol. 108, no. 5, pp. 841–852, 2001.

[3] J. M. Ruiz-Moreno, L. Arias, J. Montero, A. Carneiro, and R. Silva, "Intravitreal anti-VEGF therapy for choroidal neovascularisation secondary to pathological myopia: 4-year outcome," *The British Journal of Ophthalmology*, vol. 97, no. 11, pp. 1447–1450, 2013.

[4] J. Tombran-Tink and L. V. Johnson, "Neuronal differentiation of retinoblastoma cells induced by medium conditioned by human

RPE cells," *Investigative Ophthalmology and Visual Science*, vol. 30, no. 8, pp. 1700–1707, 1989.

[5] D. W. Dawson, O. V. Volpert, P. Gillis et al., "Pigment epithelium-derived factor: a potent inhibitor of angiogenesis," *Science*, vol. 285, no. 5425, pp. 245–248, 1999.

[6] D. S. Dhoot, S. Huo, A. Yuan et al., "Evaluation of choroidal thickness in retinitis pigmentosa using enhanced depth imaging optical coherence tomography," *British Journal of Ophthalmology*, vol. 97, no. 1, pp. 66–69, 2013.

[7] N.-K. Wang, C.-C. Lai, H.-Y. Chu et al., "Classification of early dry-type myopic maculopathy with macular choroidal thickness," *American Journal of Ophthalmology*, vol. 153, no. 4, pp. 669.e2–677.e2, 2012.

[8] H. Ohsugi, Y. Ikuno, K. Oshima, and H. Tabuchi, "3-D choroidal thickness maps from EDI-OCT in highly myopic eyes," *Optometry and Vision Science*, vol. 90, no. 6, pp. 599–606, 2013.

[9] D. G. Miller and L. J. Singerman, "Natural history of choroidal neovascularization in high myopia," *Current Opinion in Ophthalmology*, vol. 12, no. 3, pp. 222–224, 2001.

[10] N. Kara, N. Sayin, D. Pirhan et al., "Evaluation of subfoveal choroidal thickness in pregnant women using enhanced depth imaging optical coherence tomography," *Current Eye Research*, vol. 39, no. 6, pp. 642–647, 2014.

[11] N. Kitaya, S. Ishiko, T. Abiko et al., "Changes in blood-retinal barrier permeability in form deprivation myopia in tree shrews," *Vision Research*, vol. 40, no. 17, pp. 2369–2377, 2000.

[12] S. P. Becerra, R. N. Fariss, Y. Q. Wu, L. M. Montuenga, P. Wong, and B. A. Pfeffer, "Pigment epithelium-derived factor in the monkey retinal pigment epithelium and interphotoreceptor matrix: apical secretion and distribution," *Experimental Eye Research*, vol. 78, no. 2, pp. 223–234, 2004.

[13] H. E. Grossniklaus and W. R. Green, "Pathologic findings in pathologic myopia," *Retina*, vol. 12, no. 2, pp. 127–133, 1992.

[14] F. C. Delori, D. G. Goger, and C. K. Dorey, "Age-related accumulation and spatial distribution of lipofuscin in RPE of normal subjects," *Investigative Ophthalmology & Visual Science*, vol. 42, no. 8, pp. 1855–1866, 2001.

[15] N. Ogata, M. Imaizumi, M. Miyashiro et al., "Low levels of pigment epithelium-derived factor in highly myopic eyes with chorioretinal atrophy," *American Journal of Ophthalmology*, vol. 140, no. 5, pp. 937–939, 2005.

[16] Y. J. Shin, W. H. Nam, S. E. Park, J. H. Kim, and H. K. Kim, "Aqueous humor concentrations of vascular endothelial growth factor and pigment epithelium-derived factor in high myopic patients," *Molecular Vision*, vol. 18, no. 8, pp. 2265–2270, 2012.

[17] W. Chen, H. Song, S. Xie, Q. Han, X. Tang, and Y. Chu, "Correlation of macular choroidal thickness with concentrations of aqueous vascular endothelial frowth factor in high myopia," *Current Eye Research*. In press.

[18] N. Ogata, M. Wada, T. Otsuji, N. Jo, J. Tombran-Tink, and M. Matsumura, "Expression of pigment epithelium-derived factor in normal adult rat eye and experimental choroidal neovascularization," *Investigative Ophthalmology & Visual Science*, vol. 43, no. 4, pp. 1168–1175, 2002.

[19] N. M. Holekamp, N. Bouck, and O. Volpert, "Pigment epithelium-derived factor is deficient in the vitreous of patients with choroidal neovascularization due to age-related macular degeneration," *The American Journal of Ophthalmology*, vol. 134, no. 2, pp. 220–227, 2002.

[20] Y. Ikuno, Y. Jo, T. Hamasaki, and Y. Tano, "Ocular risk factors for choroidal neovascularization in pathologic myopia," *Investigative Ophthalmology & Visual Science*, vol. 51, no. 7, pp. 3721–3725, 2010.

[21] S. E. Chung, S. W. Kang, J. H. Lee, and Y. T. Kim, "Choroidal thickness in polypoidal choroidal vasculopathy and exudative age-related macular degeneration," *Ophthalmology*, vol. 118, no. 5, pp. 840–845, 2011.

[22] N. Ogata, M. Nishikawa, T. Nishimura, Y. Mitsuma, and M. Matsumura, "Unbalanced vitreous levels of pigment epithelium-derived factor and vascular endothelial growth factor in diabetic retinopathy," *American Journal of Ophthalmology*, vol. 134, no. 3, pp. 348–353, 2002.

[23] G. I. Papastergiou, G. F. Schmid, C. E. Riva, M. J. Mendel, R. A. Stone, and A. M. Laties, "Ocular axial length and choroidal thickness in newly hatched chicks and one-year-old chickens fluctuate in a diurnal pattern that is influenced by visual experience and intraocular pressure changes," *Experimental Eye Research*, vol. 66, no. 2, pp. 195–205, 1998.

[24] R. Margolis and R. F. Spaide, "A pilot study of enhanced depth imaging optical coherence tomography of the choroid in normal eyes," *American Journal of Ophthalmology*, vol. 147, no. 5, pp. 811–815, 2009.

33

Proteomic Analysis of the Vitreous following Experimental Retinal Detachment in Rabbits

Nakul Mandal,[1] **Geoffrey P. Lewis,**[2] **Steven K. Fisher,**[2,3] **Steffen Heegaard,**[4,5] **Jan U. Prause,**[5] **Morten la Cour,**[4] **Henrik Vorum,**[6] **and Bent Honoré**[7]

[1]*Department of Ophthalmology, Lund University, 22185 Lund, Sweden*
[2]*Neuroscience Research Institute, University of California, Santa Barbara, Santa Barbara, CA 93106-5060, USA*
[3]*Department of Molecular, Cellular and Developmental Biology, University of California, Santa Barbara, Santa Barbara, CA 93106-9625, USA*
[4]*Department of Ophthalmology, University of Copenhagen, 2600 Glostrup, Denmark*
[5]*Eye Pathology Institute, University of Copenhagen, 2100 Copenhagen, Denmark*
[6]*Department of Ophthalmology, Aalborg University Hospital, 9000 Aalborg, Denmark*
[7]*Department of Biomedicine, Aarhus University, 8000 Aarhus, Denmark*

Correspondence should be addressed to Nakul Mandal; nm@doctors.org.uk

Academic Editor: Ciro Costagliola

Purpose. The pathogenesis of rhegmatogenous retinal detachment (RRD) remains incompletely understood, with no clinically effective treatment for potentially severe complications such as photoreceptor cell death and proliferative vitreoretinopathy. Here we investigate the protein profile of the vitreous following experimental retinal detachment using a comparative proteomic based approach. *Materials and Methods.* Retinal detachment was created in the right eyes of six New Zealand red pigmented rabbits. Sham surgery was undertaken in five other rabbits that were used as controls. After seven days the eyes were enucleated and the vitreous was removed. The vitreous samples were evaluated with two-dimensional polyacrylamide gel electrophoresis and the differentially expressed proteins were identified with tandem mass spectrometry. *Results.* Ten protein spots were found to be at least twofold differentially expressed when comparing the vitreous samples of the sham and retinal detachment surgery groups. Protein spots that were upregulated in the vitreous following retinal detachment were identified as albumin fragments, and those downregulated were found to be peroxiredoxin 2, collagen-Iα1 fragment, and α-1-antiproteinase F. *Conclusions.* Proteomic investigation of the rabbit vitreous has identified a set of proteins that help further our understanding of the pathogenesis of rhegmatogenous retinal detachment and its complications.

1. Introduction

Rhegmatogenous retinal detachment (RRD) is characterized by the accumulation of subretinal fluid between the neurosensory retina and retinal pigment epithelium following the formation of a retinal break [1]. The pathogenesis of RRD is complex and incompletely understood, involving age-related and/or inherited structural and molecular changes of the vitreous extracellular matrix and vitreoretinal interface, and the process of posterior vitreous detachment [2]. The annual incidence of the condition has been estimated at 12.05 per 100,000, and although primary surgical reattachment is successful in the great majority of cases, photoreceptor cell death,

subretinal fibrosis, and proliferative vitreoretinopathy (PVR) continue to be significant causes of reduced visual outcomes [3, 4].

PVR involves the proliferation and migration of various cell types including retinal pigment epithelial (RPE) cells, Müller cells, inflammatory cells, and hyalocytes, which contribute to the formation of vitreal and periretinal membranes that can impede photoreceptor regeneration following surgical reattachment and cause tractional retinal detachment. The postulated epithelial-to-mesenchymal transition of RPE cells and Müller cell activation and growth onto the retinal surfaces are believed to be pivotal events in PVR [4, 5]. It appears that the exposure of such cells to the vitreous and associated growth factors as a result of RRD significantly contributes to the pathogenesis of PVR, though the basic cause as well as a clinically effective therapeutic approach for this condition remains elusive [5, 6].

Proteomics studies proteins on a large scale in pursuit of a global and integrated view of disease processes at the protein level, which may potentially lead to the identification of novel biomarkers and therapeutic targets useful in clinical practice [7–11]. RRD would likely be associated with alterations in the proteomic profiles of both the retina and vitreous. Indeed, we initially undertook the first such retinal study from which a number of potentially important proteins were identified [12]. The present study extends the proteomic investigation to the vitreous of this rabbit model of retinal detachment, building upon previous such analyses of human vitreous [13–16], in order to add further knowledge of the underlying pathophysiology [10, 17].

2. Materials and Methods

2.1. Retinal Detachment Surgery. Inferior retinal detachment was created in the right eyes of six New Zealand red pigmented rabbits. The eyes were normal with no evidence of disease on examination. Combined injections of xylazine (6.7 mg/kg) and ketamine (33.3 mg/kg) were administered intramuscularly to induce anesthesia and analgesia. The pupils were dilated with topical drops of atropine and tropicamide (1% solutions). A pipette tip, with an external diameter of approximately 100 μm, was inserted into the eye through a pars plana incision. Sodium hyaluronate (Healon, 0.25% in a balanced salt solution; Pharmacia, Piscataway, NJ) was infused via a glass pipette between the neurosensory retina and retinal pigment epithelium. Healon was necessary to prevent spontaneous retinal reattachment, and 0.25% is the most dilute solution that maintains the detachment for extended periods. Approximately 50% of the retina beneath the medullary rays, which included the central retina, was detached (Figure 1). Sham surgery was performed in the right eyes of five other rabbits that were used as controls, which involved surgical entry of the vitreous cavity without disruption of the retina. Scleral incisions were closed with 8-0 nylon suture. Seven days postoperatively the animals were euthanized by the administration of sodium pentobarbital (120 mg/kg; Butler Schein, Dublin, OH) and the eyes enucleated. After removal of the cornea and lens, the associated vitreous of the sham and detached retinas was extracted and immediately snap-frozen in liquid nitrogen within separate vials. There was no gross evidence of blood or other contamination of the vitreous samples at the time of tissue harvesting. The vitreous samples were stored at −80°C until further use.

All of the animal experiments undertaken in this study were in accordance with the standards of the National Institutes of Health Animal Care and Use Committee protocols, the ARVO Statement for the Use of Animals in Ophthalmic and Vision Research, and the guidelines of the Animal Resource Center, University of California, Santa Barbara.

2.2. Protein Extraction. The rabbit vitreous samples were homogenized and dissolved in a lysis buffer containing 9 M

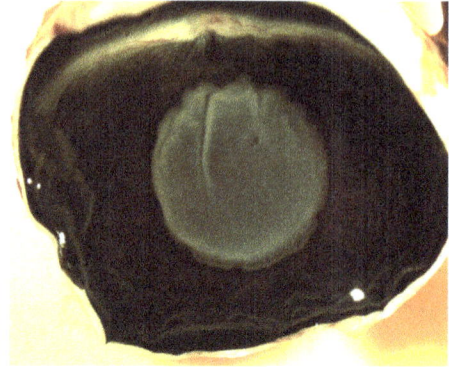

FIGURE 1: Appearance of the retinal detachment in the rabbit eye at seven days. The area of detached retina beneath the medullary rays appears grey and is surrounded by the darker attached retina. The detached retina contains a small hole where the micropipette was inserted. The retinal folds in the periphery occurred during the removal of the anterior structures.

urea, 2% (v/v) Triton X-100, 2% (v/v) immobilized pH gradient (IPG) buffer (pH 3–10 nonlinear), and 2% (w/v) dithiothreitol (DTT). The total protein content in each vitreous sample was determined with Non-Interfering Protein Assay (Calbiochem, San Diego, CA). The protein samples were stored at −80°C until further use.

2.3. Two-Dimensional Gel Electrophoresis. The extracted proteins were first fractionated by isoelectric focusing (IEF) using pH 3–10 nonlinear 18 cm IPG strips (GE Healthcare, Chalfont St. Giles, Buckinghamshire, UK). The IPG strips were rehydrated for 20 h at room temperature in 200 μL lysis buffer each containing 20 μg protein from individual vitreous samples and 150 μL rehydration buffer (8 M urea, 2% (w/v) 3-[(3-cholamidopropyl)dimethylammonio]-1-propanesulfonate (CHAPS), 0.3% (w/v) DTT, and 2% (v/v) IPG buffer), using the Immobiline DryStrip Reswelling Tray (GE Healthcare). The IEF was undertaken on a Multiphor II Electrophoresis System (GE Healthcare) at 500 V for 5 h and 3500 V in two steps for 5 h and 9.5 h in a gradient mode at 17°C with the use of a MultiTemp III Thermostatic Circulator (GE Healthcare). Before the second-dimension sodium dodecyl sulfate (SDS) polyacrylamide gel electrophoresis (PAGE), the IPG strips were equilibrated firstly for 10 min with gentle agitation in 20 mL of equilibration solution (0.6% (w/v) Tris-HCl, pH 6.8, 6 M urea, 30% (v/v) glycerol, 1% (w/v) SDS, and 0.05% (w/v) DTT) and secondly using 4.5% (w/v) iodoacetamide and bromophenol blue. The IPG strips were then transferred to 12% polyacrylamide gels for electrophoresis, which was performed at a maximum voltage of 50 V for approximately 20 h to separate the proteins vertically on the basis of molecular mass.

2.4. Protein Staining. The two-dimensional (2D) gels were silver stained using a protocol optimized for protein identification with mass spectrometry [18]. In brief, the gels were fixed overnight in 50% (v/v) ethanol, 12% (v/v) acetic acid, and 0.0185% (v/v) formaldehyde. The gels were washed 3 times for 20 min in 35% (v/v) ethanol and pretreated for 1 min in 0.02% (w/v) $Na_2S_2O_3 \cdot 5H_2O$. They were then rinsed in water and stained for 20 min in 0.2% (w/v) $AgNO_3$ and 0.028% (v/v) formaldehyde. Following further rinsing with water, development was undertaken for approximately 3 min in 6% (w/v) Na_2CO_3, 0.0185% (v/v) formaldehyde, and 0.0004% (w/v) $Na_2S_2O_3 \cdot 5H_2O$. The development was arrested in a fixative solution of 40% (v/v) ethanol and 12% (v/v) acetic acid. The 2D gels were then dried between cellophane sheets and sealed in plastic envelopes.

2.5. Image Analysis. Silver stained 2D gels were scanned on a GS-710 Calibrated Imaging Densitometer (Bio-Rad, Hercules, CA) using the Quantity One program (Bio-Rad), and the PDQuest software (Bio-Rad) was used to define, quantify, and match the protein spots on each of the 2D gels. All well-defined protein spots that were at least twofold (Mann-Whitney U test, $p < 0.05$) differentially expressed between the sham and retinal detachment vitreous groups were selected for identification with nanoliquid chromatography-electrospray ionization tandem mass spectrometry (LC-MS/MS).

2.6. Protein Identification. The 2D gels were removed from their plastic envelopes and rehydrated in water. The selected protein spots were carefully excised from the gels with a scalpel and subjected to in-gel digestion with Trypsin Gold (Mass Spectrometry Grade; Promega, Madison, WI). The peptide samples that were obtained were analyzed by LC-MS/MS as previously described [12]. In brief, peptides generated by trypsin digestion were separated on an inert nano-LC system (LC Packings, San Francisco, CA) connected to a Q-TOF Premier mass spectrometer (Waters, Milford, MA). The MassLynx 4 SP4 (Waters) was used to obtain spectra and the raw data was processed using ProteinLynx Global Server 2.1 (Waters). The processed data were used to search the total part of the Swiss-Prot database using the online version of the Mascot MS/MS Ions Search facility (Matrix Science, Ltd.). The search was undertaken with doubly and triply charged ions with up to two missed cleavages, a peptide tolerance of 50 ppm, one variable modification, carbamidomethyl-C, and a MS/MS tolerance of 0.05 Da. Contaminating peptides such as trypsin, keratin, bovine serum albumin, and all peptides originating from previous samples were disregarded. At least one "bold red" (Matrix Science Ltd., http://www.matrixscience.com/) peptide match was required in the search for protein hits. Individual peptide ions scores above approximately 36 indicated identity or extensive homology giving a less than 5% probability that the observed match was a random event. All peptides for the protein hits are reported (Table 1).

2.7. Western Blotting. In each case three micrograms of vitreous sample protein was separated on Novex 10–20% gradient Tris-Glycine polyacrylamide gels (Invitrogen Corporation, Carlsbad, CA) and subsequently transferred to nitrocellulose Hybond-C Extra membranes (GE Healthcare). The membranes were blocked overnight with 5% skimmed milk in 80 mM Na_2HPO_4, 20 mM NaH_2PO_4, 100 mM NaCl, and 0.05% Tween 20 buffer, pH 7.5. Membranes were incubated with anti-albumin (Genway Biotech, CA, USA; 1 : 5000) and anti-peroxiredoxin 2 (Abcam, Cambridge, UK; 1 : 200). No suitable antibodies were commercially available for the rabbit F isoform of α-1-antiproteinase or the rabbit collagen-Iα1 fragment that was identified with LC-MS/MS. Following washing, the membranes were further incubated with appropriate horseradish peroxidase-conjugated secondary antibodies: P0163 sheep and P0260 mouse (both 1 : 1000; DAKO, Glostrup, Denmark). Proteins were visualized with the enhanced chemiluminescence system (GE Healthcare) and imaging system (Fujifilm LAS-3000, Tokyo, Japan).

3. Results

3.1. 2D-PAGE Analysis. Up to approximately 340 protein spots were clearly resolved on each of the 11 2D gels. Ten protein spots were found to be significantly and at least twofold differentially expressed between the sham and detachment vitreous groups (Figure 2). Three protein spots were upregulated and seven spots were downregulated.

3.2. LC-MS/MS Analysis. From the three upregulated protein spots, two were identified as fragments of albumin (spots 5104 and 6101), whilst spot 6205 could not be identified. Four of the seven downregulated protein spots were identified as fragment of collagen-Iα1 (spot 0503), α-1-antiproteinase F (spots 0703 and 1707), and peroxiredoxin 2 (spot 0705). Protein spots 0102, 0815, and 1302 could not be identified (Figure 2; Table 1).

3.3. Western Blot Analysis. Western blotting developed with anti-albumin showed a heavy band at approximately 60 kDa, which is likely to represent the full length protein, whilst multiple bands below this suggest the presence of several fragments, some of which may correspond with those identified with the 2D-PAGE analysis (Figure 3, left). Peroxiredoxin 2 has a deduced molecular mass of approximately 22 kDa. However, spot 0705 containing peroxiredoxin 2 migrates with a molecular mass around 60 kDa with 2D-PAGE (Figure 2), and this size was verified by western blot analysis (Figure 3, right). Though a single and specific band was achieved with anti-peroxiredoxin 2, western blotting could not be reliably used for quantification due to a weak signal near the detection limit and variable background reaction.

4. Discussion

4.1. Albumin. Analysis with 2D-PAGE revealed fragments of albumin to be upregulated in the vitreous following retinal detachment. Albumin is the most abundant protein in plasma, aqueous, and vitreous humor, where in the latter it constitutes around 60–70% of total protein [19–21]. Serum proteins such as albumin are present in the aqueous and vitreous humor at a relatively lower level compared to the vascular circulation from where they may have in part originated [21, 22]. Western blot analysis showed an intense band at approximately 60 kDa corresponding with the full length albumin

TABLE 1: Mass spectrometric identification of the 2D-PAGE protein spots differentially expressed in the rabbit vitreous.

Spot number	Protein name (full chain length)	Peptide sequence (amino acid numbers)	Mascot Ions score	Theoretical pI; Mr kDa	Fold change RD: sham	Biological processes
5104	Albumin (608) fragment	CCSESLVDR (500–508) / TVVGEFTALLDK (570–581) / EACFAVEGPK (589–598)	52 / 14 / 28	5.67; 66.5	2.62	Transport; cellular response to starvation; maintenance of mitochondrial location; negative regulation of apoptosis; hemolysis of symbiont of host erythrocytes
6101	Albumin (608) fragment	ACVADESAANCDK (76–88) / DTYGDVADCCEK (106–117)	39 / 7	5.67; 66.5	3.13	
0503	Collagen type Iα1 (1463) fragment	GETGPAGPAGPIGPVGAR (1066–1083)	61	9.20; 94.4	0.46	Blood vessel development; collagen biosynthetic process; collagen fibril organization; leukocyte migration; platelet activation; positive regulation of cell migration, epithelial-to-mesenchymal transition, transcription, and canonical Wnt receptor signaling pathway; protein localization to nucleus; protein transport; visual perception; axon guidance
1707	α-1-antiproteinase F (413)	GDTHTQVLEGLK (89–100)	64	5.76; 43.5	0.42	Negative regulation of peptidase activity
0703	α-1-antiproteinase F (413)	IVDLVQELDAR (188–198)	70	5.76; 43.5	0.24	
0705	Peroxiredoxin 2 (198)	TDEGIAYR (120–127)	43	5.67; 21.8	0.30	Response to oxidative stress; regulation of hydrogen peroxide metabolic process; removal of superoxide radicals; positive regulation of blood coagulation; activation of MAPK; respiratory burst involved in inflammatory response; antiapoptosis; regulation of apoptotic process; negative regulation of lipopolysaccharide mediated signaling pathway; negative regulation of NF-KappaB transcription factor; T cell proliferation; homeostasis of number of cells

Protein spots 6205, 1302, 0815, and 0102 with fold changes of 2.65, 0.28, 0.27, and 0.18, respectively, could not be identified. Individual Mascot Ions scores greater than approximately 36 indicate identity or extensive homology ($p < 0.05$). Biological processes were taken from the Gene Ontology Consortium (http://geneontology.org/). RD represents retinal detachment.

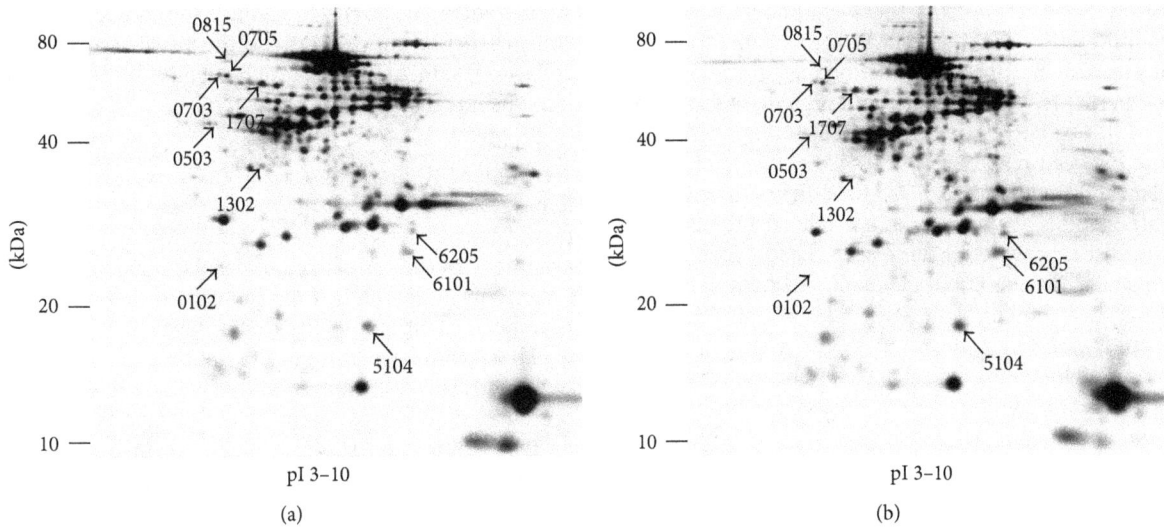

FIGURE 2: Representative 2D-PAGE images of proteins fractionated from rabbit vitreous. Ten protein spots (arrows) were found to be significantly and at least twofold differentially expressed between the sham (a) and detached (b) vitreous.

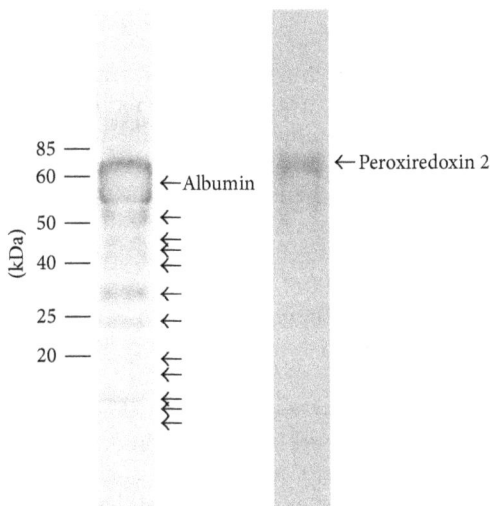

FIGURE 3: Western blot analysis of sham rabbit vitreous developed with anti-albumin and anti-peroxiredoxin 2. Labeled arrows correspond to the respective full length proteins. The unlabeled arrows for the lower molecular mass bands on the anti-albumin blot may indicate the specific cleavage fragments, which correspond with some of the differentially expressed 2D-PAGE protein spots.

protein, with multiple lower molecular mass bands that are likely its fragments. Increase of albumin and its fragments may signify increased proteolysis and the passage of albumin into the vitreous. Indeed, the breakdown of the blood-retinal barrier that occurs with retinal detachment has also been implicated in the increase of other such proteins in the vitreous [12, 23–28]. It is also possible that albumin in the vitreous may arise from de novo synthesis in the retina, similar to the reported increased gene and protein expression of albumin in the corneal epithelium during wound healing [29, 30].

Extraocular albumin is known to have diverse and important functions, which include maintenance of colloid osmotic pressure, transport of biomolecules, and inactivation of toxins through intermolecular binding [31, 32]. Albumin can also act as an antioxidant by scavenging reactive oxygen species and sequestration of metal ions and has anti-inflammatory and apoptotic regulatory abilities [32–35]. Vitreal albumin has been proposed to transport long chain fatty acids into the lens for biosynthesis of lenticular lipids [21, 31, 36]. Indeed, albumin is likely to have many such important roles in the eye, which requires further investigation.

4.2. Peroxiredoxin 2. In the present study we observed peroxiredoxin 2 to have a molecular mass above 60 kDa using both 2D-PAGE and western blot analyses. However, the predicted molecular mass of the peroxiredoxin family of proteins is approximately 22 kDa–31 kDa. This variation may represent the well-studied property of these proteins to undergo oligomerization, which can be promoted by a number of factors including overoxidation of cysteine residues of peroxiredoxin [37]. Although the present experiments were conducted in standard reducing conditions that aim to break cysteine bonds, we obtained a band well above 20 kDa. This is in keeping with another study, which also showed some peroxiredoxin 2 western blot bands appearing at molecular mass much higher than 20 kDa that was suggested to result from oligomerization or posttranslational modification [38]. Our finding could also represent a novel alternative splicing variant of peroxiredoxin 2, as reported for peroxiredoxin 5 [39].

The peroxiredoxins are a group of ubiquitous antioxidant proteins that currently comprise six members in mammals [40]. These proteins are primarily found at high levels intracellularly, mainly within the cytosol, but are also present in the mitochondria, peroxisomes, and nuclei, and they may be exported [37]. Furthermore, presence of peroxiredoxin 2 has been shown in plasma, not only as a result of hemolysis but also possibly by secretion from the T lymphocytes [41, 42]. These multifunction enzymes act as antioxidants by using redox active cysteines for the reduction and degradation of hydrogen peroxide, peroxynitrite, and organic hydroperoxides [37, 43]. Oxidative stress is thought to result from an imbalance between reactive oxygen species production and antioxidant ability and is recognized to be an important factor in the pathogenesis of a number of age-related and neurodegenerative diseases, which include age-related cataract, age-related macular degeneration, glaucoma, diabetic retinopathy, retinal detachment, and PVR [44–47]. Indeed, the present study showed a decrease in the vitreal levels of peroxiredoxin 2 following retinal detachment. This may be in keeping with reported reductions in the levels of other members of the antioxidant defense system such as glutathione and ascorbic acid both in vitreal and in blood samples of patients suffering from PVR [44, 45]. Furthermore, apart from their role as antioxidants, the peroxiredoxins can affect a diverse range of biological processes that include cellular proliferation, differentiation, and apoptosis by influencing signal transduction pathways that employ hydrogen peroxide as a secondary messenger [43, 48]. Recent studies on tears from patients with glaucoma have also identified peroxiredoxin 1 as having a possible involvement in inflammation [49, 50]. Indeed, peroxiredoxin 2 and other members of this family of proteins are liable to have a significant role in the pathophysiology of retinal detachment.

4.3. Collagen-Iα1. A fragment of collagen-Iα1 was identified in the vitreous of the rabbit; however, type I collagen has not previously been identified as a natural component of the mammalian vitreous and is rather known to be a constituent of early PVR membranes [51–53] and retinal blood vessels [54, 55]. A mixture of type II, IX, and V/XI hybrid collagen fibrils, which are separated out mainly by water and ions attracted to hyaluronan, characterizes the vitreous body [56]. Collagen, possibly with the aid of adhesive-like intermediate molecules, may provide the basis of vitreoretinal adhesion by connecting the vitreous with the retinal inner limiting membrane (ILM). This attachment is extremely strong in the vitreous base since the fibrils pass through the ILM to merge into underlying collagen networks and crypts [2, 56, 57]. Collagen is also a significant component of both epiretinal and subretinal PVR membranes [53, 58], and type I collagen is recognized to be a principal constituent during their early development [51–53]. The presence of collagen in the subretinal space, a place normally devoid of this protein, suggests that certain cells, particularly the RPE and Müller cells associated with membranes, are able to synthesize collagen under certain pathological conditions such as retinal detachment and PVR [58–61]. However, the present analysis suggests collagen-Iα1 fragment to be found in sham vitreous, which furthermore showed a decreased concentration following retinal detachment that may indicate perturbed proteolytic activity. Matrix metalloproteinases (MMP) and other proteolytic enzymes that are able to degrade and remodel vitreal collagen have been found to be increased with RRD and PVR [62–65], which could be in keeping with the decrease in α-1-antiproteinase shown in the present study. Further

studies will be necessary to confirm the source and nature of collagen-Iα1 in the vitreous and the possible mechanisms of collagen fragmentation that may be an important feature of vitreous liquefaction and RRD [2, 62, 66].

4.4. Alpha-1-Antiproteinase. 2D-PAGE showed α-1-antiproteinase (also called α-1-antitrypsin or α-1-proteinase inhibitor) at two closely positioned spots, which were largely in keeping with their predicted molecular mass but differing by their charge. Currently, four isoforms of α-1-antiproteinase have been identified in the rabbit, termed F, S1, S2, and E, which is a similar picture to the multiple variants identified in humans [67, 68]. Alpha-1-antiproteinase is an acute phase protein and archetypal member of the superfamily of serine protease inhibitors (serpin), which are involved in a wide range of biological processes that includes inflammation, angiogenesis, blood coagulation, ECM remodeling, and tumor suppression [69]. This protein has the ability to inhibit a large number of serine proteases though its principle target is neutrophil elastase [68]. Indeed, α-1-antiproteinase originally received much attention because its deficiency increases the risk of a variety of clinical conditions, such as chronic obstructive pulmonary disease, which can result from unrestrained elastase activity.

We found the F isoform of rabbit α-1-antiproteinase to be downregulated in the vitreous following retinal detachment. The F isoform of α-1-antiproteinase is the only one of the rabbit isoforms so far identified that has been shown to have the oxidizable methionine residue site that is present in human α-1-antiproteinase [67]. The oxidation of methionine to methionine sulfoxide, which can occur during episodes of inflammation as a result of oxygen-free radicals secreted by leucocytes, has an inhibiting effect upon α-1-antiproteinase function. This process is thought to enhance the ability of proteinases such as elastase to locally degrade tissue debris that occurs at sites of inflammation [67, 68].

Alpha-1-antiproteinase is primarily produced in the liver and circulated to the rest of the body tissues via the blood; however, extrahepatic sites of its synthesis have been identified, which include blood monocytes, alveolar macrophages, bronchial and gastrointestinal epithelial cells, and the cornea [70–73]. The protein has also been localized to the tear film, aqueous humor, and vitreous, where in the latter a phosphorylated form of α-1-antiproteinase has been suggested as a potential biomarker of idiopathic macular hole and rhegmatogenous retinal detachment [73–75]. It has been postulated that one of the main functions of corneal α-1-antiproteinase is to protect against the damaging effects of neutrophil elastase produced during corneal inflammation [73], and it may be expected that a similar role in addition to others is applicable to vitreal α-1-antiproteinase, though this requires further investigation.

5. Conclusion

This proteomic investigation of the rabbit vitreous has identified a set of proteins that assist our understanding of the pathogenesis of rhegmatogenous retinal detachment and its complications. Further studies will be necessary to clarify the role of these proteins. Certain proteins, such as those of low abundance and at the extremes of molecular mass, together with membrane proteins, can be difficult to resolve and detect using the 2D-PAGE technique. Therefore, complementary proteomic methods such as gel-free mass spectrometry should be considered in future work in order to help address these limitations.

Disclaimer

The authors alone are responsible for the content and writing of the paper.

Conflict of Interests

The authors report no conflict of interests.

Acknowledgments

The authors appreciate the excellent technical support provided by Mona Britt Hansen and Inge Kjærgaard and are grateful to Dr. Satpal Ahuja for the helpful suggestions for the paper. This work was supported by The Danish Society for Eye Health, The Danish Eye Research Foundation, Foreningen Østifterne, The Synoptik Foundation, The Beckett Foundation, The Danish Medical Research Council, The John and Birthe Meyer Foundation, Aarhus University Research Foundation, The National Science Foundation, USA (ITR-0331697), and National Institutes of Health, USA.

References

[1] A. Sodhi, L.-S. Leung, D. V. Do, E. W. Gower, O. D. Schein, and J. T. Handa, "Recent trends in the management of rhegmatogenous retinal detachment," *Survey of Ophthalmology*, vol. 53, no. 1, pp. 50–67, 2008.

[2] D. Mitry, B. W. Fleck, A. F. Wright, H. Campbell, and D. G. Charteris, "Pathogenesis of rhegmatogenous retinal detachment: predisposing anatomy and cell biology," *Retina*, vol. 30, no. 10, pp. 1561–1572, 2010.

[3] D. Mitry, D. G. Charteris, D. Yorston et al., "The epidemiology and socioeconomic associations of retinal detachment in Scotland: a two-year prospective population-based study," *Investigative Ophthalmology and Visual Science*, vol. 51, no. 10, pp. 4963–4968, 2010.

[4] S. K. Fisher and G. P. Lewis, "Cellular effects of detachment and reattachment on the neural retina and the retinal pigment epithelium," in *Retina*, S. J. Ryan, D. R. Hinton, A. P. Schachat, and C. P. Wilkinson, Eds., vol. 3, pp. 1991–2012, Mosby, St. Louis, Mo, USA, 2006.

[5] S. Tamiya, L. Liu, and H. J. Kaplan, "Epithelial-mesenchymal transition and proliferation of retinal pigment epithelial cells initiated upon loss of cell-cell contact," *Investigative Ophthalmology & Visual Science*, vol. 51, no. 5, pp. 2755–2763, 2010.

[6] S. Pennock, M.-A. Rheaume, S. Mukai, and A. Kazlauskas, "A novel strategy to develop therapeutic approaches to prevent proliferative vitreoretinopathy," *The American Journal of Pathology*, vol. 179, no. 6, pp. 2931–2940, 2011.

[7] N. Mandal, S. Heegaard, J. U. Prause, B. Honoré, and H. Vorum, "Ocular proteomics with emphasis on two-dimensional gel electrophoresis and mass spectrometry," *Biological Procedures Online*, vol. 12, no. 1, pp. 56–88, 2010.

[8] S. E. Coupland, H. Vorum, N. Mandal et al., "Proteomics of uveal melanomas suggests HSP-27 as a possible surrogate marker of chromosome 3 loss," *Investigative Ophthalmology & Visual Science*, vol. 51, no. 1, pp. 12–20, 2010.

[9] N. Mandal, M. Kofod, H. Vorum et al., "Proteomic analysis of human vitreous associated with idiopathic epiretinal membrane," *Acta Ophthalmologica*, vol. 91, no. 4, pp. e333–e334, 2013.

[10] L. J. Cehofski, N. Mandal, B. Honoré, and H. Vorum, "Analytical platforms in vitreoretinal proteomics," *Bioanalysis*, vol. 6, no. 22, pp. 3051–3066, 2014.

[11] L. J. Cehofski, A. Kruse, B. Kjærgaard, A. Stensballe, B. Honoré, and H. Vorum, "Dye-free porcine model of experimental branch retinal vein occlusion: a suitable approach for retinal proteomics," *Journal of Ophthalmology*, vol. 2015, Article ID 839137, 7 pages, 2015.

[12] N. Mandal, G. P. Lewis, S. K. Fisher et al., "Protein changes in the retina following experimental retinal detachment in rabbits," *Molecular Vision*, vol. 17, pp. 2634–2648, 2011.

[13] T. Shitama, H. Hayashi, S. Noge et al., "Proteome profiling of vitreoretinal diseases by cluster analysis," *Proteomics—Clinical Applications*, vol. 2, no. 9, pp. 1265–1280, 2008.

[14] J. Yu, F. Liu, S.-J. Cui et al., "Vitreous proteomic analysis of proliferative vitreoretinopathy," *Proteomics*, vol. 8, no. 17, pp. 3667–3678, 2008.

[15] J. Yu, R. Peng, H. Chen, C. Cui, and J. Ba, "Elucidation of the pathogenic mechanism of rhegmatogenous retinal detachment with proliferative vitreoretinopathy by proteomic analysis," *Investigative Ophthalmology and Visual Science*, vol. 53, no. 13, pp. 8146–8153, 2012.

[16] M. Angi, H. Kalirai, S. E. Coupland, B. E. Damato, F. Semeraro, and M. R. Romano, "Proteomic analyses of the vitreous humour," *Mediators of Inflammation*, vol. 2012, Article ID 148039, 7 pages, 2012.

[17] V. B. Mahajan and J. M. Skeie, "Translational vitreous proteomics," *Proteomics: Clinical Applications*, vol. 8, no. 3-4, pp. 204–208, 2014.

[18] E. Mortz, T. N. Krogh, H. Vorum, and A. Görg, "Improved silver staining protocols for high sensitivity protein identification using matrix-assisted laser desorption/ionization-time of flight analysis," *Proteomics*, vol. 1, no. 11, pp. 1359–1363, 2001.

[19] J. N. Ulrich, M. Spannagl, A. Kampik, and A. Gandorfer, "Components of the fibrinolytic system in the vitreous body in patients with vitreoretinal disorders," *Clinical and Experimental Ophthalmology*, vol. 36, no. 5, pp. 431–436, 2008.

[20] K. Yamane, A. Minamoto, H. Yamashita et al., "Proteome analysis of human vitreous proteins," *Molecular & Cellular Proteomics*, vol. 2, no. 11, pp. 1177–1187, 2003.

[21] J. Sabah, E. McConkey, R. Welti, K. Albin, and L. J. Takemoto, "Role of albumin as a fatty acid carrier for biosynthesis of lens lipids," *Experimental Eye Research*, vol. 80, no. 1, pp. 31–36, 2005.

[22] T. F. Freddo, "Shifting the paradigm of the blood-aqueous barrier," *Experimental Eye Research*, vol. 73, no. 5, pp. 581–592, 2001.

[23] B. C. Little and V. M. G. Ambrose, "Blood-aqueous barrier breakdown associated with rhegmatogenous retinal detachment," *Eye*, vol. 5, part 1, pp. 56–62, 1991.

[24] H. Nagasaki, K. Shinagawa, and M. Mochizuki, "Risk factors for proliferative vitreoretinopathy," *Progress in Retinal and Eye Research*, vol. 17, no. 1, pp. 77–98, 1998.

[25] C. C. Tomé, M. V. De Rojas Silva, J. Rodríguez-García, S. Rodríguez-Segade, and M. Sánchez-Salorio, "Levels of pentosidine in the vitreous of eyes with proliferative diabetic retinopathy, proliferative vitreoretinopathy and retinal detachment," *Graefe's Archive for Clinical and Experimental Ophthalmology*, vol. 243, no. 12, pp. 1272–1276, 2005.

[26] R. F. Gariano, A. K. Nath, D. J. D'Amico, T. Lee, and M. R. Sierra-Honigmann, "Elevation of vitreous leptin in diabetic retinopathy and retinal detachment," *Investigative Ophthalmology and Visual Science*, vol. 41, no. 11, pp. 3576–3581, 2000.

[27] G. E. Rose, B. M. Billington, and A. H. Chignell, "Immunoglobulins in paired specimens of vitreous and subretinal fluids from patients with rhegmatogenous retinal detachment," *The British Journal of Ophthalmology*, vol. 74, no. 3, pp. 160–162, 1990.

[28] J. E. Pederson and C. B. Toris, "Experimental retinal detachment. IX. Aqueous, vitreous, and subretinal protein concentrations," *Archives of Ophthalmology*, vol. 103, no. 6, pp. 835–836, 1985.

[29] L. Carter-Dawson, Y. Zhang, R. S. Harwerth et al., "Elevated albumin in retinas of monkeys with experimental glaucoma," *Investigative Ophthalmology & Visual Science*, vol. 51, no. 2, pp. 952–959, 2010.

[30] S. Mushtaq, Z. A. Naqvi, A. A. Siddiqui, C. Palmberg, J. Shafqat, and N. Ahmed, "Changes in albumin precursor and heat shock protein 70 expression and their potential role in response to corneal epithelial wound repair," *Proteomics*, vol. 7, no. 3, pp. 463–468, 2007.

[31] T. Peters, *All About Albumin: Biochemistry, Genetics, and Medical Applications*, Academic Press, San Diego, Calif, USA, 1996.

[32] G. J. Quinlan, G. S. Martin, and T. W. Evans, "Albumin: biochemical properties and therapeutic potential," *Hepatology*, vol. 41, no. 6, pp. 1211–1219, 2005.

[33] C. Bolitho, P. Bayl, J. Y. Hou et al., "The anti-apoptotic activity of albumin for endothelium is mediated by a partially cryptic protein domain and reduced by inhibitors of G-coupled protein and PI-3 kinase, but is independent of radical scavenging or bound lipid," *Journal of Vascular Research*, vol. 44, no. 4, pp. 313–324, 2007.

[34] E. Erkan, P. Devarajan, and G. J. Schwartz, "Mitochondria are the major targets in albumin-induced apoptosis in proximal tubule cells," *Journal of the American Society of Nephrology*, vol. 18, no. 4, pp. 1199–1208, 2007.

[35] J. Iglesias, V. E. Abernethy, Z. Wang, W. Lieberthal, J. S. Koh, and J. S. Levine, "Albumin is a major serum survival factor for renal tubular cells and macrophages through scavenging of ROS," *The American Journal of Physiology—Renal Physiology*, vol. 277, no. 5, pp. F711–F722, 1999.

[36] J. R. Sabah, H. Davidson, E. N. McConkey, and L. Takemoto, "In vivo passage of albumin from the aqueous humor into the lens," *Molecular Vision*, vol. 10, pp. 254–259, 2004.

[37] Z. A. Wood, E. Schröder, J. R. Harris, and L. B. Poole, "Structure, mechanism and regulation of peroxiredoxins," *Trends in Biochemical Sciences*, vol. 28, no. 1, pp. 32–40, 2003.

[38] G. Manandhar, A. Miranda-Vizuete, J. R. Pedrajas et al., "Peroxiredoxin 2 and peroxidase enzymatic activity of mammalian spermatozoa," *Biology of Reproduction*, vol. 80, no. 6, pp. 1168–1177, 2009.

[39] M. Sensi, G. Pietra, A. Molla et al., "Peptides with dual binding specificity for HLA-A2 and HLA-E are encoded by alternatively spliced isoforms of the antioxidant enzyme peroxiredoxin 5," *International Immunology*, vol. 21, no. 3, pp. 257–268, 2009.

[40] G. Leyens, I. Donnay, and B. Knoops, "Cloning of bovine peroxiredoxins-gene expression in bovine tissues and amino acid sequence comparison with rat, mouse and primate peroxiredoxins," *Comparative Biochemistry and Physiology B Biochemistry and Molecular Biology*, vol. 136, no. 4, pp. 943–955, 2003.

[41] J.-H. Chen, Y.-W. Chang, C.-W. Yao et al., "Plasma proteome of severe acute respiratory syndrome analyzed by two-dimensional gel electrophoresis and mass spectrometry," *Proceedings of the National Academy of Sciences of the United States of America*, vol. 101, no. 49, pp. 17039–17044, 2004.

[42] J. Fujii and Y. Ikeda, "Advances in our understanding of peroxiredoxin, a multifunctional, mammalian redox protein," *Redox Report*, vol. 7, no. 3, pp. 123–130, 2002.

[43] S. Immenschuh and E. Baumgart-Vogt, "Peroxiredoxins, oxidative stress, and cell proliferation," *Antioxidants and Redox Signaling*, vol. 7, no. 5-6, pp. 768–777, 2005.

[44] E. Cicik, H. Tekin, S. Akar et al., "Interleukin-8, nitric oxide and glutathione status in proliferative vitreoretinopathy and proliferative diabetic retinopathy," *Ophthalmic Research*, vol. 35, no. 5, pp. 251–255, 2003.

[45] S. Takano, S. Ishiwata, M. Nakazawa, M. Mizugaki, and M. Tamai, "Determination of ascorbic acid in human vitreous humor by high-performance liquid chromatography with UV detection," *Current Eye Research*, vol. 16, no. 6, pp. 589–594, 1997.

[46] M. Cederlund, F. Ghosh, K. Arnér, S. Andréasson, and B. Åkerström, "Vitreous levels of oxidative stress biomarkers and the radical-scavenger α_1-microglobulin/A1M in human rhegmatogenous retinal detachment," *Graefe's Archive for Clinical and Experimental Ophthalmology*, vol. 251, no. 3, pp. 725–732, 2013.

[47] D. N. Zacks, Y. Han, Y. Zeng, and A. Swaroop, "Activation of signaling pathways and stress-response genes in an experimental model of retinal detachment," *Investigative Ophthalmology and Visual Science*, vol. 47, no. 4, pp. 1691–1695, 2006.

[48] Z. A. Wood, L. B. Poole, and P. A. Karplus, "Peroxiredoxin evolution and the regulation of hydrogen peroxide signaling," *Science*, vol. 300, no. 5619, pp. 650–653, 2003.

[49] D. Pieragostino, S. Bucci, L. Agnifili et al., "Differential protein expression in tears of patients with primary open angle and pseudoexfoliative glaucoma," *Molecular BioSystems*, vol. 8, no. 4, pp. 1017–1028, 2012.

[50] D. Pieragostino, L. Agnifili, V. Fasanella et al., "Shotgun proteomics reveals specific modulated protein patterns in tears of patients with primary open angle glaucoma naïve to therapy," *Molecular BioSystems*, vol. 9, no. 6, pp. 1108–1116, 2013.

[51] D. G. Charteris, "Proliferative vitreoretinopathy: pathobiology, surgical management, and adjunctive treatment," *British Journal of Ophthalmology*, vol. 79, no. 10, pp. 953–960, 1995.

[52] M. Jin, S. He, V. Worpel, S. J. Ryan, and D. R. Hinton, "Promotion of adhesion and migration of RPE cells to provisional extracellular matrices by TNF-α," *Investigative Ophthalmology and Visual Science*, vol. 41, no. 13, pp. 4324–4332, 2000.

[53] J. A. Jerdan, J. S. Pepose, R. G. Michels et al., "Proliferative vitreoretinopathy membranes. An immunohistochemical study," *Ophthalmology*, vol. 96, no. 6, pp. 801–810, 1989.

[54] T. Ihanamäki, L. J. Pelliniemi, and E. Vuorio, "Collagens and collagen-related matrix components in the human and mouse eye," *Progress in Retinal and Eye Research*, vol. 23, no. 4, pp. 403–434, 2004.

[55] J. A. Jerdan and B. M. Glaser, "Retinal microvessel extracellular matrix: an immunofluorescent study," *Investigative Ophthalmology & Visual Science*, vol. 27, no. 2, pp. 194–203, 1986.

[56] M. M. Le Goff and P. N. Bishop, "Adult vitreous structure and postnatal changes," *Eye*, vol. 22, no. 10, pp. 1214–1222, 2008.

[57] S. Heegaard, O. A. Jensen, and J. U. Prause, "Structure and composition of the inner limiting membrane of the retina. SEM on frozen resin-cracked and enzyme-digested retinas of Macacca mulatta," *Graefe's Archive for Clinical and Experimental Ophthalmology*, vol. 224, no. 4, pp. 355–360, 1986.

[58] H. Laqua, "Collagen formation by periretinal cellular membranes," *Developments in Ophthalmology*, vol. 2, pp. 396–406, 1981.

[59] P. Hiscott, C. Sheridan, R. M. Magee, and I. Grierson, "Matrix and the retinal pigment epithelium in proliferative retinal disease," *Progress in Retinal and Eye Research*, vol. 18, no. 2, pp. 167–190, 1999.

[60] I. Morino, P. Hiscott, N. McKechnie, and I. Grierson, "Variation in epiretinal membrane components with clinical duration of the proliferative tissue," *British Journal of Ophthalmology*, vol. 74, no. 7, pp. 393–399, 1990.

[61] T. L. Ponsioen, M. J. A. van Luyn, R. J. van der Worp, H. H. Pas, J. M. M. Hooymans, and L. I. Los, "Human retinal Müller cells synthesize collagens of the vitreous and vitreoretinal interface in vitro," *Molecular Vision*, vol. 14, pp. 652–660, 2008.

[62] M. van Deemter, H. H. Pas, R. Kuijer, R. J. van der Worp, J. M. M. Hooymans, and L. I. Los, "Enzymatic breakdown of type II collagen in the human vitreous," *Investigative Ophthalmology and Visual Science*, vol. 50, no. 10, pp. 4552–4560, 2009.

[63] C. Symeonidis, E. Diza, E. Papakonstantinou, E. Souliou, S. A. Dimitrakos, and G. Karakiulakis, "Correlation of the extent and duration of rhegmatogenous retinal detachment with the expression of matrix metalloproteinases in the vitreous," *Retina*, vol. 27, no. 9, pp. 1279–1285, 2007.

[64] C. H. Kon, N. L. Occleston, D. Charteris, J. Daniels, G. W. Aylward, and P. T. Khaw, "A prospective study of matrix metalloproteinases in proliferative vitreoretinopathy," *Investigative Ophthalmology and Visual Science*, vol. 39, no. 8, pp. 1524–1529, 1998.

[65] C. Symeonidis, E. Papakonstantinou, E. Souliou, G. Karakiulakis, S. A. Dimitrakos, and E. Diza, "Correlation of matrix metalloproteinase levels with the grade of proliferative vitreoretinopathy in the subretinal fluid and vitreous during rhegmatogenous retinal detachment," *Acta Ophthalmologica*, vol. 89, no. 4, pp. 339–345, 2011.

[66] L. I. Los, R. J. van der Worp, M. J. A. van Luyn, and J. M. M. Hooymans, "Age-related liquefaction of the human vitreous body: LM and TEM evaluation of the role of proteoglycans and collagen," *Investigative Ophthalmology and Visual Science*, vol. 44, no. 7, pp. 2828–2833, 2003.

[67] A. Saito and H. Sinohara, "Various forms of rabbit plasma α-1-antiproteinase," *Biochemistry and Molecular Biology International*, vol. 46, no. 1, pp. 27–34, 1998.

[68] S. D. Patterson, "Mammalian α_1-antitrypsins: comparative biochemistry and genetics of the major plasma serpin," *Comparative Biochemistry and Physiology Part B: Comparative Biochemistry*, vol. 100, no. 3, pp. 439–454, 1991.

[69] G. A. Silverman, P. I. Bird, R. W. Carrell et al., "The serpins are an expanding superfamily of structurally similar but functionally diverse proteins. Evolution, mechanism of inhibition, novel functions, and a revised nomenclature," *The Journal of Biological Chemistry*, vol. 276, no. 36, pp. 33293–33296, 2001.

[70] D. H. Perlmutter, F. S. Cole, P. Kilbridge, T. H. Rossing, and H. R. Colten, "Expression of the alpha 1-proteinase inhibitor gene in human monocytes and macrophages," *Proceedings of the National Academy of Sciences of the United States of America*, vol. 82, no. 3, pp. 795–799, 1985.

[71] J. Cichy, J. Potempa, and J. Travis, "Biosynthesis of α1-proteinase inhibitor by human lung-derived epithelial cells," *Journal of Biological Chemistry*, vol. 272, no. 13, pp. 8250–8255, 1997.

[72] D. Faust, K. Raschke, S. Hormann, V. Milovic, and J. Stein, "Regulation of α1-proteinase inhibitor release by proinflammatory cytokines in human intestinal epithelial cells," *Clinical and Experimental Immunology*, vol. 128, no. 2, pp. 279–284, 2002.

[73] S. S. Twining, T. Fukuchi, B. Y. J. T. Yue, P. M. Wilson, and G. Boskovic, "Corneal synthesis of α1-proteinase inhibitor (α1-antitrypsin)," *Investigative Ophthalmology and Visual Science*, vol. 35, no. 2, pp. 458–462, 1994.

[74] M. Funding, H. Vorum, E. Nexø, and N. Ehlers, "Alpha-1-antitrypsin in aqueous humour from patients with corneal allograft rejection," *Acta Ophthalmologica Scandinavica*, vol. 83, no. 3, pp. 379–384, 2005.

[75] N. Mukai, T. Nakanishi, A. Shimizu, T. Takubo, and T. Ikeda, "Identification of phosphotyrosyl proteins in vitreous humours of patients with vitreoretinal diseases by sodium dodecyl sulphate-polyacrylamide gel electrophoresis/Western blotting/matrix-assisted laser desorption time-of-flight mass spectrometry," *Annals of Clinical Biochemistry*, vol. 45, no. 3, pp. 307–312, 2008.

Permissions

List of Contributors

Young Gun Park, Seungbum Kang and Young-Jung Roh
Department of Ophthalmology, Yeouido St. Mary's Hospital, College of Medicine, The Catholic University of Korea, No. 10, 63-ro Yeongdeungpo-gu, Seoul 07345, Republic of Korea

Ralf Brinkmann
Medical Laser Center Lübeck GmbH, Lübeck, Germany

Steven C. Schallhorn
University of California, San Francisco, 11730 Caminito Prenticia, San Diego, CA 92131, USA

Jan A. Venter and Stephen J. Hannan
Optical Express, 5 Deerdykes Road, Cumbernauld G68 9HF, UK

Keith A. Hettinger
Optical Express, 9820Willow Creek Road, Suite 260, San Diego, CA 92131, USA

Dong Yoon Kim
Department of Ophthalmology, College of Medicine, Chungbuk National University, Cheongju, Republic of Korea

Soo Geun Joe and Sung Jae Yang
Department of Ophthalmology, Gangneung Asan Hospital, College of Medicine, University of Ulsan, Gangneung 210-711, Republic of Korea

Joo Yong Lee and June-Gone Kim
Department of Ophthalmology, Asan Medical Center, College of Medicine, University of Ulsan, Seoul, Republic of Korea

Libuse Krizova
Institute of Medical Biochemistry and Laboratory Diagnostics, First Faculty of Medicine, Charles University in Prague and General University Hospital, U Nemocnice 2, 128 08 Prague 2, Czech Republic
Augenzentrum Augsburg, Prinzregentenstraße 25, 86150 Augsburg, Germany

Marta Kalousova, Ales Antonin Kubena and Tomas Zima
Institute of Medical Biochemistry and Laboratory Diagnostics, First Faculty of Medicine, Charles University in Prague and General University Hospital, U Nemocnice 2, 128 08 Prague 2, Czech Republic

Oldrich Chrapek, Barbora Chrapkova and Martin Sin
Department of Ophthalmology, Faculty of Medicine and Dentistry, Palacky University Olomouc, I. P. Pavlova 6, 775 20 Olomouc, Czech Republic

Ayong Yu, Weiqi Zhao, Fangjun Bao, Weicong Lu, Qinmei Wang and Jinhai Huang
School of Ophthalmology and Optometry, Wenzhou Medical University, 270West Xueyuan Road, Wenzhou, Zhejiang 325027, China
Key Laboratory of Vision Science, Ministry of Health of the People's Republic of China, Wenzhou, Zhejiang, China

Giacomo Savini
G. B. Bietti Foundation IRCCS, Rome, Italy

Zixu Huang
School of Ophthalmology and Optometry, Wenzhou Medical University, 270West Xueyuan Road, Wenzhou, Zhejiang 325027, China

James Lowe
Eastbourne District General Hospital, Kings Drive, Eastbourne BN21 2UD, UK

Charles R. Cleland, Evarista Mgaya and Godfrey Furahini
Kilimanjaro Christian Medical Centre Eye Department, P.O. Box 3010, Moshi, Tanzania

Clare E. Gilbert and Matthew J. Burton
International Centre for Eye Health, London School of Hygiene & Tropical Medicine, Keppel Street, LondonWC1E 7HT, UK

Heiko Philippin
Kilimanjaro Christian Medical Centre Eye Department, P.O. Box 3010, Moshi, Tanzania
International Centre for Eye Health, London School of Hygiene & Tropical Medicine, Keppel Street, LondonWC1E 7HT, UK

A. Perdicchi, D. Iacovello, A. Cutini, M. Balestrieri, M. G. Mutolo, M. T. Contestabile and S.M. Recupero
Department of Ophthalmology II, Faculty of Medicine and Psychology, "Sapienza" University of Rome, Sant'Andrea Hospital, 00100 Rome, Italy

M. Iester
Anatomical-Clinical Laboratory for the Diagnosis and Treatment of Glaucoma and Neuroophthalmology, Eye Clinic, DINOGMI, University of Genoa, Viale Benedetto XV 5, 16132 Genoa, Italy

A. Ferreras
Department of Ophthalmology, Miguel Servet University Hospital, Aragon Health Research Institute, 50009 Zaragoza, Spain

Moatasem El-Husseiny, Berthold Seitz, Elena Akhmedova, Nora Szentmary, Tobias Hager and Themistoklis Tsintarakis
Department of Ophthalmology, Saarland University Medical Center UKS, Homburg/Saar, Germany

Achim Langenbucher and Edgar Janunts
Experimental Ophthalmology, University of Saarland, Homburg/Saar, Germany

Antonella Franch, Federica Birattari and Gloria DalMas
Department of Ophthalmology, SS Giovanni e Paolo Hospital, Sestiere Castello 6777, 30122 Venice, Italy

Zala LuDnik
Fondazione Banca degli Occhi del Veneto, c/o Padiglione G. Rama, Via Paccagnella 11, Zelarino, 30174 Venice, Italy
Eye Hospital, University Medical Centre, Grablovičeva Ulica 46, 1525 Ljubljana, Slovenia

Mohit Parekh, Stefano Ferrari and Diego Ponzin
Eye Hospital, University Medical Centre, Grablovičeva Ulica 46, 1525 Ljubljana, Slovenia

Wenjing Wu and YanWang
Tianjin Eye Hospital and Tianjin Eye Institute, Tianjin Ophthalmology and Visual Science Key Laboratory, Clinical College of Ophthalmology, Tianjin Medical University, No. 4, Gansu Road, Heping District, Tianjin 300020, China

Ying Yuan
Shanghai Eye Disease Prevention & Treatment Center, Shanghai 200040, China

Zhengwei Zhang, Kelimu Jiang, Wenjing Zheng and Bilian Ke
Department of Ophthalmology, Shanghai General Hospital, Shanghai Jiao Tong University School of Medicine, Shanghai 200080, China

Jianfeng Zhu and Xiangui He
Shanghai Eye Disease Prevention & Treatment Center, Shanghai 200040, China

Ergang Du
Shanghai Eye Disease Prevention & Treatment Center, Shanghai 200040, China
Chinese Medicine Hospital of Zhejiang Province, Hangzhou, Zhejiang 310006, China

Ivan Fernandez-Bueno
Instituto Universitario de Oftalmobiologia Aplicada (IOBA), University of Valladolid, 47011 Valladolid, Spain
Centro en Red de Medicina Regenerativa y Terapia Celular de Castilla y Leon, Valladolid, Spain

Salvatore Di Lauro and Jose Carlos Pastor
Instituto Universitario de Oftalmobiologia Aplicada (IOBA), University of Valladolid, 47011 Valladolid, Spain
Department of Ophthalmology, Hospital Clinico Universitario, 47005 Valladolid, Spain

Ivan Alvarez
AJL Ophthalmic S.A., 01510 Miñano, Spain

Jose Carlos Lopez and Maria Teresa Garcia-Gutierrez
Instituto Universitario de Oftalmobiologia Aplicada (IOBA), University of Valladolid, 47011 Valladolid, Spain

Itziar Fernandez
Instituto Universitario de Oftalmobiologia Aplicada (IOBA), University of Valladolid, 47011 Valladolid, Spain
Networking Research Center on Bioengineering, Biomaterials and Nanomedicine (CIBER-BBN), Valladolid, Spain

Eva Larra
AJL Ophthalmic S.A., 01510 Miñano, Spain

Marek Rwkas and Karolina Krix-Jachym
Ophthalmology Department, Military Institute of Medicine, Szaserów Street 128, 04-141Warsaw, Poland

Tomasz garnowsk
Department of Diagnostics and Microsurgery of Glaucoma, Medical University of Lublin, Chmielna Street 1, 20-079 Lublin, Poland

Jingjing You, Li Wen and Athena Roufas
Save Sight Institute, Discipline of Clinical Ophthalmology, The University of Sydney, Sydney, NSW 2000, Australia

Chris Hodge
Save Sight Institute, Discipline of Clinical Ophthalmology, The University of Sydney, Sydney, NSW 2000, Australia
Vision Eye Institute, Chatswood, NSW2067, Australia

Gerard Sutton
Save Sight Institute, Discipline of Clinical Ophthalmology, The University of Sydney, Sydney, NSW 2000, Australia
Vision Eye Institute, Chatswood, NSW2067, Australia
Auckland University, Auckland 1010, New Zealand

Michele C. Madigan
Save Sight Institute, Discipline of Clinical Ophthalmology, The University of Sydney, Sydney, NSW 2000, Australia
School of Optometry & Vision Science, UNSW, Kensington, NSW2052, Australia

Pilar Cacho-Martínez,Mario Cantó-Cerdán, Stela Carbonell-Bonete and Ángel García-Muñoz
Departamento de Òptica, Farmacología y Anatomía, Universidad de Alicante, 03080 Alicante, Spain

Fernando A. Wilson and YangWang
College of Public Health, University of Nebraska Medical Center, 984350 Nebraska Medical Center, Omaha, NE 68198-4350, USA

JimP. Stimpson
School of PublicHealth, City University of New York, 55W. 125th Street, New York, NY 10027, USA

Shasha Gao, Tingyu Qin and Yong Lu
Department of Ophthalmology, The First Affiliated Hospital of Zhengzhou University, Zhengzhou 450052, China

Shengnan Wang
Department of Ophthalmology, Beijing Ditan Hospital, Capital Medical University, Beijing, China

Lei Liu, Song Yue, Jingyang Wu and Jiahua Zhang
Department of Ophthalmology, The First Affiliated Hospital of China Medical University, Shenyang 110001, China

Jie Lian
Department of Health center, Fengyutan Community, Shenyang 110064, China

Desheng Huang
Department of Epidemiology, School of Public Health, China Medical University, Shenyang 110122, China

Weiping Teng
Key Laboratory of Endocrine Diseases in Liaoning Province, The First Hospital of China Medical University, Shenyang 110001, China

Lei Chen
Department of Ophthalmology, The First Affiliated Hospital of China Medical University, Shenyang 110001, China
Key Laboratory of Endocrine Diseases in Liaoning Province, The First Hospital of China Medical University, Shenyang 110001, China

Keiji Inagaki
Department of Ophthalmology, St. Luke's International Hospital, 9-1 Akashi-cho, Chuo-ku, Tokyo 104-8560, Japan
Department of Ophthalmology, Juntendo University Urayasu Hospital, 1-1 Tomioka 2-chome, Urayasu-shi, Chiba 279-0021, Japan

Takuya Shuo and Kanae Katakura
Institute for Medical Innovation, St. Luke's International University, 10-1 Akashi-cho, Chuo-ku, Tokyo 104-8560, Japan

Nobuyuki Ebihara
Department of Ophthalmology, Juntendo University Urayasu Hospital, 1-1 Tomioka 2-chome, Urayasu-shi, Chiba 279-0021, Japan

AkiraMurakami
Department of Ophthalmology, Juntendo University Graduate School of Medicine, Hongo 2-1-1, Bunkyo-ku, Tokyo 113-8421, Japan

Kishiko Ohkoshi
Department of Ophthalmology, St. Luke's International Hospital, 9-1 Akashi-cho, Chuo-ku, Tokyo 104-8560, Japan

Xi Zhu, Guowei Zhang, Lihua Kang and Huaijin Guan
Eye Institute, Affiliated Hospital of Nantong University, Nantong, Jiangsu 226001, China

Masako Okura
Department of Aging Control Medicine, Juntendo University Graduate School of Medicine, 3-1-3 Hongo, Bunkyo-ku, Tokyo 113-8431, Japan
Eye Clinic Tenjin, 2-11-1 Tenjin, Chuo-ku, Fukuoka 8100001, Japan

Motoko Kawashima
Department of Ophthalmology, Keio University School of Medicine, 35 Shinanomachi, Shinjuku-ku, Tokyo 1608582, Japan

Mikiyuki Katagiri and Takuji Shirasawa
Department of Aging Control Medicine, Juntendo University Graduate School of Medicine, 3-1-3 Hongo, Bunkyo-ku, Tokyo 113-8431, Japan

Kazuo Tsubota
Department of Ophthalmology, Keio University School of Medicine, 35 Shinanomachi, Shinjuku-ku, Tokyo 1608582, Japan

Engy Mohamed Mostafa
Ophthalmology Department, Sohag University, Naser City, Sohag 82524, Egypt

Weiran Niu, Guanglin Shen, Yuanzhi Yuan and Xiaoping Ma
Department of Ophthalmology, Zhongshan Hospital of Fudan University, Shanghai 200032, China

Suming Li and Jingzhao Wang
Institute de High Performance Polymers, Qingdao University of Science and Technology, Qingdao 266042, China

Zhongyong Fan and Lan Liao
Department of Materials Science, Fudan University, Shanghai 200433, China

Tomoko Ueda-Consolvo, Mitsuya Otsuka, Yumiko Hayashi, Masaaki Ishida and Atsushi Hayashi
Department of Ophthalmology, Graduate School of Medicine and Pharmaceutical Sciences, University of Toyama, 2630 Sugitani, Toyama 930-0194, Japan

Guohong Tian, Chaoyi Feng, Mengwei Li, Yongheng Huang and Xinghuai Sun
Department of Ophthalmology, Eye, Ear, Nose, and Throat Hospital, Fudan University, Shanghai 200031, China

Zhenxin Li and Guixian Zhao
Department of Neurology, Huashan Hospital, Fudan University, Shanghai 200040, China

T. Bertelmann, C. Heun, C. Paul, E. Bari-Kacik, W. Sekundo and S. Schulze
Department of Ophthalmology, Philipps-University Marburg, Baldingerstraße, 35043 Marburg, Germany

Katsuo Tomoyose, Yuka Okada, Takayoshi Sumioka, Kumi Shirai, Tomoya Morii, Osamu Yamanaka and Shizuya Saika
Department of Ophthalmology, Wakayama Medical University, 811-1 Kimiidera, Wakayama 641-0012, Japan

Masayasu Miyajima
Laboratory Animal Center, Wakayama Medical University, 811-1 Kimiidera, Wakayama 641-0012, Japan

Kathleen C. Flanders
Laboratory of Cell Regulation and Carcinogenesis, National Cancer Institute, National Institutes of Health, Bethesda, MD, USA

Peter S. Reinach
Wenzhou Medical University School of Ophthalmology and Optometry, Wenzhou, China

Eva Charlotte Koch, Johanna Staab, Matthias Fuest and Niklas Plange
Department of Ophthalmology, RWTH Aachen University, Pauwelsstraße 30, 52072 Aachen, Germany

Katharina Witt and Andreas Voss
Department of Medical Engineering and Biotechnology, Ernst-Abbe-Hochschule Jena, 07745 Jena, Germany

Chong Chen, Xian Xu, Yuyu Miao, Gaoxin Zheng, Yong Sun and Xun Xu
Department of Ophthalmology, Shanghai Key Laboratory of Fundus Disease, Shanghai General Hospital Affiliated to Shanghai Jiao Tong University, Shanghai 200080, China

Lyubomyr Lytvynchuk
Professor Sergienko Eye Clinic, 47 A Pirogova Street, 21008 Vinnycia, Ukraine
Department of Ophthalmology, Faculty of Medicine, Albert Szent-Györgyi Clinical Center, University of Szeged, Korányi fasor Ulica 10-11, 6720 Szeged, Hungary
Stem Cells and Eye Research Laboratory, Department of Biochemistry and Molecular Biology, Faculty of Medicine, University of Debrecen, Egyetem Téren 1, 4032 Debrecen, Hungary

Andrii Sergienko
Professor Sergienko Eye Clinic, 47 A Pirogova Street, 21008 Vinnycia, Ukraine

Galina Lavrenchuk
State Institution "Research Center for Radiation Medicine of Academy of Medical Sciences of Ukraine",
Laboratory of Cell Radiobiology, 53 Melnykova Street, 04050 Kyiv, Ukraine

Goran Petrovski
Department of Ophthalmology, Faculty of Medicine, Albert Szent-Györgyi Clinical Center, University of Szeged, Korányi fasor Ulica 10-11, 6720 Szeged, Hungary
Stem Cells and Eye Research Laboratory, Department of Biochemistry and Molecular Biology, Faculty of

Sung-Cheol Yun
Department of Clinical Epidemiology and Biostatistics, Asan Medical Center, College of Medicine, University of Ulsan, Seoul 138736, Republic of Korea

Ji Wook Hong, Kyung Rim Sung and Jin Young Lee
Department of Ophthalmology, Asan Medical Center, College of Medicine, University of Ulsan, Seoul 138736, Republic of Korea

Wei Chen, Yubo Guan, Guanghui He, Hui Song, Shiyong Xie and Quanhong Han
Clinical College of Ophthalmology, Tianjin Medical University, No. 4, Gansu Road, Tianjin 300020, China

Zhiwei Li
Department of Ophthalmology, Shandong Provincial Hospital Affiliated to Shandong University, Jinan 250000, China

Nakul Mandal
Department of Ophthalmology, Lund University, 22185 Lund, Sweden

Geoffrey P. Lewis
Neuroscience Research Institute, University of California, Santa Barbara, Santa Barbara, CA 93106-5060, USA

Steven K. Fisher
Neuroscience Research Institute, University of California, Santa Barbara, Santa Barbara, CA 93106-5060, USA
Department of Molecular, Cellular and Developmental Biology, University of California, Santa Barbara, Santa Barbara, CA 93106-9625, USA

Steffen Heegaard
Department of Ophthalmology, University of Copenhagen, 2600 Glostrup, Denmark
Eye Pathology Institute, University of Copenhagen, 2100 Copenhagen, Denmark

Jan U. Prause
Eye Pathology Institute, University of Copenhagen, 2100 Copenhagen, Denmark

Morten la Cour
Department of Ophthalmology, University of Copenhagen, 2600 Glostrup, Denmark

Henrik Vorum
Department of Ophthalmology, Aalborg University Hospital, 9000 Aalborg, Denmark

Bent Honoré
Department of Biomedicine, Aarhus University, 8000 Aarhus, Denmark

www.ingramcontent.com/pod-product-compliance
Lightning Source LLC
Chambersburg PA
CBHW080508200326

41458CB00012B/4135